NLM
Class
Mark:
L.G.I.

WS
270
JOS

D1423371

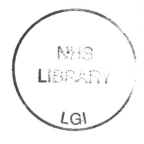
NHS
LIBRARY
LGI

Paediatric
Orthopaedics

Paediatric
Orthopaedics
A SYSTEM OF DECISION-MAKING

● Benjamin Joseph MS(Orth), MCh(Orth)
**Professor of Orthopaedics and Head of Paediatric Orthopaedic Service,
Kasturba Medical College, Manipal, India**

● Selvadurai Nayagam BSc, MCh(Orth), FRCS Ed (Trauma and Orth)
**Consultant Orthopaedic Surgeon, Royal Liverpool Children's Hospital,
Liverpool, UK**

● Randall T Loder MD
Garceau Professor of Orthopaedic Surgery, Indiana University School of Medicine
and
**Chief of Orthopaedics
James Whitcomb Riley Children's Hospital, Indianapolis, Indiana, USA**

● Ian Torode FRCS (C) FRACS
**Director of Clinical Orthopaedics and Deputy Director of Orthopaedics,
Royal Children's Hospital, Melbourne, Australia**

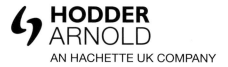
AN HACHETTE UK COMPANY

First published in Great Britain in 2009 by
Hodder Arnold, an imprint of Hodder Education, an Hachette UK company,
338 Euston Road, London NW1 3BH

http://www.hoddereducation.com

© 2009 Joseph, Nayagam, Loder and Torode

All rights reserved. Apart from any use permitted under UK copyright law, this publication may only be reproduced, stored or transmitted, in any form, or by any means with prior permission in writing of the publishers or in the case of reprographic production in accordance with the terms of licences issued by the Copyright Licensing Agency. In the United Kingdom such licences are issued by the Copyright licensing Agency: Saffron House, 6-10 Kirby Street, London EC1N 8TS.

Hachette's policy is to use papers that are natural, renewable and recyclable products and made from wood grown in sustainable forests. The logging and manufacturing processes are expected to conform to the environmental regulations of the country of origin.

Whilst the advice and information in this book are believed to be true and accurate at the date of going to press, neither the author[s] nor the publisher can accept any legal responsibility or liability for any errors or omissions that may be made. In particular, (but without limiting the generality of the preceding disclaimer) every effort has been made to check drug dosages; however it is still possible that errors have been missed. Furthermore, dosage schedules are constantly being revised and new side-effects recognized. For these reasons the reader is strongly urged to consult the drug companies' printed instructions before administering any of the drugs recommended in this book.

British Library Cataloguing in Publication Data
A catalogue record for this book is available from the British Library

Library of Congress Cataloging-in-Publication Data
A catalog record for this book is available from the Library of Congress

ISBN   978-0-340-88945-9

1 2 3 4 5 6 7 8 9 10

Commissioning Editor:	Gavin Jamieson
Project Editor:	Francesca Naish
Production Controller:	Joanna Walker
Cover Design:	Helen Townson
Indexer:	Laurence Errington

Typeset in 10/12 pt Bembo by Macmillan Publishing Solutions
Printed and bound in Spain by Graphycems

What do you think about this book? Or any other Hodder Arnold title?
Please visit our website: www.hoddereducation.com

Dedication

To my wife Susan and my children Anjali, Sunil, Santosh and Tripti for their love and support and for helping me to make the right decisions in my life.

Benjamin Joseph

To Martine, Matthew, Robert and Joshua – whose patience, understanding and continued support of a husband and dad at work has made this effort come to fruition.

Selvadurai Nayagam

To my dearest wife Christine and our three children, Andrew, Wendy, and David, whose unfailing support made this work possible.

Randall Loder

To my long suffering wife, Lyn, and my boys, Rob and Tim, who have accepted, with great tolerance and understanding, the lack of a husband and father due to firstly the demands of a medical career and secondly to help prepare this text.

Ian Torode

Contents

Foreword

The world's population of children is nearing two billion and growing, making this new Paediatric Orthopaedics textbook an important addition. An international team of authors have produced this new book, suitable for the management of all children. This book details management of musculoskeletal deformities in children regardless of their situation in life.

Eminent Paediatric Orthopaedists have pooled their experience and knowledge to provide a logical approach to the evaluation and treatment of the most common musculoskeletal deformities of childhood. The authors have thoughtfully limited the scope of the publication to 72 topics in 8 sections that cover the majority of these deformities in children. This simplifies both organization and navigation.

Paediatric Orthopaedics: A System of Decision-Making is designed for those with limited experience who most need a rational approach to management. By recommending management that is tailored to a variety of clinical situations the approach becomes comprehensive. Being comprehensive, *Paediatric Orthopaedics* will become a valuable guide for inexperienced and experienced surgeons alike.

When I was first asked by Professor Benjamin Joseph to write a preface for his new book, he described it as a guide to management. I envisioned a book with many flowcharts. Instead, the authors have created an efficient treatment table format that conveniently pairs treatment recommendations with clinical features. This approach simplifies the selection of management options by addressing important clinical findings.

The design of *Paediatric Orthopaedics: A System of Decision-Making* is both functional and attractive. The addition of a second colour enhances the drawings and helps to separate topics. The blue colour makes the book more attractive and engaging. The simple line drawings are excellent and clearly detail management procedures and the text is semi-outlined and concise. The design, format and content make this book suitable for reading either in its entirety or for quick reference. A successful book conveys information quickly and pleasantly; this book gets an excellent grade.

I predict that *Paediatric Orthopaedics: A System of Decision-Making* will not be kept in the library but rather in the clinic and will quickly show signs of overuse.

Lynn Staheli MD May 2009

On seeing the title of this new text one could be excused for asking, "What? Another one?" To be sure there have been a number of other authoritative texts published on this same subject, some with exactly the same main title, and some are much thicker than this one. It could happen that the paediatric orthopaedic surgeon who looked no further than the title might just put this text on the shelf with the other ones.

That would be a mistake. This text deserves to be read and consulted, particularly by those with some experience. The characteristic that grabs the attention with this text is not the main title, but the subtitle: *A System of Decision-Making*. Joseph, Nayagam, Loder and Torode have adopted a perspective and a structure that is not common in our textbooks. Rather than deal with either diagnostic entities or differential diagnosis they have taken an intermediate route and chosen, wherever possible, to deal with clinical problems and the strategies that can be used to solve them. For example, there is no chapter on cerebral palsy, but there is a section on decreased joint mobility. They have adopted an interesting way to present these strategies by using tables showing the links between indications and treatment and progressing from left to right with respect to age or severity. In my view this is more effective than an algorithmic representation and neatly categorizes the criteria used in the treatment decision.

Keeping authorship among the four of them gave each a monumental task, but it resulted in an extremely consistent format for the chapters and the reader is not aware of different authorship in moving from one chapter to another. They have succeeded in covering paediatric orthopaedics without succumbing to the temptation to be exhaustive and have done a good job in bringing forward the evidence available for decision support.

In considering this innovative approach it seemed to me that there are at least two circumstances in which it could prove difficult. The first is in those conditions where dependable evidence is lacking. In paediatric orthopaedics we are frequently faced with this difficulty. We have very few studies that evaluate outcomes over the lifetimes of our patients, and, in particular, very few that take into account the changing values of our patients from children to teens to adults to seniors. The authors recognize that practicing evidence-based medicine in the real world means taking the best evidence available when prospective randomized studies are not available. The best evidence could consist of observational studies, or even expert consensus, and this text handles these circumstances as well as can be expected. The chapter on 'Legg-Perthes Disease' is an example where a decision system is presented although solid evidence is scarce.

The second source of difficulty could occur when a clinical problem might result from several varied pathologies. I was particularly interested in the section on decreased joint mobility since the approaches to stiffness caused by the paralysis of polio, the spasticity of cerebral palsy, the pain of arthritis and the ankylosis of coalitions can be very different. Indeed, as one might expect, the authors are forced to deal with these different entities separately, but only after presenting the general principles of movement and its restoration.

As paediatric orthopaedic surgeons we must develop a number of skills, and no one would diminish the importance, for example, of communication skill or technical skill. I would argue that our most important skill is that of decision-making, in doing the right thing for the right patient at the right time, and this book is directed precisely at that skill.

Colin F Moseley MD May 2009

Preface

Mastering the science and art of Paediatric Orthopaedics entails acquisition of theoretical knowledge, development of surgical dexterity and learning the process of clinical decision-making. Of these three components of learning that form the foundation of Paediatric Orthopaedics, clinical decision-making is arguably the most important.

Making good decisions in Paediatric Orthopaedics can be daunting, particularly as the consequences of an inappropriate decision are far-reaching. An error in judgement could lead to disability for life. Seeking guidance from the standard sources of medical literature may be confusing; it is often replete with different ways to treat the conditions encountered in clinical practice. Orthopaedic reference books frequently list several treatments for a particular problem. How does one make the correct choices? Which option should one choose for a particular patient? What governs the surgeon's choice of a particular treatment? This book attempts to answer these questions.

In *Paediatric Orthopaedics: A System of Decision-Making* we provide a guide to management for a wide spectrum of Paediatric Orthopaedic conditions. At its inception we identified the conditions, mostly common and some occasional, that most surgeons in a Paediatric Orthopaedic practice are likely to encounter. The need to include some uncommon conditions is to provide the reader insight into decision-making trees where choices are not always made on science alone but are governed also by social issues or patient preference.

We have strived to make the book readable, clear and instructive. There will always be omissions in any textbook on a subject as vast as this and, for the sake of brevity, we have avoided detailed descriptions of surgical procedures – there are many established standard textbooks on this area. As in all other areas of medicine, each outline of management is not the only way to approach a particular clinical problem. However, we have provided the rationale for adopting the recommended treatment strategy in light of published evidence and our joint experience.

Since clinical decision-making is likely to be most difficult for those who are in training and for the junior consultant in the field, this book is specifically targeted at these two groups. We hope this book will serve as a useful starting point for the young orthopaedic surgeon to evolve a reasoned and balanced approach in his or her own practice of Paediatric Orthopaedics.

Benjamin Joseph
Selvadurai Nayagam
Randall Loder
Ian Torode

Acknowledgements

The authors acknowledge the encouragement and help received from friends and colleagues during the preparation of this book.

In particular, I thank Dr. Hitesh Shah and Dr. N.D Siddesh for the enormous effort they put in to locate suitable illustrations for the book by sifting through thousands of images.
My thanks are due to Mr. Michael Tonkin for his valuable comments regarding chapters dealing with the paralyzed hand. Dr. Bhaskaranand Kumar's comments regarding the chapters on radial club hand and absence of the thumb and the radiographs of radial club hand kindly contributed by him are all gratefully acknowledged.
A special word of thanks is due to my daughter, Dr. Anjali Benjamin Daniel who painstakingly proof-read the drafts of the manuscript.

Benjamin Joseph

I would like to thank the Radiology Film Loan personnel at Riley Children's Hospital for their support in obtaining the digital radiographic images. The assistance of our two research assistants in the Orthopaedic Division at Riley Children's Hospital, Ms. Gretchen Huffman and Ms. Elizabeth Riley, is greatly appreciated in tracking down medical references and general assistance in manuscript preparation.

Randall Loder

I wish to acknowledge the skill and dedication that Ben has contributed to convert my ramblings into readable text. I am grateful to my wife, Lyn, and my sons, Rob and Tim, for tolerating my absences to the study to put those ramblings onto the computer.

Ian Torode

SECTION 1

Deformities

General principles of treatment of deformities in children

Selvadurai Nayagam and Benjamin Joseph

Introduction

Deformity is an alteration of structure (be it length, alignment or joint position) that produces or has the potential to produce symptoms or loss of function. It is one of the commonest reasons for consulting a paediatric orthopaedic surgeon. The impact of the visible anomaly to the child and parents is of a worrisome abnormality which the treating doctor will need to distinguish as either normal variant or disease. In the event of the latter, two additional issues need resolving:

1. what is the natural history of this condition?
2. what are the consequences if it is left untreated?

Decision-making becomes a great deal simpler with both questions answered (Table 1.1).

Table 1.1 ● Decision-making based on the natural history and consequences of deformities

DECISION-MAKING ON THE BASIS OF THE NATURAL HISTORY OF THE DEFORMITY	
Natural history of the deformity	**Nature of intervention**
Deformities that tend to resolve spontaneously	Reassurance and follow-up
Deformities that tend to progress	Early intervention to correct deformity and prevent progression or recurrence (if cure is not possible, a strategy to prevent progression is warranted)
Deformities that remain static	Decision to intervene based on consequences of the deformity
DECISION-MAKING ON THE BASIS OF THE CONSEQUENCES OF THE DEFORMITY	
Consequences of the deformity	**Decision to intervene**
Deformities that are cosmetically acceptable and cause no disability	No intervention
Deformities that are cosmetically unacceptable but cause no functional disability	Consider intervention after weighing the risks of potential complications of intervention
Deformities that cause disability	Intervene
Deformities that potentially lead to long-term deleterious consequences	Intervene early to prevent onset or progression of problems
Deformities that may be beneficial	Avoid correction of the deformity

Natural history of the deformity

■ Deformities that tend to resolve spontaneously

A high proportion of children who present to the doctor have innocuous deformities that resolve spontaneously. These normal variants include physiologic genu varum and valgum, infantile flat-foot, neonatal calcaneovalgus deformity and some torsional deformities of the femur and tibia. While recognition of these diagnoses allows the doctor to reassure parents, in some children complete correction of such variants may not occur and follow up until resolution is wise.

■ Deformities that tend to progress and/or recur after surgical correction

Paralytic deformities and those caused by physeal damage tend to progress until skeletal growth stops. Unless the underlying cause is removed (e.g. muscle imbalance or physeal bar), recurrence will follow seemingly satisfactory correction. Certain deformities, such as types of scoliotic curves, may progress even after skeletal maturity.

■ Deformities that remain static

Some deformities remain static; typically these include fracture malunions that have failed to remodel completely, either from severity of the original malalignment or from the advanced age of the child.

Problems of management

Consequences of the deformity

■ **Deformities that are cosmetically acceptable and cause no functional disability**
These should be left alone.

■ **Deformities that are cosmetically unacceptable but cause no functional disability**
The threshold beyond which a deformity is cosmetically unacceptable will vary between individuals and communities. Some small deformities can cause significant angst to children who are sensitive to body image issues. The treating doctor has to be attuned to these differences.

■ **Deformities that cause functional disability**
A decision to intervene is straightforward when the disability is an obvious product of deformity.

■ **Deformities that have the potential to cause functional disability**
The need for intervention becomes less certain when no concurrent disability is present but deleterious consequences in the future suspected if left untreated. Long-term epidemiological data to support intervention are available for some conditions whereas in others intervention is based on best available current information. When supportive evidence is available, such deformities should be corrected before the disability develops. Similar to many conditions in medicine, the need for intervention evolves as more information is made available.

Appearance

This is often the impetus for seeking a medical opinion. In mild forms, which often represent normal variants, an elderly family relative is the person encouraging consultation and often quotes braces, shoe inserts or other such orthotic that has helped in the past with other children. A broad knowledge of 'deformities' that present in childhood but spontaneously resolve with age is needed to separate out disease from normal variant.

Loss of function

Deformity reduces function if, through its location or severity, it is able to influence the normal movement of joints, gait or activities of daily living.

Pain and giving way (instability)

Abnormal orientation of joints or loss of congruence between articulating surfaces will produce symptoms of pain or giving way. This applies to both upper and lower limbs; in the former it may present as painful 'clicking' or a loss of strength whereas in the lower limb it is more typically a loss of control of joint position.

Secondary adaptive or degenerative changes

The pliable skeleton of a child responds and shapes to the force vectors of weight-bearing and normal use. In the case of deformities which are present from early childhood and become long-standing, it is not unusual to find changes within the skeleton that are hallmarks of a response to abnormal force vectors. An example is the untreated clubfoot, where changes in the shape of the tarsal bones may be partly intrinsic to the condition and also due to abnormal loading of the foot.

Aims of treatment

- Improve appearance
- Improve function
- Reduce pain and instability
- Prevent the onset or progression of adaptive or degenerative changes

Principles of assessing deformity

When assessing a deformity the following are essential.

- An evaluation of the deformity in the coronal, sagittal and axial planes (which is done radiologically *and* clinically). In the event of a periarticular deformity, differentiation between soft tissue and bony components of the deformity is needed. The soft tissue problems include contracture, laxity or congenital absence of muscles or ligaments. Joint contractures are traditionally measured as degrees of loss of range within the usual planes of movement of that particular joint, although the neutral zero method[1,2] is an attractive way to standardize descriptive nomenclature.

When the origin of joint deformity is bony, this may be the result of an abnormal joint inclination or incongruence between articulating surfaces. Arthrograms and examination under anaesthesia may be necessary adjunctive investigations.

- The state of joints (contractures, range of movement, stability and the development of adaptive or degenerative changes) both proximal and distal to the deformity.
- The state of the contralateral limb.
- The impact of deformity on function – which in the lower limb may include gait, walking tolerance or the ability to participate in sports but in the upper limb may include reach, grip and activities of daily living.
- The presence, nature and efficacy of compensation mechanisms that have developed.

Many apparently solitary deformities are present with additional features that are either part of the presenting syndrome or have developed as compensation mechanisms. Examples include congenital longitudinal deficiencies of the lower limb which show a multitude of anatomical abnormalities from hip to foot or an equinus contracture of the ankle that may be accompanied by hyperextension of the knee to compensate.

Principles of analysis of deformity

It is understandable when, in a specialty so dominated by radiographic images, surgeons take the path of correcting deformity through radiograph analysis only. Deformity analysis is more than an interpretation of angles or millimetres of abnormality derived from several radiographic images or any other imaging modality, otherwise correction of deformity is reduced to simply restoring radiological parameters to within a normal range. Deformity analysis and subsequent correction is an exercise of balancing the extent of surgical interventions needed for anatomical 'normality' with the functional gains anticipated. This emphasizes that surgical correction to 'normality', while desirable in most, is not always necessary. An appropriate example is skeletal deformities accompanying neuromuscular conditions in which correction to achieve maximal functional gain is greater than that for anatomical accuracy.

Methods of deformity correction have changed over the last three decades. A revised approach to the problem has arisen through a combination of Ilizarov's work in deformity correction[3] (acute and gradual methods) using his circular external fixator, and a thorough rewriting of the rules of the analysis by Paley.[4] A comprehensive coverage of these principles is beyond the scope of this chapter but the authors recommend that surgeons are familiar with the content of the quoted references.

Modern deformity analysis gives credence to the three-dimensional basis of most deformities, whether the origin of the problem is within bone or a joint, or a combination of both. Deformity of bone exists as a deviation in the coronal or sagittal plane (or any plane in-between) where it can be measured in degrees of angulation or millimetres of translation, or in the axial plane where it can exist as degrees of rotation or millimetres of length abnormality.

Centre of rotation of angulation

Most surgeons are familiar with drawing the anatomical axes of the segment proximal and distal to a deformity in order to measure the size of the deformity in degrees at the intersection of the axes. This intersection of anatomical axes carries a greater significance in modern deformity analysis and planning; it is referred to as the centre of rotation of angulation (CORA) and can also be determined through the intersection of the mechanical axes of the segments proximal and distal to the deformity. The CORA is important for determining the axis of rotation, for determining whether there is an associated translation component in the deformity and for identifying multiapical deformities.

■ The axis of rotation for correction

The CORA indicates where an axis of rotation (named angulation correction axis or ACA by Paley) should be placed, through which the two intersecting axes of the CORA can be brought in line and hence the deformity corrected. The axis of rotation to achieve appropriate realignment of the intersecting axes is positioned on either side of the CORA but along a line termed '*the bisector*'. This is, as implied in its name, the line which bisects the angle described by the deformity (Figure 1.1a). The effect of placing the axis of rotation on the convex side of the deformity is an opening wedge correction and conversely a closing wedge if it is placed on the concave side. Moving the rotation axis further along the bisector increases or decreases the size of the opening, i.e.

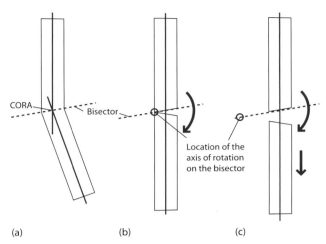

(a)   (b)   (c)

Figure 1.1 ● The anatomical (or mechanical) axes of proximal and distal segments of the deformity intersect at a centre of rotation of angulation (CORA) **(a)**. The bisector refers to a line which bisects the supplement of the angle of deformity. Placing a rotation axis on the bisector will facilitate realignment of the axes **(b)**. Placing the rotation axis further along the bisector and on the convex side of the deformity will add distraction (lengthening) to the osteotomy site **(c)**.

achieves simultaneous lengthening or shortening with the angular correction (Figure 1.1b,c). If the rotation axis is not placed on the bisector, a translation deformity will ensue.

■ Location of the CORA

■ CORA lies within the bone and coincides with the apex of angulation
When the CORA lies within the boundaries of the bone involved and coincides with the apex of angulation of the deformity, only an angular component to the deformity exists. The rotation axis to correct the deformity can be sited on the bisector and the osteotomy performed at the same level – this is equivalent to the manner in which classic deformity correction through opening or closing wedge methods was performed (Figure 1.1b).

■ CORA lies within the boundaries of the bone involved but is at a different level to that of the apex of angulation
This indicates the presence of translation in addition to the angular component (Figure 1.2a). The rotation axis should be maintained on the bisector but the osteotomy can be sited at either of the two levels (coincident with the apex of angulation of the bone or at the CORA): in the former,

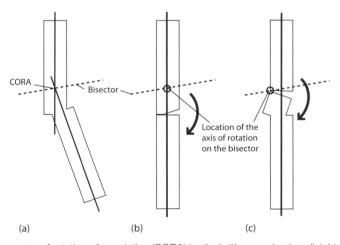

(a)   (b)   (c)

Figure 1.2 ● If the centre of rotation of angulation (CORA) is sited either proximal or distal to the apex of angulation, it indicates the presence of translation in addition to angulation within the deformity **(a)**. Placing the rotation axis on the bisector will ensure realignment of the axes, irrespective of whether the osteotomy is performed at the site of original deformity **(b)** or at the level of the CORA **(c)**.

correction of both translation and angulation is simultaneously accomplished at the site of the original deformity (Figure 1.2b); however, in the latter, a new deformity is created which correctly 'balances' the malalignment from the original site (Figure 1.2c).

■ CORA lies outside the boundaries of the involved bone

In this situation a multiapical deformity is likely to be present (and the deformity more akin to a curve). The deformity would need to be resolved through multiple osteotomies.

These features of the CORA are, in essence, the rules of osteotomy as described by Paley.[4] It explains why it is permissible to perform osteotomies away from the apex of angulation of the deformity as long as the correction is achieved through a rotation axis placed on the CORA or on its bisector. Many examples in paediatric orthopaedics illustrate this principle, e.g. performing an intertrochanteric or subtrochanteric osteotomy to correct coxa vara in a child with a slipped capital femoral epiphysis or creating lateral translation in the supracondylar osteotomy for correction of genu valgum of the distal femur.

Treatment options

Soft tissue

These problems are amenable to a variety of strategies.

- A joint contracture may be corrected by stretching, e.g. serial manipulation and casts, controlled incremental traction through a system of weights or through an external fixator, or surgical lengthening or release of the contracted tissue. These techniques are useful if the deformity is not more than moderate in degree and is of recent onset. Angular or shortening osteotomies are usually needed in addition to soft tissue procedures in long-standing or severe deformities to address adaptive bony changes that have usually occurred.
- If capsule or ligament laxity is responsible for deformity, the problem may be addressed through ligament reconstruction, surgical reefing or joint bracing. It is important to note the clinical impact of joint laxity is reduced if the mechanical axis of the limb, if originally deviated through other bony abnormality, is corrected.[5]
- Congenital absence of ligaments will produce evidence of joint laxity on formal clinical stressing but may not have a great impact on function. A decision to offer reconstruction should be based on the degree of functional compromise the anomaly produces.

Bony tissue

Osteotomies are either intra-articular, periarticular or diaphyseal. The need for intra-articular osteotomies is infrequent; examples include hemiplateau elevation in Blount's disease[6] or bending osteotomies in congenital fibula amelia.[7] Periarticular osteotomies are performed in the metaphysis and provide solutions for abnormal joint inclinations arising from metaphyseal or epiphyseal deformities. These are also performed to create an abnormal joint line inclination to counter a joint contracture that cannot be resolved through soft tissue means alone, e.g. supracondylar extension osteotomies of the femur for long-standing flexion contractures of the knee. It is often the case when metaphyseal osteotomies are performed for epiphyseal deformities, as in the previous example, that a secondary deformity is created to offset the effect of the primary deformity. This correction technique is appropriate as long as the rules of osteotomy are followed (*vide supra*). Diaphyseal osteotomies are technically easier to address as a consequence of being distant from physes and they facilitate better access for internal stabilization.

Another important surgical strategy for correction of deformity in children is guided growth. This is accomplished through bracing in some instances, or more usually by growth plate manipulation. The technique of hemiepiphyseodesis to effect change in shape or epiphyseodesis to balance limb length inequality are examples.

Strategies for preventing recurrence

The strategies needed to prevent recurrence of deformity in situations where such propensity exists will depend on the underlying cause of the deformity.

Muscle imbalance

Paralytic deformities may recur following correction unless the underlying muscle imbalance is addressed. This may entail augmenting power of the weaker side by a tendon transfer, weakening the stronger side by tendon lengthening, or through a defunctioning of the muscle by tenotomy.

Physeal damage

Asymmetric physeal damage with a resultant physeal bar should be treated by physeal bar excision or by ablation of the viable part of the physis if recurrence of the deformity is to be avoided following correction.

Metabolic bone disease

An underlying metabolic bone disorder will lead to recurrence of deformity if not addressed through medical means – in some situations this may mean lifelong treatment.

Soft tissue contracture

Fibrotic and scar tissue do not elongate sufficiently with growth and predispose to recurrence. Anticipation of and addressing the problem through long-term stretching exercises and the use of a splint during the growing years may be necessary to minimize this risk of recurrence.

References

1. Gerhardt JJ. Clinical measurements of joint motion and position in the neutral-zero method and SFTR recording: basic principles. *Int Rehabil Med* 1983; **5**: 161–4.
2. Gerhardt JJ, Rondinelli RD. Goniometric techniques for range-of-motion assessment. *Phys Med Rehabil Clin N Am* 2001; **12**: 507–27.
3. Ilizarov GA. *Transosseous Osteosynthesis*, 1st edn. Berlin: Springer-Verlag, 1992.
4. Paley D. *Principles of Deformity Correction*. Berlin: Springer, 2002.
5. Saleh M, Goonatillake HD. Management of congenital leg length inequality: value of early axis correction. *J Pediatr Orthop B* 1995; **4**: 150–8.
6. Janoyer M, Jabbari H, Rouvillain JL *et al*. Infantile Blount's disease treated by hemiplateau elevation and epiphyseal distraction using a specific external fixator: preliminary report. *J Pediatr Orthop B* 2007; **16**: 273–80.
7. Exner GU. Bending osteotomy through the distal tibial physis in fibular hemimelia for stable reduction of the hindfoot. *J Pediatr Orthop B* 2003; **12**: 27–32.

Equinus deformity

Benjamin Joseph

2

Introduction

Equinus or plantarflexion deformity of the ankle is a very common deformity that can develop in several congenital and acquired conditions encountered in paediatric orthopaedic practice.

While the term 'equinus' generally refers to a fixed plantarflexion deformity of the ankle, there are a few instances where the ankle remains in equinus while the child walks but can be passively brought to neutral or even into dorsiflexion when the child is recumbent. This phenomenon is referred to as dynamic equinus and it may be seen in some children with habitual toe-walking and when the gastrocsoleus is spastic as in cerebral palsy.

Although equinus of congenital origin may occur as an isolated deformity (Figure 2.1), it is often part of more a complex deformity such as clubfoot, convex pes valgus or equinovalgus deformity of fibular hemimelia.

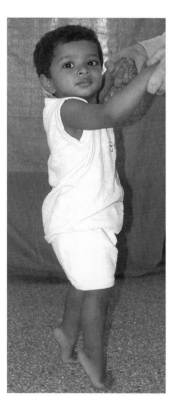

Figure 2.1 ● Equinus deformity of both feet in a child with congenital contracture of the Achilles tendons.

Equinus deformity most often develops as a consequence of contracture of the gastrocnemius, soleus or both these muscles. Much less frequently it may arise due to primary abnormality of the ankle joint or due to growth abnormality of the distal tibial growth plate. The causes of contracture of the gastrocsoleus include congenital contracture and a host of acquired conditions (Table 2.1).

Consequences of an equinus deformity

Altered gait pattern

When there is an equinus deformity, initial contact is made with the forefoot rather than the heel. During the later parts of the stance phase of gait also the heel does not come into contact with the ground and the child walks with a toe–toe sequence. This results in increased energy expenditure while walking.

Effect on the knee

When the child walks with an equinus gait the weight-bearing line and the ground reaction force passes in front of the axis of knee motion. The gastrocsoleus muscle generates a force couple that

Table 2.1 ● Causes of contracture of the gastrocsoleus

Underlying cause of contracture	Disease entity
Failure to develop normally *in utero* resulting in congenital contracture	Congenital contracture as in some cases of habitual toe-walking, multiple congenital contractures, congenital clubfoot, congenital convex pes valgus, fibular hemimelia, etc.
Postural deformity resulting in contracture	Comatose child
Failure of muscle to grow due to lack of stretch stimulus when the dorsiflexors of the ankle are paralysed	Lower motor neuron paralysis as in spina bifida, poliomyelitis, peripheral nerve injury, etc.
	Upper motor neuron paralysis as in cerebral palsy
Failure of muscle to grow due to muscle fibrosis	Volkmann's ischaemic contracture, intramuscular haemangioma, post-traumatic fibrosis or burns contracture
Primary muscle disease	Duchenne muscular dystrophy

tends to plantarflex the ankle and simultaneously extends the knee. This plantarflexor–extensor couple and the shift of the weight-bearing line anterior to the axis of knee motion can produce a recurvatum or hyperextension deformity of the knee. Such a hyperextension deformity may facilitate stabilization of the knee if the quadriceps is paralysed (see Chapter 55, The paralysed knee). However, in the absence of quadriceps muscle weakness this deformity is undesirable.

Effect on the ankle

Normally when the ankle is dorsiflexed the broader anterior part of the talus moves into the ankle mortise. In order to facilitate this, the ankle mortise has to widen in dorsiflexion and this is achieved by the lateral malleolus moving a little laterally (Figure 2.2).[1] In children with a long-standing equinus deformity the tibiofibular ligaments become contracted and will not yield sufficiently to permit movement of the anterior part of the talus into the ankle mortise.

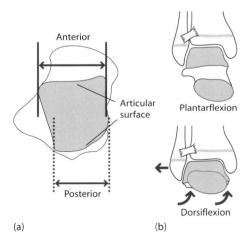

Figure 2.2 ● The anterior part of the articular surface of the talus is broader than the posterior part **(a)**. During dorsiflexion of the ankle the lateral malleolus moves laterally in order to accommodate the broader part of the talus in the ankle mortise **(b)**.

Effect on the hindfoot

A compensatory mechanism that enables the heel to rest on the ground even in the presence of an equinus deformity is the development of a valgus deformity of the hindfoot. This has been referred to as 'valgus ex-equino'.[2] The arch also collapses and a planovalgus deformity develops (see Chapter 62, The spastic foot and ankle).

Effect on the forefoot

As the child continues to walk on the toes, the forefoot broadens and the toes splay out. If the equinus remains uncorrected, metatarsalgia can develop later in adult life. If there is associated loss of sensation in the sole the increased pressure under the metatarsal heads can led to neuropathic ulceration.

Difficulty in squatting

In communities where squatting is commonplace, an equinus deformity of even a mild degree can be incapacitating as it makes it difficult to squat. In these communities an effort must be made to enable dorsiflexion of over 20–30° if possible.

Problems of management

Recurrence of deformity

Since the underlying cause for the contracture cannot be cured in many situations there is a risk of recurrence of the deformity.

Risk of overcorrection

Over-lengthening of the gastrocsoleus can cause weakness of plantarflexion and a calcaneus deformity. This is particularly disabling in cerebral palsy where it can result in a severe crouch gait (see Chapter 62, The spastic foot and ankle).

Aims of treatment

- Restore a plantigrade tread
  This is the primary aim of correcting equinus of any cause.
- Restore a heel–toe sequence of gait
  It is desirable to restore a normal heel–toe pattern of gait, although this may not always be feasible on account of the underlying disease process.
- Prevent progress of undesirable adaptive changes in the knee and foot
  Recurvatum of the knee and valgus deformity of the hindfoot should be prevented from progressing.
- Facilitate passive dorsiflexion beyond neutral if needed
  If squatting is desired, the contracture should be released sufficiently to enable dorsiflexion of at least 20°.
- Prevent recurrence of deformity
  When muscle imbalance is the underlying cause of the equinus deformity, the treatment strategy should include a tendon transfer or a long-term regimen of passive stretching exercises and bracing if a tendon transfer is not possible.
- Prevent overcorrection
  Over-lengthening of the gastrocsoleus leading to a calcaneus deformity must be avoided as this may be more disabling than the equinus deformity.

Treatment options

No intervention

The only situation where a mild fixed equinus is desirable is when there is associated weakness of the quadriceps muscle. Such children do not require any treatment for the equinus deformity.

Ankle–foot orthosis and stretching exercises

An ankle–foot orthosis can effectively correct a dynamic equinus. An orthosis should also be used post-operatively after correction of equinus in situations where there is a risk of recurrence of deformity. This should be supplemented with regular exercises that stretch the gastrocsoleus.

Wedging of plaster casts

Minor degrees of equinus deformity may be corrected by wedging of casts. This may be particularly useful in children with haemophilia where surgical intervention would require elevation of the factor VIII levels to near normal. This method is also useful to treat early recurrence of equinus deformity in clubfeet.

Tenotomy of the Achilles tendon

Percutaneous tenotomy of the Achilles tendon can be performed in situations where the foot and ankle are stiff, with little likelihood of significant motion following correction of equinus. A tenotomy is the preferred treatment in multiple congenital contractures (arthrogryposis).

Percutaneous lengthening of the Achilles tendon

For moderate degrees of equinus percutaneous techniques of tendon lengthening should suffice as correction should be obtained without having to perform a capsulotomy of the ankle joint. The Hoke's or the White's techniques of lengthening are simple and effective (Figure 2.3).[3]

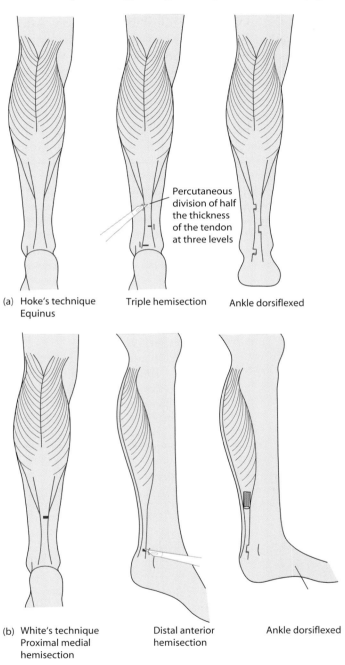

Percutaneous division of half the thickness of the tendon at three levels

(a) Hoke's technique Equinus   Triple hemisection   Ankle dorsiflexed

(b) White's technique Proximal medial hemisection   Distal anterior hemisection   Ankle dorsiflexed

Figure 2.3 ● Techniques of lengthening the Achilles tendon percutaneously. The Hoke's technique **(a)** and the White's technique **(b)** are shown.

Coronal z-plasty of the Achilles tendon

A pure severe equinus deformity can be corrected by an open coronal z-plasty combined with a posterior capsulotomy of the ankle joint.

Sagittal z-plasty of the Achilles tendon

A severe equinovarus or equinovalgus deformity should be treated by performing a sagittal z-plasty. Care should be taken to detach the medial half of the tendon from the calcaneum if there is a varus deformity and the lateral half of the tendon from the calcaneum if there is a valgus deformity.

Selective lengthening of the gastrocnemius

If it can be demonstrated that the equinus deformity is due to contracture of the gastrocnemius without involvement of the soleus, then selective lengthening of the gastrocnemius is performed. This is the preferred technique in cerebral palsy where the gastrocnemius is implicated in most instances.[4–6]

Lengthening of the Achilles tendon and tendon transfer to restore active dorsiflexion

In paralytic situations where there is demonstrable muscle imbalance, apart from lengthening the Achilles tendon a suitable tendon from the posterior compartment should be transferred to the dorsum of the foot to restore the power of dorsiflexion. Unless muscle balance is restored in this manner, the deformity will recur.

Hemitransfer of the Achilles tendon

Occasionally in children with spina bifida recurrent equinus deformity can develop even after tenotomy of the Achilles tendon despite the fact that no active contraction of the gastrocsoleus can be elicited. In these children the muscle is usually spastic and the tendon often becomes reattached to the calcaneum even after a seemingly satisfactory tenotomy. In this situation transfer of the lateral half of the Achilles tendon to the dorsum of the foot can prevent the recurrence of equinus (Figure 2.4).[7]

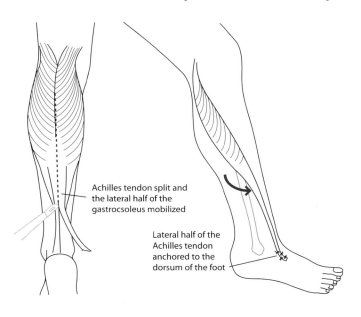

Achilles tendon split and the lateral half of the gastrocsoleus mobilized

Lateral half of the Achilles tendon anchored to the dorsum of the foot

Figure 2.4 ● Technique of transferring the lateral half of the Achilles tendon to the dorsum of the foot.

Supramalleolar osteotomy

In the older child with a stiff foot and long-standing equinus, lengthening of the Achilles tendon and a posterior capsulotomy of the ankle may not produce any appreciable correction as the talus cannot be reduced into the ankle mortise. In this situation a supramalleolar osteotomy of the tibia may be performed to make the foot plantigrade.

Triple fusion

In the skeletally mature adolescent with a severe deformity a Lambrinudi type of triple fusion would correct the equinus. Any associated varus or valgus deformity at the subtalar level could also be corrected by this procedure.

The underlying disease process

If the gastrocsoleus muscle is fibrotic and not functioning there is a risk of recurrence following tendon lengthening; a tenotomy of the Achilles tendon would be the procedure of choice. There is little risk of overcorrection following the tenotomy because of the fibrosis. On the other hand, a child with congenital contracture of the muscle with no underlying neurological problem should have a judicious lengthening of the tendon such that the muscle can function following the surgery.

Factors to be taken into consideration while planning treatment

Likelihood of recurrence of deformity

Muscle grows in response to stretch stimulus and this stretch is normally provided by the antagonistic muscles. Thus, if an equinus is associated with weakness of the dorsiflexors, adequate stretching of the gastrocsoleus will not occur. In these situations mere lengthening of the gastrocsoleus may not suffice; the stretch stimulus would have to be ensured either by augmenting the strength of dorsiflexion with a tendon transfer or by physiotherapy entailing passive stretching exercises.

Likelihood of overcorrection

While the risk of overcorrection following lengthening of the gastrocsoleus in cerebral palsy is well recognized it can occur in other clinical situations such as congenital clubfoot.

Age of the patient

Surgery on the bones as a means of correcting a long-standing equinus deformity is reserved for the older child and adolescent.

Severity of deformity

The severity of the deformity will dictate the nature of surgery.

Recommended treatment

The outline of treatment of equinus deformity is shown in Table 2.2. The treatment options shown in the table are for situations where the gastrocnemius and the soleus are contracted. If it can be demonstrated that the gastrocnemius alone is contracted, selective release of the gastrocnemius is performed. Similarly, in cerebral palsy selective release of the gastrocnemius is preferred to lengthening of the Achilles tendon.

Table 2.2 ● Outline of treatment of equinus deformity

INDICATIONS								
Mild fixed equinus + Weak quadriceps muscle	Dynamic equinus	Mild fixed equinus of recent onset + No underlying muscle imbalance	Moderate equinus + Postural deformity + No muscle imbalance + Gastrocnemius AND soleus contracted	Moderate or severe equinus + Stiff foot + High risk of recurrence + No risk of overcorrection	Severe equinus + No muscle imbalance + Gastrocnemius AND soleus contracted	Moderate or severe equinus + Muscle imbalance + No spasticity + Gastrocnemius AND soleus contracted	Recurrent equinus + Stiff scarred ankle + Long-standing deformity	Severe equinus in adolescent + Stiff foot unlikely to be corrected by soft tissue procedure
⇩	⇩	⇩	⇩	⇩	⇩	⇩	⇩	⇩
No intervention	Ankle–foot orthosis + Stretching exercises	Wedging of plaster casts	Percutaneous lengthening of Achilles tendon	Tenotomy of Achilles tendon (excise 1 cm of the tendon)	Z-lengthening of Achilles tendon + Posterior capsulotomy of the ankle joint	Z-lengthening of Achilles tendon + Tendon transfer to restore muscle balance	Supramalleolar osteotomy	Lambrinudi type of triple arthrodesis
TREATMENT								

References

1. Kapandji IA. *The Physiology of Joints*, 1st edn. Vol 2. Edinburgh: E & S Livingstone, 1870.
2. Sharrard WJW. *Paediatric Orthopaedics and Fractures*, 3rd edn. Vol 2. Oxford: Blackwell Scientific Publications, 1993.
3. Graham HK, Fixsen JA. Lengthening of the calcaneal tendon in spastic hemiplegia by the White slide technique. A long-term review. *J Bone Joint Surg Br* 1988; **70**: 472–5.
4. Yngve DA, Chambers C. Vulpius and Z-lengthening. *J Pediatr Orthop* 1996; **16**: 759–64.
5. Saraph V, Zwick EB, Uitz C, Linhart W, Steinwender G. The Baumann procedure for fixed contracture of the gastrosoleus in cerebral palsy. Evaluation of function of the ankle after multilevel surgery. *J Bone Joint Surg Br* 2000; **82**: 535–40.
6. Engsberg JR, Oeffinger DJ, Ross SA *et al.* Comparison of three heel cord surgeries in children with cerebral palsy. *J Appl Biomech* 2005; **21**: 322–33.
7. Ogilvie C, Sharrard WJ. Hemitransplantation of the tendo calcaneus in children with spinal neurological disorders. *J Bone Joint Surg Br* 1986; **68**: 767–9.

Equinovarus

Selvadurai Nayagam

3

Introduction

Equinovarus deformity is encountered most commonly as congenital clubfoot (Figure 3.1a,b). However, an identical deformity can occur in neurological conditions such as injury to the common peroneal nerve (Figure 3.1c,d), spina bifida and poliomyelitis and in association with spastic paralysis. Equinovarus deformity is occasionally seen in association with tarsal coalition when it presents as a rigid deformity, akin to teratologic types.[1]

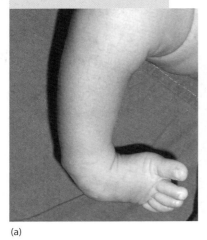 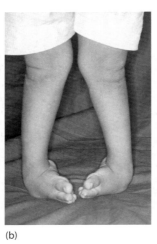 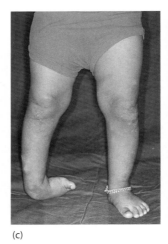 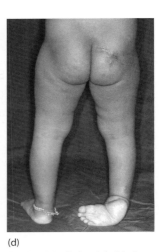

(a) (b) (c) (d)

Figure 3.1 ● Clubfoot in a neonate **(a)** and uncorrected congenital clubfoot in a toddler **(b)**. **(c,d)** Equinovarus deformity that is indistinguishable from congenital clubfoot in a child who sustained a penetrating injury to the gluteal region that severed the peroneal division of the sciatic nerve.

In congenital clubfoot, the commonest type, genetic,[2] fetal and intrauterine 'packaging' issues have been deemed responsible, as have neuromuscular conditions. There is an association with hip and spinal problems (which need to be ruled out at first assessment) and it may present with other joint contractures as in multiple congenital contractures (arthrogryposis). In the absence of an identifiable cause, it is labelled idiopathic and this represents the majority of cases. The condition is more common in males and approximately half the cases have both feet affected. It is 20–30 times more likely in siblings.

The diagnosis of the clubfoot or congenital talipes equinovarus (CTEV) can now be made antenatally by ultrasound imaging. The first consultation may therefore represent an information-gathering occasion by parents seeking guidance on prognosis and treatment. Three nuggets of information should guide the first meeting: the ultrasound test has a false positive rate if the diagnosis of clubfoot is one in isolation; as many as two-thirds of antenatally diagnosed clubfeet have other anomalies;[3–5] and the heterogeneity (especially with response to treatment) should prompt caution against overly specific predictions.

The deformity

The deformity is complex and involves the ankle, subtalar and midtarsal joints.

The hindfoot

At the ankle there is an equinus or plantarflexion deformity; at the subtalar joint there is an inversion and adduction deformity. The combined inversion and adduction deformity is referred to as hindfoot varus. It is important to be aware that inversion and adduction at the subtalar joint occur in unison because the peculiar oblique configuration of the axis of the subtalar joint dictates that as the calcaneum adducts, it inverts concomitantly (Figure 3.2a,b).

The midfoot

At the midtarsal joint the forefoot is adducted, and plantarflexed in relation to the hindfoot. Variation in severity and 'rigidity' of the deformity is commonplace.

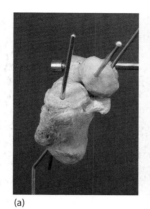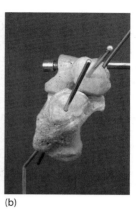

Figure 3.2 ● An articulated model of the talus and the calcaneum in the everted position of the subtalar joint **(a)** and the inverted position of the joint **(b)**. In the everted position the calcaneum is abducted, while in the inverted position the calcaneum is adducted.

(a)   (b)

Structures responsible for the deformity

Among the various structures that may be abnormal and contribute to the deformity are the gastrocsoleus and the tibialis posterior. These muscles may be contracted, working without any opposing antagonist or spastic due to an upper motor neuron paralysis. It is important to ascertain which of these mechanisms are responsible for the deformity as the strategies for dealing with each of these conditions will vary accordingly (Table 3.1).

Table 3.1 ● Origin of the deformity and intervention for equinovarus deformity in different conditions

Condition	Underlying abnormality	Intervention
Congenital clubfoot	Gastrocsoleus and tibialis posterior contractures and talus and os calcis deformities	Manual stretching with serial casts, with or without surgical elongation of the tendons of the contracted muscles will treat the majority in infancy. Additional surgery and joint releases may be needed for non-idiopathic and teratologic types
Common peroneal nerve palsy	Muscle imbalance due to unopposed action of the gastrocsoleus and the tibialis posterior (paralysed evertors and dorsiflexors)	Restore muscle balance after elimination of deformity
Cerebral palsy	Spasticity of the gastrocsoleus and the tibialis posterior	Reduce spasticity of the affected muscles

Other soft tissue contractures, including the joint capsules, develop subsequently. In long-standing cases adaptive bony changes ensue which, in the case of congenital clubfoot, add to the inherent abnormal anatomy already present in the talus and calcaneum.

Dissections of clubfeet of stillborn infants and more recent magnetic resonance imaging studies have clearly shown the structures that are contracted as well as the abnormal tarsal relationships.[6–10] This knowledge enables the surgeon to focus technique on relevant structures either during non-operative treatment or in surgical correction (Table 3.2).

While one or two of these structures would be contracted in mild cases, all structures listed can be affected in severe deformity.

Problems of management

Heterogeneity leading to variation in response to the same treatment

No universal validated classification exists but several clinical features point to increasing severity: deep or double creases, a large deformity and rigidity. The variation in morphology continues to be expressed as variation in response to treatment; many studies that appear to report a 'single' percentage success in regard to one particular treatment are thwarted by heterogeneous samples.

Recurrence

This is a possibility even when complete correction is accomplished by initial treatment. Regular follow-up until skeletal maturity will allow the supervising surgeon to diagnose mild relapse and the opportunity to intervene early with simpler modalities of treatment as opposed to more radical forms. The underlying aetiology in clubfoot is probably unaffected by treatment and this may be the basis for recurrence.

Scarring from repeated extensive open procedures

When surgical release was the primary method of treatment, those cases that recurred presented the surgeon with a rigid deformity contributed to, at least partially, by scarring. Additional surgical releases compounded the matter further.

Aims of treatment

- Restore a plantigrade foot
  A normal foot is not the objective of treatment of congenital clubfoot as this may not be possible with current methods of treatment. The deformity comprises misshapen foot bones (in particular the talus and calcaneum) and joint subluxation; correction of the latter often produces improved alignment while the abnormal shape of the bones is altered a little. The aim with treatment of all forms of equinovarus deformity is to make the foot rest flat on the ground so that weight is distributed evenly over the sole.
- Avoid a loss of suppleness through treatment
  Some degree of scarring is an inevitable consequence of surgery but it is not invariably linked to stiffness. Many clubfeet treated by open surgery remain supple. However, certain resistant forms of the deformity tend to become stiff soon after extensive open procedures and may be better approached through different treatment strategies. In clubfoot associated with multiple congenital contractures (arthrogryposis) the foot is deformed and stiff to begin with; here the aim is to make the stiff foot plantigrade.
- Ensure as near normal function of the foot as possible
  Ideally, normal range of motion coupled to normal muscle power is sought. While this may be possible in milder forms of congenital clubfoot, it is not realistic in neurogenic forms of equinovarus deformity.
- Ensure that the foot does not become painful
  Alignment compatible with normal function, without pain induced through the effects of treatment or residual deformity, is paramount. Even a little residual deformity may be tolerated if compatible with pain-free walking.
- Avoid a permanent need for orthotics
  Some form of splint usually follows the several different treatment protocols available for clubfeet. There is evidence to support protracted use in the first three to four years of life but permanent use should be justified appropriately – no significant data are available to determine whether continued protracted use actually prevents recurrence less than that of the natural history of the condition. Orthotics may be needed to avoid recurrence in neurogenic conditions if the aetiological muscle imbalance cannot be redressed.

Treatment options

Serial manipulation and casting

Serial casting is the primary method used for the newborn with a congenital clubfoot. Different techniques of manipulation have been described, including those of Kite, Ponseti and Dimeglio.[11–16] They differ in the fine detail but share common principles. There is a need to start manipulating the infant's foot as soon as possible; each being done gently and without anaesthesia. Attempts to correct equinus should be made after correction of hindfoot varus in order to avoid creating a rocker-bottom deformity.

Currently there is enthusiasm for Ponseti's technique (Figure 3.3). This method is an improvement over serial stretching and taping techniques and it is encouraging to witness the correction that can be achieved after three to five cast changes. Much of the correction is in the forefoot and 'turning' of the hindfoot into valgus; the majority will require a percutaneous tenotomy of the Achilles tendon for resolution of equinus. Correction is followed by a regime of using Denis Browne boots with a derotation bar – continuously for three months before relaxing into a night-time only protocol until the

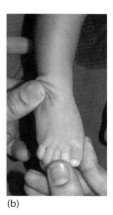
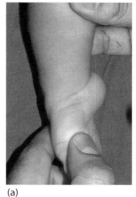

Figure 3.3 ● Technique of serial manipulation by the method of Ponseti. The foot is supinated to reduce the cavus deformity **(a)**. The foot is then abducted with counter pressure on the head of the talus to ensure that the foot moves around the head of the talus **(b)**.

(a)   (b)

age of three years.[17,18] This sequence of serial casting with or without tenotomy can be utilized for children as old as 12–14 months, with confidence in the knowledge that the divided tendon will heal. It can also be repeated if the first sequence only permits partial resolution.

Soft tissue release

Children with clubfeet that fail to respond completely after at least two applications of the Ponseti technique are potential candidates for open surgical release. They are in a minority and probably represent a different aetiological and prognostic group; often they are cases with bilateral involvement. Surgical techniques differ from the type of skin incision to degree of 'release' – from specific structures which must be freed in every case to the à la carte approach.[19–25] There are practical advantages to leaving this surgery until after the age of nine months (the surgery is technically easier and post-surgical therapy is assisted by a child who is beginning to walk by the time the cast is removed).

Children do not always present for treatment in the early post-natal period. Worldwide, particularly in poorer communities, it is not uncommon to encounter a child with clubfoot after the child has begun to walk or even later. In these older children non-operative methods may be less effective (as secondary adaptive changes are likely), leaving soft tissue release as the mainstay of correction. The severity of deformity dictates the structures that need to be released (Table 3.2).

Table 3.2 ● Soft tissue contractures contributing to individual deformity components in clubfoot

Deformity	Structures that are contracted and contributing to the deformity
Equinus	Achilles tendon and gastrocsoleus Posterior capsule of the ankle joint Posterior talofibular ligament
Hindfoot varus	Tibialis posterior Medial capsule of the subtalar joint Superficial deltoid ligament Calcaneofibular ligament
Forefoot adduction	Tibialis posterior Abductor hallucis Medial capsules of the talonavicular joint and the calcaneocuboid joints Spring ligament
Forefoot equinus (cavus)	Plantar fascia Short plantar muscles

Soft tissue surgical techniques include an isolated posterior release, a posteromedial release or a complete circumferential subtalar release. If the forefoot and hindfoot varus deformities are well corrected by serial casts and the residual deformity equinus, a posterior soft tissue release will suffice. However, in the majority of cases needing soft tissue surgery (in the event of failure or incomplete resolution from serial casts), all components of the original deformity will be present to some degree; in such feet a posterior and medial soft tissue release is necessary. In severe and stiff deformities, only a complete subtalar release will enable the calcaneum to rotate out of adduction and varus and enable adequate correction of equinus.

Gradual distraction

Gradual correction by means of external fixation is established as a powerful technique for the resistant and recurrent clubfoot.[26–29] This method appears to preserve suppleness and can be combined with foot osteotomies as an alternative to triple joint fusion in the salvage of stiff recurrent deformities in older and adolescent children. In the relapsed and stiff variants, the Ilizarov method of

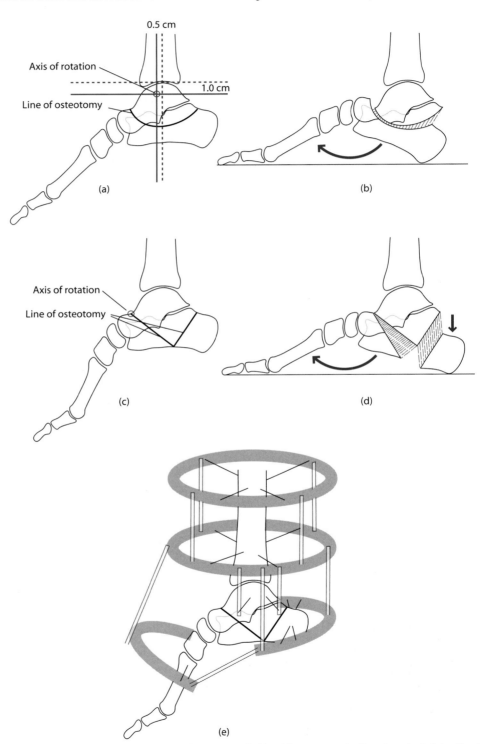

Figure 3.4 ● Techniques of performing a U osteotomy **(a,b)** or V osteotomy **(c,d)** and gradual distraction by the Ilizarov technique. The U osteotomy is performed if there is only residual equinus while a V osteotomy is used to correct equinovarus. The fixator construct is shown diagrammatically **(e)**.

gradual correction by external fixation is remarkable at salvaging these problems; full correction and some restoration of foot and ankle suppleness is possible (Figure 3.4). In older children and adolescents, this technique can be combined with calcaneal and midfoot osteotomies to create a plantigrade foot around a stiff ankle and subtalar joint. Despite its obvious strengths in achieving correction to a plantigrade foot, it incurs considerable effort and strain on behalf of the patient and family and, for the time being, should be reserved for intractable and resistant cases of deformity.

Tendon transfers

In children over the age of three years a tendon transfer can help redress some residual components of deformity and should be considered, provided the deformity is passively correctable or is corrected at the time of transfer. In neurogenic clubfeet, a tendon transfer should invariably be done as part of the index procedure so that muscle balance is restored (see Chapter 56, The paralysed foot and ankle).

■ **Tibialis anterior transfer**

■ Complete tibialis anterior transfer to the lateral aspect of the dorsum of the foot

Complete transfer of the tibialis anterior tendon (Figure 3.5a) is performed in nearly half of cases undergoing treatment by the Ponseti method. It is usual to seat the detached tendon into the lateral cuneiform. The procedure is carried out around three years of age if some return of forefoot deformity is detected and is preceded by a few serial casts.

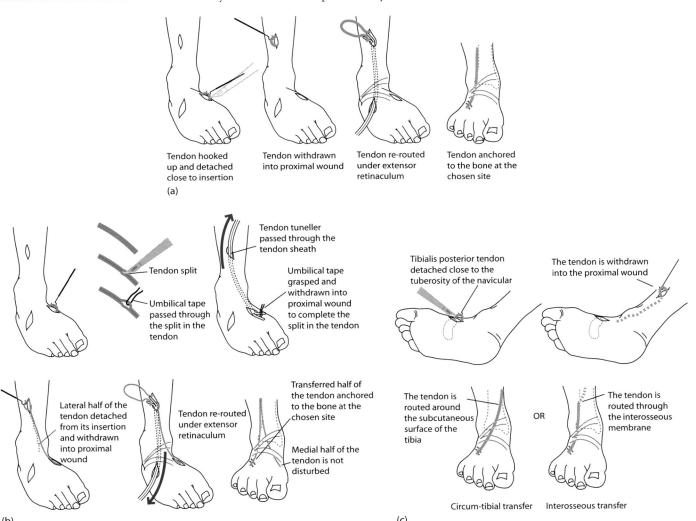

Tendon hooked up and detached close to insertion

Tendon withdrawn into proximal wound

Tendon re-routed under extensor retinaculum

Tendon anchored to the bone at the chosen site

(a)

Tendon split

Umbilical tape passed through the split in the tendon

Tendon tuneller passed through the tendon sheath

Umbilical tape grasped and withdrawn into proximal wound to complete the split in the tendon

Tibialis posterior tendon detached close to the tuberosity of the navicular

The tendon is withdrawn into the proximal wound

Lateral half of the tendon detached from its insertion and withdrawn into proximal wound

Tendon re-routed under extensor retinaculum

Transferred half of the tendon anchored to the bone at the chosen site

Medial half of the tendon is not disturbed

The tendon is routed around the subcutaneous surface of the tibia

OR

The tendon is routed through the interosseous membrane

Circum-tibial transfer   Interosseous transfer

(b)   (c)

Figure 3.5 ● Techniques of performing **(a)** a complete transfer of the tibialis anterior tendon, **(b)** a split tibialis anterior transfer and **(c)** a tibialis posterior transfer.

■ Split tibialis anterior transfer to the lateral aspect of the dorsum of the foot

Some surgeons advocate using the lateral half of the tibialis anterior which is transferred to the lateral aspect of the foot, and either anchored to the peroneus brevis tendon or to the cuboid bone (Figure 3.5b).

■ Tibialis posterior transfer

The rationale for transferring the tendon to the lateral part of the dorsum of the foot is to convert a deforming force into a corrective force (Figure 3.5c). However, the tendon is likely to be fibrotic and difficult to transfer if a previous soft issue release has already been performed.

Osteotomies

■ Osteotomies to correct forefoot adduction

Recurrence, particularly a stiff adducted forefoot deformity after previous extensive surgical release, may need further open surgery to include medial and lateral column adjusting techniques[30] if the child is of the appropriate age (four to seven years).

■ Lengthening the medial column

Open wedge osteotomy of the medial cuneiform. This operation entails placing a medially based wedge of bone graft into an osteotomy in the substance of the medial cuneiform (Figure 3.6b). The tricortical graft is harvested from the iliac crest. The graft incorporation is better after the ossific nucleus of the medial cuneiform is visible on radiographs at around four years of age.

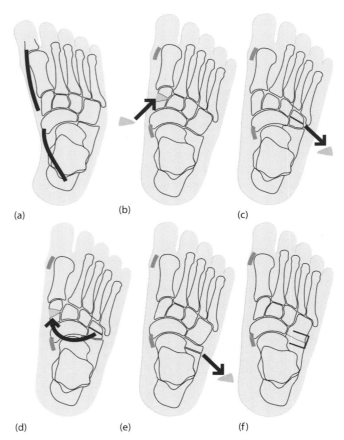

(a)   (b)   (c)

(d)   (e)   (f)

Figure 3.6 ● Osteotomies that may be performed to correct residual forefoot adduction **(a)** include an open wedge osteotomy of the medial cuneiform bone **(b)**, closed wedge osteotomy of the cuboid **(c)**, a combination of an open wedge osteotomy of the cuneiform and a closed wedge osteotomy of the cuboid **(d)**, closed wedge osteotomy of the anterior end of the calcaneum **(e)** and wedge resection and fusion of the calcaneocuboid joint **(f)**.

■ Shortening the lateral column

Closed wedge osteotomy of the cuboid. A laterally based wedge of bone is resected from the cuboid bone (Figure 3.6c). This operation can be combined with an open wedge osteotomy of the medial cuneiform (Figure 3.6d) and is a particularly attractive option since the graft for inserting into the cuneiform is available from the cuboid. If it is performed without medial column lengthening, decancellation (removing the central ossified area) of the cuboid and closing the defect acutely achieves the same effect.

Osteotomy of the anterior end of the calcaneum. A closed wedge osteotomy of the anterior end of the calcaneum achieves the same effect as an osteotomy of the cuboid. However, there is a risk that the osteotomy will run through the anterior articular facet of the calcaneum. (Figure 3.6e).

■ Osteotomies to correct hindfoot varus

These can be used to correct isolated hindfoot deformities in older children if the subtalar joint retains some movement (Figure 3.7). By translating the point of contact of the os calcis with the floor lateral to the middle of the ankle, the osteotomy restores the eversion lever through the subtalar joint. This effect can be achieved through a lateral closing wedge osteotomy of calcaneum or lateral translation osteotomy. Medial open wedge osteotomies of calcaneum achieve the same but can be fraught with wound healing problems.

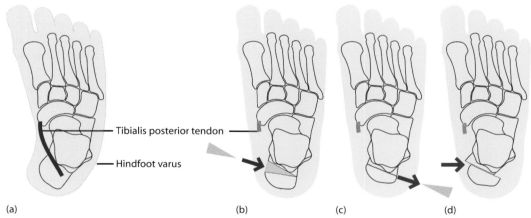

Tibialis posterior tendon

Hindfoot varus

(a)   (b)   (c)   (d)

Figure 3.7 ● Osteotomies that may be performed to correct hind foot varus include **(a)** a medial open wedge osteotomy **(b)**, a lateral closed wedge osteotomy **(c)** and a lateral displacement osteotomy of the calcaneum **(d)**.

Bone resection

Talectomy is reserved for severe cases when no other method to restore a plantigrade foot has prevailed. It has been reported to be a satisfactory choice for resistant equinovarus deformity in multiple congenital contractures (arthrogryposis), but the advent of gradual correction by the Ilizarov fixator has reduced the need of this salvage procedure. In any event, the procedure can still be followed by further recurrence of deformity, which may then prove most difficult to resolve.

Joint fusion

■ Calcaneocuboid fusion

Fusion of the calcaneocuboid joint effectively shortens the lateral column (Figure 3.6f). This was the original technique described by Evans[30] but is now modified to cuboid decancellation for the same effect.

■ Triple fusion

The triple arthrodesis is a salvage procedure; it has a place in many foot deformities involving the ankle, subtalar and midfoot joints and should ideally be performed after the age of 12 when most foot growth has already occurred. Nonetheless, it reduces the size of the foot further and may even induce degenerative changes in the ankle joint in the long term.[31]

Controversies in management

Post-correction splinting

Splinting regimes after open surgery are contentious. While the protocol in the Ponseti method is well defined (vide infra), surgeons vary in prescriptions of straight last shoes, ankle–foot orthoses and night splints following a surgical release of clubfoot. At its least intrusive, an ankle–foot orthosis for three months after the plaster of Paris support is discontinued is reasonable, if only to observe the manner of control over recurrence of deformity. Should no recurrence be evident, walking in normal last shoes should confer some protection against relapse. Residual forefoot adduction, if passively correctable, may benefit from the use of straight last shoes; stiff metatarsus adductus in straight last shoes only produces pain. Night-time splints are prescribed in the belief that control of resting foot and ankle position at a time when the child is inactive may reduce the relapse rate. In multiple congenital contractures (arthrogryposis) splinting needs to be early, protracted and well monitored.

Controversies in treating the relapsed rigid deformity

Rigidity in recurrent deformity may be related to scarring but may also be a reflection of the natural history of the condition. Salvage procedures in older children are founded on the triple arthrodesis and variants thereof but leaves the patient with a smaller, albeit better positioned foot. Techniques based on the Ilizarov method appear to provide a similar result but without diminution in foot size.

Factors to take into consideration while planning treatment

Aetiology

Idiopathic clubfeet respond well to the Ponseti method of treatment. This method can also form the initial therapy for other types of clubfeet – while the response may be variable, this approach helps reduce a large proportion of the initial presenting deformity. Persevering with the Ponseti method in the severe clubfoot deformity, especially if not of the idiopathic group, may produce pseudo-correction – the residual deformity in such cases should be amenable to open surgery.

Patient and parent circumstances

Patient (and parent) compliance with serial casting is usually good but may falter with the strict regime of Denis Brown splints in the Ponseti method.[32,33] Some anticipation of this change may prompt the surgeon to be appropriately supportive during the latter period of treatment.

Similar consideration is needed for the Ilizarov technique; supportive home circumstances are preferable if a child is undertaking a prolonged period of external fixation and gradual adjustment.

Age

The approach to the newborn with a clubfoot is understandably different from a late presenting child; serial casts may still have a role in older children but some form of open release is more likely.

Previous surgery

The Ponseti method is less likely to work in the presence of previous surgery. The scar may prevent the guided gradual correction of serial cast changes or, worse still, produce a pseudo-correction. Further open surgery or the Ilizarov technique may be better choices.

Radiological changes

Radiographs of the foot, particularly in the resistant or relapsed clubfoot, may reveal abnormal bone shape, e.g. the flat-top talus. While this 'flat-top' appearance may be due to projection obliquity in some cases, in others it is a true change. Trying to dorsiflex an ankle with a flat-top talus is likely to lead to cartilage damage over the anterior surface of the dome of the talus; corrective osteotomies are better suited in this scenario.

Muscle imbalance

Neurogenic causes, whether of upper or lower motor neuron origin, need to be assessed with regard to the imbalance of action of muscles across the ankle and foot joints. This provides the basis of correction, which needs to include both releases of contractures and appropriate tendon transfers to avert recurrence (see Chapter 53, General principles of management of lower motor neuron paralysis, Chapter 56, The paralysed foot and ankle and Chapter 62, The spastic foot and ankle).

Recommended treatment

The outlines of treatment are shown in Tables 3.3, 3.4 and 3.5.

Table 3.3 ● Treatment of equinovarus deformity in the infant and young child

INDICATIONS				
Newborn with idiopathic clubfoot + No underlying neuromuscular disease	Newborn with neurogenic clubfoot (e.g. multiple congenital contractures/arthrogryposis)	From around 9 months of age until 3 years of age + Equinovarus not responding to column 1 strategy + Predominant equinus deformity persisting (other components corrected)	From around 9 months of age until 3 years of age + Equinovarus not responding to column 1 strategy + All components of the deformity persisting + Some components are not very rigid	From around 9 months of age until 3 years of age + Equinovarus not responding to column 1 strategy + All components of the deformity persisting + All components are very rigid ⇩ Complete subtalar release + splint
⇩ Serial manipulation and casting, with or without percutaneous tendo-Achilles tenotomy, and followed by Denis Browne splint	⇩ Serial manipulation and casting to reduce the severity of deformity prior to surgery + Early (by 6 months) posterior and medial release + Cast and protracted splint use to prevent recurrence	⇩ Posterior soft tissue release + splint	⇩ Posterior and medial soft tissue release + splint	
TREATMENT				

INDICATIONS				
Residual forefoot deformity (adductus and supination) + Partially correctable passively + Aged 3–4 years	Residual forefoot deformity (adductus and supination) + Not correctable passively + Age <4 years + Ossific nucleus of cuneiform not appeared	Residual forefoot deformity (adductus and supination) + Not correctable passively + Age >4 years + Ossific nucleus of cuneiform appeared	Residual forefoot and hindfoot deformity + Not correctable passively + Previous surgery + Age >6 years (more likely in relapsed CTEV)	Forefoot adductus/supination and hindfoot equinovarus + Partially correctable passively + No previous surgery + Age >6 years (more likely seen in neurologic conditions of late onset, e.g. Duchenne muscular dystrophy, rather than relapsed congenital talipes equinovarus) ⇩
⇩	⇩	⇩	⇩	Medial soft tissue release + Tendo Achilles lengthening + Tibialis posterior tendon transfer through the interosseous membrane to the lateral border of the dorsum of the foot + Bracing after correction
Repeat serial casts + Transfer of tibialis anterior to the lateral cuneiform	Tibialis posterior lengthening + Abductor hallucis release + Talonavicular capsulotomy + Laterally based closed wedge osteotomy of cuboid/decancellation of cuboid	Tibialis posterior lengthening + Abductor hallucis release + Talonavicular capsulotomy + Laterally based closed wedge osteotomy of cuboid ± Open wedge osteotomy of the medial cuneiform	Medial soft tissue release + Posterior soft tissue release + Split tibialis anterior tendon transfer to the lateral border of the dorsum of the foot + Lateral displacement osteotomy of the calcaneal tuberosity OR Gradual correction through soft tissue distraction in an external fixator	
TREATMENT				

INDICATIONS		
Stiff forefoot and hindfoot deformity + History of previous soft tissue releases + Normal dome shape to body of talus on lateral radiograph view	Stiff forefoot and hindfoot deformity + History of previous soft tissue releases + 'Flat top' shape to body of talus on lateral radiograph view + Age >10 years	Stiff forefoot and hindfoot deformity + History of previous soft tissue releases + 'Flat top' shape to body of talus on lateral radiograph view + Changes of joint degeneration (subarticular sclerosis with joint space loss) + Age >12 years ⇩
		Triple arthrodesis OR Gradual correction through V-type osteotomy across calcaneum and midfoot with distraction in external fixation
⇩	⇩	
Gradual correction through soft tissue distraction in external fixation	Gradual correction through V-type osteotomy across calcaneum and midfoot with distraction in external fixation	
TREATMENT		

References

1. Spero CR, Simon GS, Tornetta P 3rd. Clubfeet and tarsal coalition. *J Pediatr Orthop* 1994; **14**: 372–6.

2. Dietz FR, Cole WG, Tosi LL *et al.* A search for the gene predisposing to idiopathic clubfoot. *Clin Genet* 2005; **67**: 361–2.

3. Craig S, Roberts DJB Jr,Heinsen J, Seligson D. Diagnostic ultrasonography – applications in orthopaedic surgery. *Clin Orthop Relat Res* 2002; **401**: 248–64.

4. Treadwell MC, Stanitski CL, King MR. Prenatal sonographic diagnosis of clubfoot: implications for patient counseling. *J Pediatr Orthop* 1999; **19**: 8–10.

5. Tillett RL, Fisk NM, Murphy K, Hunt DM. Clinical outcome of congenital talipes equinovarus diagnosed antenatally by ultrasound. *J Bone Joint Surg Br* 2000; **82**: 876–80.

6. Herzenberg JE, Carroll NC, Christofersen MR *et al.* Clubfoot analysis with three-dimensional computer modeling. *J Pediatr Orthop* 1988; **8**: 257–62.

7. Itohara T, Sugamoto K, Shimizu N *et al.* Assessment of the three-dimensional relationship of the ossific nuclei and cartilaginous anlagen in congenital clubfoot by 3-D MRI. *J Orthop Res* 2005; **23**: 1160–4.

8. Itohara T, Sugamoto K, Shimizu N *et al.* Assessment of talus deformity by three-dimensional MRI in congenital clubfoot. *Eur J Radiol* 2005; **53**: 78–83.

9. Saito S, Hatori M, Kokubun S, Abe Y, Kita A. Evaluation of calcaneal malposition by magnetic resonance imaging in the infantile clubfoot. *J Pediatr Orthop B* 2004; **13**: 99–102.

10. Cahuzac JP, Navascues J, Baunin C *et al.* Assessment of the position of the navicular by three-dimensional magnetic resonance imaging in infant foot deformities. *J Pediatr Orthop B* 2002; **11**: 134–8.

11. Laaveg SJ, Ponseti IV. Long-term results of treatment of congenital club foot. *J Bone Joint Surg Am* 1980; **62**: 23–31.

12. Morcuende JA, Abbasi D, Dolan LA, Ponseti IV. Results of an accelerated Ponseti protocol for clubfoot. *J Pediatr Orthop* 2005; **25**: 623–6.

13. Ponseti IV. Clubfoot management. *J Pediatr Orthop* 2000; **20**: 699–700.

14. Ponseti IV, Zhivkov M, Davis N *et al.* Treatment of the complex idiopathic clubfoot. *Clin Orthop Relat Res* 2006; **451**: 171–6.

15. Kite JH. Some suggestions on the treatment of club foot by casts. *J Bone Joint Surg Am* 1963; **45**: 406–12.

16. Dimeglio A, Bonnet F, Mazeau P, De Rosa V. Orthopaedic treatment and passive motion machine: consequences for the surgical treatment of clubfoot. *J Pediatr Orthop B* 1996; **5**: 173–80.

17. Hattori T, Ono Y, Kitakoji T, Iwata H. Effect of the Denis Browne splint in conservative treatment of congenital club foot. *J Pediatr Orthop B* 2003; **12**: 59–62.

18. Thacker MM, Scher DM, Sala DA *et al.* Use of the foot abduction orthosis following Ponseti casts: is it essential? *J Pediatr Orthop* 2005; **25**: 225–8.

19. Carroll NC, Gross RH. Operative management of clubfoot. *Orthopedics* 1990; **13**: 1285–96.

20. Turco VJ. Surgical correction of the resistant club foot. One-stage posteromedial release with internal fixation: a preliminary report. *J Bone Joint Surg Am* 1971; **53**: 477–97.

21. Turco VJ. Resistant congenital club foot – one-stage posteromedial release with internal fixation. A follow-up report of a fifteen-year experience. *J Bone Joint Surg Am* 1979; **61**: 805–14.

22. Crawford AH, Marxen JL, Osterfeld DL. The Cincinnati incision: a comprehensive approach for surgical procedures of the foot and ankle in childhood. *J Bone Joint Surg Am* 1982; **64**: 1355–8.

23. Bensahel H, Csukonyi Z, Desgrippes Y, Chaumien JP. Surgery in residual clubfoot: one-stage medioposterior release 'a la carte'. *J Pediatr Orthop* 1987; **7**: 145–8.

24. Simons GW. Complete subtalar release in club feet. Part I – a preliminary report. *J Bone Joint Surg Am* 1985; **67**: 1044–55.

25. Simons GW. Complete subtalar release in club feet. Part II – comparison with less extensive procedures. *J Bone Joint Surg Am* 1985; **67**: 1056–65.

26. Kocaolu M, Eralp L, Atalar AC, Bilen FE. Correction of complex foot deformities using the Ilizarov external fixator. *J Foot Ankle Surg* 2002; **41**: 30–9.

27. El-Mowafi H. Assessment of percutaneous V osteotomy of the calcaneus with Ilizarov application for correction of complex foot deformities. *Acta Orthop Belg* 2004; **70**: 586–90.

28. Ferreira RC, Costo MT, Frizzo GG, da Fonseca Filho FF. Correction of neglected clubfoot using the Ilizarov external fixator. *Foot Ankle Int* 2006; **27**: 266–73.

29. Utukuri MM, Ramachandran M, Hartley J, Hill RA. Patient-based outcomes after Ilizarov surgery in resistant clubfeet. *J Pediatr Orthop B* 2006; **15**: 278–84.

30. Evans D. Relapsed club foot. *J Bone Joint Surg Br* 1961; **43**: 722–33.

31. Saltzman CL, Fehrle MJ, Cooper RR, Spencer EC, Ponseti IV. Triple arthrodesis: twenty-five and forty-four-year average follow-up of the same patients. *J Bone Joint Surg Am* 1999; **81**: 1391–402.

32. Chotigavanichaya C, Scaduto AA, Snelson D, Otsuka NY. A novel orthosis for the treatment of clubfoot. *J Pediatr Orthop B* 2003; **12**: 272–6.

33. Changulani M, Garg NK, Rajagopal TS *et al.* Treatment of idiopathic club foot using the Ponseti method. Initial experience. *J Bone Joint Surg Br* 2006; **88**: 1385–7.

Calcaneus deformity

Benjamin Joseph

4

Introduction

Congenital calcaneus deformity is usually part of calcaneovalgus, either seen as an isolated deformity (Figure 4.1a) or in association with congenital posteromedial bowing of the tibia (Figure 4.1b). Congenital calcaneovalgus is a supple deformity in most instances; rarely, a rigid form may be encountered.[1] Acquired calcaneus deformity is most frequently associated with paralysis or weakness of the gastrocsoleus muscle (Figure 4.1c). Apart from neurological conditions that may cause weakness of the gastrocsoleus, excessive lengthening of the Achilles tendon in an effort to overcome an equinus deformity can result in a calcaneus deformity.[2] Less frequently, a calcaneus deformity can develop due to contracture of the muscles of the anterior compartment of the leg.

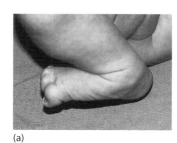
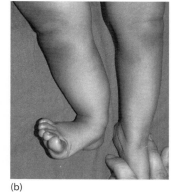
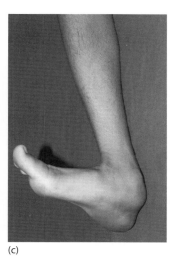

(a) (b) (c)

Figure 4.1 ● **(a)** Congenital calcaneovalgus deformity. **(b)** Calcaneovalgus deformity seen in association with congenital posteromedial bowing of the tibia. **(c)** Calcaneus deformity that has developed due to weakness of the triceps surae.

While congenital calcaneovalgus deformity usually resolves spontaneously during the first few weeks of life, all forms of paralytic calcaneus deformity tend to progress quite relentlessly throughout childhood.

Abnormality of gait

Problems of management

When there is a calcaneus deformity the normal pattern of the stance phase of gait is altered; the normal rockers are lost and the push-off is ineffective because the moment arm of gastrocsoleus is considerably reduced (Figure 4.2). This gait abnormality is even more noticeable when there is associated paralysis of the triceps surae.

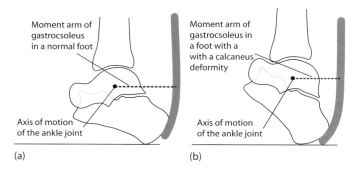

(a) (b)

Figure 4.2 ● Effect of calcaneus deformity on the moment arm of the gastrocsoleus. The normal moment arm **(a)** is significantly reduced when a calcaneus deformity develops **(b)**.

Abnormal forces under the heel

A calcaneus deformity itself results in greater loading of the heel while standing. If, in addition, the triceps surae is paralysed, shearing forces develop under the heel when uncontrolled ankle dorsiflexion occurs during the stance phase of walking. Both these factors increase the propensity for neuropathic ulceration if there is loss of sensation on the sole (e.g. in spina bifida).

Effect on the knee

Calcaneus deformity has a profound effect on the stability of the knee. In a child with a calcaneus deformity the knee can remain straight during the critical part of the stance phase when stability of the knee is essential, provided the quadriceps is functioning normally and the hamstrings are not spastic. However, if the quadriceps is not strong enough to stabilize the knee in extension, the knee will either buckle or the child will walk with a crouch gait. The latter is typically seen in children with spastic cerebral palsy in whom excessive lengthening of the gastrocsoleus has been done and who have weak quadriceps.

Effect on the forefoot

In an attempt to bring the foot down, secondarily a cavus deformity may develop (see Chapter 5, Cavus).

Aims of treatment

- Restore a plantigrade tread
- Improve the power of plantarflexion

Treatment options

Observation

Congenital calcaneovalgus deformity that is supple may be treated by gentle stretching and observation.

Tenodesis

In young children with paralytic calcaneus deformity, tenodesis of the Achilles tendon to the fibula can arrest progression of the deformity.[2,3]

Tendon transfer

Transfer of the tibialis anterior to the calcaneum can improve the muscle balance in children with weakness or paralysis of the gastrocsoleus.[4,5]

Contracture release

If the cause of the calcaneus deformity is contracture of the tibialis anterior and the toe extensors, release of the contracted tendons will correct the deformity.

Calcaneal osteotomy

An oblique osteotomy of the calcaneum with displacement of the tuberosity proximally will improve the moment arm of the gastrocsoleus (Figure 4.3).[6,7] This operation may be of benefit in patients in whom the gastrocsoleus is not paralysed but rendered weak because of altered biomechanics (depicted in Figure 4.2).

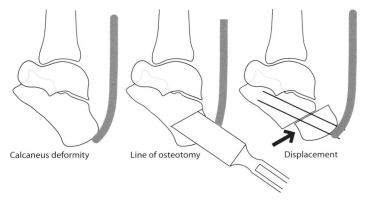

Calcaneus deformity   Line of osteotomy   Displacement

Figure 4.3 ● Proximal displacement osteotomy of the calcaneum for correcting calcaneus deformity.

Triple fusion

Triple fusion by the Elmslie technique is useful in skeletally mature patients with other hindfoot deformities in addition to the calcaneus deformity.[8]

Pantalar fusion

Iatrogenic calcaneus deformity following excessive lengthening of the Achilles tendon in cerebral palsy is difficult to treat. One option that has been suggested is a pantalar fusion.[9]

Factors to be taken into consideration while planning treatment

Recommended treatment

The factors are as follows:

- suppleness of the ankle;
- presence of muscle imbalance or muscle contracture;
- availability of functioning muscles to restore muscle balance;
- age of the child;
- presence of associated deformities in the foot.

The outline of treatment of calcaneus deformity is shown in Table 4.1.

Table 4.1 ● Treatment of calcaneus deformity

INDICATIONS						
Congenital calcaneo-valgus + Supple deformity + No muscle imbalance or contracture	Congenital or acquired calcaneovalgus + Rigid deformity + Contracture of ankle dorsiflexors	Acquired calcaneus deformity + Gastrocsoleus paralysed + No suitable strong muscle available to transfer + Young child	Acquired calcaneus deformity + Gastrocsoleus paralysed + Ankle and toes dorsiflexors are strong + Young child	Calcaneus deformity + Gastrocsoleus weak but not paralysed	Acquired calcaneus deformity + Gastrocsoleus paralysed + Adolescent	Acquired calcaneus deformity due to over-lengthening of spastic gastrocsoleus + Severe crouch + Adolescent
						⇩
						Calcaneotibial fusion
				⇩	⇩	
				Proximal displacement osteotomy of calcaneum	Triple fusion by the Elmslie technique	
			⇩			
		⇩	Transfer of tibialis anterior to the calcaneum			
	⇩	Westin's tenodesis of Achilles tendon to the fibula				
⇩	Contracture release					
Passive stretching and observation						
TREATMENT						

References

1. Edwards ER, Menelaus MB. Reverse club foot. Rigid and recalcitrant talipes calcaneovalgus. *J Bone Joint Surg Br* 1987; **69**: 330–4.
2. Wijesinha SS, Menelaus MB. Operation for calcaneus deformity after surgery for club foot. *J Bone Joint Surg Br* 1989; **71**: 234–6.
3. Westin GW, Dingeman RD, Gausewitz SH. The results of tenodesis of the tendo achillis to the fibula for paralytic pes calcaneus. *J Bone Joint Surg Am* 1988; **70**: 320–8.
4. Banta JV, Sutherland DH, Wyatt M. Anterior tibial transfer to the os calcis with Achilles tenodesis for calcaneal deformity in myelomeningocele. *J Pediatr Orthop* 1981; **1**: 125–30.
5. Fernandez-Feliberti R, Fernandez SA, Colon C *et al.* Transfer of the tibialis anterior for calcaneus deformity in myelodysplasia. *J Bone Joint Surg Am* 1992; **74**: 1038–41.

6. Badelon O, Bensahel H. Subtalar posterior displacement osteotomy of the calcaneus: a preliminary report of seven cases. *J Pediatr Orthop* 1990; **10**: 401–4.

7. Pandey AK, Pandey S, Prasad V. Calcaneal osteotomy and tendon sling for the management of calcaneus deformity. *J Bone Joint Surg Am* 1989; **71**: 1192–8.

8. Cholmeley JA. Elmslie's operation for the calcaneus foot. *J Bone Joint Surg Br* 1953; **35**: 46–9.

9. Muir D, Angliss RD, Nattrass GR, Graham HK. Tibiotalocalcaneal arthrodesis for severe calcaneovalgus deformity in cerebral palsy. *J Pediatr Orthop* 2005; **25**: 651–6.

Cavus

Benjamin Joseph

5

Introduction

Pes cavus is a deformity in which the longitudinal arch of the foot is high and does not reduce on weight-bearing. The deformity may be congenital in origin and this form of pes cavus has also been referred to as pes arcuatus. Congenital pes cavus is not associated with any muscle imbalance and does not progress. Usually there are no symptoms in children with this form of cavus, although later in life metatarsalgia may occasionally develop. Cavus deformity is far more commonly acquired and in the vast majority of instances is associated with an underlying neurological disorder.[1] The deformity tends to progress and treatment is often difficult (Figure 5.1). Among the neuromuscular diseases associated with cavus deformity are hereditary sensory motor neuropathy (e.g. Charcot–Marie–Tooth disease), spinal dysraphism, spina bifida cystica, poliomyelitis and cerebral palsy.[1,2]

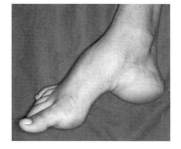

Figure 5.1 ● Severe degree of cavus deformity in an adult with polio. The deformity had progressed throughout childhood.

Problems of management

Muscle imbalance

In neurogenic pes cavus there may be muscle imbalance at the ankle, the subtalar and midtarsal joints and at the joints of the toes.[2] At the ankle there may be weakness of either the dorsiflexors or the plantarflexors. At subtalar and midtarsal joints there may be an imbalance between the invertors and the evertors of the foot. At the toes there may be an imbalance between the flexors and extensors of the metatarsophalangeal joint and the interphalangeal joints on account of intrinsic muscle paralysis.

Associated deformities

Deformities of the ankle, hindfoot and forefoot are often seen in association with the cavus deformity and these deformities develop on account of muscle imbalance (Table 5.1).

Table 5.1 ● Patterns of deformities that may be seen in neurogenic pes cavus

Joint at which muscle imbalance develops	Muscle imbalance	Deformity
Ankle	Triceps surae strong – tibialis anterior weak Tibialis anterior strong – triceps surae weak	Equinocavus Calcaneocavus
Subtalar joint	Invertors strong – evertors weak Evertors strong – invertors weak	Cavovarus Cavovalgus
Toes	Extrinsic muscles strong – intrinsic muscles of the foot weak	Claw toes

Tendency for recurrence following treatment

Recurrence of the deformity often occurs when the muscle balance is not fully restored.

Uneven pressure distribution on the sole of the foot

Excessive pressure may fall under the heads of the metatarsals in cavus feet.[3,4]

Pain

Metatarsalgia may develop on account of the excessive pressure under the metatarsal heads.

The cause of the cavus deformity varies and it is useful to understand the different ways in which the deformity may develop in order to plan the appropriate treatment.

Drop of the first metatarsal

When the tibialis anterior is weak or paralysed and the peroneus longus is functioning normally, the head of the first metatarsal is depressed owing to the unopposed action of the peroneus longus (Figure 5.2). This is referred to as 'dropping' of the first metatarsal. Plantarflexion of the first metatarsal accentuates the medial longitudinal arch of the foot and a cavus deformity develops. In Charcot–Marie–Tooth disease there is also weakness of the peroneus brevis while the tibialis posterior remains strong and this causes a varus deformity of the hindfoot.

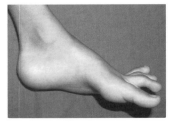

Figure 5.2 ● Drop of the first metatarsal seen in a child with paralysis of the tibialis anterior. The peroneus longus was functioning normally.

Calcaneus deformity

Paralysis of the triceps surae will lead to a calcaneus deformity due to unopposed action of the ankle dorsiflexors. This pattern of paralysis is often seen in spina bifida and poliomyelitis. The angle between the long axis of the calcaneum and the first metatarsal is reduced to less than 150°, the heel moves anteriorly and a cavus deformity develops (Figure 5.1). The deformity tends to progress relentlessly and may become very severe by skeletal maturity.

Contracture of the plantar fascia

If the metatarsophalangeal joints are hyperextended the plantar fascia tightens up and the arch of the foot is accentuated (Figure 5.3). When there is paralysis of the intrinsic muscles of the foot, the metatarsophalangeal joints hyperextend and a cavus develops secondarily. Similarly, when a patient with an equinus deformity walks on the forefoot with the metatarsophalgeal joint extended secondary cavus deformity develops.

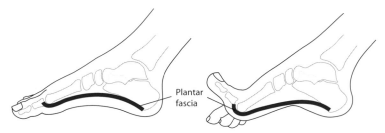

Plantar fascia

Figure 5.3 ● Diagram demonstrating how tightening of the plantar fascia results in accentuation of the arch of the foot.

- Correct the deformity
- Minimize the risk of recurrence
- Relieve pain

Treatment options

Shoe modification

Shoes modified to accommodate the high arched foot with a wide toe box to prevent pressure on the dorsum of the interphalangeal joints may suffice in milder degrees of pes cavus if there is no significant muscle imbalance.

Plantar fascia release

If the plantar fascia is contracted it should be released and this will correct mild degrees of cavus (Figure 5.4a). Even in more severe degrees of pes cavus where bony surgery is being contemplated, a plantar fascia release should be undertaken.[5,6] This will facilitate correction by removal of a smaller wedge of bone than when bony surgery is undertaken without a plantar fascia release.

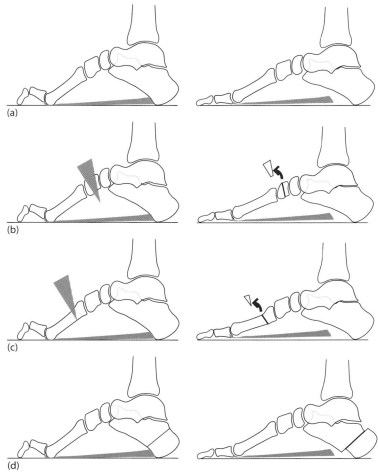

Figure 5.4 ● Diagram illustrating how a cavus deformity can be corrected by a plantar fascia release **(a)**, a midtarsal osteotomy **(b)**, a basal metatarsal osteotomy **(c)** and a calcaneal displacement osteotomy **(d)**.

Midtarsal osteotomy

A dorsally based wedge of bone is excised from the cuboid and the cuneiforms. A truncated wedge should be excised when the deformity is more severe (Figure 5.4b).[7]

Extension osteotomy of the base of the first metatarsal

If the primary pathology is a dropped first metatarsal, an extension osteotomy of the base of the first metatarsal will facilitate correction of the cavus deformity (Figure 5.4c).

Displacement osteotomy of the calcaneum

If the primary pathology is a calcaneus deformity, a displacement osteotomy of the calcaneum may be performed. The tuberosity of the calcaneum is displaced proximally after the plantar fascia and the muscles taking origin from the calcaneum are released (Figure 5.4d).[6,8]

Triple arthrodesis

In the adolescent with a complex deformity such as a calcaneocavovalgus or an equinocavovarus, a triple fusion may be needed to make the foot plantigrade. The Elmslie–Cholmley technique is useful for dealing with a calcaneocavovalgus while a traditional triple fusion will correct an equinocavovarus.[9]

Tendon transfers

Appropriate tendon transfers should be performed in addition to any of the operations listed above while correcting neurogenic pes cavus.[5]

Age of the child

In a young child with a mild cavus deformity, soft tissue operations such as release of the plantar fascia and tendon transfers may correct the deformity. However, bony operations are necessary in the older child.

Rigidity of the deformity

If the deformity is supple, soft tissue operations may suffice but bony procedures are necessary for correction of rigid deformities.

Presence and nature of associated deformities

If the cavus deformity is associated with a varus deformity of the hindfoot it is important to determine whether the varus deformity is a compensatory deformity that may correct once the primary cause of the cavus is addressed. In children who have weakness of the tibialis anterior with normal power of the peroneus longus, the first metatarsal drops and the forefoot pronates. Coleman demonstrated that the varus deformity may develop as a compensatory mechanism in such situations to enable the child to place the pronated forefoot on the ground (Figure 5.5). The Coleman's block test may help to identify whether the hindfoot varus is rigid or supple and compensatory. In the latter situation no surgery is necessary for the hindfoot varus as it should resolve if the normal forefoot alignment is restored (Figure 5.6). If the cavus deformity is associated with a rigid hindfoot deformity, correction of the hindfoot deformity is necessary in addition to any procedure that deals with the cavus.

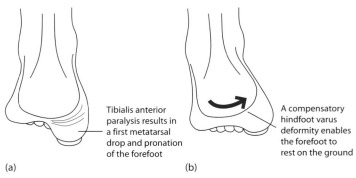

Tibialis anterior paralysis results in a first metatarsal drop and pronation of the forefoot

A compensatory hindfoot varus deformity enables the forefoot to rest on the ground

(a)   (b)

Figure 5.5 ● **(a,b)** Diagram illustrating how a compensatory hindfoot varus can enable a pronated forefoot to rest on the ground.

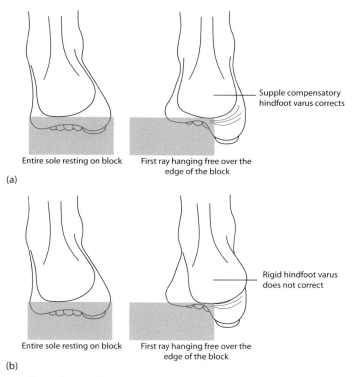

Figure 5.6 ● Diagram illustrating the Coleman's block test. The patient initially stands with the entire sole resting on the block (left). The hindfoot varus is noted. The patient then stands on the block with the first ray unsupported and hanging over the edge of the block (right). If the hindfoot varus corrects, the hindfoot deformity is supple **(a)** while if it remains unchanged it is rigid **(b)**.

Nature of muscle imbalance

The precise nature of the muscle imbalance at the ankle, subtalar and midtarsal joints and at the metatarsophalangeal joints should be identified and the appropriate tendon transfers must be performed (see Chapter 56, The paralysed foot and ankle).

Primary deformity that caused the secondary cavus deformity

In the younger child, addressing the primary deformity that led to development of the cavus will often improve the cavus deformity. For example, in a young child with paralysis of the gastrocsoleus, the cavus deformity can be prevented from progressing and may even be corrected by performing a tenodesis of the Achilles tendon (a procedure aimed at correcting the calcaneus deformity; see Chapter 56, The paralysed foot and ankle). Similarly, if the primary problem is weakness of the tibialis anterior and drop of the first metatarsal, prompt restoration of muscle balance by transfer of the extensor hallucis longus to the neck of the first metatarsal with tenodesis of the interphalangeal joint can prevent the cavus from progressing.

The choice of bony surgery may also be governed by the underlying cause of the cavus. A rigid cavus caused by a dropped first metatarsal can be improved by a basal metatarsal extension osteotomy, while a proximal displacement osteotomy of the calcaneum should be considered for a rigid cavus secondary to a calcaneus deformity.

An outline of treatment of cavus deformity is shown in Table 5.2.

Recommended treatment

Table 5.2 ● Outline of treatment of cavus deformity

INDICATIONS					
Mild cavus + Negligible muscle imbalance + Young child	Mild cavus + Supple deformity + Muscle imbalance + Young child	Moderate cavus + Rigid deformity + Muscle imbalance + Older child	Moderate cavus + Rigid deformity + Muscle imbalance predominantly of first ray with drop of the first metatarsal + Older child	Moderate cavus + Rigid deformity + Muscle imbalance predominantly of the ankle with calcaneus deformity + Older child	Severe cavus + Rigid deformity + Associated deformities at ankle, subtalar and midtarsal joints + Adolescent
⇩	⇩	⇩	⇩	⇩	⇩
Shoe modification and follow-up to note whether progression of the deformity occurs	Plantar fascia release + Tendon transfer to restore muscle imbalance	Plantar fascia release + Midtarsal osteotomy + Tendon transfer to restore muscle imbalance	Plantar fascia release + Extension osteotomy of the base of the first metatarsal + Transfer of extensor hallucis longus to the neck of the first metatarsal	Plantar fascia release + Proximal displacement osteotomy of the calcaneum + Tendon transfer to provide plantarflexor power	Triple fusion + Tendon transfers to restore muscle balance
TREATMENT					

References

1. Schwend RM, Drennan JC. Cavus foot deformity in children. *J Am Acad Orthop Surg* 2003; **11**: 201–11.
2. Mann RA, Missirian J. Pathophysiology of Charcot–Marie–Tooth disease. Clin Orthop Relat Res 1988; 234: 221–8.
3. Metaxiotis D, Accles W, Pappas A, Doederlein L. Dynamic pedobarography (DPB) in operative management of cavovarus foot deformity. *Foot Ankle Int* 2000; **21**: 935–47.
4. Chan G, Sampath J, Miller F *et al.* The role of the dynamic pedobarograph in assessing treatment of cavovarus feet in children with Charcot–Marie–Tooth disease. *J Pediatr Orthop* 2007; **27**: 510–6.
5. Roper BA, Tibrewal SB. Soft tissue surgery in Charcot–Marie–Tooth disease. *J Bone Joint Surg Br* 1989; **71**: 17–20.
6. Dekel S, Weissman SL. Osteotomy of the calcaneus and concomitant plantar stripping in children with talipes cavo-varus. *J Bone Joint Surg Br* 1973; **55**: 802–8.
7. Olney B. Treatment of the cavus foot. Deformity in the pediatric patient with Charcot–Marie–Tooth. *Foot Ankle Clin* 2000; **5**: 305–15.
8. Parsons SW, Duckworth T, Betts RP, Rowley DI. Os calcis osteotomy in the management of deformities of the hindfoot in spinal dysraphism. *Z Kinderchir* 1986; **41** (Suppl 1): 30–2.
9. Mann DC, Hsu JD. Triple arthrodesis in the treatment of fixed cavovarus deformity in adolescent patients with Charcot–Marie–Tooth disease. *Foot Ankle* 1992; **13**: 1–6.

Congenital vertical talus

Selvadurai Nayagam

6

Introduction

Congenital vertical talus is a relatively rare foot deformity that has often been considered to be a rigid form of flatfoot. However, in severe cases the medial longitudinal arch is not merely collapsed but is reversed such that the sole of the foot is convex. This has led to the condition also being called congenital convex pes valgus. The latter term is probably more appropriate as it describes the deformity more precisely. It is also important to be aware that in some flatfeet the talus may be aligned somewhat vertically when the ankle is in the neutral position; the tarsal alignment becomes restored on plantarflexion of the ankle. This should not be confused with the true vertical talus.

Congenital vertical talus is characterized by a dislocation of the talonavicular joint, with the navicular displaced dorsally and the head of the talus pointing plantarward. The heel is in equinus and valgus, the forefoot dorsiflexed and abducted producing, in severe cases, a convex border to the sole or a 'rocker bottom' foot (Figure 6.1). It is bilateral in about 50 percent of patients and is linked to arthrogryposis, neural tube defects and chromosome anomalies such as trisomy 18.[1,2]

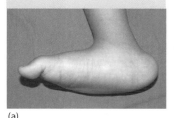
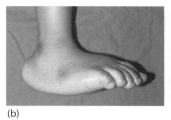
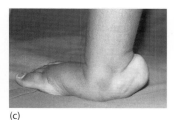
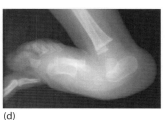

(a) (b) (c) (d)

Figure 6.1 ● The foot of a child with vertical talus viewed from the medial **(a)** and lateral **(b)** aspects clearly shows the convex 'rocker bottom' appearance of the sole. The deformity is accentuated on weight-bearing **(c)**. The lateral radiograph of the foot **(d)** shows the components of the deformity clearly.

Problems of management

Appearance

There is no mistaking the rocker bottom foot and an early consultation is often requested by parents. In subtler forms however, the problem is not recognized until the child stands and the foot arch noted to be non-existent. When the condition is unilateral, the asymmetry may bring the problem to attention sooner.

Abnormal foot loading

Occasionally when the child presents late a hard callosity is noted beneath the head of the talus which is directed into the sole of the foot on the medial side. The callosity develops in response to the high contact pressures beneath the head of the talus. Pain on walking may develop in due course.

Footwear

Unless a total contact insole is used, it is difficult to find off-the-shelf footwear that relieves the discomfort of walking on a rocker bottom foot. The problem is an issue in late presentations which occur in areas where access to medical care is restricted.

Aims of treatment

- To reduce a joint dislocation
  Restoring the anatomy improves the appearance of the foot and should produce a return towards more normal foot biomechanics. However, the foot may remain stiff in children with arthrogryposis.
- To improve the foot contact profile and reduce pain from walking
  It is imperative that the abnormal loading of the foot is remedied and thereby reduce foot pain if it is present.

Treatment options

Serial casts and percutaneous surgery

Until recently, this was thought not to be helpful. The technique of casting is specific and is usually followed by percutaneous Achilles tenotomy and fractional lengthening of the tibialis anterior, extensor digitorum communis and peroneus brevis tendons, if needed. The talonavicular joint is reduced by the serial casts or, if incomplete, openly reduced (through a small medial incision) and held with a Kirschner wire. Aftercare following cast and Kirschner wire removal involves stretching exercises performed by the child's parents and the use of a night-time brace consisting of two shoes held parallel by a connecting metal bar until the child has learnt to walk. Thereafter, a solid ankle–foot orthoses moulded in 15° plantarflexion and 15° adduction is used until the age of two.[3]

Open soft tissue releases

This is the mainstay of treatment in many centres. It is usually performed around 10–12 months, just before the child begins to walk. The objectives of surgery are to openly reduce the talonavicular joint, correct hindfoot equinus by lengthening the tendo Achilles and capsulotomies of the posterior ankle and subtalar joints and realign the calcaneocuboid joint, if necessary (Figure 6.2).[2,4,5] The procedure can be performed through a single circumferential incision (Cincinatti) or through multiple longitudinal ones.

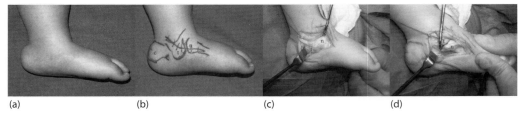

(a) (b) (c) (d)

Figure 6.2 ● The flat medial border of the sole is visible in **(a)**. The calcaneum [c], talus [t] and navicular [n] are palpated and drawn on the skin **(b)**. In **(c)** the talus and navicular are labelled and clearly show the navicular lying dorsal to the head of the talus. A blunt hook is used to lift the head of the talus and reduce the talonavicular joint in **(d)**; the navicular and a Z-lengthened portion of the tibialis posterior tendon are visible.

Tibialis anterior transfer to the neck of the talus

Supplementary procedures may include transfer of the tibialis anterior tendon into the neck of talus to maintain reduction by preventing the talus from plantarflexing.[4,5]

Excision of the navicular

Occasionally, in the older child reduction of the talonavicular dislocation may not be achieved even after adequate release of contracted soft tissue. Excision of the navicular has been recommended in older children when the head of talus cannot be reduced.[6]

Triple fusion

Residual deformities that are present in the adolescent may be corrected by a triple arthrodesis.

Factors to be taken into consideration while planning treatment

Flatfoot or vertical talus?

When the plantar profile of the foot is truly rocker bottom, as is the case in severe examples, the diagnosis is straightforward. However, when the presentation is flatfoot, the diagnosis may be missed if not carefully assessed. A lateral foot radiograph with the ankle in plantarflexion should discriminate between a flexible flatfoot and oblique talus from vertical talus; in the latter, the talonavicular joint remains dislocated on this radiograph whereas it is seen to reduce in the other conditions (Figure 6.3). Interpretation of the radiograph can be tricky as only the calcaneum, talus, cuboid (sometimes the lateral cuneiform) and metatarsal shafts are visible in the young infant; the reduction of the talonavicular joint is inferred from the position of the talar axis in relation to the shaft of the first metatarsal.

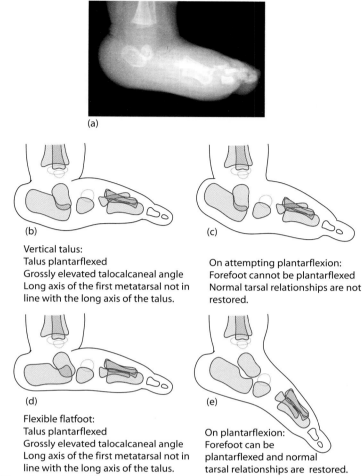

(a)

(b)

Vertical talus:
Talus plantarflexed
Grossly elevated talocalcaneal angle
Long axis of the first metatarsal not in
line with the long axis of the talus.

(c)

On attempting plantarflexion:
Forefoot cannot be plantarflexed
Normal tarsal relationships are not
restored.

(d)

Flexible flatfoot:
Talus plantarflexed
Grossly elevated talocalcaneal angle
Long axis of the first metatarsal not in
line with the long axis of the talus.

(e)

On plantarflexion:
Forefoot can be
plantarflexed and normal
tarsal relationships are restored.

Figure 6.3 ● The talus is plantarflexed in the lateral radiograph of this foot **(a)**. The plantarflexed position of the talus can be seen in vertical talus and flatfoot. In order to distinguish between the two conditions a lateral radiograph must be taken when passive plantarflexion is being attempted. In vertical talus **(b)** the abnormal tarsal relationships are not restored to normal by plantarflexing the foot **(c)**. In flatfoot **(d)** the normal tarsal relationships are restored in plantarflexion **(e)**.

Age at presentation

Similar to the clubfoot, manipulation and serial casts should be considered as initial treatment. While it is preferable to start manipulation and serial casts as soon as possible after birth, successful non-operative treatment has occasionally been reported in children as late as four years of age.[3,7] However, late presentations at this age are more likely to be handled with open soft tissue releases.

Syndrome association

The diagnosis of vertical talus should prompt the orthopaedic surgeon to look for neural tube defects or arthrogryposis. The results of treatment are more gratifying if vertical talus is not associated with these conditions (Figure 6.4). The possibility of associated chromosome anomalies makes referral to a clinical geneticist advisable, particularly as heterogeneous gene defects and autosomal dominant transmission have been reported in some series.[8–10]

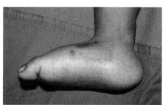

Figure 6.4 ● Satisfactory post-operative appearance of vertical talus in a child, corrected by soft tissue surgery. There was no underlying neurological or chromosomal anomaly.

Recommended treatment

The outline of treatment of vertical talus is summarized in Table 6.1.

Table 6.1 ● Outline of treatment of congenital vertical talus

INDICATIONS				
Vertical talus (confirmed by lateral radiograph in plantarflexion) + Neonate	Vertical talus (confirmed by lateral radiograph in plantarflexion) + Infant or young child + Not responding to manipulations and casting	Vertical talus (confirmed by lateral radiograph in plantarflexion) + Infant or young child + Tendency for talus to plantarflex even after open reduction and tendon releases	Vertical talus + Older child + Reduction of talonavicular dislocation not achieved even after release of all contracted tendons and capsules	Adolescent with untreated vertical talus OR Residual deformities after previous surgery for vertical talus ⇩ Triple arthrodesis as salvage procedure
⇩ Manipulation and serial casts + Percutaneous Achilles tenotomy + Fractional lengthening of tibialis anterior, extensor digitorum communis and peroneus brevis + Kirschner wire fixation of reduced joint	⇩ Lengthening of the Achilles tendon, tibialis anterior, extensor digitorum and peroneus brevis + Posterior ankle and subtalar capsulotomies + Lateral calcaneocuboid capsulotomy + Open reduction of talonavicular joint + Kirschner wire fixation	⇩ Lengthening of the Achilles tendon, tibialis anterior, extensor digitorum and peroneus brevis + Posterior ankle and subtalar capsulotomies + Lateral calcaneocuboid capsulotomy + Open reduction of talonavicular joint + Kirschner wire fixation + Transfer of tibialis anterior to neck of the talus	⇩ Excision of navicular bone to facilitate dorsiflexion of the talus + Kirschner wire fixation + Transfer of tibialis anterior to neck of the talus	
TREATMENT				

Rationale of treatment suggested

As with other congenital foot anomalies, there is a spectrum of presentation ranging from the true rocker bottom to flatfoot. Early use of non-operative treatment (usually manipulation and serial casts) in combination with limited surgery appears to be an evolving general principle in the management of some of the more enigmatic congenital foot conditions, for example clubfoot, and now with congenital vertical talus.[7,11] To enable this aim, surgeons need to be able to distinguish subtler forms of congenital vertical talus from flexible flatfoot or the oblique talus and apply the strategy appropriately. Open reduction of the talonavicular, ankle and subtalar joints to correct the deformity is an extensive surgical dissection with inevitable scarring leading to stiffness in some; leaving this option to late presentations or those failing to respond to the more limited surgical methods is wise.

References

1. Lloyd-Roberts GC, Spence AJ. Congenital vertical talus. *J Bone Joint Surg Br* 1958; **40**: 33–41.
2. Kodros SA, Dias LS. Single-stage surgical correction of congenital vertical talus. *J Pediatr Orthop* 1999; **19**: 42–8.
3. Dobbs MB, Purcell DB, Nunley R, Morcuende JA. Early results of a new method of treatment for idiopathic congenital vertical talus. Surgical technique. *J Bone Joint Surg Am* 2007; **89** (Suppl 2): 111–21.

4. Duncan RD, Fixsen JA. Congenital convex pes valgus. *J Bone Joint Surg Br* 1999; **81**: 250–4.
5. Zorer G, Bagatur AE, Dogan A. Single stage surgical correction of congenital vertical talus by complete subtalar release and peritalar reduction by using the Cincinnati incision. *J Pediatr Orthop B* 2002; **11**: 60–7.
6. Clark MW, D'Ambrosia RD, Ferguson AB. Congenital vertical talus: treatment by open reduction and navicular excision. *J Bone Joint Surg Am* 1977; **59**: 816–24.
7. Dobbs MB, Purcell DB, Nunley R, Morcuende JA. Early results of a new method of treatment for idiopathic congenital vertical talus. *J Bone Joint Surg Am* 2006; **88**: 1192–200.
8. Dobbs MB, Schoenecker PL, Gordon JE. Autosomal dominant transmission of isolated congenital vertical talus. *Iowa Orthop J* 2002; **22**: 25–7.
9. Dobbs MB, Gurnett CA, Pierce B *et al.* HOXD10 M319K mutation in a family with isolated congenital vertical talus. *J Orthop Res* 2006; **24**: 448–53.
10. Gurnett CA, Keppel C, Bick J, Bowcock AM, Dobbs MB. Absence of HOXD10 mutations in idiopathic clubfoot and sporadic vertical talus. *Clin Orthop Relat Res* 2007; **462**: 27–31.
11. Mukerjee KB, Ippolito E, Farsetti P, Caterini R, Tudisco C. Long-term comparative results in patients with congenital clubfoot treated with two different protocols. *J Bone Joint Surg Am* 2004; **86**: 1830–1; author reply 1831–2.

Planovalgus deformity

Benjamin Joseph

7

Introduction

Planovalgus and pes planus are other descriptive terms for flatfoot, which is very frequently encountered in paediatric orthopaedic practice. Although the vast majority of children with planovalgus deformity are asymptomatic and function quite normally, many of them present to the paediatric orthopaedic clinic, presumably because there is a notion that all flatfeet are pathological and will not function normally in later life. This view may have become widespread since, in many countries in the past, potential recruits for the armed forces were rejected if they had flatfeet.

The deformity involves the hindfoot and the forefoot; the hindfoot is in valgus; the forefoot is in abduction and the medial longitudinal arch is collapsed (Figure 7.1).[1] It is important to recognize that all three of these components are part of the flatfoot deformity and that these components are interrelated. As will be come apparent in the later part of this chapter, adequate correction of one of these components will correct the other two components.

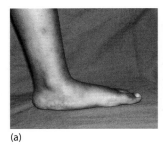 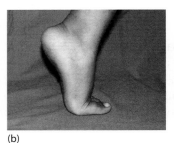 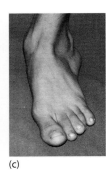

(a) (b) (c)

Figure 7.1 ● The components of flatfoot: the medial longitudinal arch has collapsed **(a)**, the hindfoot is in valgus **(b)** and the forefoot is abducted **(c)**.

The flatfoot is regarded as being mobile or flexible if the medial longitudinal arch can be restored either by standing on tiptoe or on performing the Jack's test (Figure 7.2).[2] If the arch cannot be restored the deformity is regarded as rigid.

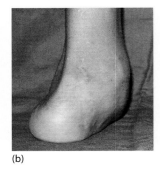 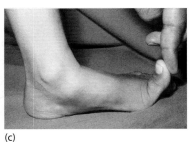

(a) (b) (c)

Figure 7.2 ● Mobile flatfoot in a child **(a)**; the arch is restored on standing on tip-toe **(b)**. The Jack's test – the collapsed medial arch on weight-bearing is restored when the great toe is passively dorsiflexed **(c)**.

Mobile flatfoot is very common in toddlers; the frequency reduces quite dramatically in the pre-school years. This implies that the medial longitudinal arch develops by the time the child is around five or six years of age.[3] However, the prevalence of flatfoot remains high among older children with hypermobile joints and obesity. The prevalence is low among communities where wearing shoes is uncommon.[4,5] This suggests that walking barefoot may actually facilitate development of the arch.

A rigid flatfoot is always pathological and should be investigated further. The commonest cause of a rigid flatfoot is tarsal coalition, which is discussed elsewhere in this book (see Chapter 51, Tarsal coalition).

In this chapter the issues related to treatment of mobile flatfoot alone will be discussed.

Apart from flatfoot associated with hypermobile joint syndrome there are a few other causes of mobile flatfoot. Isolated paralysis of the tibialis posterior muscle can result in a planovalgus deformity. Contracture of the gastrocsoleus is another cause of flatfoot.

The severity of the deformity varies, and a useful classification of the severity has been suggested by Tachdjian.[6] Mild flatfoot is one where the arch is depressed on standing but just visible. In moderate flatfeet the arch is obliterated on standing but is present when the child is not weight-bearing. In severe flatfeet the arch is not present even while recumbent, the medial border of the foot is convex and the head of the talus is palpable in the sole.

Problems of management

Appearance

The appearance of the foot is often disconcerting for the parents although the child is seldom aware of the deformity.

Distortion and wearing out of footwear

The heel counter of shoes becomes distorted and the medial aspect of the heel wears out faster than normal and thus shoes need to be replaced more frequently (Figure 7.3). Often, this is what parents find distressing.

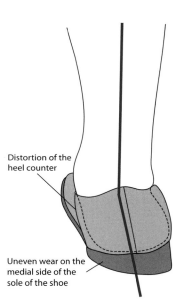

Distortion of the heel counter

Uneven wear on the medial side of the sole of the shoe

Figure 7.3 ● Distortion of the heel counter and wearing down of the medial aspect of the heel of the shoe that can be seen in footwear used by children with flatfeet.

Pain

It is exceedingly uncommon to encounter foot pain in young children with mobile flatfeet. However, occasionally, in the older child, symptoms of foot strain may develop especially if the child stands or walks for a long time. Persistent or severe pain in the foot needs to be investigated more carefully with appropriate imaging to ensure that occult tarsal coalition is not the cause of symptomatic flatfoot.

Aims of treatment

- Reassurance of the parents
  In the vast majority of instances all that is required is reassurance to the parents that no active treatment is needed and that asymptomatic flatfoot may be ignored.
- Correct the deformity, if justified
  In the rare instance in which the deformity is severe and there are persistent symptoms, an attempt should be made to correct the deformity.
- Reduce the early wearing out of shoes
  If the child wears out shoes very fast an effort must be made to prevent this. It is important to emphasize to the parents that whatever is being done is solely to prevent damage to footwear rather than actually treating the foot itself.
- Relieve pain, if present
  A painful flatfoot warrants treatment.

Treatment options

Reassurance

Shoe inserts and shoe modifications

Numerous shoe inserts have been devised for 'correcting' flatfoot; the UCBL insert,[7] the Helfet heel cup[8] (Figure 7.4) and the arch support are among the more well known. It needs to be emphasized that many of these inserts will improve the arch and prevent the heel from going into valgus as long as the insert or orthosis is worn in the shoe but the foot will revert to its original position as soon as the insert is removed. There is no convincing evidence in the literature that any of these devices actually alters the natural history of flatfoot. On the contrary, there is evidence that the use of shoe inserts does not cure flatfoot.[9] Nevertheless, use of shoe inserts can reduce the rate of wearing down of shoes and for this reason they may be justifiably recommended. An arch support may also help in reducing symptoms of foot strain.

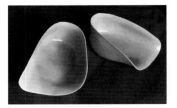

Figure 7.4 ● Helfet heel cups used as shoe inserts to control the hindfoot valgus and to support the arch of the foot.

Surgery that aims at restoring the medial longitudinal arch

The musculotendinous, capsular and ligamentous structures that normally support the arch may be stretched or ineffective. These include the tibialis posterior tendon and the spring ligament. Operations have been devised to attempt to either reef these structures or to reconstruct them.[10] Another approach has been to fuse intertarsal joints in the midfoot to prevent the arch from collapsing.[2,11]

Surgery that aims to correct the hindfoot valgus

If the hindfoot can be prevented from going into valgus at the subtalar joint, the flatfoot can be controlled. The surgical options for controlling subtalar valgus are discussed in detail in Chapter 8, Valgus deformity of the ankle and subtalar joint.

Surgery that aims at correcting the forefoot abduction

Lengthening of the lateral column of the foot has been advocated as a means of correcting the forefoot abduction (Figure 7.5).[12] By correcting this component of the deformity alone satisfactory correction of the entire planovalgus deformity has been reported. The osteotomy should run between the anterior and middle articular facets of the calcaneum. However, a significant proportion of individuals are likely to have fused anterior and middle facets on the calcaneum.[13] In these individuals such an osteotomy would run through the articular cartilage which could result in pain.

Restoring muscle balance

If the underlying cause of flatfoot is paralysis of the tibialis posterior muscle balance can be restored by a tendon transfer or by performing a medial displacement osteotomy of the tuberosity of the calcaneum (see Chapter 56, The paralysed foot and ankle). A displacement osteotomy of the calcaneum will improve the hindfoot valgus even if there is no weakness of the tibialis posterior.[14,15]

Lengthening of the Achilles tendon

Lengthening of the Achilles tendon is indicated when the cause of flatfoot is contracture of the gastrocsoleus.

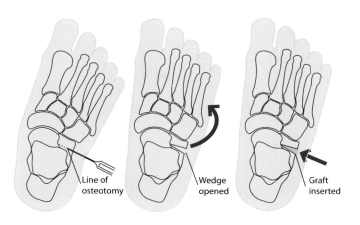

Line of osteotomy

Wedge opened

Graft inserted

Figure 7.5 ● Diagram showing the technique of lengthening the lateral column of the foot.

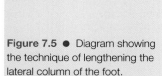

Factors to be taken into consideration while planning treatment

Severity of the deformity

Surgical intervention is justified only for severe degrees of flatfoot.

Age of the child

Since there is the possibility that flatfoot will resolve with development of the arch as the child grows older, no intervention is necessary for the young child.

Table 7.1 ● Outline of treatment of mobile flatfoot in children

INDICATIONS				
Mild or moderate flatfoot + Young child + No symptoms + No excessive wearing out of shoes	Moderate or severe flatfoot + Young child + No symptoms + Excessive and rapid wearing out of shoes	Moderate or severe flatfoot + Older child + Symptoms of foot strain on standing + No excessive wearing out of shoes	Severe flatfoot + Older child + No symptoms + Excessive and rapid wearing out of shoes + Unacceptable appearance + Child not keen on prolonged use of shoe insert	Severe flatfoot + Older child + Pain
			⇩	
			Medial displacement osteotomy of the calcaneum	⇩
				Exclude tarsal coalition + Subtalar fusion
		⇩		
		Insole arch support, Helfet heel cup or UCBL insert		
	⇩			
	Helfet heel cup or UCBL insert			
⇩				
Reassure parents + Encourage barefoot activity if local weather conditions permit				
Should account for over 90% of children with flatfeet				
TREATMENT				

Symptoms

If the child has foot pain that can be attributed to the flatfoot, intervention is necessary.

Effect on footwear

An effort must be made to minimize wearing out of footwear.

An outline of treatment of mobile flatfoot is shown in Table 7.1.

Recommended treatment

Rationale of treatment suggested

Why are shoe inserts only recommended if there are symptoms of foot strain or if the wearing down of footwear is excessive?
Since shoe inserts do not alter the natural history of flatfoot,[9] there is no justification in prescribing them for children who have no symptoms and if wearing down of shoes is not excessive.

Why is calcaneal osteotomy recommended as the method for improving the appearance of the foot?
The calcaneal osteotomy is an extra-articular procedure and does not reduce the mobility of the foot as in an arthrodesis. It also alters the mechanics of the hindfoot by increasing the inverter lever arm, thus facilitating correction.

Why is subtalar fusion preferred to lengthening of the lateral column of the foot?
Although lateral column lengthening appears to have good long-term results in a good proportion of patients,[12,16] there is a risk of pain developing if the osteotomy runs through the articular facet.[13] The author has personally seen this happen. For this reason subtalar fusion is recommended although it entails loss of motion at the hindfoot.

References

1. Bordelon RL. Hypermobile flatfoot in children. Comprehension, evaluation, and treatment. *Clin Orthop Relat Res* 1983; **181**: 7–14.
2. Jack EA. Naviculo-cuneiform fusion in the treatment of flat foot. *J Bone Joint Surg Br* 1953; **35**: 75–82.
3. Pfeiffer M, Kotz R, Ledl T, Hauser G, Sluga M. Prevalence of flat foot in preschool-aged children. *Pediatrics* 2006; **118**: 634–9.
4. Rao UB, Joseph B. The influence of footwear on the prevalence of flat foot. A survey of 2300 children. *J Bone Joint Surg Br* 1992; **74**: 525–7.
5. Sachithanandam V, Joseph B. The influence of footwear on the prevalence of flat foot. A survey of 1846 skeletally mature persons. *J Bone Joint Surg Br* 1995; **77**: 254–7.
6. Tachdjian MO. *The Child's Foot*. Philadelphia: WB Saunders.
7. Bleck EE, Berzins UJ. Conservative management of pes valgus with plantar flexed talus, flexible. *Clin Orthop Relat Res* 1977; **122**: 85–94.
8. Helfet AJ. A new way of treating flat feet in children. *Lancet* 1956; **i**: 262–4.
9. Wenger DR, Mauldin D, Speck G, Morgan D, Lieber RL. Corrective shoes and inserts as treatment for flexible flatfoot in infants and children. *J Bone Joint Surg Am* 1989; **71**: 800–10.
10. Fraser RK, Menelaus MB, Williams PF, Cole WG. The Miller procedure for mobile flat feet. *J Bone Joint Surg Br* 1995; **77**: 396–9.
11. Ford LA, Hamilton GA. Naviculocuneiform arthrodesis. *Clin Podiatr Med Surg* 2004; **21**: 141–56.
12. Mosca VS. Calcaneal lengthening for valgus deformity of the hindfoot. Results in children who had severe, symptomatic flatfoot and skewfoot. *J Bone Joint Surg Am* 1995; **77**: 500–12.
13. Ragab AA, Stewart SL, Cooperman DR. Implications of subtalar joint anatomic variation in calcaneal lengthening osteotomy. *J Pediatr Orthop* 2003; **23**: 79–83.
14. Koutsogiannis E. Treatment of mobile flat foot by displacement osteotomy of the calcaneus. *J Bone Joint Surg Br* 1971; **53**: 96–100.
15. Marcinko DE, Lazerson A, Elleby DH. Silver calcaneal osteotomy for flexible flatfoot: a retrospective preliminary report. *J Foot Surg* 1984; **23**: 191–8.
16. GE Phillips. A review of elongation of os calcis for flat feet. *J Bone Joint Surg Br* 1983; **65**: 15–18.

Valgus deformity of the ankle and subtalar joint

8

Benjamin Joseph

Benjamin Joseph

Introduction

Valgus deformity of the hindfoot may be seen as an isolated deformity or in association with either an equinus or a calcaneus deformity. Valgus of the hindfoot is also an integral part of flatfoot or planovalgus deformity, which is discussed in Chapter 7, Planovalgus deformity.

The valgus deformity of the hindfoot may be at the ankle joint, the subtalar joint or both these joints may be contributing to the deformity (Table 8.1). It is important to identify the site of pathology as it will influence the treatment.

Table 8.1 ● Causes of hindfoot valgus due to abnormalities at the ankle and subtalar joints

Joint	Abnormality	Site of pathology	Nature of pathology and conditions where it is seen
Ankle joint	Tilt of ankle mortise	Distal tibia	Incomplete remodelling of distal tibial fracture Incomplete remodelling of congenital posteromedial bowing of the tibia[1]
		Distal tibial physis	Asymmetric growth following physeal damage after trauma or osteomyelitis
		Distal tibial epiphysis	Abnormal growth as in Trevor's disease or skeletal dysplasia[2]
		Fibula	Lack of support from lateral malleolus in fibular hemimelia Proximally situated lateral malleolus seen in spina bifida,[3] congenital pseudarthrosis of the tibia,[4] congenital pseudarthrosis of the fibula, hereditary multiple osteochondromatosis or following harvesting of fibula as bone graft[5] Proximal migration of the lateral malleolus during tibial lengthening
		Ligament	Deltoid ligament injury
Subtalar joint	Excessively everted position of subtalar joint	Muscles acting on the joint	Muscle imbalance – evertors stronger than invertors Muscle contracture – contracture of peroneal muscles, contracture of gastrocsoleus
		Ligaments and capsule	Hypermobile joints in joint laxity syndromes, overcorrection following subtalar capsular release for congenital clubfoot

Problems of management

Locating the site of the deformity

The exact site of the deformity needs to be identified in order to plan appropriate treatment. Apart from careful clinical examination, it is important to obtain anteroposterior radiographs of the ankle joint to determine whether the distal articular surface of the tibia is perpendicular to the long axis of the tibial shaft. In children with valgus inclination of the articular surface, the lateral malleolus may be proximally located (the distal fibular physis should normally be at the level of the ankle joint) and the distal tibial epiphysis may be wedge shaped (Figure 8.1a). An anteroposterior radiograph of the foot taken with the foot plantarflexed by 30° and with a cranial tilt of 30° of the radiograph tube will show the alignment of the talus and calcaneum. Excessive divergence of these bones with a high talocalcaneal angle suggests that there is valgus at the subtalar joint (Figure 8.1b).

Aim of treatment

● To make the foot plantigrade

Treatment options for correcting subtalar valgus

Orthosis

An ankle–foot orthosis can effectively prevent the hindfoot from everting if the deformity is supple. This would be the option of choice in a child who is too young for other surgical options to be considered.

Soft tissue balancing operations

If the underlying cause for the valgus deformity at the subtalar joint is muscle power imbalance between the invertors and evertors an appropriate tendon transfer may correct the deformity if it is still supple (see Chapter 56, The paralysed foot and ankle).

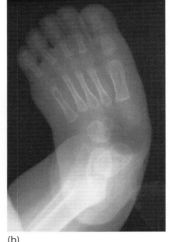
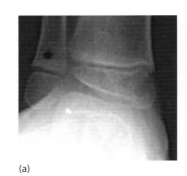

Figure 8.1 ● (a) Radiograph of the ankle of a child with a valgus deformity showing a wedge-shaped distal tibial epiphysis. **(b)** Anteroposterior radiograph of the foot taken with 30° plantarflexion of the ankle and the radiograph tube directed 30° cranially shows wide divergence of the talus and calcaneum with a high talocalcaneal angle. This implies that there is valgus at the subtalar joint.

(a)　　　　　　　　　　(b)

If the valgus deformity is on account of contracture of either the peronei or the gastrocsoleus, lengthening of the tendon should facilitate correction.

Subtalar arthroereisis

The principle of the operation is that as long as the sinus tarsi is prevented from closing, eversion of the subtalar joint can be prevented. Placing an implant in the sinus tarsi to restrict eversion of the subtalar joint is called arthroereisis (Figure 8.2). This procedure was developed to treat hindfoot valgus of flatfoot in children[6] and then extended to other neuromuscular conditions.[7] A technique involving placement of a staple across the subtalar joint without any attempt to achieve bony fusion has also been tried. The procedure is not effective in a small proportion of cases and complications are not infrequent.[8]

Figure 8.2 ● Diagram illustrating the technique of performing an arthroereisis. The hindfoot valgus **(a)** is corrected by inverting the subtalar joint; this opens the sinus tarsi **(b)**. An implant is placed into the sinus tarsi to keep it open **(c)**, thereby preventing hindfoot valgus.

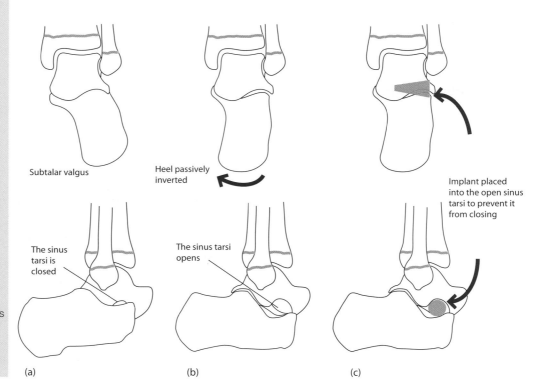

Subtalar valgus

Heel passively inverted

Implant placed into the open sinus tarsi to prevent it from closing

The sinus tarsi is closed

The sinus tarsi opens

(a)　　　　　　　　　　(b)　　　　　　　　　　(c)

Subtalar arthrodesis

Fusion of the subtalar joint will prevent the hindfoot from everting and this is an effective method of correcting hindfoot valgus at the subtalar joint. However, this is at the cost of permanently losing all subtalar motion.

Calcaneal osteotomy

Displacing the tuberosity of the calcaneum medially improves the appearance of the hindfoot although it does not actually correct the deformity at the subtalar joint if it is a rigid deformity (Figure 8.3). However, if the deformity is supple, the calcaneal osteotomy can facilitate dynamic correction of the deformity by shifting the Achilles tendon further from the axis of subtalar motion and thereby augmenting the invertor moment of the muscle (see Chapter 56, Figure 56.4f).

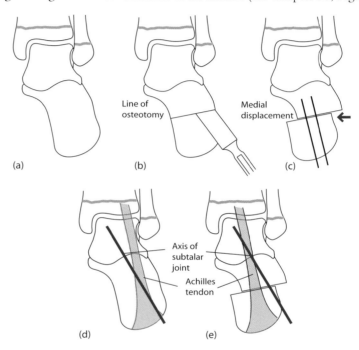

Figure 8.3 ● Diagram illustrating the technique of performing a medial displacement osteotomy of the calcaneum **(a–c)**. Medial displacement of the tuberosity increases the invertor moment of the gastrocsoleus by virtue of shifting the Achilles tendon medially in relation to the axis of the subtalar joint **(d,e)**.

Treatment options for correcting ankle valgus

Screw epiphyseodesis of the distal tibia

When there is asymmetric growth at the distal tibial physis with a wedge-shaped epiphysis, epiphyseodesis with a single screw passed obliquely from the medial malleolus across the growth plate has been found to be effective.[9–11] However, sufficient remaining growth must be present to achieve correction of the deformity. It has been estimated that the rate of correction of the valgus tilt after a screw epiphyseodesis is about 0.6° per month.[11] If the deformity is severe and it seems unlikely that the entire deformity will be corrected by this procedure alone, it may have to be combined with a supramalleolar osteotomy (Figure 8.4).

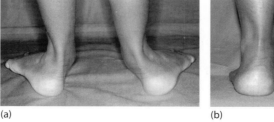
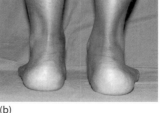

Figure 8.4 ● Severe valgus deformity of the ankle in a girl with a mesomelic skeletal dysplasia **(a)**. The factors that contributed to the valgus deformity at the ankle joint included a high-riding lateral malleolus, a wedge-shaped distal tibial epiphysis and an inclined articular surface. A combination of a supramalleolar osteotomy, lengthening of the fibula and screw epiphyseodesis of the medial malleolus resulted in complete correction of the deformity. The appearance of the ankle **(b)** after seven years is very satisfactory.

Supramalleolar osteotomy

A simple closed wedge osteotomy may not suffice when there is severe deformity and, in such instances, Wiltse's[12] technique is a good option (Figure 8.5).

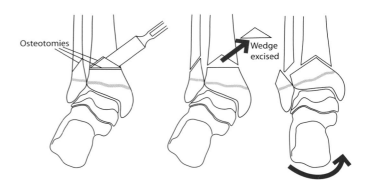

Osteotomies

Wedge excised

Figure 8.5 ● Diagram illustrating the technique of performing a Wiltse osteotomy for a valgus deformity of the ankle.

Reconstruction of the lateral malleolus

Reconstruction of the lateral malleolus has been attempted in children with fibular hemimelia (see Chapter 35, Fibular hemimelia).[13]

Lengthening the fibula (see Chapter 45)

Lengthening of the fibula as a means of pulling the lateral malleolus distally has been recommended (see Chapter 45, Discrepancies of length in the fibula).[14]

Tibiofibular synostosis

Creation of a synostosis between the distal tibia and fibula can prevent proximal migration of the lateral malleolus in conditions where there is such a propensity (as in congenital pseudarthrosis of the fibula or after harvesting of fibula as bone graft[15]). Similarly, a synostosis can be performed during tibial lengthening as a means of preventing proximal migration of the lateral malleolus and a valgus deformity of the ankle.

Factors to be taken into consideration while planning treatment

The site of the deformity

At the outset it is necessary to determine the site of the deformity as the treatment will depend on whether the ankle joint or the subtalar joint is at fault.

Suppleness of the deformity

If the valgus deformity is at the subtalar joint and can be passively corrected, the treatment is directed at simply preventing the subtalar joint from everting. Orthotic measures or surgical measures that prevent excessive eversion of the subtalar joint will be effective in correcting such a deformity. However, if the deformity is rigid these measures will not succeed.

Presence of underlying muscle imbalance

Restoration of muscle imbalance may help in correcting a paralytic valgus deformity of the subtalar joint.

Presence of underlying growth abnormality

Ankle valgus deformity on account of abnormal growth of the distal tibial epiphysis needs to be treated by attempting to restore symmetrical physeal growth. Merely correcting the deformity without addressing the growth abnormality will lead to recurrence of the deformity.

Recommended treatment

The treatment of subtalar valgus and ankle valgus is shown in Tables 8.2 and 8.3, respectively.

Table 8.2 ● Outline of treatment of subtalar valgus

INDICATIONS				
Supple deformity (passively correctable) + Child <5 years of age	Supple deformity (passively correctable) + Muscle imbalance present and appropriate tendon available for transfer	Supple deformity (passively correctable) + Muscle imbalance present and no appropriate tendon available for transfer OR Hypermobile joint with no muscle imbalance	Rigid deformity (passively not correctable) + Contracture of peronei or gastrocsoleus	Rigid deformity (passively not correctable) + No contracture of peronei or gastrocsoleus
⇩ Ankle–foot orthosis	⇩ Tendon transfer	⇩ Subtalar arthrodesis (extra-articular technique if the child is skeletally immature)	⇩ Lengthening of contracted tendon	⇩ Medial displacement osteotomy of the calcaneal tuberosity
TREATMENT				

Table 8.3 ● Treatment outline of ankle valgus

INDICATIONS				
Mild or moderate ankle valgus + Wedge-shaped distal tibial epiphysis + Sufficient growth remaining to achieve correction	Mild or moderate ankle valgus + Wedge-shaped distal tibial epiphysis + Sufficient growth remaining to achieve correction + Lateral malleolus proximally situated	Severe ankle valgus + Wedge-shaped distal tibial epiphysis + Insufficient growth remaining to achieve correction + Lateral malleolus proximally situated	Mild, moderate or severe ankle valgus + Distal tibial epiphysis NOT wedged + Lateral malleolus normally situated	Severe ankle valgus + Fibula absent
⇩ Screw epiphyseodesis	⇩ Screw epiphyseodesis + Lengthening of fibula	⇩ Screw epiphyseodesis + Lengthening of fibula + Supramalleolar osteotomy of tibia	⇩ Supramalleolar osteotomy of the tibia	⇩ Attempt reconstruction of a lateral malleolus If unsuccessful and ankle is unstable, consider ankle fusion (see Chapter 35, Fibular hemimelia)
TREATMENT				

References

1. Shah H, Siddesh ND, Joseph B. Congenital postero-medial bowing of the tibia. A retrospective analysis of growth abnormalities in the leg. *J Pediatr Orthop B* 2009 May; **18**(3): 120–8.
2. Bhatia M, Joseph B. A variant of Reinhardt-Pfeiffer mesomelic skeletal dysplasia. *Pediatr Radiol* 2000; **30**: 184–5.
3. Malhotra D, Puri R, Owen R. Valgus deformity of the ankle in children with spina bifida aperta. *J Bone Joint Surg Br* 1984; **66**: 381–5.
4. Joseph B, Somaraju VVJ, Shetty SK. Management of congenital pseudarthrosis of the tibia in children under 3 years of age. Effect of early surgery on union of the pseudarthrosis and growth of the limb. *J Pediatr Orthop* 2003; **23**: 740–6.
5. Kanaya K, Wada T, Kura H, Yamashita T, Usui M. Valgus deformity of the ankle following harvesting of a vascularized fibular graft in children. *J Reconstr Microsurg* 2002; **18**: 91–6.
6. Smith SD, Millar EA. Arthrorisis by means of subtalar polyethylene peg implant for correction of hindfoot pronation in children. *Clin Orthop Relat Res* 1983; **181**: 15–23.
7. Vedantam R, Capelli AM, Shoenecker PL. Subtalar arthroereisis for the correction of planovalgus deformity in children with neuromuscular disorders. *J Pediatr Orthop* 1988; **18**: 294–8.
8. Sanchez AA, Rathjen KE, Mubarak SJ. Subtalar staple arthroereisis for planovalgus foot deformity in children with neuromuscular disease. *J Pediatr Orthop* 1999; **19**: 34–8.
9. Beals RK. The treatment of ankle valgus by surface epiphysiodesis. *Clin Orthop Relat Res* 1991; **266**: 162–9.
10. Stevens PM, Belle RM. Screw epiphysiodesis for ankle valgus. *J Pediatr Orthop* 1997; **17**: 9–12.
11. Davids JR, Valadie AL, Ferguson RL, Bray EW 3rd, Allen BL Jr. Surgical management of ankle valgus in children: use of a transphyseal medial malleolar screw. *J Pediatr Orthop* 1997; **17**: 3–8.
12. Wiltse LL. Valgus deformity of the ankle: a sequel to acquired or congenital abnormalities of the fibula. *J Bone Joint Surg Am* 1972; **54**: 595–606.
13. Weber M, Siebert CH, Goost H, Johannisson R, Wirtz D. Malleolus externus plasty for joint reconstruction in fibular aplasia: preliminary report of a new technique. *J Pediatr Orthop B* 2002; **11**: 265–73.
14. Snearly WN, Peterson HA. Management of ankle deformities in multiple hereditary osteochondromata. *J Pediatr Orthop* 1989; **9**: 427–32.
15. Fragnière B, Wicart P, Mascard E, Dubousset J. Prevention of ankle valgus after vascularized fibular grafts in children. *Clin Orthop Relat Res* 2003; **408**: 245–51.

Metatarsus adductus and skewfoot

Selvadurai Nayagam

Introduction

Forefoot adduction is one of the most common foot deformities that prompt a consultation with a paediatric orthopaedic surgeon. Forefoot adduction may be seen in three different conditions: clubfoot (both congenital and acquired), metatarsus adductus and skewfoot. The site of the forefoot deformity and the alignment of the hindfoot vary in these three conditions and it is important that these factors are clearly recognized in order to plan appropriate treatment (Table 9.1 and Figure 9.1).

Table 9.1 ● Pattern of deformities in the three different conditions presenting with forefoot adduction

Condition	Site and nature of forefoot deformity		Hindfoot deformity
	Tarsometatarsal joints	Midtarsal joint (talonavicular and calcaneocuboid joints)	
Metatarsus adductus	Adducted	Normal	None
Clubfoot	Normal	Adducted	Varus and equinus
Skewfoot	Adducted	Abducted	Valgus and equinus

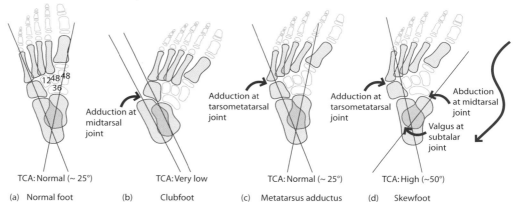

(a) Normal foot (b) Clubfoot (c) Metatarsus adductus (d) Skewfoot

Figure 9.1 ● These drawings depict the differences between forefoot adduction of clubfoot, metatarsus adductus and skewfoot when assessed from an anteroposterior radiograph. In a normal foot **(a)**, the talocalcaneal angle (TCA) is approximately 25°. The ossific nuclei of the calcaneum, talus and the cuboid and the metatarsal shafts that are ossified at birth are shaded. The timing of appearance of the remaining tarsal bones is indicated in months. In a clubfoot **(b)**, the talocalcaneal angle is reduced and there is near parallelism of the axes. The forefoot is adducted at the midtarsal joint. In metatarsus adductus **(c)**, the talocalcaneal angle is normal and the forefoot is medially deviated at the tarsometatarsal joint. In skewfoot **(d)**, the talocalcaneal angle is increased. The metatarsals are adducted at the tarsometatarsal joints, and in severe examples, the navicular, cuboid and cuneiforms are laterally translated. This produces the S-shaped contour and the term 'serpentine foot' which is sometimes used for the condition.

Metatarsus adductus

Metatarsus adductus is sometimes synonymously referred to as metatarsus varus or forefoot adductus; some authors distinguish between metatarsus adductus and metatarsus varus by the degree of rigidity of the deformity, the latter being the stiffer type. An association with hip dysplasia and internal tibial torsion has also been reported.[1,2]

The natural history of metatarsus adductus is one of spontaneous improvement in the great majority.[3] However, a careful diagnosis before adopting a nihilistic approach (no treatment) is wise because both clubfeet and skewfeet present with similar looking forefoot deformities but require very different management strategies (Figure 9.2).

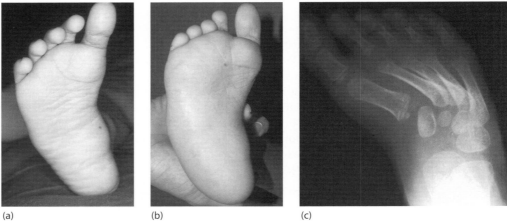

(a)   (b)   (c)

Figure 9.2 ● Forefoot adduction seen in metatarsus adductus **(a)** may appear very similar to forefoot adduction of congenital or paralytic clubfoot **(b)**; however, the anteroposterior radiograph of the foot with metatarsus adductus shows a normal midtarsal alignment and adduction at the tarsometatarsal joints **(c)**.

Skewfoot

Skewfoot is a rare deformity that is difficult to treat due to the complex pathoanatomy of the condition. The deformity includes an adducted and often plantarflexed forefoot, a laterally and dorsally displaced navicular on the head of the talus, a plantarflexed talus and a valgus calcaneum. There is often a concomitant contracture of the Achilles tendon.

Problems of management

Deformity

This is the most frequent reason for consultation. Parents or relatives notice the curved appearance of the foot in the young infant and seek medical advice – usually because of anxiety over progression of the deformity or that it will interfere with the child's ability to walk.

In-toeing gait

In those who present later in childhood, the complaint is in-toeing. Careful prone examination of the thigh–foot angle will distinguish metatarsus adductus from internal tibial torsion (Figure 9.3). A careful look at the hip is mandatory because of an association with developmental dysplasia of the hip (DDH).

Shoe-fitting problems

When a child presents with local pressure problems in footwear owing to metatarsus adductus, the deformity is likely to be of the rigid variety or the diagnosis one of the rare skewfoot. The pressure is usually over the base of the fifth metatarsal although complaints are directed sometimes at the great toe and nearby metatarsophalangeal joint.

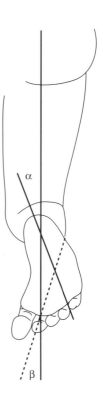

Figure 9.3 ● The thigh–foot angle in the prone position allows a measure of tibial torsion. In metatarsus adductus, the overall axis of the forefoot needs to be assessed with reference to the thigh axis (angle β). The calcaneal axis (angle α) represents tibial torsion, and both calcaneal and metatarsal axes are collinear when metatarsus adductus is absent.

Aims of treatment

- Avoid treating a deformity which spontaneously improves
  Most cases of metatarsus adductus improve; those that improve need no active treatment.
- Reduce problems with shoe fitting
  A stiff metatarsus adductus or a skewfoot can cause local pressure problems in an unmodified shoe.
- Correct persistent deformity to improve the appearance of the foot and gait
  Correction of the deformity should be considered for cases that do not resolve, particularly if the deformity is severe.

Treatment options

Observation

This is recommended for the majority once it is confirmed that the metatarsus adductus is present alone and there is no associated hindfoot deformity. Some record of progress can be made by photocopying the feet while the child is supported standing on the glass platen of a photocopier.

Serial casts

This is indicated in a minority of cases of metatarsus adductus which are either severe or appear not to be resolving as the child gets older. It is also needed in the stiffer varieties that produce local pressure problems in footwear. If serial reviews suggest little improvement and stiffness in the deformity is found, starting serial cast treatment by six months will allow correction in most with three to five cast changes.

Unlike cast treatment for clubfeet, the fulcrum for applying an external rotation torque when moulding the cast is located over the cuboid (Figure 9.4). The cast is also carefully moulded over the os calcis to prevent it drifting into excessive valgus.[1,4] Application of serial casts for a late presentation is also successful in treating persistent metatarsus adductus but is more difficult to carry out in the larger, more active child.

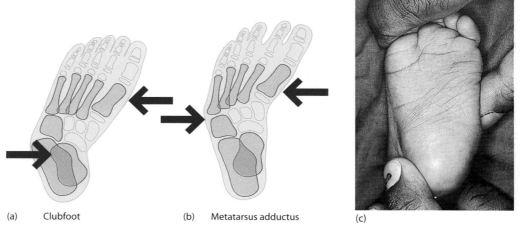

(a)   Clubfoot   (b)   Metatarsus adductus   (c)

Figure 9.4 ● In manipulation and serial cast moulding of congenital clubfoot **(a)**, the fulcrum is over the lateral aspect of the neck of talus for a laterally directed torque over the medial border of the foot (dark arrows). While correcting metatarsus adductus **(b,c)**, the fulcrum is placed over the cuboid instead of neck of talus for manipulation and serial casting (dark arrows).

The skewfoot can, in some cases, and particularly if the presentation is early, be improved by serial casts but the danger is converting the deformity into a flatfoot owing to the already present valgus hindfoot deformity.

Shoe modification

Denis Browne splints and rigid shoes with a straight medial border have been tried for correcting metatarsus adductus but there is no strong evidence that they alter the natural history of the condition.[5] However, shoes modified to accommodate the deformity may relieve pressure symptoms.

Soft tissue surgery

Persistence of deformity after attempted correction through serial casts may lead to surgery. Contracture of the abductor hallucis muscle and abnormal insertion of the tibialis anterior or tibialis posterior have been implicated as factors that contribute to the deformity. Consequently, release of the abductor hallucis and the abnormal insertion of the tibialis posterior have been advocated.[6–8] Since capsular contractures on the medial aspect of the foot are likely to be present in the more rigid feet that require surgery, a combination of capsular release and tendon release may be required. In its simplest form, surgery for metatarsus adductus will involve release of the naviculo-cuneiform and cuneiform-metatarsal joints together with lengthening of the abductor hallucis.[9] Complete tarsometatarsal joint releases advocated in the past[10] are not currently recommended.[11]

Basal metatarsal osteotomies

In the older child with metatarsus adductus, soft tissue surgery may not suffice and osteotomies of the bases of all five metatarsals may be needed[12] (Figures 9.5 and 9.6).

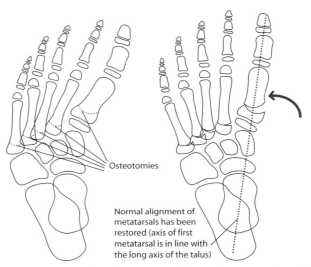

Osteotomies

Normal alignment of metatarsals has been restored (axis of first metatarsal is in line with the long axis of the talus)

Figure 9.5 ● Diagram depicting correction of metatarsus adductus by osteotomies of the bases of the metatarsals.

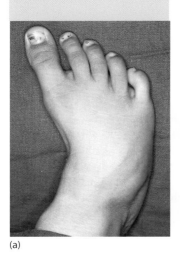

(a)

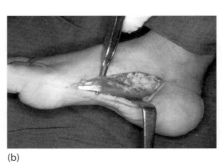

(b)

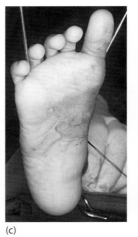

(c)

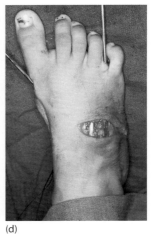

(d)

Figure 9.6 ● Uncorrected metatarsus adductus in a six-year-old boy **(a)** was treated by release of the abductor hallucis tendon and osteotomy of the bases of all five metatarsals. The tightness of the abductor hallucis was confirmed during surgery **(b)**. The appearance of the sole of the foot following osteotomy of the metatarsals and Kirschner wire stabilization of the first and the fifth metatarsals **(c,d)** shows a straight lateral border. The pre-operative appearance of the sole of the foot is shown in Figure 9.2(a).

Combined calcaneal osteotomy and cuneiform osteotomy

A surgical approach for skewfoot involves a calcaneal lengthening osteotomy, medial cuneiform opening wedge osteotomy and lengthening of the Achilles tendon[13] (Figure 9.7).

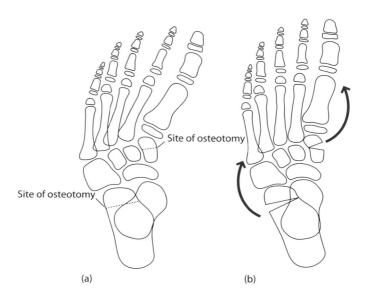

Figure 9.7 ● Diagram illustrating the technique of correction of skew foot deformity. Open wedge osteotomies of the medial cuneiform and the anterior end of the calcaneum correct the forefoot adduction and the midfoot abduction.

(a)   (b)

Factors to be taken into consideration while planning treatment

Age at presentation

The age at presentation is important. If the first presentation is when the child is older, further spontaneous improvement in metatarsus adductus is unlikely. This would prompt a treatment protocol starting with serial casts. In comparison, a more reserved approach is wise when dealing with the young infant; the odds are in favour of the metatarsus adductus being simple and likely to resolve spontaneously. Ideally, serial cast treatment should start before walking age but this may not be possible in all cases.

Severity and stiffness

In mild and flexible deformities, reassurance and an offer to review can be provided. However, in the presence of stiffness in the deformity, closer follow-up is wise. This allows the surgeon to institute non-operative treatment early for those noted not to improve. An attempt at subjectively 'grading' the degree of stiffness may help estimate the likelihood of spontaneous correction and the number of cast changes needed for treatment, if this should prove necessary.

The type of forefoot and hindfoot deformity

Metatarsus adductus in the infant is a clinical diagnosis. It is important to distinguish clubfeet and skewfeet from metatarsus adductus. Clubfeet will reveal elements of forefoot supination and hindfoot equinovarus; treatment by serial casts soon after birth is recommended. In contrast, the skewfoot is a rigid form of metatarsus adductus accompanied by a valgus and equinus hindfoot. The valgus hindfoot and forefoot adduction give the appearance of a flatfoot in the child who is already standing.

Radiographs are not routinely indicated in flexible metatarsus adductus in the infant as their interpretation is fraught with inaccuracy[14] because many of the ossification centres are not visible. There is the added difficulty that many reference angles alter with age.[15] On account of these limitations it may not always be possible to differentiate metatarsus adductus and skewfoot on the evidence of radiographs.[13]

Syndrome association

A possible link of metatarsus adductus to DDH and internal tibial torsion has been noted and must be looked for at clinical examination. Skewfoot is often bilateral and may be associated with recognized syndromes or systemic conditions (diastrophic dwarfism, osteogenesis imperfecta, cerebral palsy, spinal dysraphism).

Recommended treatment

An outline of treatment is shown in Table 9.2.

Table 9.2 ● Outline of treatment of metatarsus adductus and skewfoot

INDICATIONS				
Metatarsus adductus + Flexible + Infant	Metatarsus adductus OR Skewfoot + Stiff (unable to passively correct with ease) + Infant	Metatarsus adductus + Stiff (unable to passively correct with ease) + Poor response to serial casting	Metatarsus adductus + Stiff deformity + Older child	Skewfoot + Stiff deformity + Older child
⇩	⇩	⇩	⇩	⇩
Reassurance and periodic review	Serial casting	Release of abductor hallucis and medial capsules of naviculocuneiform and first tarsometatarsal joints	Abductor hallucis release and basal metatarsal osteotomies	Calcaneal osteotomy (lateral column lengthening) + Medial cuneiform open wedge osteotomy + Achilles tendon lengthening
TREATMENT				

Rationale of treatment suggested

A foot deformity which improves spontaneously in the great majority of children needs little more than reassurance and an offer to review. However, the pitfall is mistaking a clubfoot or skewfoot for metatarsus adductus. Clubfeet should undergo serial cast treatment soon after birth whereas metatarsus adductus, if such treatment is necessary, can commence before walking age. The vast majority of cases of metatarsus adductus are thus resolved, leaving operative intervention for the few resistant cases that continue to produce symptoms, usually with footwear. The surgeon needs to be satisfied that non-operative measures have been fully tried, including shoe wear modification, before embarking on surgery.

The skewfoot is a rare and altogether different deformity. Surgery is needed more often and reflects the stiffness and resistance to serial cast treatment. Even so, non-operative management should be tried but with the caveat that the surgeon avoids exaggerating the existing valgus hindfoot deformity and producing a flatfoot.

References

1. Ponseti IV, Becker JR. Congenital metatarsus adductus: the results of treatment. *J Bone Joint Surg Am* 1966; **48**: 702–11.
2. Kumar SJ, MacEwen GD. The incidence of hip dysplasia with metatarsus adductus. *Clin Orthop Relat Res* 1982; **164**: 234–5.
3. Rushforth GF. The natural history of hooked forefoot. *J Bone Joint Surg Br* 1978; **60**: 530–2.
4. Berg EE. A reappraisal of metatarsus adductus and skewfoot. *J Bone Joint Surg Am* 1986; **68**: 1185–96.
5. Tracey HW. Treatment of congenital metatarsus varus with Denis Browne splints. *South Med J* 1968; **61**: 939–42.
6. Lichtblau S. Section of the abductor hallucis tendon for correction of metatarsus varus deformity. *Clin Orthop Relat Res* 1975; **110**: 227–32.
7. Mitchell GP. Abductor hallucis release in metatarsus varus. *Int Orthop* 1980; **3**: 299–304.
8. Browne RS, Paton DF. Anomalous insertion of the tibialis posterior tendon in congenital metatarsus varus. *J Bone Joint Surg Br* 1979; **61**: 74–6.

9. Asirvatham R, Stevens P. Idiopathic forefoot-adduction deformity: medial capsulotomy and abductor hallucis lengthening for resistant and severe deformities. *J Pediatr Orthop* 1997; **17**: 496–500.

10. Heyman CH, Herndon CH, Strong JM. Mobilization of the tarsometatarsal and intermetatarsal joints for the correction of resistant adduction of the fore part of the foot in congenital club-foot or congenital metatarsus varus. *J Bone Joint Surg Am* 1958; **40**: 299–309.

11. Stark JG, Johanson JE, Winter RB. The Heyman-Herndon tarsometatarsal capsulotomy for metatarsus adductus: results in 48 feet. *J Pediatr Orthop* 1987; **7**: 305–10.

12. Berman A, Gartland JJ. Metatarsal osteotomy for correction of adduction of the fore part of the foot in children. *J Bone Joint Surg Am* 1971; **53**: 498–506.

13. Mosca VS. Flexible flatfoot and skewfoot. *J Bone Joint Surg Am* 1995; **77**: 1937–45.

14. Cook DA, Breed AL, Cook T, DeSmet AD, Muehle CM. Observer variability in the radiographic measurement and classification of metatarsus adductus. *J Pediatr Orthop* 1992; **12**: 86–9.

15. Vanderwilde R, Staheli LT, Chew DE, Malagon V. Measurements on radiographs of the foot in normal infants and children. *J Bone Joint Surg Am* 1988; **70**: 407–15.

Anterolateral bowing of the tibia and congenital pseudarthrosis of the tibia

10

Benjamin Joseph

Benjamin Joseph

Introduction

Congenital anterolateral bowing of the tibia is a potentially troublesome deformity, particularly when it is associated with either neurofibromatosis or fibrous dysplasia. The bowed tibia may fracture and the fracture may fail to unite, progressing on to a frank pseudarthrosis. The fracture usually develops once the child begins to walk although it can occur in infancy (Figure 10.1b). If the limb is adequately protected from angular and torsional stresses, the fracture may be prevented in a proportion of children (Figure 10.1c).

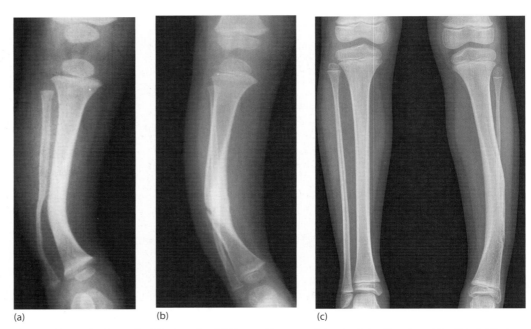

(a) (b) (c)

Figure 10.1 ● Radiograph of the leg of a child born with congenital anterolateral bowing of the tibia **(a)** that fractured after a trivial fall **(b)**. No form of bracing had been used prior to the fracture. Radiograph of a child with neurofibromatosis and anterolateral bowing that has been protected in a brace since infancy **(c)**.

Problems of management of established pseudarthrosis

Obtaining union

Obtaining union of an established pseudarthrosis is difficult.[1] In the past, numerous operations have been tried with dismal results.[2] It is important to be aware of the procedures that have a poor chance of success in order to avoid them as inappropriate surgery may further compromise the chance of a satisfactory outcome.[3,4]

Shortening of the limb

At birth itself the affected tibia is slightly shorter than the normal side. Progressive shortening of the leg occurs as long as the pseudarthrosis remains ununited.[5] Repeated unsuccessful operations further hamper normal growth of the leg.

Tendency for refracture following union

There is a tendency for the tibia to refracture even after sound union is achieved. This tendency diminishes after skeletal maturity. However, some patients do sustain refractures in adult life.

Growth abnormalities of the tibia, fibula and femur

In addition to the three primary problems listed above, there are other growth abnormalities of the tibia, fibula and the ipsilateral femur that may need to be taken into consideration while planning treatment.[5] These include abnormal inclination of the proximal tibial physis, posterior bowing of the proximal third of the tibial diaphysis, proximal migration of the lateral malleolus, fibular hypoplasia, fibular pseudarthrosis, ankle valgus and calcaneus deformity (Figure 10.2). Several of these growth abnormalities develop if the tibial pseudarthrosis remains ununited and they become more severe as the child grows. This implies that the sooner union of the pseudarthrosis is achieved the less pronounced these growth abnormalities will be.[5]

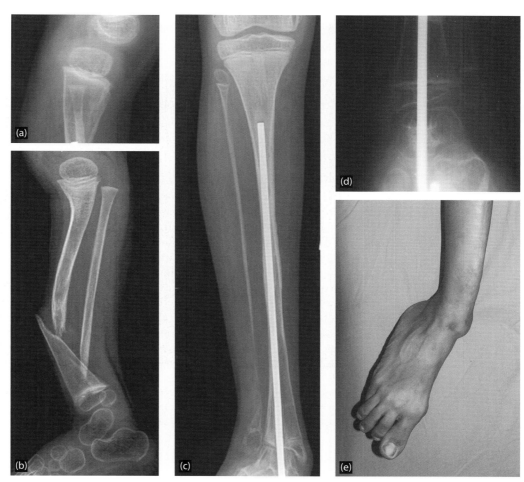

Figure 10.2 ● Growth abnormalities of the tibia and fibula noted in children with congenital pseudarthrosis of the tibia include abnormal inclination of the proximal tibial physis **(a)**, posterior bowing of the proximal third of the tibia **(b)**, fibular hypoplasia **(c)**, proximal migration of the fibular physis **(d)** and valgus deformity of the ankle **(e)**.

Ankle deformity and arthritis

Valgus deformity of the ankle and degenerative arthritis are seen in a significant proportion of adults with healed pseudarthrosis of the tibia.[1]

Aims of treatment

- Achieve union
- Prevent refracture
- Correct limb length inequality
- Correct associated growth abnormalities
- Prevent ankle deformity and arthritis

Treatment strategies

Strategies to achieve union

Among the various procedures that have been performed, only three have reported union rates of over 70 percent and, currently, they are the only options worth considering. They are microvascular free fibular transfer,[6–8] the Ilizarov technique[1,3,8,9] and bone grafting with intramedullary nailing.[4,5,10,11] Irrespective of the method adopted it is recommended that excision of the pseudarthrosis should be an integral part of the procedure.[1,4,10]

Strategies for minimizing the risk of refracture
- Splint the limb in an orthosis until skeletal maturity.
- Retain an intramedullary nail until skeletal maturity.

Strategies for dealing with shortening of the limb
- Minimize the extent of shortening by obtaining union of the pseudarthrosis as early as possible.
- Established shortening can be addressed by limb equalization procedures (see Chapter 44, Length discrepancy of the tibia).

Strategies for minimizing valgus deformity of the ankle
- Ensure union of the fibular pseudarthrosis.
- Retaining an intramedullary rod that crosses the ankle joint can also prevent ankle deformity although the motion is lost.

Treatment options

Intramedullary rodding and cortical bone grafting

The exact details of how the procedure is done vary from report to report. However, there are three essential steps to the operation: excision of the pseudarthrosis, bone grafting and intramedullary rodding (Figure 10.3). Excision of the pseudarthrosis involves excising the tapered ends of the bone until fresh bleeding is encountered. In addition, the thick periosteum surrounding the entire area of the pseudarthrosis is excised. There is general agreement that autogenous bone grafting facilitates union. However, some surgeons use cancellous graft while others recommend cortical graft.[4,5] The author prefers cortical graft harvested from the subcutaneous surface of the opposite tibia. Three struts of cortical bone are placed around the site of the excised pseudarthrosis after ensuring that the fragments are well apposed. No attempt is made to anchor the grafts to the tibia. The types of intramedullary rods that have been used vary.[4,11,12] The author uses a Rush rod which is passed from the heel into the tibia. A rod of sufficient length must be selected to ensure that the tip of the rod reaches the proximal tibial metaphysis. The tip of the rod

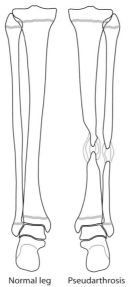
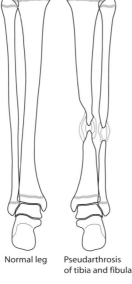
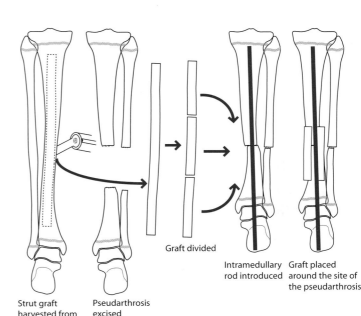

Figure 10.3 ● Technique of cortical bone grafting and intramedullary rodding.

Normal leg

Pseudarthrosis of tibia and fibula

Strut graft harvested from subcutaneous surface of tibia

Pseudarthrosis excised

Graft divided

Intramedullary rod introduced

Graft placed around the site of the pseudarthrosis

will gradually recede distally as the child grows. Since the region of the pseudarthrosis needs to be supported until skeletal maturity, the rod will have to be changed and a longer rod put in once the original rod tip has receded to the middle of the tibial shaft.

Microvascular free fibular transfer

The procedure entails harvesting a long segment of the opposite fibula along with its vascular pedicle.[6,10,11] This is transferred into the gap created after radical excision of the pseudarthrotic segment. The vessels of the transferred fibula are anastomosed to the local vessels (Figure 10.4). The transferred fibula is fixed securely to the tibia. It is important to ensure that the method of fixation does not compromise the circulation of the transferred fibula and the distal tibia. For this reason some surgeons do not recommend the use of an intramedullary rod. The operation is demanding and the operating time can be over six hours with two teams of surgeons.

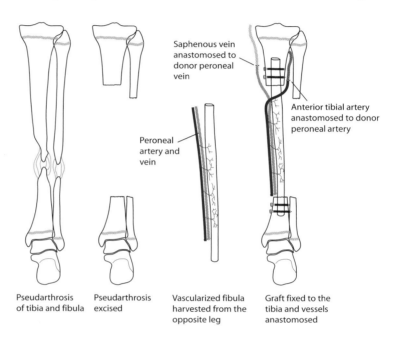

Saphenous vein anastomosed to donor peroneal vein

Peroneal artery and vein

Anterior tibial artery anastomosed to donor peroneal artery

Pseudarthrosis of tibia and fibula

Pseudarthrosis excised

Vascularized fibula harvested from the opposite leg

Graft fixed to the tibia and vessels anastomosed

Figure 10.4 ● Diagram showing the technique of microvascular free fibular transfer for pseudarthrosis of the tibia.

The Ilizarov technique

The Ilizarov frame is applied, the pseudarthrosis is excised and the fragments are compressed. The compression can be applied in different ways including closed longitudinal compression, side-to-side compression, segmental bone transport and resection with acute compression.[7] Resection and acute compression is recommended as bone grafting can also be combined with the procedure. A metaphyseal osteotomy is also performed and tibial lengthening is begun after seven to ten days (Figure 10.5). The highest union rates have been reported for this approach as opposed to longitudinal compression, side-to-side compression or segmental bone transport.

Age of the child

The age of the child is an important factor that can influence the choice of treatment. The chances of obtaining union following the Ilizarov procedure are low in children under three or four years of age.[1,3]

Similarly, it is technically difficult to perform a microvascular free fibular transfer in a very young child.[6] However, intramedullary rodding and cortical bone grafting has been shown to be effective even in children under the age of three years.[4,5]

Chances of obtaining union

It is imperative that the method that is chosen has a high chance of facilitating union for the particular age of the child.

Factors to be taken into consideration while planning treatment

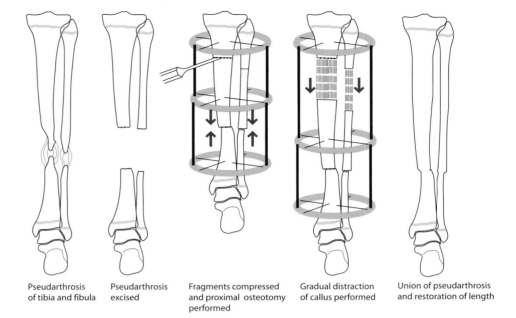

Figure 10.5 ● Diagram showing the technique of treating congenital pseudarthrosis of the tibia with the Ilizarov ring fixator.

Pseudarthrosis of tibia and fibula

Pseudarthrosis excised

Fragments compressed and proximal osteotomy performed

Gradual distraction of callus performed

Union of pseudarthrosis and restoration of length

Simplicity and ease of the procedure

The microvascular free fibular transfer is a highly demanding and complex procedure and should only be attempted by surgeons with sufficient expertise.

Cost

The cost of microvascular surgery is likely to be a great deal more than other procedures because the operating time required is so much longer.

Feasibility of addressing associated deformities and limb length issues along with obtaining union

A procedure that can address all these problems should be considered if the child has significant shortening and deformities other than the anterolateral bow.

Table 10.1 summarizes the factors that need to be considered while selecting the procedure.

Table 10.1 ● Factors to be taken into consideration while choosing the primary procedure

Factors to be considered	Microvascular free fibular transfer	Ilizarov technique	Intramedullary rodding and bone grafting
Reported union rate	>70%	>70%	>70%
Success in children under the age of 3 years	Poor	Poor	Good
Ability to reduce risk of refracture	Does not reduce risk	Does not reduce risk	Reduces risk
Simultaneous correction of limb length inequality	Not possible	Possible	Not possible
Simultaneous correction of all deformities	Not possible	Possible	Not possible
Prevention of late ankle valgus	Not possible	Not possible	Possible
Complexity of the procedure	Very complex	Complex	Simple
Cost	Very high	High	Low

Recommended treatment

The outline of treatment recommended is shown in Table 10.2.

Table 10.2 ● Treatment of anterolateral bowing and pseudarthrosis of the tibia

INDICATIONS			
Anterolateral bow without fracture	Established pseudarthrosis + Skeletally immature child (1–13 years of age) + Shortening <10% + No gross deformities of the tibia or ankle other than anterolateral bowing	Established pseudarthrosis + Child over 5 years of age + Intramedullary (IM) nailing and bone grafting has failed OR consider as primary option if Shortening >10% + Deformities of the tibia or ankle other than anterolateral bowing that need correction	Established pseudarthrosis + Child over 5 years of age + IM nailing and bone grafting and Ilizarov technique have failed
	⇩	⇩	⇩
⇩ Knee–ankle–foot orthosis	Excision of pseudarthrosis + Autogenous cortical bone grafting + Transarticular Rush rodding + Bracing till skeletal maturity after union	Ilizarov technique that includes: Excision of pseudarthrosis + Autogenous cortical bone grafting + Compression of fragments + Metaphyseal osteotomy and tibial lengthening + Concomitant correction of tibial deformities + Bracing until skeletal maturity after union	Radical excision of pseudarthrosis + Microvascular free fibular transfer
TREATMENT			

Rationale of treatment suggested

Why has intramedullary nailing and bone grafting been recommended as the first choice?
The operation has a good chance of success even in children less than three years of age. This is a distinct advantage because growth abnormalities and shortening of the tibia can be minimized if union can be achieved in the young child. Retaining the intramedullary rod until skeletal maturity may minimize the risk of refractures. The procedure is relatively simple, is the cheapest option available and can be done without sophisticated equipment or very specialized training.

Why has transarticular rodding been advocated?
Rod exchange is easy when the hook is in the heel, and if the transarticular rod is retained until skeletal maturity it may prevent ankle and subtalar valgus. This, however, is at the expense of persistent ankle stiffness. In a long-term review it was noted that valgus deformity and degenerative arthritis of the ankle were very common and less than 30 percent of patients had normal ankles even when the ankle was not transfixed.[1] Thus the disadvantage of a stiff, normally aligned ankle must be weighed against the risk of ankle valgus and painful arthritis.

Why has cortical bone graft been recommended?
Evidence from the literature shows that among procedures used in the past, those that used cortical graft fared better than those with cancellous graft. Furthermore, cortical graft can resist resorption longer than can cancellous graft.

68 ANTEROLATERAL BOWING AND CONGENITAL PSEUDARTHROSIS OF THE TIBIA

References

1. Grill F, Bollini G, Dungl P *et al.* Treatment approaches for congenital pseudarthrosis of tibia: results of the EPOS multicenter study. European Paediatric Orthopaedic Society (EPOS). *J Pediatr Orthop* 2000; **9**: 75–89.

2. Hardinge K. Congenital anterior bowing of the tibia. The significance of the different types in relation to pseudarthrosis. *Ann R Coll Surg Engl* 1972; **51**: 17–30.

3. Wientroub S, Grill F. Congenital pseudarthrosis of the tibia: Part 1. European Pediatric Orthopaedic Society multicenter study of congenital pseudoarthrosis. *J Pediatr Orthop B* 2000; **9**: 1–2.

4. Joseph B, Mathew G. Management of congenital pseudarthrosis of the tibia by excision of the pseudarthrosis, onlay grafting, and intramedullary nailing. *J Pediatr Orthop B* 2000; **9**: 16–23.

5. Joseph B, Somaraju VV, Shetty SK. Management of congenital pseudarthrosis of the tibia in children under 3 years of age: effect of early surgery on union of the pseudarthrosis and growth of the limb. *J Pediatr Orthop* 2003; **23**: 740–6.

6. Anderson DJ, Schoenecker PL, Sheridan JJ, Rich MM. Use of an intramedullary rod for the treatment of congenital pseudarthrosis of the tibia. *J Bone Joint Surg Am* 1992; **74**: 161–8.

7. Baker JK, Cain TE, Tullos HS. Intramedullary fixation for congenital pseudarthrosis of the tibia. *J Bone Joint Surg Am* 1992; **74**: 169–78.

8. Romanus B, Bollini G, Dungl P *et al.* Free vascular fibular transfer in congenital pseudoarthrosis of the tibia: results of the EPOS multicenter study. European Paediatric Orthopaedic Society (EPOS). *J Pediatr Orthop B* 2000; **9**: 90–3.

9. de Boer HH, Verbout AJ, Nielsen HK, van der Eijken JW. Free vascularized fibular graft for tibial pseudarthrosis in neurofibromatosis. *Acta Orthop Scand* 1988; **59**: 425–9.

10. Ghanem I, Damsin JP, Carlioz H. Ilizarov technique in the treatment of congenital pseudarthrosis of the tibia. *J Pediatr Orthop* 1997; **17**: 685–90.

11. Grill F. Treatment of congenital pseudarthrosis of tibia with the circular frame technique. *J Pediatr Orthop B* 1996; **5**: 6–16.

12. Johnston CE II. Congenital pseudarthrosis of the tibia. Results of technical variations in the Charnley-Williams procedure. *J Bone Joint Surg Am* 2002; **84**: 1799–1810.

Posteromedial bowing of the tibia

Benjamin Joseph

11

Introduction

Congenital posteromedial bowing of the tibia is a relatively uncommon condition. It is usually unilateral and is associated with a calcaneovalgus deformity of the foot at birth (Figure 11.1). Its natural history is distinctly different from congenital anterolateral bowing. Posteromedial bowing tends to resolve, to a great extent, spontaneously as the child grows.[1-3] Unlike anterolateral bowing, in children with posteromedial bowing there is no risk of the tibia fracturing and a pseudarthrosis developing. Nor is the condition associated with neurofibromatosis or fibrous dysplasia.

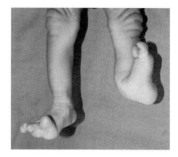

Figure 11.1 ● Appearance of the limb of a newborn infant with congenital posteromedial bowing of the tibia. The calcaneovalgus deformity of the foot and the shortening of the leg are clearly seen.

Problems of management

Tibial deformity

Although spontaneous resolution of the bowing does occur to a great extent, in children with more severe degrees of bowing some residual deformity may persist, warranting correction (Figure 11.2a).

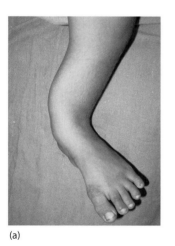
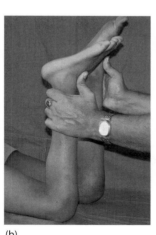
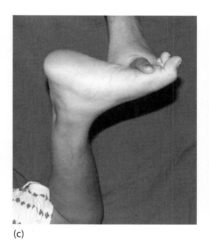
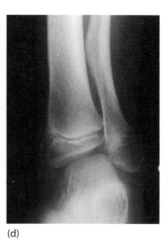

(a)   (b)   (c)   (d)

Figure 11.2 ● **(a)** Persistent posteromedial bowing of the tibia in a six-year-old girl. **(b)** Reduction in the range of plantarflexion of the left ankle in an eight-year-old boy who had posteromedial bowing of the tibia. **(c)** Weakness plantarflexion of the ankle is demonstrated in a 12-year-old girl as she attempts to plantarflex against resistance offered by the examiner. **(d)** Radiograph of the ankle of a boy showing a wedge-shaped distal tibial epiphysis and a valgus deformity of the ankle.

Shortening

Some degree of shortening of the tibia is invariably present in this condition and the degree of shortening appears to be proportionate to the severity of bowing. While the degree of shortening may often be quite mild, significant shortening may occasionally occur.

Foot and ankle deformity

The calcaneovalgus deformity of the foot that may be quite severe at birth improves quite rapidly. However, in some instances the range and strength of ankle movement is never fully regained and some deformity may persist (Figures 11.2b,c). The valgus deformity of the ankle may persist on account of residual medial bowing of the distal tibia. In some children physeal growth abnormalities may be present and may contribute to persistence of deformity (Figure 11.2d).

Aims of treatment

- Correct residual deformities of the tibia
  Ideally, all residual deformities of the tibia in both the sagittal and coronal planes should be corrected. Apart from improving the appearance of the limb this will help in restoring the normal alignment of the ankle.
- Equalize the limb lengths
  It is desirable to equalize limb lengths or at least reduce the discrepancy to a level that may be managed with an inconspicuous sole raise.
- Correct deformities of the foot and ankle
  Since the ankle is a weight-bearing joint it is important to ensure that the tibial plafond is parallel to the knee and the ground and any deformity that is present should be corrected in order to achieve this aim.

Treatment options

No intervention

No intervention is necessary if adequate resolution of the deformity of the foot and the tibia has occurred and if the limb length inequality is less than 2 cm at skeletal maturity.

Limb length equalization

If the anticipated shortening at skeletal maturity is likely to exceed 2 cm, limb length equalization is needed. The technique of limb length equalization will depend on whether tibial deformity correction is also concomitantly required and on the degree of shortening. The degree of shortening encountered in this condition is usually only of moderate degree and limb length equalization can easily be achieved by shortening the longer limb. However, if residual tibial deformity is present, it is more appropriate to correct the deformity and concomitantly lengthen the tibia.

Deformity correction

■ Correction of tibial deformity

Angulation of the tibia at the junction of the middle and lower thirds of the tibia can be corrected by a diaphyseal osteotomy. If concomitant limb lengthening is being undertaken, a fixator may be used (Figure 11.3) or else the osteotomy may be fixed with a plate.

■ Correction of ankle deformity

A valgus deformity of the ankle may persist on account of the bowing of the distal tibia or due to abnormal physeal inclination and asymmetric growth. A supramalleolar osteotomy will correct the former problem while arrest of the medial side of the growth plate is necessary to deal with the latter. The epiphyseodesis can be performed by passing a single screw obliquely from the medial malleolus (Figure 11.4).[4]

Factors to be taken into consideration while planning treatment

Degree of spontaneous resolution of the tibial deformity

If complete or near-complete resolution of the tibial deformity occurs, no active intervention is needed in this regard. However, if the residual deformity is clinically visible, correction may be justified.

Degree of spontaneous resolution of the foot and ankle deformity

If the distal tibial articular surface is not horizontal, correction of the deformity needs to be undertaken.

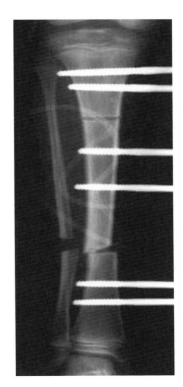

Figure 11.3 ● Radiograph showing correction of the tibial bowing and concomitant lengthening of the tibia in a boy with congenital posteromedial bowing of the tibia.

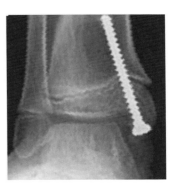

Figure 11.4 ● Screw epiphyseodesis of the distal tibia was performed to correct ankle valgus in a boy with posteromedial bowing of the tibia.

Extent of limb length inequality at skeletal maturity

The extent of tibial shortening will determine the strategies for equalizing the limb lengths (see Chapter 44, Length discrepancy of the tibia).

Level of deformity of the tibia

If the bow in the tibia is in the distal third and is contributing to the ankle deformity, a supramalleolar osteotomy is appropriate whereas if the deformity is at the junction of the distal and middle thirds of the tibia the osteotomy should be performed at this level.

Site of ankle deformity

If the ankle deformity is caused by abnormal physeal growth with a wedge-shaped distal epiphysis, a temporary epiphyseodesis is needed whereas if a distal tibial deformity is present correction should be at the supramalleolar level.

<table>
</table>

Recommended treatment

The outline of management of posteromedial bowing of the tibia is shown in Table 11.1.

Table 11.1 ● Outline of treatment of posteromedial bowing of the tibia

INDICATIONS					
Anticipated leg length inequality at skeletal maturity <2 cm + Complete or near-complete resolution of tibial deformity + No ankle deformity ⇩ No intervention	Anticipated leg length inequality at skeletal maturity 2–4 cm + Complete or near-complete resolution of tibial deformity + No ankle deformity ⇩ Contralateral proximal tibial epiphyseodesis at optimal time to equalize limb lengths at skeletal maturity	Anticipated leg length inequality at skeletal maturity >4 cm + Complete or near-complete resolution of tibial deformity + No ankle deformity ⇩ Tibial lengthening to equalize limb lengths	Anticipated leg length inequality at skeletal maturity >2 cm + Residual deformity of the tibial shaft ⇩ Tibial metaphyseal lengthening + Diaphyseal osteotomy to correct tibial bowing	Ankle valgus deformity at supramalleolar level + NO wedging of the distal tibial physis ⇩ Supramalleolar corrective osteotomy + Intervention as shown in columns 2/3/4 as indicated	Ankle valgus deformity at physeal level with wedging of the distal tibial physis ⇩ Screw epiphyseodesis of distal tibia + Intervention as shown in columns 2/3/4 as indicated
TREATMENT					

References

1. Hofmann A, Wenger DR. Posteromedial bowing of the tibia. Progression in leg lengths. *J Bone Joint Surg Am* 1981; **63**: 384–8.
2. Pappas AM. Congenital posteromedial bowing of the tibia and fibula. *J Pediatr Orthop* 1984; **4**: 525–31.
3. Heyman CH, Herndon CH, Heiple KG. Congenital posterior angulation of the tibia with talipes calcaneus. A long-term report of eleven patients. *J Bone Joint Surg Am* 1959; **41**: 476–88.
4. Stevens PM, Belle RM. Screw epiphysiodesis for ankle valgus. *J Pediatr Orthop* 1997; **17**: 9–12.

Tibial torsion

Benjamin Joseph

12

Introduction

The axis of the knee joint and the axis of the ankle joint are not in the same plane and during normal walking there is a mild degree of out-toeing even though the knee faces forwards. In other words, the angle between the long axis of the foot and the line of progression (the foot-progression angle) is about 10° outwards normally. This is on account of some degree of normal lateral or external torsion of the tibia. If the external torsion of the tibia is excessive there is an out-toeing gait, whereas if there is no lateral torsion or if there is internal tibial torsion, there will be an in-toeing gait (Figure 12.1). Torsional deformities of the tibia may be either congenital or developmental and may be present either in association with angular deformities or as an isolated deformity. Torsional deformities of the tibia may also be seen as part of a more widespread rotational malalignment of the limb involving the femur, tibia and the foot.[1,2]

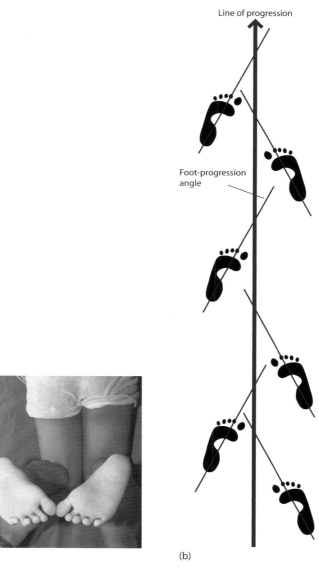

(a)   (b)

Figure 12.1 ● Bilateral tibial torsion in a child **(a)**; tracings of the feet show the foot progression angles **(b)**. The in-toeing is clearly evident.

Problems of management

Cosmetic problems

While in the vast majority of instances torsional deformities of the tibia may only be of concern because of the peculiar gait, in a few situations there may be more adverse implications.

Aggravation of foot deformities

In children with paralysis of the foot and ankle, an associated torsional deformity can aggravate the disability on account of paralysis. For example, a paralytic valgus deformity of the hindfoot can get worse in the presence of excessive external tibial torsion as the child drags the foot while walking (Figure 12.2). In cerebral palsy, external tibial torsion makes the foot an ineffective lever for normal walking.[3] In clubfoot, internal tibial torsion will make in-toeing caused by residual forefoot adduction appear more pronounced.

Anterior knee pain

Excessive femoral anteversion associated with severe compensatory external tibial torsion (miserable malalignment syndrome) may result in anterior knee pain.

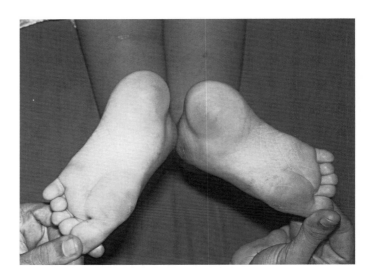

Figure 12.2 ● This child with spina bifida had a grossly abnormal out-toeing gait due to marked external tibial torsion. She also has valgus deformities of both hindfeet.

Aims of treatment

- Improve appearance
  If there is no anterior knee pain or foot deformity that may be aggravated by the torsional abnormality no intervention is required and the parents must be counselled accordingly. However, if the child and the parents feel strongly that the gait is unsightly and request correction, an attempt may be made to improve cosmesis and gait after explaining clearly the potential complications and risks of surgery.
- Correct torsional deformity if it contributes to foot deformity
  Torsional abnormality of the tibia must be corrected if it contributes to aggravation of a deformity of the foot or if it hampers efficient gait.
- Relieve anterior knee pain
  If there is significant anterior knee pain associated with a miserable malalignment syndrome the torsional abnormalities of both the femur and the tibia need to be addressed.

Treatment options

Observation

In the young child, if there is a possibility of spontaneous resolution of the deformity it is appropriate to wait and watch.

Orthotic management

Various forms of shoe modifications and orthotic devices incorporating twister cables have been used in an attempt to correct torsional abnormalities, but none of them have been shown to be effective.[2]

Derotation osteotomy of the tibia

If the torsional deformity needs to be corrected, derotation osteotomy of the tibia will be required. The osteotomy may be performed in the supramalleolar region, in the diaphysis or in the proximal metaphyseal region.

■ Supramalleolar osteotomy

An osteotomy in the supramalleolar region is relatively easy to perform and is less likely to be complicated by injury to the vessels or a compartment syndrome. If an associated varus or valgus deformity of the ankle is present it can also be corrected at this level. Internal fixation with two crossed Kirschner wires is adequate (Figure 12.3). Even if only one side needs to be corrected, both legs should be draped free. This enables the surgeon to ensure that symmetry is restored.

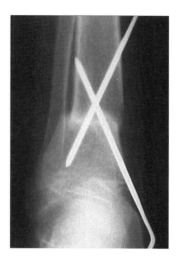

Figure 12.3 ● Post-operative radiograph of a child showing the technique of performing a supramalleolar derotation osteotomy of the tibia to correct abnormal tibial torsion.

■ Proximal metaphyseal osteotomy

If there is associated tibia vara a proximal metaphyseal osteotomy will be required in the older child despite the higher risks of neurovascular injury.

■ Diaphyseal osteotomy

In the younger child with Langenskiöld stage I, II or III Blount's disease, correction of the tibia vara and the internal tibial torsion can be achieved simultaneously by performing an oblique osteotomy in the upper third of the tibia (Figure 12.4). The oblique osteotomy runs from the anterior cortex distally to the posterior cortex proximally[4] (see Chapter 67, Blount's disease).

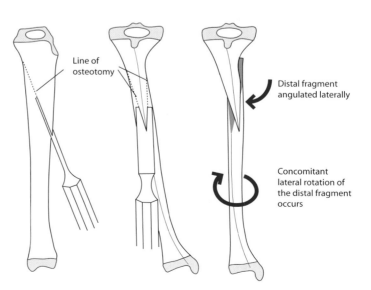

Line of osteotomy

Distal fragment angulated laterally

Concomitant lateral rotation of the distal fragment occurs

Figure 12.4 ● Diagram showing the technique of performing an oblique tibial osteotomy in order to correct tibia vara and internal tibial torsion.

Factors to be taken into consideration while planning treatment

Unilateral or bilateral involvement

A torsional deformity that is unilateral is unsightly even if it is of a moderate degree and thus would need to be corrected (Figure 12.5).

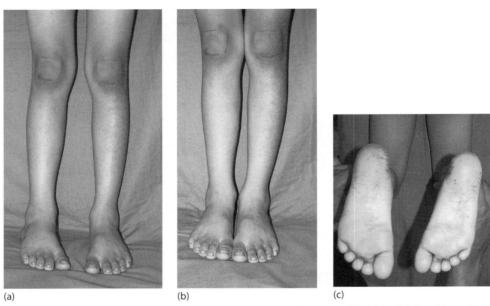

(a)　　　　　　　　　　　　　(b)　　　　　　　　　　　　　(c)

Figure 12.5 ● Unilateral internal tibial torsion in a child; the internal torsion of the right tibia is evident when the child stands with both patellae facing forwards **(a)**. With both feet facing forwards, the right patella faces laterally **(b)**. When the child lies prone with the knee flexed the abnormal thigh–foot angle confirms internal tibial torsion on the right **(c)**.

Age of the child

Symmetrical internal tibial torsional deformities tend to resolve partially or completely as the child grows and thus correction should not be considered before the child is at least ten years of age.

Disability and appearance

If the functional limitation due to the deformity is minimal and the appearance is not unsightly, no intervention is necessary. On the other hand, if the disability or the appearance is unacceptable the deformity may be corrected.

Propensity for spontaneous resolution or progression of the deformity

Since the tibia twists laterally during normal growth, external tibial torsion is unlikely to resolve spontaneously whereas internal tibial torsion has the potential to resolve as the child grows. However, internal tibial torsion associated with angular deformities such as tibia vara of Blount's disease is likely to progress unlike torsion associated with physiological genu varum which resolves as the genu varum improves. Torsional abnormalities seen in paralytic situations also tend to progress and may become quite severe (Figure 12.6).

Presence of associated deformity at the knee or foot and ankle

The presence of associated deformities will influence the need for correction of the torsional deformity and may also influence the surgical technique used for correction. Correction of isolated tibial torsion will entail a derotation osteotomy, but in a situation like Blount's disease an osteotomy that can correct both the angular and the torsional deformities should be chosen if possible.

Tendency for the torsion to aggravate associated deformity

If the torsional deformity is likely to contribute to aggravation of an angular deformity such as a varus or valgus deformity of the foot, both deformities must be corrected.

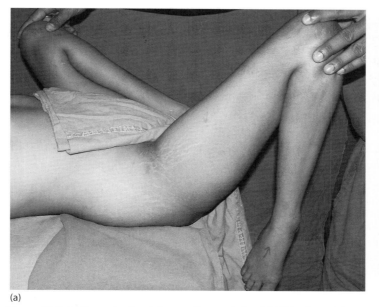
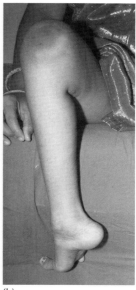

(a)   (b)

Figure 12.6 ● Severe torsional abnormality seen in the right tibia of an adolescent with post-polio paralysis who also has flexion deformities of the hip and knee.

Assessment of the child

Determining the severity of the deformity

Estimating the degree of torsion of the tibia may be done by clinical measurement or by imaging. Clinical estimates are less accurate, but may be sufficient when the deformity is bilateral and symmetrical. The clinical assessment of a child with a torsional deformity of the tibia should include assessment of the torsional profile examination described by Staheli *et al.*[1] to confirm that the deformity is restricted to the tibia alone. Measurement of the thigh–foot angle will provide a good clinical estimate of the magnitude of the deformity in the tibia (Figure 12.7). The thigh–foot angle can also be measured intra-operatively at the time of surgical correction.

When more complex torsional deformities involving the whole limb are involved, either ultrasound[5] or computed tomography scan measurement[6] of tibial torsion is necessary to determine the contribution of the tibia in the overall torsional malalignment.

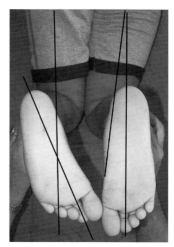

Figure 12.7 ● Measurement of the thigh–foot angle is done with the child prone and with the knee flexed to 90°. Care should be taken to avoid holding the foot.

Assessing the functional limitations

Children with excessive internal tibial torsion tend to trip more frequently and parents are often concerned about this. The parents need to be reassured that children grow out of this tendency as they become older. Torsional deformities can make some muscles work very inefficiently because of alteration in the lever-arms. This is particularly important in children with cerebral palsy. Correction of the lever-arm dysfunction entails correction of the torsional deformity.[3]

Identifying associated deformities

Angular deformities at the knee (e.g. genu varum), the proximal tibia (e.g. tibia vara) or at the ankle and foot (e.g. valgus or varus) need to be identified. Similarly, if a torsional deformity of the femur is present it should be identified and measured.

Recommended treatment

The outline of treatment of tibial torsion is shown in Table 12.1.

Table 12.1 ● Outline of treatment of torsional deformities of the tibia in children

INDICATIONS							
Isolated bilateral symmetrical internal tibial torsion + Child <10 years of age	Isolated bilateral symmetrical internal tibial torsion in child >10 years of age + Excessive in-toeing (foot-progression angle >30° internal) + Parents concerned about appearance of the child	Isolated unilateral internal OR external tibial torsion >20° as compared to the opposite side	Internal tibial torsion + Paralytic varus deformity of the hindfoot OR External tibial torsion + Paralytic valgus deformity of the hindfoot	Internal tibial torsion + Early Blount's disease (stage I, II or III) In a young child	Internal tibial torsion + Advanced Blount's disease (stage IV, V, VI) In an adolescent	Internal tibial torsion + Excessive femoral anteversion with excessive in-toeing	External tibial torsion + Excessive femoral anteversion (miserable malalignment syndrome)
⇩ Observe until 10 years of age for spontaneous resolution of deformity	⇩ Consider bilateral supramalleolar derotation osteotomy	⇩ Unilateral supramalleolar derotation osteotomy	⇩ Supramalleolar derotation osteotomy + Correction of hindfoot deformity	⇩ Rab's oblique osteotomy of the proximal tibial diaphysis	⇩ Proximal tibial metaphyseal osteotomy	⇩ Supramalleolar external rotation osteotomy ± Femoral external rotation osteotomy	⇩ Supramalleolar internal rotation osteotomy + Femoral external rotation osteotomy
TREATMENT							

References

1. Staheli LT, Corbett M, Wyss C, King H. Lower extremity rotational problems in children. Normal values to guide management. *J Bone Joint Surg Am* 1985; **67**: 39–47.
2. Staheli LT. Rotational problems of the lower extremities. *Orthop Clin North Am* 1987; **18**: 508–12.
3. Gage JR. Novachek TF. An update on the treatment of gait problems in cerebral palsy. *J Pediatr Orthop B* 2001; **10**: 265–74.
4. Rab GT. Oblique tibial osteotomy for Blount's disease (tibia vara). *J Pediatr Orthop* 1988; **8**: 715–20.
5. Joseph B, Carver RA, Bell MJ *et al.* Measurement of tibial torsion by ultrasound. *J Pediatr Orthop* 1987; **7**: 317–23.
6. Jakob RP, Haertel M, Stussi E. Tibial torsion calculated by computerized tomography and compared to other methods of measurement. *J Bone Joint Surg Br* 1980; **62**: 238–42.

Flexion deformity of the knee

Benjamin Joseph

13

Introduction

Flexion deformity of the knee is frequently encountered in paediatric orthopaedic practice. It may occur in a variety of conditions including congenital anomalies such as congenital dislocation of the patella, tibial hemimelia or popliteal pterygium syndrome, paralytic conditions such as multiple congenital contractures, spina bifida, polio and cerebral palsy and following trauma to the bone or growth plates in the vicinity of the knee. Flexion deformity of the knee can also develop following any form of acute or chronic arthritis. It is important to be aware of the underlying pathology that resulted in the deformity as treatment will have to be planned accordingly.

A flexed knee is a major impediment to normal walking and this is particularly so in the presence of weakness of the quadriceps muscle (see Chapter 55, The paralysed knee). On the other hand, flexion deformity of up to 90° is of little consequence in a child who is wheelchair bound. More severe degrees of flexion deformity can make it difficult to sit comfortably in a chair.

Pathogenesis of flexion deformity

Contractures of soft tissue at the back of the knee

This is the most common cause of flexion deformity and the soft tissues that are contracted and responsible for the deformity vary (Table 13.1). It is essential that the offending tissue is recognized and appropriately released in order to correct the deformity. It is also of paramount importance to be aware of associated contracture of the neurovascular structures which will dictate the procedure to adopt and the limits of correction that may be done safely.

Table 13.1 ● Tissues that are contracted in different conditions

Tissue that is contracted	Conditions where contractures occur
Skin	Burns Popliteal pterygium syndrome
Fascia	Polio Popliteal pterygium syndrome
Muscles and tendons	Polio Spina bifida Cerebral palsy Multiple congenital contractures (MCC) Popliteal pterygium syndrome Arthritis
Posterior capsule of knee	Primarily in MCC Secondarily in long-standing flexion deformity of any cause
Sciatic nerve and its branches	Popliteal pterygium syndrome

Muscle imbalance

In neuromuscular diseases where weakness of the quadriceps occurs, unopposed action of the hamstring muscles can result in a flexion deformity of the knee. Initially, the deformity may be dynamic but, in due course, contracture of the hamstrings will develop.

Spasticity or protective spasm of the hamstrings

Spasticity of the hamstrings in upper motor neuron paralysis often produces flexion deformity of the knee. Initially, the deformity will be dynamic but if the spasticity is not controlled contracture of the hamstring muscles will occur in due course.

Protective muscle spasm due to a painful condition affecting the knee can produce a flexion deformity. This is seen in children with septic arthritis, tubercular arthritis, haemophilic arthropathy and following trauma. In more chronic conditions the muscles that are in spasm may become contracted.

Altered orientation of muscles crossing the knee

If there is an aberrant low insertion of anomalous hamstring muscles, the tendon of the muscle will bowstring and this effectively increases the flexor moment arm of the muscle quite considerably. In congenital dislocation of the patella the quadriceps mechanism may be shifted posterior to the axis of movement of the knee and when this occurs the quadriceps will function as a perverted flexor of the knee.

Growth plate damage

Asymmetric damage to the posterior part of the growth plate of either the femur or the tibia will result in a flexion deformity of the knee.

Bony deformity

Malunion of a fracture of the distal femoral metaphysis or the proximal tibial metaphysis can result in a flexion deformity. Since the deformity is in the plane of movement of the knee and since the site of malunion is close to the growth plate, the conditions are favourable for remodelling. Consequently, in the vast majority of instances the deformity should reduce with remodelling, particularly following a fracture that has occurred in early childhood.

Problems of management

Correcting the deformity and improving the range of movement of the knee

Apart from flexion deformities secondary to bony deformity, virtually all other instances of flexion deformity will involve some degree of contracture of soft tissues that cross the back of the knee. In order to overcome the soft tissue contracture three strategies are available. The first entails elongating the contracted soft tissue by stretching it, surgically lengthening it or by surgically dividing it. The second strategy entails performing an osteotomy of the femur and removing a wedge of the same angle as the degree of flexion deformity from the anterior surface of the distal femur. The third option entails shortening the femur sufficiently to enable the knee to extend fully in the presence of the contracted soft tissue (Figure 13.1). Each of these options has their merits and disadvantages and in some situations a combination of two of these strategies may need to be used to effectively deal with the deformity.

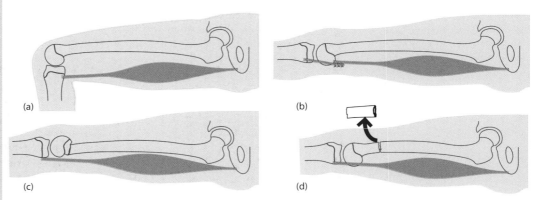

Figure 13.1 ● The strategies for correcting a flexion deformity of the knee **(a)** include stretching or lengthening of the hamstrings **(b)**, supracondylar extension osteotomy **(c)** and femoral shortening **(d)**.

If soft tissues that are contracted can be completely stretched, the range of movement of the knee can be restored to normal. On the other hand, if the deformity is corrected by performing an extension osteotomy of the femur in the supracondylar region, the arc of motion does not increase but is merely shifted, and range of flexion of the knee will reduce by exactly the same degree of extension obtained at the osteotomy site. If the femur is shortened to such an extent that the knee can be extended fully, the range of motion can then be restored to normal (Figure 13.2). While it is desirable to restore full range of motion of the knee, there are instances where shortening of the femur or lengthening of the soft tissue may not be feasible, and one may have to accept the limitations of flexion and perform a supracondylar extension osteotomy.

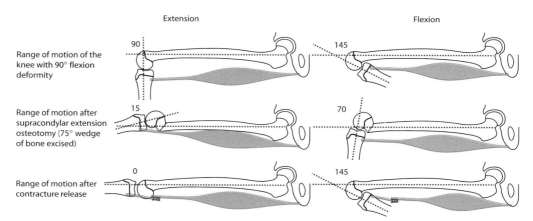

Figure 13.2 ● The effect of hamstring lengthening and supracondylar extension osteotomy on the range of motion of the knee

Stretch of neurovascular structures

The neurovascular structures may be stretched quite considerably when a severe flexion deformity of the knee is corrected.[1] Similarly, in popliteal pterygium syndrome, the sciatic nerve may actually bow string across the knee and occupy the posterior part of the pterygium making it extremely vulnerable to excessive stretch and damage during correction of the flexion deformity. Apart from actual nerve damage, stretch of the sciatic nerve may cause systemic hypertension;[2] all patients undergoing correction of flexion deformity by traction should be regularly monitored for hypertension.

Recurrence of deformity

Flexion deformity of the knee is notoriously prone to recurrence following initial correction in multiple congenital contractures and popliteal pterygium syndrome.[3–5] Recurrence of deformity often occurs in the presence of active inflammatory arthritis. One needs to be aware of conditions where there is a high chance of recurrence and adopt strategies that reduce the risk of recurrence or at least delay or minimize the severity of recurrent deformity if possible.

Aims of treatment

- Correct the deformity without causing neurovascular damage
  The popliteal vessels and the sciatic nerve may be excessively stretched when severe flexion deformities are being corrected. This must be anticipated and avoided by shortening the femur sufficiently to relieve tension on the neurovascular structures.[6]
- Increase the range of movement of the knee, if possible
  It is desirable if the range of movement of the knee can be fully restored and, at the same time, full correction of the deformity can be obtained.
- If the range of movement cannot be increased, alter the arc into a more functional range
  The arc of motion should be such that the child can stand erect without flexion of the knee and also sit comfortably in a chair.
- Prevent recurrence of deformity
  Following correction of the deformity, bracing and tendon transfers may need to be considered as measures to prevent recurrence of the deformity.

Treatment options

Wedging of plaster casts

Minor degrees of flexion may be corrected quite easily with serial wedging of plaster casts.[7] The two methods of wedging are by removing a wedge of the cast from the front of the knee and closing the gap or by cutting the cast across the popliteal fossa and opening out a wedge posteriorly. Care should be taken to avoid pressure sores; the risk of a pressure sore is greater when closing a wedge anteriorly.

Traction

Skin traction is an effective means of correcting a mild flexion deformity of recent onset. More severe degrees of deformity and long-standing deformity may not yield to skin traction; in such situations skeletal traction is indicated. One of the well-recognized risks of correcting a flexion deformity of the knee is posterior subluxation of the tibia (Figure 13.3a). This can be avoided by applying two-pin traction, as illustrated in Figure 13.3b. The proximal tibial pin enables anterior translation of the tibia while the distal pin corrects the flexion deformity. Quite severe degrees of deformity can be corrected by traction[8] but it must be emphasized that several weeks of traction may be needed to achieve correction. Traction may be used as the primary method of correction or may be used to correct residual deformity following soft tissue release.

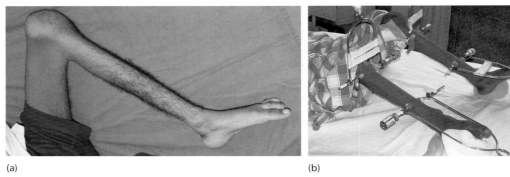

(a)
(b)

Figure 13.3 ● If longitudinal traction alone is applied to correct a severe flexion deformity of the knee, as in this adolescent **(a)**, posterior subluxation of the tibia can occur. This complication can be avoided by application of two-pin traction as seen here **(b)**. The traction on the proximal pin is to avoid posterior subluxation of the knee while the distal pin is for longitudinal traction.

Soft tissue release

Soft tissue release involves lengthening or dividing the soft tissue structure that is contributing to the deformity. Most frequently the hamstring tendons need to be released. If the hamstring muscles are paralysed, simple tenotomy of the tendons will suffice. On the other hand, if hamstring function is to be retained, the tendons should be lengthened.

Release of the posterior capsule of the knee joint may be needed in multiple congenital contractures and in severe flexion deformity of any cause.[9]

Soft tissue distraction

An attractive alternative to soft tissue release is to stretch the soft tissues with the help of an external fixator.[10] In reality, the effect is exactly the same as that of traction; the advantage, however, is that the child can remain mobile and does not necessarily have to remain in hospital until the deformity is corrected. As in the case of traction, subluxation of the knee can occur and the fixator should be appropriately modified to prevent this complication.

Restoring muscle balance

If the underlying cause for the flexion deformity is imbalance between the quadriceps and the hamstrings, muscle balance should be restored. If the hamstring power is normal and the quadriceps is paralysed, the feasibility of transferring the hamstrings to the front of the knee should be considered (see Chapter 55, The paralysed knee).

Supracondylar femoral osteotomy

Extension osteotomy of the femur in the supracondylar region is often performed to correct flexion deformity of the knee.[11] As indicated earlier, if this operation is performed to correct deformity caused by soft tissue contracture, the range of movement of the knee will not increase and there will be loss of terminal flexion following the operation. However, the range of movement will improve if this operation is done to correct a flexion deformity due to malunion of a fracture.

In children, internal fixation can be dispensed with if the spike osteotomy technique[12] is followed (Figure 13.4). This avoids the need for a second operation to remove an implant. If it is desirable to avoid using a plaster cast post-operatively, formal internal fixation will be needed.

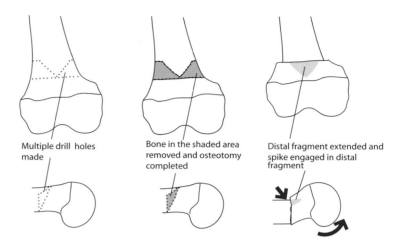

Multiple drill holes made

Bone in the shaded area removed and osteotomy completed

Distal fragment extended and spike engaged in distal fragment

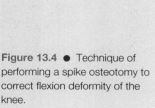

Figure 13.4 ● Technique of performing a spike osteotomy to correct flexion deformity of the knee.

Femoral shortening

This option is particularly useful when there is severe bilateral symmetrical flexion deformity. The femur is divided in the supracondylar region and the knee is extended. The extent to which the fragments overlap with full correction of the deformity is the amount of femoral shortening that is needed.

Physeal bar excision

If the deformity is due to a physeal bar, excision of the bar would help in correcting the deformity. However, access to a physeal bar in the back of the distal femur or the proximal tibia can be very awkward and technically difficult.

Epiphyseodesis

Arrest of growth of the anterior part of the distal femoral epiphysis has been attempted as a measure to deal with recurrent flexion deformity of the knee in difficult situations where other options have failed.[13]

Factors to be taken into consideration while planning treatment

Severity of the deformity

The most important factor that determines the treatment is the severity of deformity.

Underlying cause

The treatment will be influenced by the underlying cause of the deformity; bony deformity will need to be addressed by bony surgery while soft tissue causes primarily have to be treated by soft tissue release.

Unilateral or bilateral deformity

While femoral shortening is quite acceptable for dealing with bilateral deformity, it is less desirable for treating unilateral deformity. However, if the deformity is severe and there is risk of neurovascular compromise, femoral shortening may be justified, even for unilateral deformity.

Recommended treatment

The outline of treatment of flexion deformity of the knee is shown in Table 13.2.

Table 13.2 ● Treatment of flexion deformity of the knee

INDICATIONS

Flexion deformity due to bony deformity	Flexion deformity + Muscle imbalance with quadriceps paralysis + Skeletally immature	<20° flexion deformity + Muscle imbalance with quadriceps paralysis + Skeletally mature	<20° flexion deformity + No underlying bone or growth plate abnormality + No muscle imbalance + Unilateral OR bilateral	20–40° flexion deformity + No underlying bone or growth plate abnormality + No muscle imbalance + Unilateral OR bilateral	40–60° flexion deformity + No underlying bone or growth plate abnormality + No muscle imbalance + Unilateral OR bilateral	>60° flexion deformity + No underlying bone or growth plate abnormality + No muscle imbalance + Unilateral	>60° flexion deformity + No underlying bone or growth plate abnormality + No muscle imbalance + Bilateral	Recurrent flexion deformity
⇩	⇩	⇩	⇩	⇩	⇩	⇩	⇩	⇩

TREATMENT

| Supracondylar femoral osteotomy OR Proximal tibial osteotomy (if deformity is in the tibia) | Hamstring transfer (if all other criteria for transfer are fulfilled – see Chapter 55) | Supracondylar femoral extension osteotomy sufficient to create 10° of recurvatum (to stabilize the paralysed knee) | Skin traction OR Wedging of plaster casts | Hamstring lengthening | Hamstring lengthening + Supracondylar femoral extension osteotomy to correct residual deformity | Hamstring lengthening followed by skeletal traction OR Gradual distraction with an external fixator | Hamstring lengthening followed by skeletal traction OR Bilateral femoral shortening | Anterior epiphyseodesis of distal femoral growth plate |

Rationale of treatment suggested

Why is gradual distraction or femoral shortening, rather than supracondylar extension osteotomy, recommended for correction of severe degrees of flexion deformity?

Femoral shortening and gradual distraction reduce the risk of nerve damage. There is a great risk of producing irreversible nerve damage by acutely correcting severe flexion deformity.[1] This is why supracondylar extension osteotomy is not recommended as a means of correcting severe flexion deformity.

Why is hamstring lengthening recommended prior to supracondylar extension osteotomy for moderate deformity?

If a supracondylar osteotomy alone is performed to correct a moderately severe flexion deformity, the range of knee movement will not increase. Lengthening of the hamstrings will increase the range of motion. The supracondylar osteotomy merely corrects any residual deformity after hamstring lengthening.

Why is femoral shortening recommended for severe bilateral deformity?

Femoral shortening is a simple and quick way of achieving correction of flexion deformity and since both femora are shortened, limb length inequality will not occur.

References

1. Aspden RM, Porter RW. Nerve traction during correction of knee flexion deformity. A case report and calculation. *J Bone Joint Surg Br* 1994; **76**: 471–3.
2. Shah A, Asirvatham R. Hypertension after surgical release for flexion contractures of the knee. *J Bone Joint Surg Br* 1994; **75**: 358–61.
3. Oppenheim WL, Larson KR, McNabb MB, Smith CF, Setoquchi Y. Popliteal pterygium syndrome: an orthopaedic perspective. *J Pediatr Orthop* 1990; **10**: 58–64.
4. Brunner R, Hefti F, Tgetgel JD. Arthrogrypotic joint contracture at the knee and the foot: correction with a circular frame. *J Pediatr Orthop B* 1997; **6**: 192–7.
5. Murray C, Fixen JA. Management of knee deformity in classical arthrogryposis multiplex congenita (amyoplasia congenita). *J Pediatr Orthop B* 1997; **6**: 186–91.
6. de Moraes barros Fucs PM, Svartman C, de Assumpção PM. Knee deformity from poliomyelitis treated by supracondylar femoral extension osteotomy. *Int Orthop* 2005; **29**: 380–4.
7. Westberry DE, Davids JR, Jacobs JN, Pugh LI, Tanner SL. Effectiveness of serial stretch casting for resistant or recurrent flexion contractures following hamstring lengthening in children with cerebral palsy. *J Pediatr Orthop* 206; **26**: 109–14.
8. Parekh PK. Flexion contracture of the knee following poliomyelitis. *Int Orthop* 1983; **7**: 165–72.
9. Heydarian K, Akbarnia BA, Jabalameli M, Tabador K. Posterior capsulotomy for treatment of severe flexion contracture of the knee. *J Pediatr Orthop* 1984; **4**: 700–4.
10. Damsin JP, Ghanem I. Treatment of severe flexion deformity of the knee in children and adolescents using Ilizarov technique. *J Bone Joint Surg Br* 1996; **78**: 140–4.
11. Asirvatham R, Mukherjee A, Agarwal S *et al*. Supracondylar femoral extension osteotomy: its complications. *J Pediatr Orthop* 1993; **13**: 642–5.
12. Deitz FR, Weinstein SL. Spike osteotomy for angular deformities of long bones in children. *J Bone Joint Surg Am* 1988; **70**: 848–52.
13. Kramer A, Stevens PM. Anterior femoral stapling. *J Pediatr Orthop* 2001; **21**: 804–7.

Genu recurvatum

Benjamin Joseph

14

Introduction

Hyperextension of the normal knee is prevented by two mechanisms: the integrity of the strong posterior capsule and ligament complex of the knee and the orientation of the articular surfaces of the femur and tibia. It follows that whenever there is a genu recurvatum deformity, either or both these mechanisms are abnormal and ineffective.

If the articular surfaces of the femur and tibia are normally aligned and there is laxity of the posterior capsule and ligaments, the knee will have a normal range of passive flexion, but extension of the knee will be excessive (Figure 14.1a). When the posterior capsule and ligaments are normal and there is abnormal inclination of the articular surface of the tibia, there will be limitation of terminal flexion of the knee and a comparable degree of hyperextension (Figure 14.1b). This clinical feature can help to identify the underlying cause.

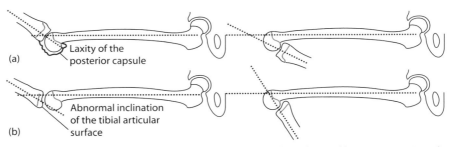

(a)   Laxity of the posterior capsule

(b)   Abnormal inclination of the tibial articular surface

Figure 14.1 ● Diagram illustrating the range of motion of the knee in patients with genu recurvatum due to posterior capsular laxity **(a)** and genu recurvatum due to a forward inclination of the tibial articular surface **(b)**.

If abnormal inclination of the articular surfaces is suspected, a true lateral view radiograph can confirm the abnormality. Normally, the tibial articular surface is inclined 14° (±3.6°) backwards. If the anterior part of the tibial growth plate is damaged the articular surface will tilt progressively forwards and a recurvatum deformity will develop (Figure 14.2). Among the causes for proximal tibial growth plate damage are Osgood–Schlatter's disease,[1] osteomyelitis and trauma. Iatrogenic causes include prolonged traction or cast immobilization,[2] damage to the growth plate by skeletal pin traction[3] or damage at the time of surgery. Often no specific cause can be attributed to the physeal damage and growth arrest.

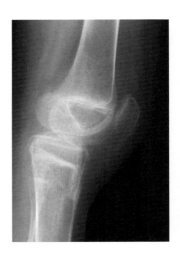

Figure 14.2 ● Lateral radiograph of the knee of an adolescent with genu recurvatum that developed due to inclination of the tibial articular surface following growth plate damage.

Genu recurvatum is seen in children with hypermobile joint syndromes.[4] In these children the deformity is usually mild and is symmetrical; no treatment is warranted as this deformity should not be considered as being pathological.

Genu recurvatum associated with congenital contracture of the quadriceps and congenital dislocation of the knee is discussed in Chapter 29, Congenital dislocation of the knee. The management of acquired genu recurvatum is discussed in this chapter.

Problems of management

Identifying the underlying problem

It is imperative that the underlying cause of the deformity is identified and addressed. Treatment will differ according to the underlying cause.

Pain

Pain can develop in some patients with genu recurvatum; the pain may be at the back of the knee where the capsule is excessively stretched or in the front of the knee.

Risk of recurrence

Recurrence of the deformity can occur in two situations. When there has been damage to the growth plate and the child is still skeletally immature, mere correction of the deformity will invariably be followed by recurrence of the deformity. The second situation is where forces that produced the genu recurvatum continue to act following plication of the lax posterior capsule. For example, an uncorrected equinus deformity can lead to recurrence of recurvatum following capsular plication as the ground reaction force in the stance phase produces a hyperextension moment at the knee in every gait cycle.

Aims of treatment

- Correct the deformity
  Apart from the instance mentioned earlier, where genu recurvatum deformity may be ignored, all children with genu recurvatum need to be treated. It is ideal if the deformity can be permanently corrected. However, in instances where permanent correction may not be feasible, an attempt needs to be made to prevent the knee from hyperextending while the child walks.
- Relieve pain if present
  If pain develops due to excessive stretch of the posterior capsule, this must be addressed.
- Prevent recurrence
  If the underlying problem is growth plate damage, appropriate intervention should be taken to avoid recurrence after surgery. Similarly, if the recurvatum developed due to abnormal stresses, those stresses must be removed before embarking on corrective surgery.

Treatment options

Bracing

Braces that immobilize the knee can prevent hyperextension; however, this results in a stiff knee gait. Ankle foot orthoses that hold the ankle in 5–10° of dorsiflexion have been shown to effectively control genu recurvatum in cerebral palsy.[5] A Lehneis modification of a floor-reaction orthosis is also effective in controlling genu recurvatum (see Chapter 55, The paralysed knee).

Acute correction by anterior open wedge osteotomy of the tibia

An anterior open wedge osteotomy has been used to correct genu recurvatum;[6,7] however, wound healing can be a problem (Figure 14.3a).

Acute correction by posterior closed wedge osteotomy of the tibia

Posterior closed wedge osteotomy of the proximal tibia has also been used;[8] the frequency of complications is low and there is the added advantage of being able to ablate the posterior part of the physis simultaneously. This ensures that recurrence of the deformity does not occur. Some anterior translation of the distal fragment can be added to restore the contour of the tibial tuberosity (Figure 14.3b).

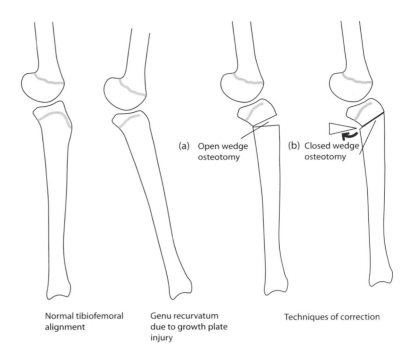

(a) Open wedge osteotomy

(b) Closed wedge osteotomy

Normal tibiofemoral alignment

Genu recurvatum due to growth plate injury

Techniques of correction

Figure 14.3 ● Diagram demonstrating how genu recurvatum can be corrected by an open wedge osteotomy or a closed wedge osteotomy.

Flexion supracondylar osteotomy of the femur

Flexion osteotomy of the distal femur is appropriate if the primary pathology is in the femur.[9] However, a deformity in the femur producing genu recurvatum is infrequent.

Gradual correction with an external fixator

If the deformity is unilateral there is usually an element of shortening. This can be addressed along with correction of the deformity by techniques of gradual correction involving callotasis with an external fixator (Figure 14.4). The technique permits correction of any associated angular deformity in another plane if a ring fixator is used.[10]

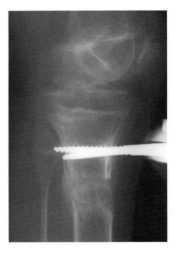

Figure 14.4 ● Radiograph of an adolescent with genu recurvatum and shortening treated by gradual callus distraction and lengthening.

Epiphyseodesis

In a skeletally immature child with genu recurvatum secondary to physeal damage, correction of the deformity must be combined with a posterior epiphyseodesis in order to prevent recurrence of the deformity.

Reefing of the posterior capsule of the knee joint

Tightening the lax posterior capsule is technically demanding and recurrence of the deformity may be seen in a proportion of patients.[11] An elaborate operation described by *Perry et al.*[11] entails proximal advancement of the posterior capsule, construction of a check-rein in the midline posteriorly with the tendons of the semitendinosis and gracilis and fashioning of two diagonal bands posteriorly using the biceps femoris and the iliotibial band. The authors caution that a rigid brace that prevents hyperextension of the knee must be worn for at least a year following the operation.

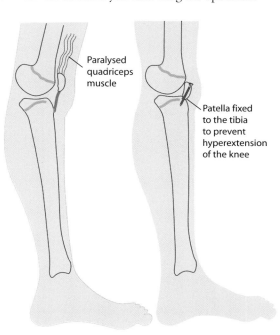

Paralysed quadriceps muscle

Patella fixed to the tibia to prevent hyperextension of the knee

Figure 14.5 ● Diagram illustrating the method of performing a patella bone block to prevent genu recurvatum in the skeletally mature patient.

Anterior patellar bone block

In skeletally mature individuals with genu recurvatum and quadriceps paralysis, a bone block in the front of the tibia can prevent the hyperextension of the knee (Figure 14.5).[12]

No intervention

No intervention is justified in children with bilateral genu recurvatum of a mild degree secondary to hypermobile joint syndrome. Mild genu recurvatum of up to 10–15° in children with quadriceps paralysis should not be corrected as this enables the knee to remain stable (see Chapter 55, The paralysed knee).

Factors to be taken into consideration while planning treatment

The underlying condition

The treatment varies with the underlying condition and hence it is essential that the underlying condition is identified. Treatment of 15° of recurvatum in a child with lower motor neuron paralysis is totally different from the same degree of deformity following a traumatic anterior growth plate arrest.

The cause of the deformity (capsular laxity or bony deformity)

It is also imperative that a distinction is made between recurvatum due to capsular laxity and recurvatum due to bony deformity as the treatment differs in these two situations.

The age of the child

In children with physeal damage, treatment will vary according to whether the child is skeletally mature or not.

Recommended treatment

An outline of treatment of genu recurvatum is shown in Table 14.1.

Table 14.1 ● Treatment of genu recurvatum

INDICATION	TREATMENT
Genu recurvatum associated with hypermobile joint syndrome + Mild deformity + Bilateral and symmetrical ⇩	No intervention (not required)
Genu recurvatum of 10–15° + Lower motor neuron quadriceps paralysis ⇩	No intervention (intervention contraindicated as recurvatum will help to stabilize the knee)
Genu recurvatum >15° + Lower motor neuron quadriceps paralysis ⇩	Lehneis modification of floor-reaction orthosis
Genu recurvatum due to rigid equinus deformity ⇩	Correct equinus deformity
Genu recurvatum in cerebral palsy + No equinus contracture ⇩	Rigid ankle-foot orthosis molded in 10° of dorsiflexion
Genu recurvatum due to posterior capsular laxity ⇩	Capsular reefing + Bracing to prevent hyperextension
Genu recurvatum due to anterior physeal damage of proximal tibia + Adolescent ⇩	Osteotomy and gradual correction of deformity with external fixator + Limb lengthening if there is limb length inequality
Genu recurvatum due to anterior physeal damage of proximal tibia + Young child ⇩	Epiphyseodesis of posterior part of the growth plate + Corrective closed wedge osteotomy + Limb lengthening OR Contralateral epiphyseodesis

Rationale of treatment suggested

Why is gradual correction with an external fixator recommended in the adolescent with physeal damage?
Precise correction of the deformity and concomitant correction of the limb length inequality can be achieved by this method.

Why is closed wedge osteotomy recommended for the skeletally immature with physeal arrest?
The closed wedge osteotomy has a lower risk for complications than an open wedge osteotomy. The posterior part of the physis can be ablated at the same time. If the distal fragment is displaced anteriorly by a few millimetres the contour of the tibial tuberosity can also be restored.

References

1. Zimbler S, Merkow S. Genu recurvatum: a possible complication after Osgood–Schlatter disease. Case report. *J Bone Joint Surg Am* 1984; 66: 1129–30.
2. Ishikawa H, Abraham LM Jr, Hirohata K. Genu recurvatum: a complication of prolonged femoral skeletal traction. *Arch Orthop Trauma Surg* 1984; 103: 215–8.
3. Bjerkreim I, Benum P. Genu recurvatum: a late complication of tibial wire traction in fractures of the femur in children. *Acta Orthop Scand* 1975; 46: 1012–19.
4. Remvig L, Jensen DV, Ward RC. Epidemiology of general joint hypermobility and basis for the proposed criteria for benign joint hypermobility syndrome: review of the literature. *J Rheumatol* 2007; 34: 804–9.
5. Rosenthal RK, Deutsch SD, Miller W, Schumann W, Hall JE. A fixed-ankle below-the-knee orthosis for the management of genu recurvatum in spastic cerebral palsy. *J Bone Joint Surg Am* 1975; 57: 545–7.
6. Irwin CE. Genu recurvatum following poliomyelitis: a controlled method of operative correction. *J Am Med Assn* 1942; 120: 277–80.
7. Moroni A, Pezzuto V, Pompili M, Zinghi G. Proximal osteotomy of the tibia for treatment of genu recurvatum in adults. *J Bone Joint Surg Am* 1992; 74: 577–86.
8. Bowen JR, Morley DC, McInerny Y, MacEwen GD. Treatment of genu recurvatum by proximal tibial closing wedge/anterior displacement osteotomy. *Clin Orthop Relat Res* 1983; 179: 194–9.
9. Mehta SN, Mukherjee AK. Flexion osteotomy of the femur for genu recurvatum after poliomyelitis. *J Bone Joint Surg Br* 1991; 73: 200–2.
10. Choi IH, Chung CY, Cho TJ, Park SS. Correction of genu recurvatum by the Ilizarov method. *J Bone Joint Surg Br* 1999; 81: 769–74.
11. Perry J, O'Brien JP, Hodgson AR. Triple tenodesis of the knee: a soft tissue operation for paralytic genu recurvatum. *J Bone Joint Surg Am* 1976: 58: 978–85.
12. Men HX, Bian CH, Yang CD *et al.* Surgical treatment of the flail knee after poliomyelitis. *J Bone Joint Surg Br* 1991; 73: 195–9.

Genu varum

Selvadurai Nayagam

15

Introduction

The task of deciding between physiological and pathological bow legs can be sometimes be difficult. Symmetrical genu varum before the age of two years is rarely pathological (Figure 15.1a). Thereafter, some degree of genu valgum is seen until the adult tibiofemoral angle of about 6° (although this value may differ slightly with different populations) is reached at six to seven years of age (Figure 15.2).[1,2]

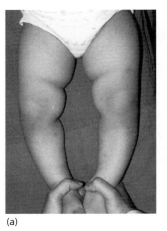 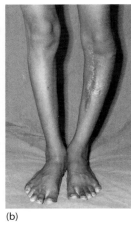 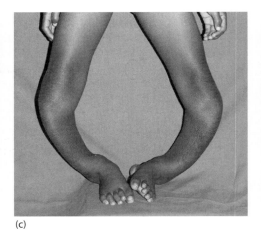 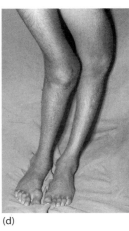

(a)   (b)   (c)   (d)

Figure 15.1 ● **(a)** Symmetrical genu varum in this infant is physiological. **(b)** Unilateral genu varum in this adolescent has developed following trauma. **(c)** This boy with severe genu varum has a form of skeletal dysplasia. There is a varus deformity of the distal tibia in addition to the proximal deformity. His elder sibling had a wind-swept deformity with genu varum on the left and genu valgum on the right **(d)**.

Genu varum is more likely to be pathological if it is:

● present after two years of age;
● unilateral;
● associated with shortening (of the limb or of stature);
● severe;
● in a child with obesity.

Mild deformities after the age of two years may resolve spontaneously and probably represent extreme variants of physiological bowing but moderate deformities are likely to be pathological, caused by:

● trauma or infection (including meningococcal) producing a bony bar at the proximal tibial physis (Figure 15.1b);
● rickets (including the vitamin D-resistant variety);
● Blount's disease (tibia vara): two varieties, infantile and adolescent, are usually described depending upon the age of presentation;
● generalized or focal osteochondrodysplasias, e.g. hereditary multiple exostoses, achondroplasia, focal fibrocartilaginous dysplasia (Figure 15.1c);
● tibial hemimelia.

A family history of bow legs should raise suspicions of hypophosphataemic rickets, hereditary multiple exostoses or of a bone or cartilage dysplasia (Figure 15.1d).

Clinical examination poses traps for the unwary. A young toddler may appear bow-legged if both knees and hips are flexed when walking; a gentle repositioning of the hips and knees with

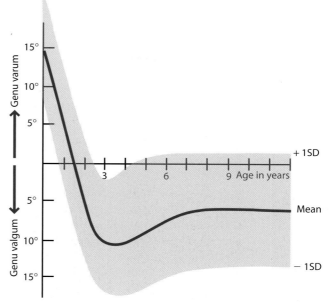

Figure 15.2 ● The tibiofemoral angle changes as the child grows; the alignment of the knee passes from genu varum in early childhood to some degree of genu valgum before assuming the normal adult alignment around six years of age.

the child lying down will clarify this. Internal tibial torsion or an angular deformity arising from the tibial shaft or distal metaphysis may mimic genu varum. Both these conditions produce a widening of the intercondylar distance at the knee – simply to facilitate each foot clearing the other when standing straight or walking.

Radiographs are useful; they document the size of deformity and enable the aetiology to be diagnosed in some cases, for example Blount's disease, physeal arrest from trauma, multiple exostoses.

Progression of deformity

The follow-on of diagnosing a pathological genu varum is deciding whether progression of the deformity is likely. The following indicators are helpful:

● In tibia vara, progression is linked to the size of deformity at presentation (Figure 15.3) and obesity. Specifically, a body mass index ⩾22 together with a metadiaphyseal angle ⩾10° is strongly suggestive of progression.[3] If size of deformity alone is used as a prognostic arbiter, then a metadiaphyseal angle ⩾16° and a tibial varus contributing to more than half of the total deformity (the genu varum is often a combination of tibial and femoral varus) are useful.[4]

Problems of management

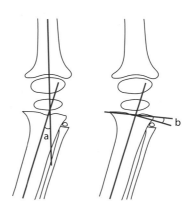

Figure 15.3 ● Measures of severity of genu varum include the tibiofemoral angle **(a)** and the metaphyseo-diaphyseal angle **(b)**.

- Varus deformities from bony bars across the physis will progress, as will deformities produced by focal lesions lying in close proximity to the growth plate, e.g. osteochondromas or enchondromas. If the physeal tether is not removable, consideration should be given to completing the physeal arrest at the time of deformity correction and performing a proximal fibula epiphyseodesis. This will prevent recurrence and the residual problem of leg length discrepancy is dealt with accordingly.
- In achondroplasia genu varum is controversially linked to fibula overgrowth and lateral collateral ligament laxity in the knee.[5–7] There is often a component of distal tibial varus as well. Spontaneous improvement is unlikely.
- The diagnosis of focal fibrocartilaginous dysplasia is important and made on the radiograph – the appearance is typical. Spontaneous resolution is likely if the varus is less than 30°.[8,9]

Alignment of the lower limb

Plain radiographs of Blount's disease often give an impression of a depressed medial tibial condyle – an appearance recognized as one of the more advanced Langenskiöld stages of tibia vara.[10] The tibial joint line has the appearance of a tilted 'pitched roof' but the radiograph may be misleading – the 'incomplete' medial tibial condyle may represent unossified cartilage. Magnetic resonance imaging (MRI) and arthrography will show the true joint level on the medial side – these investigations are important lest an unwary surgeon attempts to 'elevate' the medial side.[11] If there is a true underdevelopment of the medial tibial condyle on MRI (clinical suspicion is raised if there is significant laxity to valgus stressing), treatment would then need to include an elevation of the hemiplateau.[12]

Nearly one-third of the overall varus deformity may arise in the distal femur in adolescent tibia vara.[13] Similarly, in achondroplasia and some other skeletal dysplasias distal tibial varus is often present (see Figure 15.1c). Correction needs to address all components contributing significantly to the genu varum deformity.[14]

Associated features related to the underlying aetiology

Associated limb shortening or abnormal bone biochemistry needs to be addressed.

Aims of treatment

- Restoration of limb alignment
- Arrest of progression
- Prevention of recurrence post-correction

Treatment options

Orthotic correction

This is a mainstay of treatment for the infantile variety of tibia vara (Blount's disease) for Langenskiöld stages I and II (see Chapter 67, Blount's disease). An above-knee orthosis which is custom moulded to provide three-point correction is used.[15] Most will take 12–18 months of brace use to resolve, and success rates of 90 percent are reported when the presenting deformity is of a mild to moderate degree.[15] Bracing is ineffective if the underlying cause is a physeal tether. Some mild cases of rickets respond to bracing as long as medical treatment of the abnormal bone turnover is provided.

Surgical correction

■ Growth manipulation through hemiepiphyseal arrest

Permanent hemiepiphyseodesis had to be timed with reference growth charts in order to accomplish angular correction by the time the child reaches skeletal maturity. Fortunately, newer techniques have allowed the 'braking effect' of a hemiepiphyseodesis to be reversible and as such used earlier in childhood. Hemiepiphyseal arrest will not work if the opposite side of the physis is not growing normally – as in physeal bar obstruction or in Ollier's disease (multiple enchondromatosis).[16] Hemiepiphyseal arrest can be achieved using staples,[17] oblique screws[18] or tension-band plates[19] (Figure 15.4). Success with these techniques lies with preservation of the periosteum overlying the perichondrial ring during insertion and removal of the implant. Timing the insertion of these implants according to growth charts is no longer necessary and neither is delaying the procedure until adolescence. Good results can be achieved for deformities early in childhood and can be repeated should the deformity recur after removal of the implant.[17] Tibia vara in adolescence is also amenable to the technique provided sufficient growth remains and the deformity is mild to moderate in severity (Figure 15.5).[20,21]

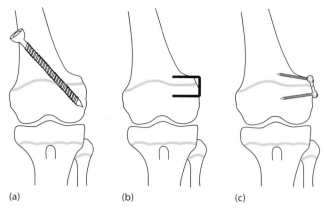

(a) (b) (c)

Figure 15.4 ● Hemiepiphyseal arrest may be achieved by inserting oblique screws **(a)**, staples **(b)** or tension-band plates **(c)**.

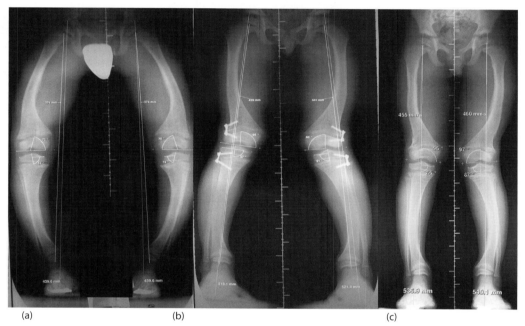

(a) (b) (c)

Figure 15.5 ● **(a)** Symmetrical genu varum arising in a child with hypophosphataemic rickets, **(b)** treated by distal femoral and proximal tibial 8-plates which act as temporary and reversible tethers to growth on the side of application. **(c)** Correction after 24 months with removal of plates to prevent overcorrection.

■ Acute correction by osteotomy

Deformity correction by hemiepiphyseodesis proceeds at approximately 1° per month, with large deformities taking two to three years to correct. Consequently, hemiepiphyseodesis is inappropriate if the child is near skeletal maturity. In this case and for those deformities precipitated by abnormalities of the growth plate (physeal bars, juxtaphyseal enchondromas), corrective osteotomy is the better alternative. Depending on the age and size of the child, the method of stabilization can vary from crossed Kirschner wires and a long leg cast to internal and external fixation (Figure 15.6). The corrective osteotomy can be combined with an attempt at removing the precipitating cause, e.g. epiphysiolysis in the case of bony tethers.

■ Gradual correction by osteotomy

Gradual correction by external fixation (the Ilizarov method) is suitable if the genu varum is associated with tibial shortening. The proximal tibial osteotomy serves as a site of both deformity correction and lengthening. In achondroplasia the technique can be used not only to increase stature but to tighten the lateral collateral ligament.[14]

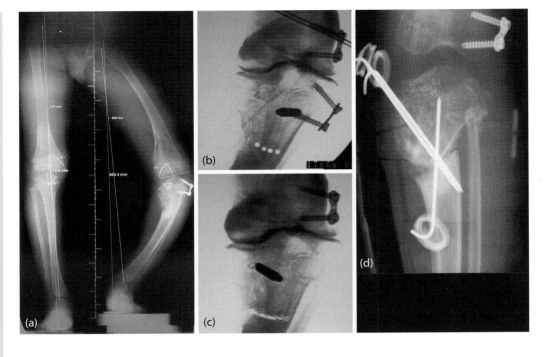

Figure 15.6 ● **(a)** Unilateral genu varum from Ollier's disease with failure to correct with tibial 8-plate. **(b)** Focal dome osteotomy with multiple drill holes (femoral 8-plate applied to correct femoral deformity). **(c)** Drill hole connected by osteotome; 8-plate removed. **(d)** Acute correction along focal dome osteotomy with Kirschner wire fixation.

Factors to be taken into consideration while planning treatment

Severity of the deformity
The severity of the deformity is one of the important factors that will determine the type of treatment.

The age of the child
Orthotic management is reserved for the young child with mild genu varum.

Physiological or pathological genu varum
Physiological genu varum needs no active treatment while pathological genu varum does require treatment.

Tendency for progression
If there is a tendency for progression, appropriate measures need to be taken to correct the underlying cause or the deformity will recur following apparently satisfactory correction.

The presence of a depressed medial plateau
If it is confirmed that there is true depression of the medial tibial condyle, elevation of the tibial plateau is needed in order to restore the alignment of the articular surface.

Contribution of a distal femoral or distal tibial component to the deformity
It is imperative that the femur and the tibia's contributions to the deformity are recognized and treatment directed accordingly to each component of the deformity.

Presence of concomitant tibial shortening
This is more likely if tibia vara is unilateral and presents in adolescence. Some degree of shortening is also present in a physeal arrest, enchondromatosis, osteochondromatosis and tibial hemimelia, and needs to be accounted for in the overall management.

Is there an underlying problem with bone turnover?
A routine biochemical profile of calcium and bone turnover will diagnose metabolic bone disorders – coincident medical treatment at the time of deformity correction will reduce the risk of recurrence.

The outline of treatment of genu varum is shown in Table 15.1.

Recommended treatment

Table 15.1 ● Treatment of genu varum

INDICATIONS						
Metaphyseal-diaphyseal angle <11° + Young child	Metaphyseal-diaphyseal angle 11–16° + Young child	Metaphyseal-diaphyseal angle >16° + Young child	Metaphyseal-diaphyseal angle >11° + Older child with sufficient growth remaining + No limb length inequality	Severe deformity (correction not likely with hemiepiphyseodesis) + Older child + No limb length inequality	Metaphyseal-diaphyseal angle >11° + Older child + Limb length inequality OR Fibular collateral ligament laxity	Recurrent deformity + Large physeal tether not amenable to resection
⇩	⇩	⇩	⇩	⇩	⇩	⇩
Observe for resolution or progression	Orthotic use and monitor for resolution or progression	Hemiepiphyseal arrest by reversible technique OR Proximal tibial osteotomy (acute correction)	Hemi-epiphyseal arrest by reversible technique	Proximal tibial osteotomy (acute OR gradual correction)	Proximal tibial osteotomy by gradual correction + Tibial lengthening + Tightening of fibular collateral ligament (if needed)	Proximal tibial osteotomy + Epiphyseodesis of viable lateral half of tibial physis + Proximal fibula epiphyseodesis + Elevation of medial tibial plateau (if needed) + Correction of limb length inequality

TREATMENT

Remove any underlying cause, if present (e.g. epiphysiolysis of physeal bar or treatment of rickets)

Rationale of treatment suggested

Observation of mild degrees of genu varum is wise, particularly if the child is just over two years of age and there is no identifiable cause. Many will improve. Non-surgical treatment is recommended where it works best – in mild to moderate degrees of infantile tibia vara and rickets. In contrast, surgery should be considered when the deformity is severe or presents in late childhood or adolescence. There are broadly two types of surgical treatment available: growth manipulation by temporary hemiepiphyseal arrest or osteotomy. The first technique has the advantages of being minimally invasive at surgery and minimally intrusive in the manner of post-operative recovery. It is suitable for those with sufficient growth remaining and if the cause of deformity is not an abnormality of the physis itself, e.g. a physeal bar. For the other problems, osteotomy works well. The choice of acute over gradual correction largely depends on whether the deformity is too large to correct intra-operatively without risk of traction injury to neurovascular structures or if lengthening or collateral ligament tightening is envisaged as part of treatment.

References

1. Salenius P, Vankka E. The development of the tibiofemoral angle in children. *J Bone Joint Surg Am* 1975; **57**: 259–61.
2. Arazi M, Ogun TC, Memik R. Normal development of the tibiofemoral angle in children: a clinical study of 590 normal subjects from 3 to 17 years of age. *J Pediatr Orthop* 2001; **21**: 264–7.
3. Scott AC, Kelly CH, Sullivan E. Body mass index as a prognostic factor in development of infantile Blount disease. *J Pediatr Orthop* 2007; **27**: 921–5.
4. Bowen RE, Dorey FJ, Moseley CF. Relative tibial and femoral varus as a predictor of progression of varus deformities of the lower limbs in young children. *J Pediatr Orthop* 2002; **22**: 105–11.
5. Ain MC, Shirley ED, Pirouzmanesh A, Skolasky RL, Leet AI. Genu varum in achondroplasia. *J Pediatr Orthop* 2006; **26**: 375–9.
6. Bailey JA, II. Orthopaedic aspects of achondroplasia. *J Bone Joint Surg Am* 1970; **52**: 1285–301.
7. Lee ST, Song HR, Mahajan R *et al*. Development of genu varum in achondroplasia: relation to fibular overgrowth. *J Bone Joint Surg Br* 2007; **89**: 57–61.
8. Choi IH, Kim CJ, Cho TJ *et al*. Focal fibrocartilaginous dysplasia of long bones: report of eight additional cases and literature review. *J Pediatr Orthop* 2000; **20**: 421–7.
9. Dusabe JP, Docquier PL, Mousny M, Rombouts JJ. Focal fibrocartilaginous dysplasia of the tibia: long-term evolution. *Acta Orthop Belg* 2006; **72**: 77–82.
10. Langenskiold A, Riska EB. Tibia vara (osteochondrosis deformans tibiae): a survey of seventy-one cases. *J Bone Joint Surg Am* 1964; **46**: 1405–20.
11. Stanitski DF, Stanitski CL, Trumble S. Depression of the medial tibial plateau in early-onset Blount disease: myth or reality? *J Pediatr Orthop* 1999; **19**: 265–9.
12. Janoyer M, Jabbari H, Rouvillain JL *et al*. Infantile Blount's disease treated by hemiplateau elevation and epiphyseal distraction using a specific external fixator: preliminary report. *J Pediatr Orthop B* 2007; **16**: 273–80.
13. Gordon JE, King DJ, Luhmann SJ, Dobbs MB, Schoenecker PL. Femoral deformity in tibia vara. *J Bone Joint Surg Am* 2006; **88**: 380–6.
14. Beals RK, Stanley G. Surgical correction of bowlegs in achondroplasia. *J Pediatr Orthop B* 2005; **14**: 245–9.
15. Raney EM, Topoleski TA, Yaghoubian R, Guidera KJ, Marshall JG. Orthotic treatment of infantile tibia vara. *J Pediatr Orthop* 1998; **18**: 670–4.
16. Shapiro F. Ollier's disease. An assessment of angular deformity, shortening, and pathological fracture in twenty-one patients. *J Bone Joint Surg Am* 1982; **64**: 95–103.
17. Mielke CH, Stevens PM. Hemiepiphyseal stapling for knee deformities in children younger than 10 years: a preliminary report. *J Pediatr Orthop* 1996; **16**: 423–9.
18. Khoury J, Tavares J, McConnell S, Zeiders G, Sanders J. Results of screw epiphysiodesis for the treatment of limb length discrepancy and angular deformity. *J Pediatr Orthop* 2007; **27**: 623–8.
19. Stevens PM. Guided growth for angular correction: a preliminary series using a tension band plate. *J Pediatr Orthop* 2007; **27**: 243–59.
20. Park SS, Gordon JE, Luhmann SJ, Dobbs MB, Schoenecker PL. Outcome of hemiepiphyseal stapling for late-onset tibia vara. *J Bone Joint Surg Am* 2005; **87**: 2259–66.
21. Henderson RC, Kemp GJ, Greene WB. Adolescent tibia vara – alternatives for operative treatment. *J Bone Joint Surg Am* 1992; **74**: 342–50.

Genu valgum

Selvadurai Nayagam

16

Introduction

Children may have knock knees between the ages of three and six years. This natural femoral–tibial alignment was subject to many 'treatments' until the natural progression to a normal adult shape was appreciated to occur spontaneously in the vast majority.[1-3] However, an abnormal alignment persists in some (when it is termed idiopathic) whereas in others a specific disease process is responsible; the important causes are a previous proximal tibial fracture,[4-6] hypophosphataemic rickets,[7,8] obesity[9] and multiple hereditary osteochondromatosis.[10-12] Genu valgum can also exist as part of a longitudinal deficiency of the lower limb because of hypoplasia of the lateral femoral condyle (Figures 16.1 and 16.2). Less frequent causes include Ellis-van Creveld syndrome[13] (Figure 16.3a,b), spondyloepimetaphyseal dysplasia[14,15] (Figure 16.3c) and focal fibrocartilaginous dysplasia.[16,17]

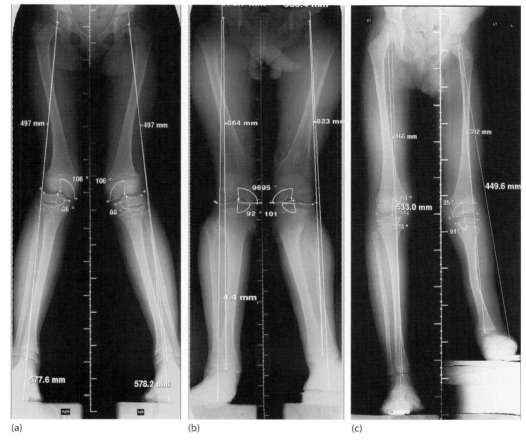

Figure 16.1 ● Genu valgum can present as bilateral symmetrical **(a)** or unilateral deformities **(b,c)**. In **(a)**, this has arisen from hypophosphataemic rickets. An osteochondroma near the physis in a patient with hereditary multiple exostoses has caused a unilateral deformity in **(b)** whereas hypoplasia of the lateral femoral condyle associated with a congenital longitudinal deficiency has produced the genu valgum in **(c)**.

(a) (b) (c)

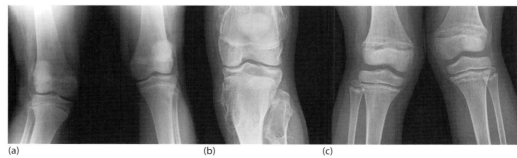

(a) (b) (c)

Figure 16.2 ● The physis can be influenced by different factors leading to a genu valgum deformity. Obesity can produce large forces that exaggerate the natural femorotibial valgus alignment leading to physeal distraction on the medial side **(a)**; an osteochondroma in close proximity to a physis can influence longitudinal growth **(b)**; and hypophosphataemic rickets is a generalized disorder producing defective mineralization at the physis **(c)**.

Problems of management

Appearance

This often represents the main reason for consultation. Reassurance and an offer to follow up the child is all that is necessary if the deformity is bilateral, not severe (an intermalleolar distance of less than 15 cm) and present under the age of six years. The surgeon needs to be aware of hyperextension at the knee (or a proximal tibial recurvatum deformity) mimicking a genu valgum. If the deformity is severe, unilateral or present in older children, a detailed past and family history, serum biochemical profile of bone metabolism and radiographs may reveal the cause.

Circumduction gait and difficulty running

Knee valgus produces changes in gait; there is increased hip adduction, a varus internal moment at the knee with the knee joint centre shifted medially.[18] The child runs in an awkward manner and this may trigger teasing in school. There is some evidence to suggest these children walk with a slower cadence in comparison to children without the deformity.[19] These parameters are reduced to normal after correction.[18]

Anterior knee pain and patellofemoral instability

Mechanical factors, e.g. patella maltracking, instability and lateral facet overload in association with genu valgum have been thought responsible for anterior knee pain in adolescents but the evidence is contradictory.[20] There are several reasons for anterior knee pain in the adolescent. In a small number, maltracking may be responsible and the symptoms eased through correction of the knee deformity.[21] Frank persistent dislocation of the patella may occur in association with more severe degrees of genu valgum.

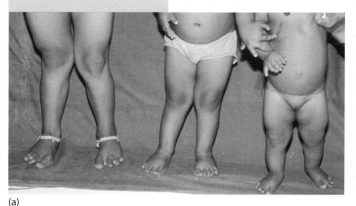
(a)

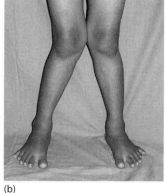
(b)

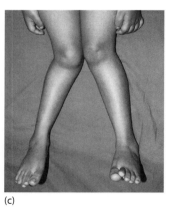
(c)

Figure 16.3 ● Genu valgum in Ellis van Creveld syndrome begins in early childhood. These three siblings have Ellis van Creveld syndrome; genu valgum is evident in two of the siblings **(a)**. If untreated, the deformity can progress to a severe degree **(b)**. Severe genu valgum in a child with another form of skeletal dysplasia **(c)**.

Assessment

Determining the site of the deformity

In the majority of instances the deformity is in the distal femur. However, there are some situations where the pathology is in the proximal tibia. It is important that the site of deformity is identified. Genu valgum due to distal femoral pathology is generally masked when the knee is flexed while the deformity persists on knee flexion if the proximal tibia is at fault (Figure 16.4).

Determining the severity of the deformity

If the deformity is bilateral and symmetrical the intermalleolar distance may be measured clinically and this can be used as a guide to treatment. Unilateral or asymmetrical deformities need to be measured more accurately with the help of full-length standing radiographs.

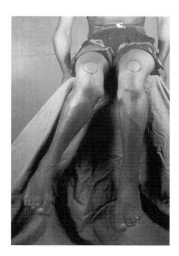

Figure 16.4 ● Genu valgum due to pathology in the proximal tibia in an adolescent; the deformity is not masked on flexion of the knee.

Aims of treatment

- Restoration of limb alignment
- Prevention of recurrence post-correction

Treatment options

Observation

Most children who present for an orthopaedic opinion are likely to have physiologic genu valgum. The child has a symmetrical and mild to moderate deformity and is usually under six years of age. Documenting progression (or improvement) is important. Clinical measurements suffice and the intermalleolar distance can be used. If the deformity appears to worsen or persists after six to seven years of age, further documentation can be added through standing hip-to-ankle radiographs.

Guided growth

This is eminently useful, simple to perform and is reversible should overcorrection occur. The correction is accomplished by creating a temporary tether in the physis on the convex side of the deformity (usually the medial aspects of the distal femoral and/or proximal tibial physes) which allows faster growth on the lateral side to effect an improvement in alignment. The tether is created using staples, screws or tension band plates[21–25] (Figure 16.5). Previously, the technique of hemiepiphyseodesis was irreversible and had to be performed in accordance with growth charts so that correction was achieved when skeletal maturity was reached. If an overcorrection was observed to start occurring, the surgeon had to promptly perform a hemiepiphyseodesis of the contralateral side of the physis. With the newer implants and improved surgical techniques, the physeal arrest is reversible and does not need to be timed.[23] When correction is accomplished, the tether (implant) is removed.

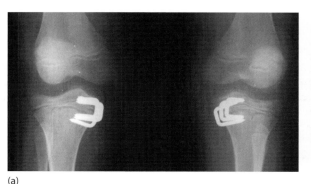 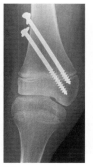 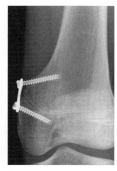

(a) (b) (c)

Figure 16.5 ● Growth of the physis can be guided to correct genu valgum by using staples **(a)**, screws **(b)** or a tension-band plate **(c)**.

Corrective osteotomy

If there is insufficient growth remaining or the child is skeletally mature and if the cause of the genu valgum deformity is a disorder of the physis, hemiepiphyseodesis is unlikely to work. Corrective osteotomies will produce the desired improved alignment but need to be performed with previous deformity analysis (Figure 16.6). In younger children simple methods of fixation will suffice (crossed Kirschner wires and long leg casts) but in older children more substantial implants or external fixators may be needed.

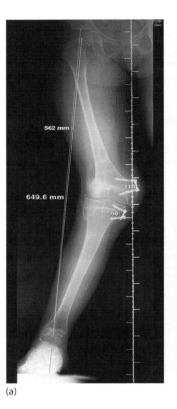 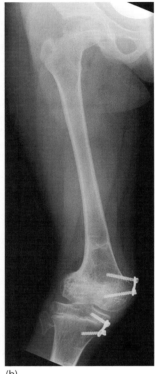 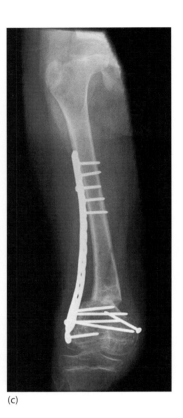

(a)   (b)   (c)

Figure 16.6 ● Attempted guided growth for correction of this unilateral genu valgum deformity was unsuccessful owing to a faulty physis on the lateral side of the distal femur **(a)**. Corrective osteotomy provides the solution; here performed with lateral translation in accordance with the rules of osteotomy for deformity correction (see Chapter 1, General principles of treatment of deformities in children) and held with internal fixation **(a,b)**.

Combination of corrective osteotomy and hemiepiphyseodesis

If the deformity is due to abnormal physeal growth and if the deformity is severe, a combination of these techniques may be warranted in order to achieve correction and to prevent recurrence of the deformity.

Decompression of the peroneal nerve

The common peroneal nerve may be stretched when an acute correction of severe genu valgum is performed. In order to minimize the risk of nerve damage a prophylactic decompression of the nerve down to the neck of the fibula has been recommended[26] (Figure 16.7).

Factors to be taken into consideration while planning treatment

Severity of the deformity

If the deformity is mild and symmetrical, mere observation is justified, while more severe degrees of deformity may warrant intervention. Severe genu valgum may not correct fully by modulating physeal growth and then an osteotomy is required.

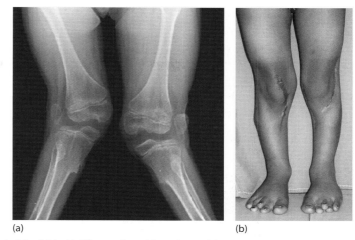

(a)   (b)

Figure 16.7 ● In this child with Ellis van Creveld syndrome **(a)** corrective osteotomy of the proximal tibia, medial tibial epiphyseal stapling, decompression of the common peroneal nerve and realignment of the patella were performed in order to correct the deformity **(b)**.

Number of years of remaining growth and the state of the physis

It is preferable to have at least two years of remaining growth and for the physis to be normal for hemiepiphyseodesis to work.

Site of pathology (femoral or tibial)

The decision to perform femoral or tibial hemiepiphyseodesis (or both) will depend on where the deformity arises, and this is usually the femur. Deformity analysis by radiograph will indicate the appropriate physis to treat. If the period of remaining growth is short, both distal femoral and proximal tibial physes can be treated to achieve an improved limb axis at the expense of mild joint inclination.[27]

Focal lesions responsible for deformity

If the deformity has been caused by a physeal arrest from trauma or infection, or if there are bone lesions (osteochondromata) near the physis which exert an influence on growth, further imaging of these lesions is warranted and, if possible, these should be removed.

Associated limb shortening

A shortened deformed limb is likely if there is an underlying longitudinal deficiency of the limb or the cause of deformity was a disturbance of the physis (arrest, infection). Rarely, the limb may be longer (Figure 16.8). In these situations, limb length equalization may be necessary and should be included with treatment of the deformity.

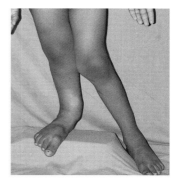

Figure 16.8 ● This boy with Ollier's disease has genu valgum of the left knee. The limb length inequality also needs to be addressed along with correction of the deformity.

Recommended treatment

The outline of treatment of genu valgum is shown in Table 16.1.

Table 16.1 ● Outline of treatment of genu valgum

INDICATIONS			
Bilateral, symmetrical genu valgum in a child 3–6 years + Intermalleolar distance less than 15 cm ⇩ Observe for resolution or progression If unresolved and significant in degree after age 7, offer to treat by hemiepiphyseodesis	Bilateral, symmetrical genu valgum in a child 3–6 years + Intermalleolar distance greater than 15 cm ⇩ Obtain serum biochemistry of bone metabolism Obtain radiographs to exclude local lesions near physis Check BMI Observe initially If unresolved and significant in degree after age 7, offer to treat by hemiepiphyseodesis	Asymmetrical genu valgum in a child 3–6 years ⇩ Obtain imaging of physis and surrounding bone to exclude local lesions Check BMI Rule out possible associated syndromes (*see Introduction*) Observe initially If unresolved and significant in degree after age 7, offer to treat: by hemiepiphyseodesis if physis is normal; by osteotomy if not	Asymmetrical genu valgum in a child (after 7 years) ⇩ Obtain imaging of physis and surrounding bone to exclude local lesions Check BMI Rule out possible associated syndromes (*see Introduction*) If unresolved and significant in degree after age 7, offer to treat: by hemiepiphyseodesis if physis is normal and sufficient growth remaining; by osteotomy if not
		In addition, consider: 1 Decompression of the peroneal nerve at the time of deformity correction 2 Soft tissue stabilization of the patella if there is patellar instability 3 Limb length equalization if limb length inequality is present 4 Removal of the underlying cause of deformity is possible	
Treatment should be directed to the femur or tibia or both, depending on the site of the deformity			
TREATMENT			

Rationale of treatment suggested

While most children tend to adopt adult femoral–tibial alignment by the age of six years, the rate and size of improvement can vary between children of different racial groups.[28,29] An expectant approach is justified with a symmetrical deformity that is not severe in a child under six years because the deformity is likely to be physiologic. In the event that spontaneous improvement has not occurred by nine to ten years of age, treatment by hemiepiphyseodesis can be undertaken. It is the simplest method for producing the desired correction when the physis is normal. Osteotomies for this group of children are inappropriate as they are more invasive and not without complications; an exception are children with severe deformities which interfere markedly with gait and need correcting promptly.[29]

In deformities that have arisen from physeal damage, worsening with growth is likely and attempts to remove the underlying cause recommended. This is undertaken at the time of deformity correction which is by osteotomy. Osteotomy is also needed for skeletally mature children with deformity as guided growth methods are redundant.

References

1. Kling TJ, Hensinger R. Angular and torsional deformities of the lower limbs in children. *Clin Orthop Relat Res* 1983; **176**: 136–47.
2. Salenius P, Vankka E. The development of the tibiofemoral angle in children. *J Bone Joint Surg Am* 1975; **57**: 259–61.
3. White GR, Mencio GA. Genu valgum in children: diagnostic and therapeutic alternatives. *J Am Acad Orthop Surg* 1995; **3**: 275–83.

4. Currarino G, Pinckney LE. Genu valgum after proximal tibial fractures in children. *AJR Am J Roentgenol* 1981; **136**: 915–8.

5. Jackson DW, Cozen L. Genu valgum as a complication of proximal tibial metaphyseal fractures in children. *J Bone Joint Surg Am* 1971; **53**: 1571–8.

6. Muller I, Muschol M, Mann M, Hassenpflug J. Results of proximal metaphyseal fractures in children. *Arch Orthop Trauma Surg* 2002; **122**: 331–3.

7. Davids JR, Fisher R, Lum G, Von Glinski S. Angular deformity of the lower extremity in children with renal osteodystrophy. *J Pediatr Orthop* 1992; **12**: 291–9.

8. Omoloja AA, Kumar K, Crawford AH, Strife CF. Epiphyseal stapling and recombinant human growth hormone for correction of genu valgum in children with chronic renal insufficiency. *J Pediatr Orthop* 2003; **23**: 639–42.

9. de Sa Pinto AL, de Barros Holanda PM, Radu AS, Villares SM, Lima FR. Musculoskeletal findings in obese children. *J Paediatr Child Health* 2006; **42**: 341–4.

10. Nawata K, Teshima R, Minamizaki T, Yamamoto K. Knee deformities in multiple hereditary exostoses. A longitudinal radiographic study. *Clin Orthop Relat Res* 1995; **313**: 194–9.

11. Peterson HA. Multiple hereditary osteochondromata. *Clin Orthop Relat Res* 1989; **239**: 222–30.

12. Miura H, Noguchi Y, Mitsuyasu H *et al.* Clinical features of multiple epiphyseal dysplasia expressed in the knee. *Clin Orthop Relat Res* 2000; **380**: 184–90.

13. Lichiardopol C, Militaru C. Ellis-van Creveld syndrome. *Rom J Morphol Embryol* 2006; **47**: 363–6.

14. Amirfeyz R, Taylor A, Smithson SF, Gargan MF. Orthopaedic manifestations and management of spondyloepimetaphyseal dysplasia Strudwick type. *J Pediatr Orthop B* 2006; **151**: 41–4.

15. Miura H, Noguchi Y, Mitsuyasu H *et al.* Clinical features of multiple epiphyseal dysplasia expressed in the knee. *Clin Orthop Relat Res* 2000;**380**: 184–90.

16. Ruchelsman DE, Madan SS, Feldman DS. Genu valgum secondary to focal fibrocartilaginous dysplasia of the distal femur. *J Pediatr Orthop* 2004; **24**: 408–13.

17. Choi IH, Kim CJ, Cho TJ *et al.* Focal fibrocartilaginous dysplasia of long bones: report of eight additional cases and literature review. *J Pediatr Orthop* 2000; **20**: 421–7.

18. Stevens PM, MacWilliams B, Mohr RA. Gait analysis of stapling for genu valgum. *J Pediatr Orthop* 2004; **24**: 70–4.

19. Pretkiewicz-Abacjew E. Knock knee and the gait of six-year-old children. *J Sports Med Phys Fitness* 2003; **43**: 156–64.

20. Fairbank JC, Pynsent PB, van Poortvliet JA, Phillips H. Mechanical factors in the incidence of knee pain in adolescents and young adults. *J Bone Joint Surg Br* 1984; **66**: 685–93.

21. Stevens PM, Maguire M, Dales MD, Robins AJ. Physeal stapling for idiopathic genu valgum. *J Pediatr Orthop* 1999; **19**: 645–9.

22. Khoury J, Tavares J, McConnell S, Zeiders G, Sanders J. Results of screw epiphysiodesis for the treatment of limb length discrepancy and angular deformity. *J Pediatr Orthop* 2007; **27**: 623–8.

23. Stevens PM. Guided growth for angular correction: a preliminary series using a tension band plate. *J Pediatr Orthop* 2007; **27**: 243–59.

24. Mielke CH, Stevens PM. Hemiepiphyseal stapling for knee deformities in children younger than 10 years – a preliminary report. *J Pediatr Orthop* 1996; **16**: 423–9.

25. Pistevos G, Duckworth T. The correction of genu valgum by epiphysial stapling. *J Bone Joint Surg Br* 1977; **59**: 72–6.

26. Paley D, Herzenberg JE. *Principles of Deformity Correction*. Berlin: Springer, 2002, 504.

27. Heath CH, Staheli LT. Normal limits of knee angle in white children – genu varum and genu valgum. *J Pediatr Orthop* 1993; **13**: 259–62.

28. Arazi M, Ogun TC, Memik R. Normal development of the tibiofemoral angle in children: a clinical study of 590 normal subjects from 3 to 17 years of age. *J Pediatr Orthop* 2001; **21**: 264–7.

29. Steel HH, Sandrow RE, Sullivan PD. Complications of tibial osteotomy in children for genu varum or valgum. Evidence that neurological changes are due to ischemia. *J Bone Joint Surg Am* 1971; **53**: 1629–35.

Coxa vara

Randall Loder

17

Introduction

Coxa vara is a deformity of the proximal femur that results in a reduction of the normal neck–shaft angle and it includes a wide spectrum of types with varying pathologies and differing sites of deformity.[1] The different types of coxa vara are developmental, congenital, dysplastic and acquired (Figure 17.1). The deformity may occur at the physis, the metaphyseal region of the femoral neck or subtrochanteric region depending on the underlying pathology (Table 17.1). Determination of the type and location of the coxa vara is of utmost importance as treatment planning is dependent upon these two factors.

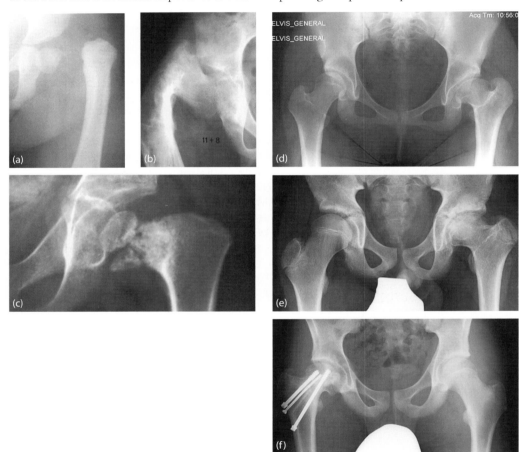

Figure 17.1 ● Examples of different types of coxa vara: **(a)** congenital coxa vara with a subtrochanteric pseudarthrosis; **(b)** dysplastic coxa vara, in this case due to fibrous dysplasia; **(c)** developmental coxa vara, with the hallmark triangular fragment in the inferior femoral neck; **(d)** acquired coxa vara following Perthes' disease; **(e)** coxa vara following osteomyelitis of the left femur resulting in physeal damage; and **(f)** coxa vara following non-union of a femoral neck fracture.

Table 17.1 ● Types of coxa vara, the underlying pathology and the natural history of each type

Type of coxa vara	Underlying pathology	Site of deformity	Propensity for progression or resolution
Congenital	Dysgenesis	Subtrochanteric	Progression occurs
Developmental	Growth abnormality	Physis	May progress/remain static/resolve
Dysplastic	Metabolic: *Rickets*	Physis	May progress if disease process is not arrested
	Dysplasia: *Fibrous dysplasia*	Metaphysis	Progression occurs
Acquired	Avascularity: *Sepsis, Perthes' disease*	Physis and epiphysis	Progression occurs
	Trauma: *Malunion of fracture*	Physis: *Epiphyseal slip*	May partially resolve
		Metaphysis: *Fracture neck of femur*	
		Subtrochanteric: *Subtrochanteric fracture*	

Types of coxa vara

Congenital coxa vara

Congenital coxa vara is the type associated with a congenital short femur and proximal femoral focal deficiency.[2,3] It is more commonly unilateral and presents with an out-toeing gait and an external rotation deformity of the hip due to retroversion of the femoral neck. Varying degrees of shortening of the limb are usually present and later genu valgum frequently develops. It can also be associated with fibular deficiency.

Developmental coxa vara

Developmental coxa vara has, in the past, been known as congenital coxa vara. However, it is now termed developmental coxa vara, as most are not diagnosed at birth but rather present when the child begins to ambulate with a Trendelenburg limp. The pathognomonic radiographic sign is the inferior and posterior bony metaphyseal fragment in the femoral neck.[4,5] Developmental coxa vara is bilateral in up to one half of cases.

Dysplastic coxa vara

Dysplastic coxa vara is due to an underlying bony abnormality such as fibrous dysplasia, vitamin D-resistant rickets, osteopetrosis and various generalized skeletal dysplasias (e.g. spondylometaphyseal, spondyloepiphyseal and cleidocranial dysplasias). These are frequently bilateral deformities, except in the case of fibrous dysplasia.

Acquired coxa vara

Acquired coxa vara can develop following trauma; the trauma may be perinatal epiphyseal separation or a femoral neck fracture in an older child. Malunion of either of these injuries can lead to coxa vara. Excessive varus angulation while performing a varus osteotomy for Perthes' disease or for hip subluxation is an iatrogenic cause for coxa vara. Acquired coxa vara can also be due to vascular insults, such as Perthes' disease or proximal femoral growth disturbance associated with developmental hip dysplasia.

Finally, acquired coxa vara may be the result of septic processes. Infantile septic arthritis may be complicated by a vascular insult resulting in a Perthes'-like process and coxa vara.

Site of deformity

Congenital coxa vara is usually subtrochanteric, and may range from a varus deformity with sclerotic features to a complete pseudarthrosis. In the older child plain radiographs will be sufficient to make this determination; in younger children arthrography or magnetic resonance imaging (MRI) may be needed.

Developmental coxa vara occurs at the inferior and posterior areas of the proximal femoral metaphysis, immediately adjacent to the physis. Typically, plain radiographs are sufficient to determine this location; computed tomography or MRI may occasionally be necessary.

Dysplastic coxa vara occurs at the level of involvement of the underlying bony process. For example, vitamin D-resistant rickets, being a failure of mineralization process, occurs at the physis and proximal metaphysis (primary spongiosa). The radiographic changes in renal osteodystrophy are not unlike a slipped capital femoral epiphysis. Fibrous dysplasia is typically metaphyseal and can vary from minimal varus to a massive shepherd's crook deformity. In skeletal dysplasias the varus develops at the physeal level in epiphyseal dysplasias and at the metaphyseal level in metaphyseal dysplasias. In epiphyseal dysplasias delayed and fragmented ossification of the epiphysis may be noted.

The level of involvement in acquired coxa vara is obviously dependent upon the level of the initial pathology. Post-traumatic coxa vara may occur either at the physis (neonatal physeal separation) or the metaphysis (malunion of a femoral neck fracture). Coxa vara from vascular compromise following development dysplasia of the hip treatment or Perthes' results in coxa vara at the physis with impaired physeal growth and continued normal trochanteric growth (Figure 17.2). This, in due course, gives the appearance of an apparent trochanteric overgrowth. Coxa vara caused by sepsis can occur at the physeal or the metaphyseal level.

The use of the articulotrochanteric distance (ATD) is often helpful in older children to localize the level of pathology. In those children with a decreased ATD, the location of the deformity is at the physeal or intertrochanteric level. If the ATD is equal to the normal side, then the coxa vara is occurring at the subtrochanteric level, although in a severe subtrochanteric shepherd's crook deformity due to fibrous dysplasia the ATD may be a negative value.

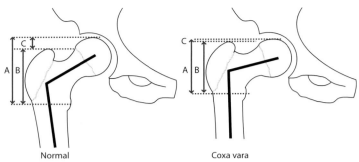

Normal   Coxa vara

Figure 17.2 ● Coxa vara due to impaired growth of the capital femoral physis is measured by comparing the growth of the femoral physis and the trochanteric physis. The measurement from the lesser trochanter to the top of the femoral head (A) reflects the growth of the capital physis, and the measurement from the lesser trochanter to the top of the greater trochanter (B) reflects trochanteric growth. In the normal left hip, the distance from the top of the greater trochanter to the top of the femoral head (C) is about 20 ± 5 mm. In the hip with coxa vara due to impaired growth of the capital femoral physis in the right hip, A decreases and B is normal, thereby decreasing C.

Progression or resolution of deformity

If there is discontinuity of the neck or subtrochanteric pseudarthrosis as in proximal femoral deficiency, the coxa vara tends to progress with increasing abductor weakness and leg length discrepancy. The propensity for progression in developmental coxa vara can often be predicted by the Hilgenreiner epiphyseal angle (HEA).[5] If the HEA is >60°, all will progress, those between 45 and 60° may or may not progress and <45° often correct spontaneously (Figure 17.3). In dysplastic and acquired coxa vara, progression is unpredictable and close observation is required. Traumatic coxa vara may spontaneously improve if there is enough remaining growth and thus greater remodelling can be anticipated in the younger child.

Problems of management

Altered mechanics of the hip resulting in abductor muscle weakness and a Trendelenburg gait

There are two mechanisms by which the abductor mechanism of the hip can be rendered ineffective. They are a reduction in the neck-shaft angle and relative 'overgrowth' of the greater trochanter due to impaired growth of the femoral neck. Both result in the point of insertion of the hip abductor muscles to the greater trochanter moving higher than the centre of rotation of the hip joint, which usually corresponds to the centre of the femoral head. This disrupts the lever arm of the hip abductors and a Trendelenburg gait ensues.

Risk of progression of the deformity and potential for recurrence of the deformity

If the deformity develops on account of an abnormality of physeal growth, the deformity is likely to progress until skeletal maturity and unless the underlying pathology can be remedied there is a risk of recurrence of the deformity once it has been surgically corrected. There is evidence to suggest that in developmental coxa vara, if the HEA is <45° the deformity may resolve and conversely if the angle is >60° it tends to progress. While correcting this type of coxa vara an attempt is made to reduce the HEA to 30° in order to minimize the risk of recurrence of the deformity.

Associated femoral retroversion

Developmental coxa vara is associated with retroversion of the femur. This may not be of consequence if the degree of retroversion is not marked and if there is bilateral involvement. However, even a moderate degree of retroversion in unilateral cases and more severe degrees of retroversion in bilateral cases need to be corrected.

Associated acetabular dysplasia

Acetabular dysplasia is sometimes associated with developmental coxa vara. It is important to appreciate this and deal with the acetabular dysplasia prior to performing a valgus osteotomy to avoid the risk of creating an unacceptable degree of uncovering of the femoral head.

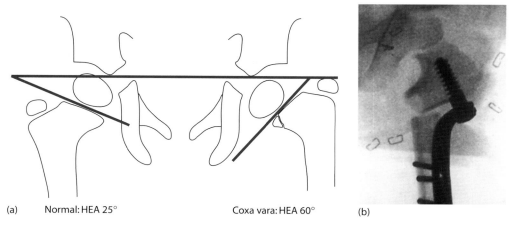

(a)   Normal: HEA 25°   Coxa vara: HEA 60°   (b)

Figure 17.3 ● **(a)** The Hilgenreiner epiphyseal angle (HEA) is created by the intersection of two lines on an anteroposterior pelvis radiograph. The first line is drawn through the triradiate cartilage of both hips. The second line is a line drawn through the physis and that intersects with the triradiate cartilage line. The extent of reduction of the HEA following surgery is an estimate of the adequacy of correction. **(b)** The intra-operative radiograph of a child with developmental coxa vara after proximal femoral valgus osteotomy. Note that the HEA is quite low. The lateral femoral cortex of the proximal fragment is in contact with the transverse osteotomy surface of the distal fragment in order to obtain adequate correction.

Associated limb length discrepancy

In unilateral cases limb length inequality is often present and may be quite significant. Apart from the inherent shortening of the limb associated with the underlying condition, a phenomenon of early proximal femoral physis closure after valgus osteotomy in children with developmental coxa vara has been documented.[4] One needs to be aware of this phenomenon and look for further shortening of the limb that may develop following a valgus osteotomy to correct the coxa vara.

Associated deformities of the knee

Genu valgum tends to progress in the presence of coxa vara on account of the abnormal stresses on the knee created by the malalignment of the limb. Children who have a genu valgum need to have early correction of the coxa vara to prevent progression of the knee deformity.

Aims of treatment

- Halt progression of the deformity
  First and foremost it is necessary to halt progression of the deformity if this is possible.
- Improve proximal femoral anatomy
  This entails surgical restoration of the neck-shaft angle to normal and ensuring that the tip of the greater trochanter is at or below the level of the centre of the femoral head. As mentioned earlier, in the young child with developmental coxa vara the risk of recurrence needs to be minimized by restoring a normal HEA. Surgery is necessary in those deformities whose natural history is not one of gradual remodelling. Surgery is also needed in the types that show partial improvement when the child approaches skeletal maturity and no further resolution can be expected.
- Appropriately adjust leg length inequality
  If the projected limb length discrepancy at skeletal maturity is not acceptable, then appropriate limb length equalization is desirable. If there is residual abductor weakness at maturity it is best to leave the involved limb slightly short to accommodate the swing phase of gait.

Treatment options

Halting deformity progression

If the deformity is due to an underlying metabolic condition, then appropriate medical management is needed first, such as in the case of vitamin D-resistant rickets or renal osteodystrophy. Unfortunately, most aetiologies of childhood coxa vara do not lend themselves to medical management alone.

Correcting proximal femoral pathologic anatomy
■ Proximal femoral valgus osteotomy

The mainstay of treatment is valgus osteotomy. However, knowing the location of the deformity is paramount in planning the osteotomy level. For children with coxa vara due to physeal or metaphyseal deformity (e.g. developmental coxa vara, Perthes' disease, septic sequel), a valgus intertrochanteric osteotomy is desirable. For those with subtrochanteric deformity (e.g. congenital coxa vara), a subtrochanteric osteotomy is more appropriate (Figure 17.4).

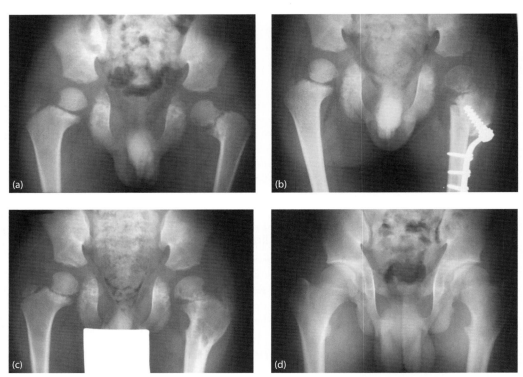

Figure 17.4 ● The anteroposterior pelvis radiograph of a boy with cleidocranial dysostosis and left coxa vara at six years of age **(a)**. A valgus osteotomy was performed using a screw and side plate method of fixation, correcting the Hilgenreiner epiphyseal angle. Note the healed osteotomy at age six years two months **(b)**; correction was maintained as shown in radiographs at the ages of eight years **(c)** and 15 years **(d)**.

When planning a proximal femoral osteotomy the status of any potentially pseudarthrotic areas must be known. In those with deformity due to infantile sepsis, it is possible that the entire femoral head and neck has disappeared, or that there is simply a pseudarthrosis between the basilar neck and more proximal metaphyseal area. The same exists in children with proximal femoral focal deficiency. There may be a complete pseudarthrosis at the subtrochanteric level, or simply a fibrous or cartilaginous anlage that has not yet ossified. In order to obtain the necessary information it may be necessary to perform an MRI and an arthrogram before the definitive surgical procedure.

As developmental coxa vara may be accompanied by retroversion, internal rotation is combined with the valgus correction while performing the osteotomy. This may also be necessary in those with dysplastic coxa vara. Correction of the HEA to <30° is suggested to minimize the risk of recurrence in those with developmental coxa vara.[4,5,6,7]

The fixation device should not cross the physis unless the child is almost skeletally mature. Careful templating with the surgeon's personal preference of fixation device is necessary before surgery to ensure that the necessary equipment and devices are available. The peculiar anatomy to each case mandates careful planning of the osteotomy and its internal fixation. Potential fixation devices include hip screw with side plate constructs, blade plates, external fixators and in younger children simple wires if performing the Pauwel's type of osteotomy. If the underlying aetiology is fibrous dysplasia, intramedullary fixation and cortical bone fibular grafting should be considered.

■ Greater trochanteric epiphyseodesis

When there is inadequate abductor power after valgus osteotomy, or if valgus osteotomy is not needed owing to only a mild element of coxa vara, then greater trochanteric repositioning can be considered to improve hip abductor strength. If the child is younger than eight or nine years, an epiphyseodesis of the greater trochanter can be performed (Figure 17.5).[8] After this age, there is inadequate remaining growth from the greater trochanteric physis to obtain adequate increase in the ATD with a simple epiphyseodesis. In this instance formal greater trochanteric transfer is necessary.

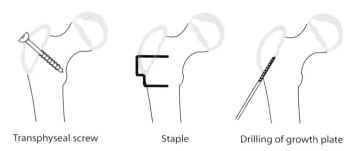

Transphyseal screw   Staple   Drilling of growth plate

Figure 17.5 ● Techniques of performing a trochanteric epiphyseodesis.

■ Greater trochanteric transfer

Distal and lateral transfer of the greater trochanter is done close to or after skeletal maturity. The entire greater trochanter with the gluteal muscle attachment is detached and transferred distally and fixed with two screws (Figure 17.6). The mechanics of the hip improves quite dramatically and the Trendelenburg gait disappears if the trochanter has been shifted sufficiently distally (Figure 17.7) and laterally.

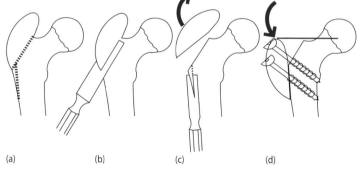

(a)   (b)   (c)   (d)

Figure 17.6 ● Diagram illustrating the technique of trochanteric advancement. The tip of the trochanter must be brought to the level of the centre of the femoral head in order to abolish the Trendelenburg sign.

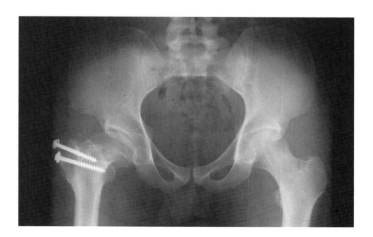

Figure 17.7 ● The tip of the greater trochanter has been brought down to the level of the centre of the femoral head by transfer of the trochanter. The Trendelenburg sign was abolished by the surgery.

If a combination of a valgus osteotomy and a trochanteric transfer is being contemplated, this author recommends that transfer of the greater trochanter be done as a secondary procedure and not at the same time as the valgus osteotomy. This is to minimize the number of moving parts and potential complications that could occur with inadequate fixation of so many fragments.

Factors to be taken into consideration while planning treatment

Age of the child

In a young child with a type of coxa vara that has the propensity to progress, early correction of the deformity is indicated. The choice of whether to perform a trochanteric apophyseodesis or trochanteric transfer again depends on the age of the child.

Unilateral or bilateral involvement

The issue of limb length equalization arises only in children with unilateral involvement.

Severity of the deformity

If the deformity is severe enough to produce weakness of the hip abductor muscles and a Trendelenburg gait, surgical intervention is justified.

Type of coxa vara and the risk of progression

The type of coxa vara determines the behaviour of the deformity. If the type has a tendency to progress, intervention is needed.

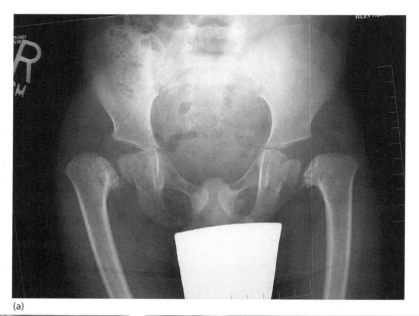

(a)

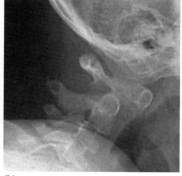

(b)

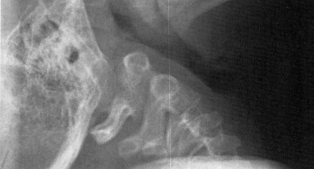

(c)

Figure 17.8 ● A child with spondyloepiphyseal dysplasia presented with a limp and abductor lurch. Radiographs at age three years demonstrated bilateral coxa vara (a) with a low Hilgenreiner epiphyseal angle. By age six years, progressive hip pain and fatigue was due to instability of the cervical spine as demonstrated on lateral flexion (b) and extension (c) radiographs. There is a significant increase in the atlanto-dens interval on the flexion radiograph.

Table 17.2 ● Outline of treatment of coxa vara

INDICATIONS							
Young child + Coxa vara NOT likely to progress + No abductor weakness + No hip pain	Any age + Coxa vara NOT likely to progress + Hip abductor weakness OR Hip pain	Young child + Coxa vara likely to progress (OR progress documented) ± Hip abductor weakness ± Hip pain	Any age + Coxa vara likely to progress (OR progress documented) + Retroversion of femur	Any age + Coxa vara likely to progress (OR progress documented) + Acetabular dysplasia	Older child + Sufficient growth remaining before skeletal maturity + Coxa vara at physeal level + Hip abductor weakness	Adolescent + Mild/moderate coxa vara + Trochanteric 'overgrowth'	Adolescent + Severe coxa vara + Trochanteric overgrowth
⇩	⇩	⇩	⇩	⇩	⇩	⇩	⇩
Periodic observation for: status of coxa vara and limb-length inequality in unilateral cases	Valgus osteotomy	Valgus osteotomy (attempt to reduce Hilgenreiner epiphyseal angle to <30°)	Valgus + Internal rotation osteotomy	Valgus osteotomy + Correction of acetabular dysplasia	Trochanteric apophyseodesis alone if coxa vara is mild OR Trochanteric apophyseodesis + Valgus osteotomy if coxa vara is severe	Distal and lateral transfer of the greater trochanter	Valgus osteotomy + Distal and lateral transfer of the greater trochanter (staged procedure)
TREATMENT							

Presence of associated deformities

■ Femoral retroversion

If retroversion is present, it can be corrected along with the correction of the coxa vara.

■ Acetabular dysplasia

If acetabular dysplasia is present it needs to be addressed concomitantly.

■ Limb length inequality

The limb length inequality needs to be addressed after dealing with the coxa vara.

■ Genu valgum

The presence of genu valgum increases the urgency of correction of the coxa vara since the hip deformity can aggravate the knee deformity.

Other associated medical issues

In children with skeletal dysplasias, anaesthetic considerations and potential cervical spine instabil-ity must be considered (Figure 17.8). In those with underlying metabolic disease, appropriate medical evalu-ation is necessary.

The outline of treatment of coxa vara is shown in Table 17.2.

Recommended treatment

Rationale of treatment choice

Why is it necessary to determine the aetiology of the coxa vara?
The natural history of spontaneous resolution is markedly dependent upon the aetiology. Coxa vara caused by trauma will often spontaneously improve, bypassing the need for an osteotomy. Developmental and dysplastic coxa vara often progress, and will either need surgery at presentation or later. Congenital coxa vara may or may not be progressive. This information is needed to counsel the parents appropriately.

Why is it necessary to determine the location of the coxa vara?
This is needed to plan the correct valgus osteotomy at the level of pathology and maximize mechanical axis correction.

References

1. Beals RK. Coxa vara in childhood: evaluation and management. *J Am Acad Orthop Surg* 1998; **6**: 93–9.
2. Ring PA. Congenital short femur: simple femoral hypoplasia. *J Bone Joint Surg Br* 1959; **41**: 73–9.
3. Gillespie R. Classification of congenital abnormalities of the femur. In: Herring JA, Birch JG (eds). *The Child with a Limb Deficiency*. Rosemont, IL: American Academy of Orthopaedic Surgeons, 1998: 63–72.
4. Desai SS, Johnson LO. Long-term results of valgus osteotomy for congenital coxa vara. *J Pediatr Orthop* 1993; **294**: 204–10.
5. Weinstein JN, Kuo KN, Millar EA. Congenital coxa vara: a retrospective review. *J Pediatr Orthop* 1984; **4**: 70–7.
6. Cordes S, Dickens DRV, Cole WG. Correction of coxa vara in childhood. *J Bone Joint Surg Br* 1991; **73**: 3–6.
7. Carroll K, Coleman S, Stevens PM. Coxa vara: surgical outcomes of valgus osteotomies. *J Pediatr Orthop* 1997; **17**: 220–4.
8. Gage JR, Cary JM. The effects of trochanteric epiphyseodesis on growth of the proximal end of the femur following necrosis of the capital femoral epiphysis. *J Bone Joint Surg Am* 1980; **62**: 785–94.

Femoral anteversion

Randall Loder

18

Introduction

Each human femur has a particular torsion and the vast majority of femora demonstrate a wide range of torsion, typically anteversion. Femoral anteversion reduces as the child grows. The normal average femoral anteversion is around 40° at birth, and as the child matures into adulthood it decreases to around 10–15°.[1] Femoral anteversion is around 5° higher in females than in males.

Increased femoral anteversion can be idiopathic, or associated with other conditions such as developmental hip dysplasia and cerebral palsy. Femoral retroversion is much less common; it is rarely idiopathic apart from in obese adolescents but is frequently associated with developmental coxa vara and slipped capital femoral epiphysis.

Femoral anteversion results in an in-toeing gait (Figure 18.1) and this is often of significant concern to parents. However, idiopathic femoral anteversion does not predispose the individual to lower extremity functional deficits[2] or an increased risk of hip osteoarthritis.[3] Most children with increased femoral anteversion slowly resolve their in-toeing. In a few children there is significant residual femoral anteversion and in-toeing gait in early adolescence.[4,5]

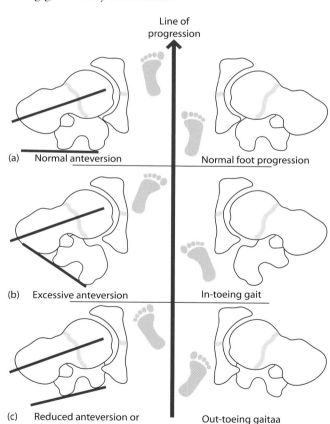

Figure 18.1 ● Diagram showing normal anteversion **(a)**, excessive femoral anteversion **(b)** and reduced anteversion **(c)**. The angle the long axis of the foot makes with the line of progression (foot–progression angle) changes with the degree of femoral anteversion.

Problems of management

Cosmetic problems

For most parents the particular area of concern is the cosmetic aspect of the in-toeing gait.

Anterior knee pain

Increased femoral anteversion may be part of the miserable malalignment syndrome (Figure 18.2) which is accentuated femoral anteversion associated with a large compensatory external tibial torsion.[6,7] This can result in an extremely awkward gait and, more importantly, significant anterior knee pain and patellar malalignment as these children get older, heavier and more active.[6–8]

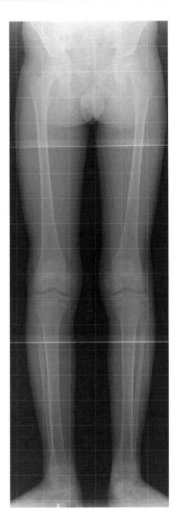

Figure 18.2 ● Appearance of a full-length standing radiograph of the lower limbs of a child with miserable malalignment syndrome. The radiograph has been taken with the patellae facing forwards. The child has femoral anteversion (this gives a false impression of increase in the neck–shaft angle) and external tibial torsion (the radiographic projection of the ankles is not a true anteroposterior view on account of the tibial torsion).

Contribution to hip instability in potentially unstable hips

In developmental dysplasia of the hip and in paralytic hip dislocations of cerebral palsy, polio and spina bifida, one of the factors contributing to the instability of the hip in some cases is increased femoral anteversion. Hence the differentiation between idiopathic and pathologic anteversion is very important. If the anteversion is associated with developmental hip dysplasia or paralytic hip dysplasia then the therapy must follow the guidelines for that particular problem and correction of the anteversion constitutes only one part of the overall treatment.

Aims of treatment

- Improve cosmesis of gait
  If the gait is so unsightly as to cause concern to the child, correction of the anteversion may be considered.
- Relieve anterior knee pain in the miserable malalignment syndrome
  In this relatively rare situation, the aim of treatment is to relieve the child's anterior knee pain by improving the normal anatomic relationship between the femur and tibia with respect to torsion.
- Improve stability of the unstable hip
  In situations where the increased femoral anteversion is contributing to hip instability, the stability needs to be improved by correcting the anteversion.

Treatment options

Observation

Observation of the in-toeing gait is the most widely selected option. Since the natural history is one of gradual resolution, the aim of observing the child over time is to simply document this natural improvement. Shoe wear modifications (wedges), orthotics (Denis Browne splints or twister cables) and physiotherapy have no effect on the natural history of the disorder.[9,10]

Rotational osteotomy

This is the only method by which the abnormal bony torsion can be corrected. Since most children do not demonstrate functional deficits, it is rarely indicated. Similarly, since most children resolve their in-toeing gait by mid- to late childhood, osteotomy is not indicated until the child has passed the age beyond which spontaneous resolution will no longer occur, typically 10–12 years of age.[11–13]

At this age the child can also become involved in the discussion and decision-making regarding the significantly invasive treatment of osteotomy and the expected rehabilitation and outcome.

If the diagnosis is simple femoral anteversion, then femoral rotational osteotomy is indicated in the child over 10 or 12 years of age if internal rotation is ≥80° and external rotation is ≤10°, and if there are associated functional issues. These can be difficult to sort out from the cosmetic concerns of the parents. Consultation with teachers and athletic coaches can sometimes be helpful.

The osteotomy can be performed at the intertrochanteric level with blade-plate fixation, at the mid-diaphysis with intramedullary nail fixation or at the distal metaphyseal level with dynamic compression plate fixation. The type of fixation depends upon the surgeon's familiarity with the fixation technique, whether the proximal femoral physes are closed or open, and the role of potential patellofemoral abnormalities.

If the proximal femoral physes are still open, rigid antegrade intramedullary nailing is contraindicated due to the risk of avascular necrosis of the femoral head. In children with open proximal femoral physes, the majority of the osteotomies will be performed at the proximal level, usually intertrochanteric with blade-plate type of fixation.

If there are significant patellofemoral malalignment issues, and if they can be corrected by a more distal osteotomy, then the procedure should occur at that level.

In the presence of the miserable malalignment syndrome, tibial rotational osteotomy should also be performed (Figure 18.3). This is performed at the supramalleolar level unless there is an associated proximal tibial varus or valgus angular deformity (see Chapter 12, Tibial torsion).[6–8]

Femoral osteotomy for medial torsion is not a benign procedure, with complication rates of around 15 percent. These complications include infection, avascular necrosis, loss of fixation, nonunion, malunion and nerve palsies.[14,15]

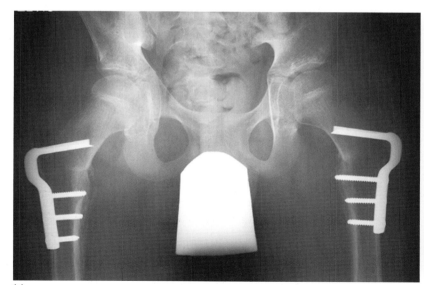
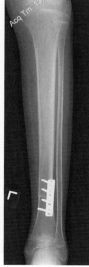

Figure 18.3 ● Radiographs of the child in Figure 18.2 who underwent bilateral femoral **(a)** and tibial **(b)** rotational osteotomies. The femoral neck–shaft angle appears normal, indicating correction of the anteversion of the femur. The knee and ankle joints also appear properly oriented indicating correction of the external tibial torsion.

(a)   (b)

Pre-operative assessment

Differentiating between idiopathic and associated disorders

This is the most important factor to consider. If the abnormal femoral torsion is associated with an underlying pathologic process (e.g. hip dysplasia, cerebral palsy, developmental coxa vara) then the treatment must address the primary pathology.

Anatomic location of torsional pathology

It is important to emphasize that there are several causes for in-toeing and the torsional abnormality is at a different site in each condition. Hence it is imperative that the site of the torsional pathology is clearly identified.

The torsional profile is used to determine the location of the torsional abnormality which causes the in-toeing gait. The torsional profile consists of four components[12]: gait progression, hip rotation, thigh–foot angle and foot border profiles. The gait progression angle simply describes the deviation of the child's gait from a straight ahead pattern; a negative angle indicates an in-toeing gait, and a positive angle indicates an out-toeing gait relative to a completely straight ahead gait. Passive hip rotation assessment involves measurement of both internal and external rotation; as femoral anteversion increases, internal rotation increases at the expense of external rotation. The passive ranges of hip rotation measured with the hips in extension and also in flexion can be recorded on a grid[16] for documenting change in the movement as the child grows (Figure 18.4). The thigh–foot angle indicates the amount of tibial torsion; an external thigh–foot angle indicates relative external tibial torsion, while an internal thigh–foot angle indicates relative internal tibial torsion. This is extremely important when the physician is considering the possibility of a miserable malalignment syndrome. The foot borders indicate whether there is a torsional component from the foot itself. A concave medial border indicates the likelihood of metatarsus adductus; a concave lateral border indicates the likelihood of a significant pes valgus.

Factors to be taken into consideration while planning treatment

Age of the child

If the child is young, there is ample time to observe the maturation and changes of gait during growth. If the child is in their early teens or older, there will probably be much less natural resolution, which will impact on the selected treatment.

State of the proximal femoral physes

If a decision has been made to perform a derotation osteotomy, the choice of the technique will be influenced by the status of the physes. If the proximal femoral physes are still open, rigid antegrade nailing would not be considered as the method of internal fixation.

The presence of patellar malalignment

If there is evidence of patellar maltracking and realignment of the patella is indicated, a distal femoral osteotomy is preferred to a proximal femoral osteotomy.

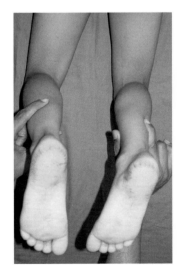

Figure 18.4 ● Clinical assessment of the torsional profile which includes measurement of tibial torsion **(a)** and passive rotation of the hips is done with the child lying prone. The ranges of internal rotation **(b)** and external rotation **(c)** of the hips are recorded and can be marked on a grid **(d)**.

(a)

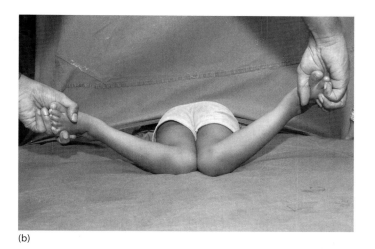

(b)

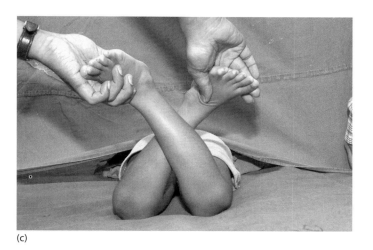

(c)

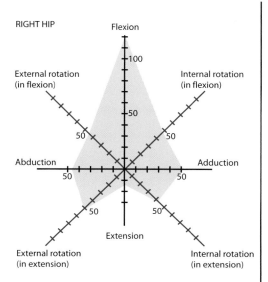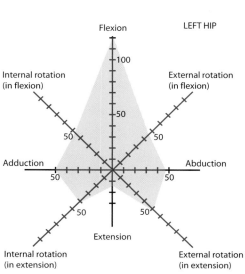

(d)

Recommended treatment

The recommended outline of treatment of femoral anteversion is shown in Table 18.1.

Table 18.1 ● Treatment of femoral anteversion

INDICATIONS					
Bilateral idiopathic femoral anteversion in a child OR Miserable malalignment syndrome + <10 years of age	Bilateral idiopathic femoral anteversion in a child >10 years of age + Unacceptable in-toeing + External rotation of the hip <10°	Miserable malalignment syndrome in a child >10 years of age + No patellar instability	Miserable malalignment syndrome in a child >10 years of age + Patellar instability warranting patellar stabilization	Unilateral OR bilateral femoral anteversion + Hip instability (congenital or paralytic)	Unilateral OR bilateral femoral anteversion + Coxa valga + Hip instability (congenital or paralytic)
⇩	⇩	⇩	⇩	⇩	⇩
Observe for resolution	Intertrochanteric derotation osteotomy (avoid rigid intramedullary (IM) nail if proximal femoral physes are still open)	Intertrochanteric derotation osteotomy (avoid rigid IM nail if proximal femoral physes are still open) + Supramalleolar tibial internal rotation osteotomy	Supracondylar femoral derotation osteotomy + Patellar realignment + Supramalleolar tibial internal rotation osteotomy	Intertrochanteric OR Subtrochanteric derotation osteotomy + Hip stabilization procedure	Intertrochanteric OR Subtrochanteric derotation combined with varus osteotomy + Hip stabilization procedure
TREATMENT					

References

1. Shands Jr AR, Steele MK. Torsion of the femur. A follow-up report on the use of the Dunlap method for its determination. *J Bone Joint Surg Am* 1958; **40**: 803–16.
2. Staheli LT, Lippert F, Denotter P. Femoral anterversion and physical performance in adolescent and adult life. *Clin Orthop Relat Res* 1977; **129**: 213–16.
3. Hubbard DD, Staheli LT, Chew DE, Mosca VS. Medial femoral torsion and osteoarthritis. *J Pediatr Orthop* 1988; **8**: 540–2.
4. Svenningsen S, Apalset K, Terjesen T, Anda S. Regression of femoral anteversion. A prospective study of intoeing children. *Acta Orthop Scand* 1989; **60**: 170–3.
5. Staheli LT, Corbett M, Wyss C, King H. Lower-extremity rotational problems in children. *J Bone Joint Surg Am* 1985; **67**: 39–47.
6. Bruce WD, Stevens PM. Surgical correction of miserable malalignment syndrome. *J Pediatr Orthop* 2004; **24**: 392–6.
7. Delgado ED, Schoenecker PL, Rich MM, Capelli AM. Treatment of severe torsional malalignment syndrome. *J Pediatr Orthop* 1996; **16**: 484–8.
8. Cooke TDV, Price N, Fisher B, Hedden D. The inwardly pointing knee. An unrecognized problem of external rotational malalignment. *Clin Orthop Relat Res* 1990; **260**: 56–60.
9. Fabry G, MacEwen GD, Shands Jr AR. Torsion of the femur. A follow-up study in normal and abnormal conditions. *J Bone Joint Surg Am* 1973; **55**: 1726–38.
10. Knittel G, Staheli LT. The effectiveness of shoe modifications for intoeing. *Orthop Clin North Am* 1976; **7**: 1019–25.
11. Staheli LT. Rotational problems in children. *J Bone Joint Surg Am* 1993; **75**: 939–49.
12. Staheli LT. Torsional deformity. *Pediatr Clin North Am* 1977; **24**: 799–811.
13. Shim JS, Staheli LT, Holm BN. Surgical correction of idiopathic medial femoral torsion. *Int Orthop* 1995; **19**: 220–3.
14. Staheli LT, Clawson DK, Hubbard DD. Medial femoral torsion: experience with operative treatment. *Clin Orthop Relat Res* 1980; **146**: 222–5.
15. Svenningsen S, Apalset K, Terjesen T, Anda S. Osteotomy for femoral anteversion. Complications in 95 children. *Acta Orthop Scand* 1989; **60**: 401–5.
16. Rao KN, Joseph B. Value of measurement of hip movements in childhood hip disorders. *J Pediatr Orthop* 2001; **21**: 495–501.

Cubitus varus and valgus

Benjamin Joseph

19

Introduction

Abnormally high or low carrying angles with obvious cubitus valgus or varus are seen in children with sex chromosomal anomalies. In general, children with chromosomal anomalies that result in short stature have higher carrying angles whereas those with a tall stature have low carrying angles.[1] Cubitus valgus is most marked in the XO phenotype and cubitus varus is seen with multiple supernumerary sex chromosomes (Figure 19.1). Cubitus varus and valgus are seen more commonly following trauma, disease or as part of a congenital anomaly affecting the distal humerus.

The commonest cause of cubitus varus is malunion of a supracondylar fracture. It can also develop following damage to the distal humeral growth plate. Very occasionally, a varus deformity may develop following a lateral humeral condylar fracture.[2] Developmental cubitus varus can occur in skeletal dysplasias and in children with hereditary multiple osteochondromatosis.[3]

Cubitus valgus frequently follows lateral condylar fractures of the humerus and may be seen in some skeletal dysplasias. It is also often seen in association with nail–patella syndrome. The deformity in nail–patella syndrome can be quite severe on account of hypoplasia of the lateral humeral condyle and the radial head[4] that are characteristic of this condition.

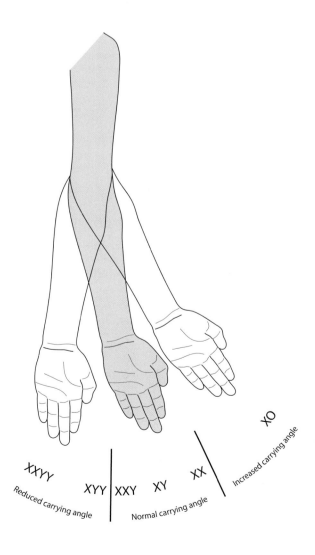

Figure 19.1 ● The carrying angle in sex chromosomal anomalies.

Problems of management

Cosmetic defect

Since cubitus varus and valgus do not limit elbow function unless the deformity is so severe as to make the joint unstable, the main issue in most instances is that of an unacceptable appearance. The deformity is particularly conspicuous if it is unilateral and of a moderate or severe degree (Figure 19.2).

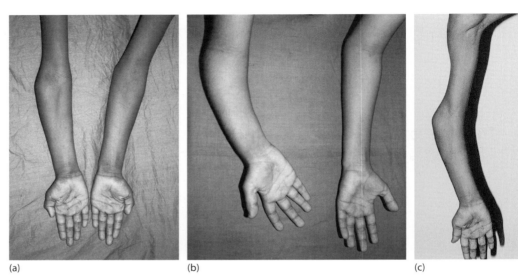

(a) (b) (c)

Figure 19.2 ● Examples of mild **(a)**, moderate **(b)** and severe **(c)** unilateral cubitus varus; the causes include malunion of a supracondylar fracture **(a and c)** and hereditary multiple osteochondromatosis **(b)**. The moderate and severe deformities warrant correction.

Progression of the deformity and nerve damage

Cubitus valgus due to non-union of a lateral condylar fracture is progressive. Over a period of time it may become severe enough to stretch the ulnar nerve as it courses over the elbow and cause tardy ulnar nerve palsy. Surprisingly, cubitus varus has also been implicated as predisposing to tardy ulnar nerve palsy due to recurrent subluxation of the nerve and entrapment neuropathy.[5]

Progression of deformity and joint instability

If progressive cubitus varus or valgus become very severe, instability of the elbow may ensue. Apart from the instability in the coronal plane, two other forms of instability may develop following cubitus varus. Long-standing cubitus varus can result in tardy rotatory instability of the elbow[6] and recurrent posterior dislocation of the radial head. The latter problem usually follows a fresh episode of trauma.[7] These reports suggest that cubitus varus may not be merely a cosmetic problem and highlight the need to correct the deformity to prevent complications that may arise in the long term.

Predilection for lateral condylar fracture following cubitus varus

Children with uncorrected cubitus varus appear to be more prone to develop fractures of the lateral condyle of the humerus if they fall on the outstretched arm.[8] This has been attributed to altered anatomy resulting in abnormal stresses on the lateral condyle.

Aims of treatment

- Improve cosmetic appearance
  The majority of children with cubitus varus present for treatment because the parents are concerned about the appearance. Surgery to improve the appearance is justified if the deformity is unilateral; however, correction of bilateral cubitus varus in a child with a chromosomal

abnormality is not. The parents need to be reminded that a scar will be created and this itself may mar the appearance. Most correction techniques for cubitus varus employ incisions on the lateral aspect or the posterior aspect of the elbow and both these regions are exposed areas that are very visible. A simple closed wedge osteotomy of the distal radius produces a prominence on the lateral aspect of the elbow and, again, this may look unsightly.[9] Several modifications of the osteotomy that attempt to minimize the lateral prominence have been described in the literature.

- Prevent or limit nerve damage
  The risk of nerve damage is far greater with cubitus valgus and therefore correction of cubitus valgus should be undertaken early.
- Prevent or correct joint instability
  Progressive cubitus varus and valgus should be corrected before the deformities become severe and lead to joint instability.

Treatment options for cubitus varus

If correction of the deformity is considered necessary, an osteotomy is needed. The type of osteotomy, the surgical approach and the type of fixation may vary.

Lateral closed wedge osteotomy

A simple closed wedge osteotomy fixed with wires or screws, which corrects the varus angulation, has been widely used. One criticism of this osteotomy is that it creates a lateral prominence that is ugly.[9] However, not all patients are aware of the prominence and many do not consider it to be ugly.[10] Although most surgeons use a lateral approach when performing this operation, the very visible scar on the outer aspect of the elbow can be avoided by using a medial approach.[11]

Lateral closed wedge osteotomy with medial displacement

If, in addition to performing a closed wedge osteotomy the distal fragment is displaced medially, the prominence on the lateral aspect of the elbow is minimized (Figure 19.3).

Medial open wedge osteotomy with gradual correction with the help of an external fixator

Gradual correction of the deformity with the help of an external fixator can be done by opening out a wedge medially. The advantages are that the prominence on the lateral aspect of the elbow seen after a lateral closed wedge osteotomy is avoided and the scar will be obscured from view as it will be on the medial aspect of the elbow.

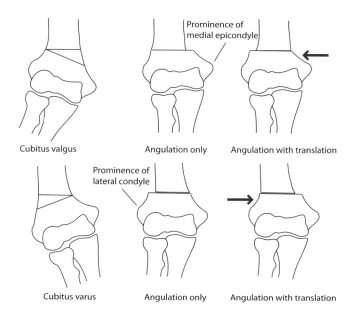

Figure 19.3 ● Diagram showing how translation of the distal fragment improves the appearance when closed wedge osteotomies for correction of cubitus varus and valgus are performed.

Corrective osteotomy

A simple closed wedge osteotomy will result in prominence of the medial epicondyle, and lateral translation of the distal fragment is recommended so this may be avoided.[12] The osteotomy may be done in conjunction with internal fixation and bone grafting if there is an associated non-union of the lateral condyle.

Ulnar nerve transposition

If any symptoms or objective signs of ulnar nerve stretch are present, transposition of the ulnar nerve to the front of the elbow is necessary. This relaxes the nerve and further progression of neurological deficit is prevented. There is no consensus on whether prophylactic ulnar nerve transposition is necessary in all children with cubitus valgus.

Factors to be taken into consideration while planning treatment

Is the deformity progressive?

If there has been progression of the deformity there is a risk of recurrence following correction. One way to avoid recurrence is to wait until skeletal maturity to correct the deformity. However, this may result in severe deformity and may put the ulnar nerve at risk. The second option is to correct the deformity and monitor the patient to see whether the deformity recurs.

Is there associated nerve damage that can be attributed to the deformity?

Surgical correction of the deformity must be undertaken as soon as impairment of nerve function is detected.

How severe is the deformity?

If the deformity is severe an attempt must be made to avoid prominence of the condyle following corrective osteotomy by displacing the distal fragment appropriately.

Recommended treatment

An outline of treatment of cubitus varus and valgus is shown in Table 19.1.

Table 19.1 ● Outline of treatment of cubitus varus and valgus

INDICATIONS				
Bilateral cubitus varus or valgus in child with chromosomal anomaly	Unilateral cubitus varus or valgus + Mild deformity + No risk of progression (no growth plate damage) + Parents or child very concerned about deformity	Unilateral cubitus varus or valgus + Moderate or severe deformity + No risk of progression (no growth plate damage)	Unilateral cubitus varus or valgus + Mild or moderate deformity + Progression present (growth plate damage present)	Unilateral cubitus valgus + Impairment of ulnar nerve function
⇩	⇩	⇩	⇩	⇩
No intervention	Closed wedge supracondylar osteotomy	Closed wedge supracondylar osteotomy + Displacement of distal fragment (medially while correcting varus OR laterally while correcting valgus)	Defer surgery until close to skeletal maturity and follow guidelines as in column 2 or 3 *Intervene earlier if deformity becomes severe or if joint instability develops*	Early corrective osteotomy as in column 2 or 3 depending on severity of the deformity + Anterior transposition of ulnar nerve
TREATMENT				

References

1. Baughman FA Jr, Higgins JV, Wadsworth TG, Demaray MJ. The carrying angle in sex chromosome anomalies. *JAMA* 1974; **230**: 718–20.
2. So YC, Fang D, Leong JC, Bong SC. Varus deformity following lateral humeral condylar fractures in children. *J Pediatr Orthop* 1985; **5**: 569–72.
3. Joseph B. Elbow problems in children. In: Gupta A, Kay SPJ, Scheker LR (eds). *The Growing Hand*. London: Harcourt, 2000: 769–82.
4. Sharrard WJW. *Paediatric Orthopaedics and Fractures*, 3rd edn. Oxford: Blackwell Scientific, 1993: 152–3.
5. Abe M, Ishizu T, Shirai H, Okamoto M, Onomura T. Tardy ulnar nerve palsy caused by cubitus varus deformity. *J Hand Surg Am* 1995; **20**: 5–9.
6. O'Driscoll SW, Spinner RJ, McKee MD *et al.* Tardy posterolateral rotatory instability of the elbow due to cubitus varus. *J Bone Joint Surg Am* 2001; **83**: 1358–69.
7. Abe M, Ishizu T, Nagaoka T, Onomura T. Recurrent posterior dislocation of the head of the radius in post-traumatic cubitus varus. *J Bone Joint Surg Br* 1995; **77**: 582–5.
8. Davids JR, Maguire MF, Mubarak SJ, Wenger DR. Lateral condylar fracture of the humerus following posttraumatic cubitus varus. *J Pediatr Orthop* 1994; **14**: 466–70.
9. Wong HK, Lee EH, Balasubramaniam P. The lateral condylar prominence: a complication of supracondylar osteotomy for cubitus varus. *J Bone Joint Surg Br* 1990; **72**: 859–61.
10. Barrett IR, Bellemore MC, Kwon YM. Cosmetic results of supracondylar osteotomy for correction of cubitus varus. *J Pediatr Orthop* 1998; **18**: 445–7.
11. Hui JH, Torode IP, Chatterjee A. Medial approach for corrective osteotomy of cubitus varus: a cosmetic incision. *J Pediatr Orthop* 2004; **24**: 477–81.
12. Lins RE, Waters PM. Fractures and dislocations of the elbow. In: Gupta A, Kay SPJ, Scheker LR (eds). *The Growing Hand*. London: Harcourt, 2000: 545–66.

Varus and valgus deformity of the wrist

Benjamin Joseph

20

Introduction

Varus and valgus deformities of the wrist are relatively uncommon. Severe radial deviation of the wrist (valgus deformity) is characteristically seen in children with radial club hand (see Chapter 39, Radial club hand) and severe ulnar deviation (varus deformity) is seen in children with ulnar club hand (see Chapter 40, Ulnar club hand). Less severe deformities of the wrist may develop due to abnormal growth at the distal radial physis or secondary to disparity in lengths of the radius and ulna (Figure 20.1). These mechanisms lead to a varus deformity of the wrist in children with hereditary multiple osteochondromatosis and as part of Madelung's deformity. These two conditions are discussed in greater detail in this chapter.

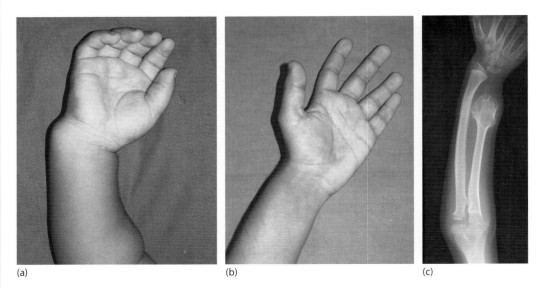

(a)   (b)   (c)

Figure 20.1 ● Valgus deformity of the wrist in a child with skeletal dysplasia **(a)**; varus deformity of the wrist in a child with hereditary multiple osteochondromatosis **(b)**; and radiograph of forearm of a child with hereditary multiple osteochondromatosis showing the ulna with an osteochondroma in the distal metaphysis **(c)**. The ulna is short but the radial head is not dislocated.

Deformity of the wrist in hereditary multiple osteochondromatosis

Osteochondromata can interfere with normal linear growth of long bones. In the upper limb, deformities of wrist, forearm and elbow may develop in children with hereditary multiple osteochondromatosis.[1–5] The pattern of deformities is determined by the location of the osteochondroma[5] (Table 20.1). Among the different deformities that may develop, varus deformity of the wrist is common; valgus deformity is less frequently seen. The primary cause of varus deformity of

Table 20.1 ● Patterns of deformities of the forearm and wrist in hereditary multiple osteochondromatosis

Site of osteochondroma	Deformity
Distal ulna	Short ulna – moderate or severe shortening
	Tilt of distal radial articular surface
	Bowing of the radius
	Late dislocation of the radial head
Distal radius	Mild shortening of radius
	Mild valgus deformity of the wrist
Proximal radius	Early dislocation of the radial head
Proximal radius and distal ulna	Early dislocation of the radial head
	Short ulna

the wrist is disproportionate shortening of the ulna as a result of growth arrest due to an osteochondroma situated on the distal ulna. The short ulna, in turn, causes compensatory deformities of the less severely affected radius. These secondary radial deformities include diaphyseal bowing and ulnar deviation of the distal articular surface. In addition, the radial head may dislocate. While the wrist deformity may be the most obvious, the abnormalities of the entire limb including the forearm, elbow and wrist need to be addressed if the appearance and function of the limb are to improve.

Problems of management

Shortened ulna
The primary cause of varus deformity at the wrist is the short ulna.

Ulnar deviation of the distal radial articular surface
This develops later and aggravates the varus deformity of the wrist.

Carpal slip
As the inclination of the articular surface increases, the carpus begins to slip ulnarwards.

Bowing of the radius
The disparity in lengths of the radius and ulna results in bowing of the shaft of the radius. The severity of bowing appears to be related to the extent of ulnar shortening. However, the radial bow is less severe if the radial head dislocates.

Limitation of pronation
Loss of pronation of the forearm may develop.

Subluxation or dislocation of the radial head
In a proportion of children the radial head dislocates; initially, the dislocation may not cause any symptoms but pain may develop later. It has been suggested that the risk of radial head dislocation is high if shortening of the ulna exceeds 8 percent.[6]

Aims of treatment

- Improve the appearance of the limb
  Often children are only concerned about the appearance of the deformed wrist and forearm and complain of little functional disability. In these children an attempt must be made to improve the appearance of the limb.[2]
- Relieve pain
  If pain develops following radial head dislocation the pain must be relieved.
- Restore motion
  Usually wrist and elbow motion is near normal in these children; however, pronation may be quite significantly restricted.[2] Although it is desirable to improve pronation, a great deal of improvement in the range of motion cannot be expected[2] and hence it is important that the child and the parents are informed about this prior to surgery.

Treatment options

Hemiepiphyseal stapling of the distal radial epiphysis
Stapling of the radial side of the distal radial epiphysis has been recommended as a means of correcting the abnormal inclination of the radial articular surface.[1–3] However, as Masada *et al.*[5] point out, this will further shorten the forearm.

Excision of osteochondroma of the distal ulna
It is generally accepted that the distal ulnar osteochondroma is responsible for the retarded growth of the ulna and, consequently, all surgeons advocate excision of this offending osteochondroma.

Radial osteotomy

Masada *et al.*[5] have demonstrated significant improvement of the tilt of the articular surface and the carpal slip by performing a corrective osteotomy of the distal radius. The advantage of this operation over epiphyseal stapling is that further shortening of the radius will not occur.

Acute lengthening of the ulna

Acute lengthening of the ulna can be done either by doing a step cut osteotomy of the ulna, manually distracting the fragments and fixing the fragments in the distracted position with screws[1] or by a transverse osteotomy and an intercalary graft (Figure 20.2).

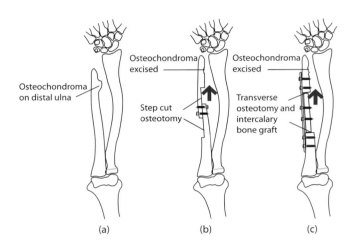

Figure 20.2 ● Osteochondroma on distal ulna **(a)**. Techniques of acute lengthening of the ulna. No graft is required when a step cut osteotomy is performed **(b)**, but an intercalary graft is required when a transverse osteotomy is performed **(c)**.

Gradual lengthening of the ulna

Gradual lengthening of the ulna can be performed with the help of an external fixator (see Chapter 48, Discrepancies of length in the forearm). The author prefers to use a monolateral fixator as mounting it on the subcutaneous ulna is easy (Figure 20.3).

Excision of the head of the radius

Excision of the radial head is reserved for the chronically dislocated radial head that has become painful. Ideally, this operation should be delayed until skeletal maturity is almost reached.

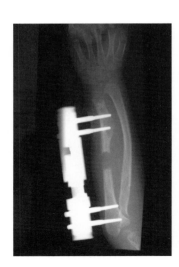

Figure 20.3 ● Radiograph of a child with hereditary multiple osteochondromatosis undergoing lengthening of the ulna with a monolateral fixator.

Factors to be taken into consideration while planning treatment

Location of the offending osteochondroma

An osteochondroma located at the metaphyseal region of the distal ulna needs to be excised if progression of the deformity is to be arrested.

Extent of shortening of the ulna

When shortening of the ulna approaches 8 percent there is a risk of radial head subluxation. Restoring the length of the ulna at this stage could prevent the radial head from subluxating.

Inclination of the distal radial articular surface and carpal slip

Tilt of the distal radial articular surface in excess of 30° and carpal slip greater than 60 percent have been suggested as indications for surgical intervention.[1]

Presence of pain

Pain from a dislocated radial head requires early surgical intervention.

Age of the child

Radial head excision should be deferred until adolescence if possible.

Recommended treatment

The outline of treatment of varus deformity of the wrist in hereditary multiple osteochondromatosis is shown in Table 20.2.

In a child with an osteochondroma in the distal radius and shortening of the radius with a valgus deformity of the wrist, excision of the radial osteochondroma is recommended.

Table 20.2 ● Outline of treatment of varus deformity of the wrist and the associated problems in hereditary multiple osteochondromatosis

INDICATIONS					
Distal ulnar osteochondroma present + No ulnar shortening + No tilt of distal radial articular surface + No carpal slip ⇩ Observation	Distal ulnar osteochondroma present + Ulnar shortening <8% + Tilt of distal radial articular surface <30° + Carpal slip <60% ⇩ Excision of ulnar osteochondroma	Distal ulnar osteochondroma present + Ulnar shortening approaching 8% + Tilt of distal radial articular surface <30° + Carpal slip <60% ⇩ Excision of ulnar osteochondroma + Gradual lengthening of the ulna	Distal ulnar osteochondroma present + Ulnar shortening <8% + Tilt of distal radial articular surface >30° + Carpal slip <60% ⇩ Excision of ulnar osteochondroma + Gradual lengthening of the ulna + Distal radial osteotomy	Distal ulnar osteochondroma present + Ulnar shortening >8% + Radial head subluxating OR Radial head dislocation of recent onset ⇩ Excision of ulnar osteochondroma + Gradual lengthening of the ulna + Indirect reduction of radial head	Distal ulnar osteochondroma present + Ulnar shortening >8% + Long-standing radial head dislocation + Pain in elbow + Adolescent ⇩ Excision of the radial head
TREATMENT					

Rationale of treatment suggested

Why is gradual lengthening of the ulna preferred to acute lengthening?
Gradual lengthening will enable the surgeon to lengthen the requisite amount precisely, while the amount of lengthening that can be achieved by acute lengthening will be determined by the soft tissue tension. Furthermore, no internal fixation or bone grafting is required when gradual lengthening is performed.

Why is a distal radial osteotomy preferred to hemiepiphyseal stapling to correct tilt of the distal articular surface of the radius and carpal slip?
Complete correction of the deformity can be obtained by an osteotomy of the radius, whereas a hemiepiphyseodesis is less predictable. The epiphyseodesis will result in further shortening of the forearm, which to begin with is usually shorter than normal.

The wrist in Madelung deformity

Madelung deformity is a rare entity caused by an inherited condition called dyschondrosteosis which is transmitted by an autosomal dominant gene.[7] The deformity at the wrist is due to an abnormality of growth of the ulnar half of the distal radial physis brought about by a soft tissue tether.[7] The soft tissue tether is usually a strong abnormal ligament that links the proximal pole of the lunate to the palmar and ulnar cortex of the distal radius.

The deformity in classical Madelung deformity is an ulnar and volar deviation of the wrist with prominence of the lower end of the ulna. However, there are variants, such as reverse Madelung deformity and the 'chevron carpus'.[8] The nature of the deformity depends on the exact site of physeal arrest (Table 20.3). The deformity is more frequently seen in girls, usually appearing at around 12 years of age and gradually progressing until skeletal maturity.

Table 20.3 ● Pattern of deformity in Madelung deformity and its variants

Type	Site of physeal growth arrest	Deformity
Madelung deformity	Ulnar and volar part of physis	Ulnar tilt of articular surface of radius
		Volar tilt of articular surface of radius
		Dorsal prominence of ulna
		Instability of inferior radio-ulnar joint
Reverse Madelung deformity	Ulnar and dorsal part of physis	Ulnar tilt of articular surface of radius
		Dorsal tilt of articular surface of radius
		Volar prominence of ulna
		Instability of inferior radio-ulnar joint
Chevron carpus	Ulnar and central part of the physis	Little or no deformity of wrist
		Wedge-shaped carpus
		No instability of inferior radio-ulnar joint

Problems of management

Deformity

The prominence of the distal end of the ulna is what draws the attention of most patients initially. In late untreated cases obvious deformity of the wrist is also evident.

Instability of the wrist and the inferior radio-ulnar joint

Instability of the inferior radio–ulnar joint develops if treatment is delayed.

Pain

Pain after physical exertion is often an early feature in Madelung deformity; pain is most severe in children with a chevron carpus.

Aims of treatment

- Prevent progression of the deformity
- Correct pre-existing deformity
- Relieve pain

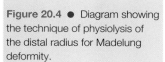

Treatment options

Physiolysis

Early physiolysis has been recommended by Vickers and Nielsen,[7,8] who have shown that the procedure can arrest progression of the deformity and restore normal growth of the radius quite effectively (Figure 20.4). The operation entails resection of a sliver of bone from the ulnar aspect of the distal radius, identifying the growth plate, ensuring that any bone bridge is removed and placing fat graft astride the growth plate to prevent a bridge from reforming. A volar approach is used for Madelung deformity while a dorsal approach is used for reverse Madelung deformity in order to gain the best access to the site of physeal arrest.

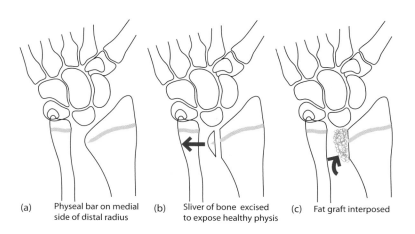

(a) Physeal bar on medial side of distal radius   (b) Sliver of bone excised to expose healthy physis   (c) Fat graft interposed

Figure 20.4 ● Diagram showing the technique of physiolysis of the distal radius for Madelung deformity.

Resection of the soft tissue tether

Resection of the soft tissue tether should be done whenever physiolysis is undertaken. The wrist joint has to be opened as the abnormal ligament is attached to the lunate. When done in conjunction with physiolysis, the entire ligament can be followed to its proximal attachment to the radius and excised. When mere excision of the tether is performed for a chevron carpus, excision of 1 cm of the ligament should suffice.[8]

Corrective osteotomy of the distal radius

An established deformity in a long-standing case can be improved by an osteotomy of the distal radius.[9]

In classical Madelung deformity a dorsal- and lateral-based wedge of bone is excised from the distal radius close to the articular surface. In reverse Madelung deformity the wedge must be volar- and lateral-based (Figure 20.5).

Excision of the distal ulna

Excision of the distal ulna can remove the unsightly prominence in the older patient with established deformity. This may be combined with the osteotomy of the distal radius.

Factors to be taken into consideration while planning treatment

Age of the child

If the child has sufficient growth remaining, a procedure that attempts to restore normal growth may be tried. However, after skeletal maturity the aim is to correct any established deformity.

Pattern of deformity

The approach and the type of correction vary depending on whether the deformity is a Madelung deformity, a reverse Madelung deformity or a chevron carpus.

Severity of deformity

If the deformity is mild in a skeletally immature child, surgery may be directed to preventing progression. On the other hand, more severe deformity needs to be corrected.

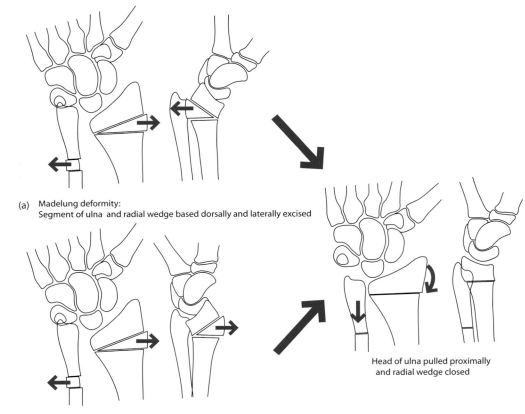

(a) Madelung deformity:
Segment of ulna and radial wedge based dorsally and laterally excised

(b) Reverse Madelung deformity:
Segment of ulna and radial wedge based ventrally and laterally excised

Head of ulna pulled proximally
and radial wedge closed

Figure 20.5 ● Diagram showing the techniques of distal radial osteotomy for Madelung **(a)** and reverse Madelung deformity **(b)**.

Recommended treatment

The recommended treatment is shown in Table 20.4.

Table 20.4 ● Outline of treatment of Madelung deformity and its variants

INDICATIONS					
Madelung deformity pattern + Skeletally immature + Wrist deformity mild	Reverse Madelung deformity pattern + Skeletally immature + Wrist deformity mild	Chevron wrist deformity pattern + Skeletally immature + Wrist deformity mild	Any pattern of deformity + Skeletally immature + Wrist deformity moderate	Madelung deformity pattern + Skeletally mature ± Pain ⇩	Reverse Madelung deformity pattern + Skeletally mature ± Pain ⇩
					Volar and radial based closed wedge osteotomy + Excision of the lower end of ulna
			⇩	Dorsal and radial based closed wedge osteotomy + Excision of the lower end of ulna	
		⇩	Corrective osteotomy of distal radius + Respective treatment as in column 1, 2 or 3		
⇩	⇩	Excision of soft tissue tether ONLY			
Excision of soft tissue tether + Physiolysis via a volar approach	Excision of soft tissue tether + Physiolysis via a dorsal approach				
TREATMENT					

References

1. Fogel GR, McElfresh EC, Peterson HA, Wicklund PT. Management of deformities of the forearm in multiple hereditary osteochondromas. *J Bone Joint Surg Am* 1984; **66**: 670–80.

2. Wood VE, Sauser D, Mudge D. The treatment of hereditary multiple exostosis of the upper extremity. *J Hand Surg* 1985; **10**: 505–13.

3. Siffert RS, Levy RN. Correction of wrist deformity in diaphyseal aclasis by stapling. Report of a case. *J Bone Joint Surg Am* 1965; **47**: 1378–80.

4. Pritchett JW. Lengthening of the ulna in patients with hereditary multiple exostosis. *J Bone Joint Surg Br* 1986; **68**: 561–5.

5. Masada K, Tsuyuguchi Y, Kawai H *et al.* Operations for forearm deformity caused by multiple osteochondromas. *J Bone Joint Surg Br* 1989; **71**: 24–9.

6. Burgess RC, Cates H. Deformities of the forearm in patients who have multiple cartilaginous exostosis. *J Bone Joint Surg Am* 1993; **75**: 13–18.

7. Vickers DW. Madelung deformity. In: Gupta A, Kay SPJ, Scheker LR (eds). *The Growing Hand*. London: Harcourt, 2000: 791–8.

8. Vickers D, Nielsen G. Madelung deformity: Surgical prophylaxis (physiolysis) during the late growth period by resection of the dyschondrosteosis lesion. *J Hand Surg Br* 1992; **17**; 401–7.

9. Ranawat CS, DeFiore J, Straub LR. Madelung's deformity. An end-result study of surgical treatment. *J Bone Joint Surg Am* 1975; **57**: 772–5.

Scoliosis

Ian Torode

21

Introduction

A scoliotic deformity of the spine can be defined as one where the principal deformity is in the coronal plane. The deformity, however, is commonly more complex with deformity components in the sagittal and transverse planes (Figure 21.1). In idiopathic scoliotic curves in particular, the deformity in the transverse plane is of major importance.

Since the clinical evaluation and treatment differs depending on the aetiology of the deformity, idiopathic, neuromuscular and congenital scoliosis are considered separately.

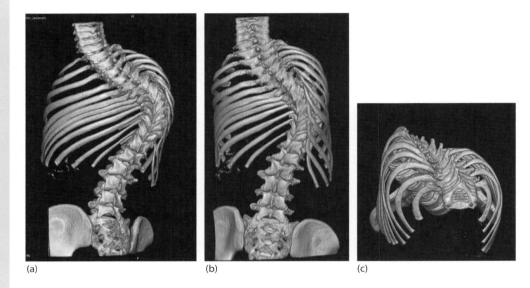

(a)　　　　　　　　(b)　　　　　　　　(c)

Figure 21.1 ●　(a–c) 3-D CT reconstruction images of a case of severe scoliosis showing that there are components of the deformity in the coronal, sagittal and transverse planes.

Idiopathic scoliosis

Classification

Idiopathic scoliosis is commonly classified according to age at onset and the anatomical location of the curves; the apex of the curve being the point of reference (Figure 21.2).

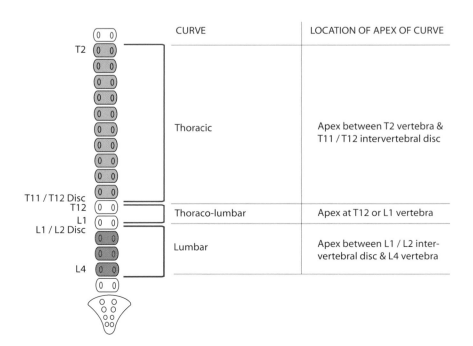

CURVE	LOCATION OF APEX OF CURVE
Thoracic	Apex between T2 vertebra & T11 / T12 intervertebral disc
Thoraco-lumbar	Apex at T12 or L1 vertebra
Lumbar	Apex between L1 / L2 intervertebral disc & L4 vertebra

Figure 21.2 ● Classification of scoliosis on the basis of the location of the apex of the curve suggested by the Scoliosis Research Society.

Three categories of deformity based on the age at onset have been defined:

- Infantile – onset up to three years of age
- Juvenile – onset three to ten years of age
- Adolescent – onset after ten years of age.

Alternatively, the onset may be described as *early* (includes infantile and juvenile) or *late*. However, the difference in behaviour of infantile curves, treated early as described by Mehta,[1] justifies considering those children as a separate group.

Infantile idiopathic scoliosis

The incidence is uncommon and may represent less than 1 percent of all idiopathic curves.[2] The deformity is commonly a left thoracic curve and is seen more frequently in boys. There is an associated incidence of plagiocephaly and hip dysplasia and, because these curves commonly resolve, the possibility exists that this is a positional deformity.

Problems of management

Progression of deformity

Not all curves resolve; some progress and hence it is necessary to identify the curves that are likely to resolve and those that have the propensity to progress. Mehta[3] used radiographic criteria to differentiate these two groups. She measured the rib-vertebra angle on the convex and concave sides of the curve on the apical vertebra. She noted that if the difference between the angles on the convex and concave sides (rib-vertebra angle difference or RVAD) is >20° the curve runs the risk of progression. She also noted the position of the rib heads in relation to the vertebral body. She suggested that if the rib heads overlap the vertebral body (phase II configuration) there is a likelihood of progression (Figure 21.3).

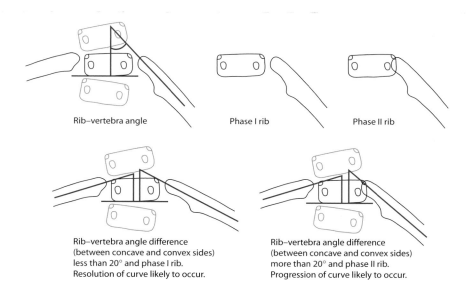

Rib–vertebra angle　　　　Phase I rib　　　　Phase II rib

Rib–vertebra angle difference (between concave and convex sides) less than 20° and phase I rib. Resolution of curve likely to occur.

Rib–vertebra angle difference (between concave and convex sides) more than 20° and phase II rib. Progression of curve likely to occur.

Figure 21.3 ● Method of measuring the rib–vertebra angle difference and the factors that predict the natural history of the curve in infantile idiopathic scoliosis.

Aim of treatment

- Facilitate resolution of the curve when spontaneous resolution does not occur.

Treatment options

Observation

Children with flexible curves that are <20° are observed at regular intervals. Most of these curves resolve spontaneously.

Casting under general anaesthesia

If the curve is stiff and >20° and if the RVAD is >20°, the child is placed in a corrective cast under general anaesthesia. This is done on a Risser or Cotrel table. The cast is changed after six to eight weeks.

Bracing

If the curve is reduced to <20° an underarm brace is then employed and the spine monitored.

Surgery

Children who have curves that are not controlled by repeated casts will need surgical intervention as outlined for juvenile idiopathic scoliosis.

- Rib-vertebra angle difference
- Rigidity of the curve
- Response to conservative measures

If the curve does not resolve either spontaneously or following casting, the child should be examined with magnetic resonance imaging (MRI) to look for the presence of a Chiari malformation and syringomyelia. Scoliosis secondary to syringomyelia is described under neuromuscular scoliosis.

An outline of treatment of idiopathic infantile scoliosis is shown in Table 21.1.

Table 21.1 ● Outline of treatment of idiopathic infantile scoliosis

INDICATIONS			
Onset <36 months + RVAD <20° + Phase I rib	Onset <36 months + RVAD >20° + Phase II rib	Onset <36 months + RVAD >20° + Phase II rib + Good response to casting (curve reduced to <20°)	Onset <36 months + RVAD >20° + Phase II rib + Poor response to casting or bracing (no resolution of deformity) + MRI excludes syringomyelia[a]
⇩	⇩	⇩	⇩
Observe for resolution of deformity If resolution occurs – maintain follow-up OR If progression occurs, treat as in column 2	Risser/Cotrel cast If deformity reduces to <20° treat as in column 3 OR If deformity does not reduce treat as in column 4	Brace (underarm brace if apex below T7 and Milwaukee brace if apex at T7 or above)	Treat with surgery as for juvenile idiopathic scoliosis
TREATMENT			

[a]If syringomyelia is present treat as for neuromuscular scoliosis.

In these children the gender ratios start to favour girls as age increases. Most curves require intervention because of progression. Severe curves and progressive deformities warrant investigation with MRI to ensure that there is no underlying neurological abnormality.

Progression of deformity

Most curves progress and if prompt treatment is not instituted the curves may become very severe.

Growth arrest after spinal fusion

Spinal fusion in the young child will arrest growth of the vertebral column and this may result in the trunk being very short. On account of this an attempt must be made to avoid very early fusion. However, this needs to be balanced against the risk of unacceptable progression of the deformity.

Aim of treatment

• Control the deformity until the child is old enough for definitive spinal fusion
In children with juvenile onset scoliosis, *control* of the deformity rather than resolution is the goal.

Treatment options

Observation

All children with curves <30° are kept under observation with serial radiographs taken in the erect posteroanterior position.

Bracing

Children with curves that exceed 30° at presentation or who have progressive curves >20° and with an apex below T7 are candidates for brace treatment with an underarm orthosis (Figure 21.4).

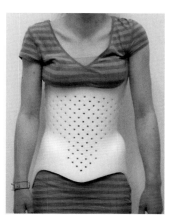

Figure 21.4 ● An underarm brace used for treatment of moderate degrees of scoliosis with the apex below the T7 vertebra.

Casting

Children with more severe curves are treated with manipulation and casts under general anaesthetic as previously described to try to reduce the curve to a level suitable for bracing (Figure 21.5).

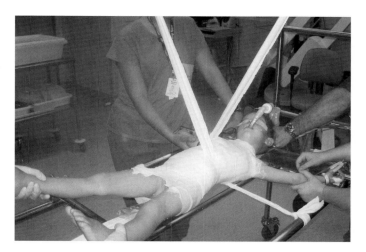

Figure 21.5 ● Technique of application of a corrective cast under anaesthesia.

Instrumentation without fusion

In these young children, if the deformity can be reduced to and kept below 40°, then continued non-operative treatment is appropriate. However, if the curve exceeds 40° surgical intervention becomes necessary.

■ **Posterior instrumentation without fusion**

Numerous techniques have been employed using various hook and pedicle screw configurations or sublaminar wires. While there has been some success with these techniques the results utilizing a dual rod construct with a combination of hooks and pedicle screws have been shown to be more stable with a marked reduction in complications.[4]

■ **Vertebral expanding prosthetic titanium rib**

This device was developed to address chest wall deformities in asphyxiating thoracic dystrophies;[5] however, it has also been shown to have some application in the control of childhood spinal deformities. It needs to be adjusted to accommodate and promote growth of the spine. Its disadvantage is that it corrects the spine by acting on the ribs and thus not directly acting on the spine. However, because the spine has not been instrumented there are advantages when the time for definitive fusion is reached and, should infection be an issue, the later surgery is not through a previously contaminated field.

■ **SHILLA procedure**

This technique, involves the insertion of multiple pedicle screws. The screws are not locked to the rods in order to allow for growth. Lengthening procedures are also employed. This technique is in its infancy and long-term results are not available.

Anterior apical fusion

This procedure, performed via a thoracotomy, was done in the past to control progression of the curve by fusing only the apex of the deformity. It was hoped that progression of the curve could be prevented without jeopardizing the growth of the rest of the spine. However, observation of these children has shown this procedure is not successful and it is no longer advocated.

Definitive spinal fusion

At some point in time a decision must be reached to perform a definitive spinal fusion as the final step in the management of these deformities. That time will depend on the success and tolerance of the lengthening procedures, combined with an appropriate assessment of the growth of the child. The goal of reaching maturity before performing a definitive fusion is inappropriate as the natural history in these children is to develop a spontaneous fusion in the concavity of the curve posteriorly around 10 to 12 years of age. This leads to cessation of posterior growth and acts as an unsegmented bar which results in a crankshaft phenomenon worsening the deformity; therefore, a planned fusion at that time is more appropriate.

These children will all have further growth ahead of them, and continued observation even after fusion is mandatory to monitor progression or adding on phenomena.

Factors to be taken into consideration while planning treatment

Age of the child

In children between the ages of three and ten every effort must be made to control the deformity and defer fusion. Between the ages of 10 and 12 years definitive fusion should be undertaken.

Severity of the curve

If the curve can be kept to below 40° conservative measures are justified while more severe curves warrant surgical intervention.

Location of the curve

Curves with the apex below T7 may be controlled with an underarm brace while higher curves will require a Milwaukee brace.

Response to conservative measures

If there is no favourable response to conservative treatment with a brace, surgery is needed to achieve control of the deformity.

Presence of neurological abnormalities

An underlying Chiari malformation or syringomyelia will need to be dealt with by the neurosurgeons. Once this is done, there may be some spontaneous resolution of the curve.

Recommended treatment

An outline of treatment of juvenile idiopathic scoliosis is shown in Table 21.2.

Table 21.2 ● Outline of treatment of juvenile idiopathic scoliosis

INDICATIONS					
3–10 years of age + Curve at presentation >30° OR >20° with documented progression of curve + Apex below T7 vertebra	3–10 years of age + Curve >40°	3–10 years of age + Curve reduced from 40° to <30° by casting	3–10 years of age + Curve progression despite casting or bracing + Features of Chiari malformation on MRI	3–10 years of age + Curve progression despite casting or bracing + No evidence of Chiari malformation on MRI	10–12 years of age + Uncontrolled deformity (curve >40°) OR Deformity controlled by bracing OR by dual rods (curve <40°)
⇩	⇩	⇩	⇩	⇩	⇩
Underarm brace	Manipulation and casting under GA + Assess response to casting (if curve reduces treat as in column 3) (if curve does not reduce treat as in column 4, 5, 6)	Underarm brace (if apex below T7) + Monitor for progression + Continue bracing as long as curve stays under 40°	Neurosurgical decompression + Monitor for resolution of curve (if curve does not resolve treat as in column 5)	Dual growing rod without spinal fusion + Rod lengthening every 6 months until 10 years of age (then treat as in column 6)	Definitive spinal fusion (DO NOT wait until skeletal maturity) + Continue monitoring until skeletal maturity for progression or add on phenomena
TREATMENT					

Adolescent idiopathic scoliosis

Children presenting with a scoliotic deformity beyond the first decade will have a distinct gender bias in favour of girls. Adolescent boys with scoliosis should be viewed with relative suspicion of an underlying pathology although boys will make up approximately 20 percent of cases of adolescent idiopathic scoliosis. Detection of the deformity in adolescents in a timely manner remains problematic. This is an age at which parents no longer get to see their children undressed and the concern is often raised by a third party, such as a dance teacher or swimming instructor. While school screening by trained health professionals has merit, the economic costs seem to outweigh the benefits to individual children.

Classification

The King classification of scoliosis was widely utilized in the Harrington era but has now largely been replaced in usage by the Lenke classification (Figure 21.6). This system has six curve types with modifiers. Its benefit is that the surgical management of a particular curve can be derived from its curve type.[6]

Examination

The examination in the first instance must exclude any signs of spinal dysraphism, i.e. skin lesions, hairy patches, absence of abdominal reflexes, etc. Second, the examination must include an appreciation of spinal imbalance in both the coronal and sagittal planes and leg length discrepancy. The examination then should look at the clinical features that may dictate treatment and these include the shoulder asymmetry, rib hump, waist line asymmetry and flexibility of both the thoracic and lumbar regions.

Investigations

If the child has features of typical idiopathic scoliosis, special investigations are not necessary. All children with a visible spinal deformity should have erect posteroanterior and lateral full-length

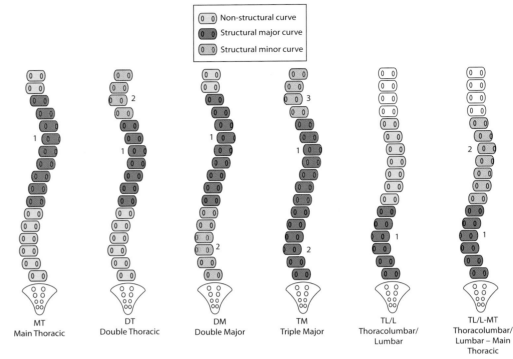

Non-structural curve
Structural major curve
Structural minor curve

MT	DT	DM	TM	TL/L	TL/L-MT
Main Thoracic	Double Thoracic	Double Major	Triple Major	Thoracolumbar/ Lumbar	Thoracolumbar/ Lumbar – Main Thoracic

Structural curve: Cobb angle on lateral bending film >25°
Major curve: Structural curve with greatest Cobb angle

Figure 21.6 ● Lenke classification of adolescent idiopathic scoliosis.

radiographs of the spine. A bone age assessment is often useful to assess skeletal maturity. However, if the deformity is severe enough to contemplate surgery, then the patient's lung function, blood profile, cardiac status and spinal cord should be examined.

Problems of management

Progression of deformity
The curve tends to progress especially during growth spurts; the rate of progression varies from patient to patient.

Loss of spinal balance
Compensatory curves develop above or below the primary curve in order to maintain the alignment of the head above the pelvis. However, if the primary curve progresses beyond a certain point the compensatory mechanisms cannot cope and there is a loss of spinal balance.

Cosmetic issues
The majority of the curves are in the thoracic region and these curves are associated with an unsightly rib hump (Figure 21.7).

Pain
In a small proportion of children pain develops.

Aims of treatment

- Prevent progression of the deformity
- Improve spinal balance
- Improve cosmetic appearance
- Reduce pain

Treatment options

Observation or no active treatment
A curve that is not severe enough to cause any cosmetic problems (usually below 20°) and is not progressing can be simply observed.

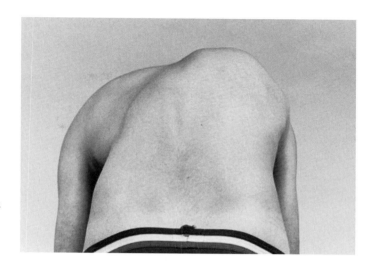

Figure 21.7 ● A rib hump that is best visualized when the patient bends forward is often cosmetically unacceptable.

Bracing

Children with a curve in the 20–40° range with significant growth remaining may be candidates for brace treatment. Prescription of a brace demands the availability of a skilled orthotist and the compliance of the patient to wear a brace. Climatic factors can play a major role in wearability of a brace. Most curves can be controlled by an underarm orthosis.

Surgery

There are essentially only three surgical approaches and one or more may be utilized.

■ Anterior discectomy and fusion without instrumentation

This can be performed by an open thoracotomy or by thoracoscopy. For exposure of the lumbar spine, division of the diaphragm may be necessary. This approach is used for large rigid curves and also for the relatively immature spine to prevent the crankshaft phenomenon and recurrent deformity.

■ Anterior approach with instrumentation and fusion

In the thoracic spine this procedure can be via thoracoscopy or open thoracotomy. In the lumbar spine an open procedure is necessary. The combination of mobilization of the spine by complete discectomy and removal of cartilaginous endplates coupled with instrumentation can provide a large correction with a relatively short fusion (Figure 21.8). Fixation is via single or double screws in each vertebral body. Single or dual rod systems are available.

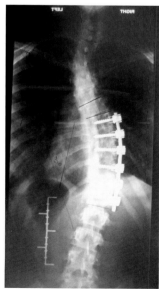
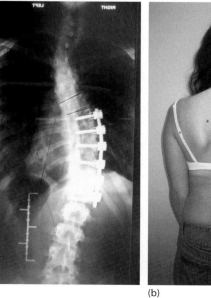

Figure 21.8 ● Post-operative radiograph of the spine following anterior instrumentation and fusion **(a)** and a very satisfactory appearance following surgery **(b)**.

(a)

(b)

■ Posterior instrumentation and fusion

The posterior approach is versatile with regard to the number of levels that can be exposed. Mobilization and correction can be improved by removal of the facet joints, both inferior and superior (Ponte osteotomy), pedicle subtraction osteotomy and complete vertebrectomy. Fixation can be via hooks, pedicle screws or sublaminar wires or cables, or a combination of these devices (Figure 21.9).

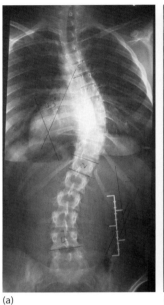 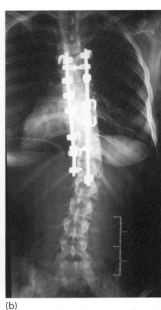

(a)   (b)

Figure 21.9 ● Adolescent idiopathic scoliosis **(a)** treated by posterior instrumentation and fusion **(b)**.

- The age of the child and skeletal growth remaining
- The curve type
- The severity of the curve
- Rate of progression of the curve.

- The surgeon's skill
- Operation facilities available to the surgeon
- The implants that are available.

Curve type and surgery

■ Lenke 1 (main thoracic curve)

These patients can be addressed by either posterior or anterior instrumentation with fusion. More severe curves will direct the surgeon to a posterior approach, possibly combined with traction and/or anterior discectomies.

■ Lenke 2 (double thoracic curves)

By definition both curves are structural and hence warrant fusion. However, the upper thoracic curve can be left alone if the affected shoulder is not elevated and the upper thoracic curve is modest in degree. Instrumentation is via a posterior approach.

■ Lenke 3 (double major)

If both curves are severe and similar in magnitude then both curves will need to be included in the fusion. In less severe curves, particularly if one curve is relatively flexible, then consideration should be given to selective fusion of one curve to shorten the fusion. Usually a posterior approach is used, although in some cases a combined anterior instrumentation of the thoracolumbar component followed by posterior instrumentation can save a level at the lower end of the fusion.

■ Lenke 4 (triple major)

The approach is as per Lenke 3 curves.

■ Lenke 5 (thoracolumbar/lumbar)

It is the opinion of the author that these curves are best addressed via an anterior approach with internal fixation. Using this approach, removal of the intervertebral discs within the curve can result in excellent correction and a very high rate of fusion. Some surgeons advocate a posterior approach with pedicle screws at all levels but too often this results in a longer fusion in an area where having some residual mobility is very important.

■ Lenke 6 (structural thoracolumbar and thoracic)

These curves need careful assessment to see what approach can maintain the most unfused lumbar discs. Often a combination of an anterior approach with fixation of the thoracolumbar curve followed by posterior instrumentation of both curves will provide the best outcome. This approach will usually save a level when compared with a pure posterior approach even if pedicle screws are inserted at all levels.

Rationale of treatment suggested

Children whose curves have progressed beyond 40° despite wearing a brace or children who present with a deformity beyond the brace range with a progressive deformity should be considered for surgical intervention.

However, not all patients with that degree of curvature need surgical intervention. For example, a girl with a well-balanced spine, who is close to skeletal maturity having had her menarche three years before, and whose radiographs do not show progression and who does not have a significant cosmetic deformity may not benefit functionally from a spinal fusion.

Neuromuscular scoliosis

There is a multitude of conditions that can fall under the heading of neuromuscular scoliosis. This chapter covers some of the major groups, i.e. cerebral palsy, spina bifida, Duchenne muscular dystrophy and syringomyelia. Each of these groups has distinctly different physical attributes or deficiencies.

Children with cerebral palsy have retained sensation and motor power; however, they have little or no control over what are often powerful muscle actions that can cause deformity. These children are often severely handicapped in communication and therefore cannot express their pain, which must add to the frustration and misery of the condition.

Spina bifida patients often have deficiencies of both power and sensation and sometimes a variable degree of spasticity in some muscle groups. While intellect may be impaired, communication is usually not a problem; however, the absence of sensation can result in the painless development of decubitus ulcers of which the patient is unaware.

Children with Duchenne muscular dystrophy have retained sensation but gradually diminishing muscle power. Communication is not an issue. Spinal deformities usually develop after the boys are confined to wheelchairs at a stage when they are too weak to lift themselves, hence painful areas are felt but the boys need assistance to be repositioned to relieve pain.

Syringomyelia patients usually have no neurological signs to indicate any spinal cord pathology. The diagnosis is confirmed by the use of MRI in cases of atypical scoliosis. These are patients with either early onset progressive curves or left-sided thoracic curves, or both. Abdominal reflexes may be absent but this is not pathognomonic of syringomyelia.

Cerebral palsy

Spastic cerebral palsy

Scoliosis is not uncommon in cerebral palsy and may develop in approximately 5 percent of hemiplegic patients and in 60–70 percent of quadriplegic patients; the overall incidence is approximately 25 percent.[7]

Intrathecal baclofen plays a significant role in the management of spasticity but there is increasing concern about a possible relationship with the development of spinal deformity.

Athetoid cerebral palsy

In this group of patients there is a good chance of normal intellect being poorly recognized because of communication difficulties. The concerns are of deformities secondary to movement disorders rather than spasticity. These children commonly develop a single lumbar curve with pelvic obliquity rather than the long 'c' curve or double curves of spastic cerebral palsy. These children are more likely to be independent and keen to be able to transfer themselves rather than depend on carers.

Problems of management

Unfavourable natural history

Compared with idiopathic scoliosis, in cerebral palsy the scoliosis is likely to have an earlier onset, be more progressive, less responsive to orthotic treatment, more likely to progress after skeletal maturity and more likely to require surgical stabilization.

Compromised sitting balance

One of the major consequences of scoliosis in cerebral palsy is compromised sitting position and balance.

Pelvic obliquity

Pelvic obliquity is frequently seen in these children. Pelvic obliquity increases the potential for ischial decubiti, can compromise hip stability and complicates the treatment of hip deformities. Any instrumentation of the spine must be coordinated with surgical treatment of hip pathology.

Problems for the carer

The spinal deformity may result in difficulties for parents and carers in seating, toileting and feeding.

Pulmonary complications

Pulmonary compromise is less commonly seen.

Aims of treatment

- Maintain the functional level of the child
  The principal aim of treatment is to maintain the patient's functional level. Usually this means maintaining sitting comfort although occasionally it is to protect walking ability.
- Improve or prevent the effects of pelvic obliquity
  This means avoidance of ischial decubitus and improvement of hip alignment.
- Improve the ability of the patient to sit
  Enabling the child to sit for meals and toileting is an important aim.
- Make the task of carers less arduous

Treatment options

An assessment of treatment options should be preceded by the statement that there is no evidence that non-operative methods of treatment of scoliosis in cerebral palsy will alter the functional outcome or alter the natural history.

Anterior instrumentation alone

This may be considered in athetoid cerebral palsy with modest deformities.

Anterior discectomy without instrumentation

This procedure is seldom done in isolation but is commonly performed prior to posterior instrumentation for severe curves in spastic cerebral palsy.

Posterior release of joints and soft tissues followed by anterior instrumentation

This is useful for lumbar curves where the pelvis is not part of the scoliosis and where independence in transfers or ambulation is important.

Posterior instrumentation and fusion

Posterior instrumentation is the most common procedure with or without extension to the sacrum or pelvis for spastic cerebral palsy patients with pelvic obliquity and where the sacrum is in the curve. However, this option should be used with caution where the hip is dysplastic or if hip degeneration exists.

Decision-making questions

- Which children should undergo surgical intervention for scoliosis?
- Should the approach be purely anterior or posterior alone or should the posterior approach be followed by anterior instrumentation?
- Should the fusion extend to the sacrum and pelvis?

Factors to be taken into consideration while planning treatment

- The type of cerebral palsy.
- The severity and rigidity of the curves.
- The extent of the distal extent of the deformity (i.e. are the sacrum and pelvis involved?).
- The degree of independence: if there is a possibility of independence it is important to try to fuse shorter (fewer) segments to retain independent movement as compared with the case of a spastic quadriplegic propped up in a chair who will be moved by carers.
- The level of intellect: if a child has normal intellect he or she is more likely to be independent.

Recommended treatment

There are some children who are not candidates for spinal surgery. This includes children who are not aware of their surroundings but can be made to sit without skin problems or pain despite a large curve. It is also inappropriate to intervene in children with other severe co-morbidities such as pulmonary disease and those who frequently need intensive care.

The recommended treatment for most cerebral palsy curves is for a combined procedure with anterior discectomies, usually from the thoracolumbar and lumbar levels, followed by long posterior instrumentation but avoiding involvement of the sacrum where possible. For children with athetoid cerebral palsy with principally a lumbar curve, posterior releases of both joints and soft tissues followed by anterior instrumentation to L4 is the treatment of choice.

Rationale of treatment suggested

Most cerebral palsy patients with severe scoliosis are intellectually impaired and the goals of treatment are to reduce deformity, maintain sitting balance and make the handling of the patients easier. Commonly, there is pelvic obliquity but hip pathology is also common in these patients and, where possible, maintenance of motion across the lumbosacral junction and across the sacroiliac joints should be entertained. Luque instrumentation to the pelvis with the Galveston technique has been commonly employed. Frequently, there is loosening of the rods within the pelvis seen on follow-up radiographys which reflects the demands placed on the lumbosacral junction by the patient and by carers in lifting. More secure fixation into the pelvis can be obtained by the use of iliac screws and S1 pedicle screws, but a more rational approach would be to use pedicle screws in the lumbar spine for improved correction and avoid fixation to the sacrum and pelvis. Furthermore, the presence of actual or potentially painful hip pathology should suggest caution in loading the hips by eradicating all spine and pelvic movement.

Spina bifida

By virtue of the aetiology of spina bifida the spine is commonly involved in the pathology and disabilities that ensue. Owing to the spinal cord involvement, paralytic or neurogenic scoliosis is commonly seen but both congenital deformities and neurogenic deformities can coexist. Congenital anomalies are common with all forms of anomalies being recorded. Defects in formation can coexist with defects in segmentation.

Problems of management

Risk of decubitus ulceration

The combination of lack of sensation and the propensity to develop pelvic obliquity leads to a real risk of decubitus ulcers.

Early onset of spinal deformity

Deformities often develop at a relatively young age in children with spina bifida.

Higher risk of post-operative complications

Posterior spinal surgery is associated with a high risk of post-operative infection and failure of fusions.

Problems following fusion to the sacrum or pelvis

Long fusions to the sacrum in immature children can result in subluxation of the sacroiliac joints. Fusions to the pelvis result in rigidity over regions with deficient sensation which increases the risk of skin breakdown.

Difficulties with use of orthoses

Only occasionally are orthoses the definitive treatment. Even in these instances difficulties with urinary diversions, other health issues and the need for additional orthoses for the lower extremities should not be underestimated.

Aims of treatment

Preservation of spinal motion in ambulant children

Some children remain walkers throughout life and every effort must be made to preserve spinal motion segments in these children with the potential to remain as walkers.

- Correct spinal deformity and reduce or eliminate pelvic obliquity
- Preserve some intervertebral, lumbosacral or sacroiliac motion wherever possible
- Maintain ambulation

Treatment options

- Orthoses: Milwaukee or Boston brace
- Anterior discectomies and fusion
- Anterior instrumentation and fusion
- Posterior instrumentation and fusion
- Traction: halo femoral.

Factors to be taken into consideration while planning treatment

Level of anticipated ambulatory and sport activity

The level of ambulation expected in adolescence, combined with the intellectual drive and the wish to do wheelchair sports or equivalent, can influence the treatment decision.

Level of the curve

The level of the curvature and the involvement of the sacrum in the deformity are important issues that need to be considered.

Neurological level of involvement

The neurological level and the need to preserve neurological function also need to be considered while planning treatment. In particular, a child with low-level neurological deficit has a good chance of remaining as a community ambulator and in these children mobility of as many motion segments as possible needs to be retained.

Age and skeletal maturity

Definitive fusion is usually deferred until skeletal maturity.

Recommended treatment

The recommended treatment is outlined in Table 21.3.

Rationale of treatment suggested

Orthotic use is feasible in selected patients if it is thought that this may be the definitive treatment. In more severely involved younger patients braces may be used to try and buy time but generally speaking this is difficult and has the additional hazards of urinary diversions and sensory issues.

Ambulant patients and wheelchair athletes are usually not willing to risk losing mobility and independence by fusion of the lumbar spine to the pelvis. Numerous patients with broken Harrington rods *in situ* and pseudarthroses would prefer to avoid returning to the surgeon rather than lose the motion gained by the surgical failure.

Long fusions to the sacrum should be delayed if possible to allow for maturation of the sacroiliac joints. In the immature patient a successful fusion to the pelvis may eventually lead to subluxation through the sacroiliac joints. Spina bifida patients clearly have more infections and pseudarthroses by posterior instrumentation compared with anterior instrumentation. Therefore, a long posterior instrumentation, if needed, should almost always be preceded by an anterior fusion with or without instrumentation.

Duchenne muscular dystrophy

Scoliosis is common in Duchenne muscular dystrophy (DMD), although most boys do not have a significant curve prior to losing ambulatory ability. The most common deformity pattern is a lumbar or thoracolumbar curve associated with pelvic obliquity. The pelvic obliquity leads to unequal loading across the ischial tuberosities and therefore pain and/or skin breakdown may result (Figure 21.10). However, some boys develop a balanced double curve and then pelvic obliquity is less of an issue. A third pattern exists where the boys sit with the trunk out of balance but with an essentially level pelvis and therefore weight is reasonably evenly distributed and pain is not an issue.

Table 21.3 ● Outline of treatment of scoliosis in spina bifida

INDICATIONS				
Modest curve + Progression noted + Ambulant child + Skeletally immature + Urinary diversion and/or lower limb bracing does not interfere with spinal bracing ⇩ Boston brace (if apex of curve below T7) OR Milwaukee brace (if apex of curve is above T7)	Moderate curve + Ambulant child + Close to skeletal maturity + No pelvic obliquity ⇩ Anterior instrumentation and fusion	Moderate curve + Non-ambulant child keen on wheelchair sports + Close to skeletal maturity + No pelvic obliquity ⇩ Anterior instrumentation and fusion	Severe curve + Skeletally immature (too young for definitive fusion) ⇩ Dual growing rods without spinal fusion	Severe curve + Skeletally mature + With or without pelvic obliquity ⇩ Halo femoral traction + Anterior discectomies + Posterior instrumentation (try to avoid fusion to the sacrum or pelvis)
TREATMENT				

Duchenne muscular dystrophy is one of the muscular dystrophies where medical treatment has been shown to be effective in preventing deformity. The use of steroids in DMD has altered the natural history of the condition.[8]

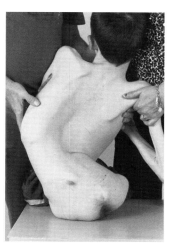

Figure 21.10 ● Pelvic obliquity can lead to uneven loading of the ischial tuberosity. This can result in pain or ulceration.

Compromised pulmonary function

Pulmonary function becomes severely compromised as the disease progresses and this precludes the use of anterior procedures. There is a relatively small window of opportunity where the spinal deformity of a pattern that is likely to cause misery can be demonstrated to be worsening and where the pulmonary function is still adequate for surgery. It is essential that this interval is identified and surgery undertaken before pulmonary function deteriorates too much. The pulmonary compromise also demands early mobilization to maintain respiratory function and avoid atelectasis.

Poor cardiac function

Cardiomyopathy often coexists in these boys. The use of trans-oesophageal echocardiography has proved useful in monitoring fluid balance and cardiac output during surgery. Hypotension due to poor cardiac output will be worsened by fluid loading. In that setting, blood losses need to be replaced by blood rather than crystalloid fluids.

Altered body weight

The boys fall into one of two groups by weight; some are quite underweight and are then more affected by the deformity of the spine, others are obese and well padded across the buttocks. Obesity makes the surgery longer and thus more risky but, on the other hand, gives a better padded bottom on which to sit and pain is often not an issue. This can make the selection of patients for surgery difficult.

Intra-operative bleeding

These patients will start to bleed profusely after approximately 100 minutes of surgery. The surgery should be completed within three hours; it is imperative that techniques that take more time to complete are avoided. Failure to expeditiously complete the task will result in excessive morbity and potential mortality.

Osteopenia

Pedicle screws alone in osteopenic bone seen in these children are subject to reduced pullout strength.

Associated deformities of the hip and knee

Hip flexion contractures are often present. A deformity of approximately 45° is not an issue; however, in some boys the combination of a hip flexion deformity and correction of their lumbar lordosis may result in a flexed pelvis and an unhappy boy. Knee flexion contractures and ankle equinus should not be ignored. Hip flexion deformities predispose these boys to distal femoral fractures and feet deformities preclude the wearing of shoes. Both should be addressed surgically.

Pre-operative assessment

- Each child must be individually assessed for their own particular natural history of the disease. In some the disease pattern will have been modified by steroids.
- The spinal deformity needs to be assessed to try and predict if pelvic obliquity and spinal imbalance is likely to make sitting miserable.
- Pulmonary and cardiac function needs to be carefully reviewed and monitored so that a window of opportunity is not missed.

Aims of treatment

- To correct the pelvic obliquity and spinal imbalance
- To complete the surgery within an operative time of three hours
- To mobilize the patients by the third post-operative day sitting in their wheelchairs
- To avoid pulmonary infections

Treatment options

- Posterior instrumentation with Luque rods and wires and with Galveston fixation to the pelvis.
- Posterior instrumentation with pedicle screws or hybrid instrumentation.

Factors to be taken into consideration while planning treatment

- Procedure that is likely to take least time to perform as surgery time is of critical importance
- The need to include the pelvis in the fixation.

Recommended treatment

In most boys the use of a Luque rod with Galveston fixation to the pelvis is the most expeditious method of completing the task in a reasonable time. It is also the most cost-effective. Formal bone graft harvesting is not necessary. In some boys pedicle screw fixation to the lumbar spine and sublaminar cables proximally will avoid the need to include the pelvis in the fixation (Table 21.4). Pedicle screw fixation of the entire spine will, in most surgeons' hands, result in too long a surgical exposure time.

Table 21.4 ● Outline of treatment of scoliosis in Duchenne muscular dystrophy

INDICATIONS	
Severe curve with pelvic obliquity + Curve extending to sacrum ⇩	Less severe curve with pelvic obliquity + Curve not extending to sacrum ⇩
Segmental sublaminar instrumentation with Luque rods with Galveston fixation to the pelvis	Pedicle screw fixation of lumbar spine with segmental sublaminar wires proximally
TREATMENT	

Rationale of treatment suggested

In most boys the pelvic obliquity is the key issue with regard to pain. Usually this means inclusion of the pelvis in the fixation. Occasionally with less severe curves that do not extend to the sacrum, the use of pedicle screws in the lumbar spine, protected by sublaminar cables, will obviate the need to fix to the pelvis.

Syringomyelia

Syringomyelia is well recognized as a causative factor in the development of scoliosis (Figure 21.11). The lesion is often associated with a Chiari malformation. In the otherwise well child this is likely to be a Chiari 1 malformation; in children with spina bifida a Chiari 2 malformation may be seen. The typical patient is a boy with a left thoracic curve of early onset. However, these lesions can also be seen in girls with early onset scoliosis.

In the presence of a Chiari malformation and a large syrinx, the appropriate treatment is surgical decompression at the level of the occiput–C1 junction with a duroplasty.

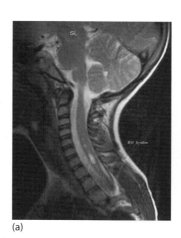 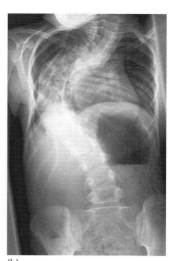

Figure 21.11 ● Magnetic resonance imaging showing a syrinx in the cervical region **(a)** and the severe degree of scoliosis in the same child **(b)**.

(a)   (b)

A reduction in syrinx size usually results in a reduction or stabilization of the spinal deformity. These children are then observed and a planned definitive fusion at 12–14 years of age is performed as the natural history is one of curve progression at puberty, even if there has been a good initial response to the surgical decompression.

If the syrinx is not reduced the scoliotic curve can be expected to worsen. Further neurosurgical procedures may be appropriate but spinal fusion may need to be considered. If MRI demonstrates a dilated canal without a Chiari malformation, neurosurgical decompression may not be indicated but this is not a good prognostic sign for the likelihood of improvement of the deformity with casting. Surgical intervention is usually necessary.

Congenital scoliosis

Congenital scoliosis refers to a spinal deformity in the coronal plane due to the presence of a congenital anomaly of the spine. It does not relate to the presence or absence of a clinically demonstrable deformity at birth.

As these anomalies have their origin in fetal somite formation, abnormalities in other organ systems should be suspected. All children thus recognized should have a renal ultrasound, an examination of the heart by a paediatrician and, ultimately, MRI examination of the spine.

Congenital scoliosis can be due to vertebral anomalies alone or due to the presence of congenital rib fusions with or without vertebral anomalies. The anomalies may be due to failure of formation or failure of segmentation, or a combination of both pathologies.

Failure of formation

Hemivertebrae can be classified in the following ways (Figure 21.12).

Fully segmented hemivertebra

There is a normal disc space above and below the hemivertebra; the growth imbalance is likely to lead to progression of the deformity which usually occurs slowly at the rate of 1–2° a year.[9] A fully segmented hemivertebra at the lumbosacral junction can produce a significant truncal imbalance and a long secondary scoliosis.

Semi-segmented hemivertebra

This form has no major growth imbalance and the deformity induced is essentially due to the mass of the hemivertebra. Often the deformity does not warrant surgical intervention although there may be a significant imbalance with a lesion at the lumbosacral junction.

Non-segmented hemivertebra

Without growth plates between the vertebrae there is no growth imbalance and no deformity. Thus no intervention is required.

Incarcerated hemivertebra

With a fully incarcerated hemivertebra the deformity induced is usually modest and no intervention is required.

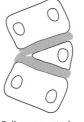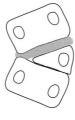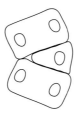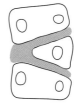

| Fully segmented hemivertebra | Semi-segmented hemivertebra | Non-segmented hemivertebra | Incarcerated hemivertebra |

Figure 21.12 ● Diagram showing the different types of congenital hemivertebra.

Failure of segmentation

Failure of segmentation can result in an unsegmented bar that may manifest as vertebral fusions, rib fusions or both. An unsegmented bar will produce a significant and progressive deformity as growth on the contralateral side progresses.

Progression of the curve in infancy is often quite slow and it may take some time to document change that is also apparent to the parents. This slow progression does afford time to allow the child to grow, which will make the surgery slightly less difficult and the anaesthetic risks less.

Problems of management

Associated visceral anomalies

A vertebral anomaly may be only one component of the failure in embryogenesis and hence other organ systems must be examined

Abnormal growth of adjacent vertebrae

Growth of an abnormal vertebra is unpredictable and adjacent vertebrae may have less than normal growth but appear normal early in life.

Secondary growth retardation

Secondary growth retardation of anomalous vertebrae can develop due to abnormal loading. These secondary effects on growth due to deformity may worsen the underlying problem.

Stunting of growth of the spine after fusion

Surgical fusions may control the deformity but will also worsen the stunting effect on vertebral growth due to the spinal anomaly.

Aims of treatment

- Prevent progression
- Improve spinal imbalance and deformity
- Prevent or correct neurological compression
- Improve thoracic cage volume

Treatment options

Hemiepiphyseodesis on the convexity

Prophylactic growth plate arrest on the convexity of the curve is performed through separate anterior and posterior approaches. The surgery is relatively simple and the risk to neurological structures is minimal. However, the correction takes place over time and the degree of correction is unpredictable.

In this age of instant gratification and hardware, the simplicity of this procedure may be overlooked.

Hemivertebra resection

There are three techniques by which this can be achieved: staged anterior and posterior approaches, posterior resection only with fusion and simultaneous anterior and posterior resection and fusion.

■ Staged anterior and posterior resection and fusion

The surgical technique involves an anterior retroperitoneal approach and identification of the offending lesion. The hemivertebra is removed back to the pedicle. The adjacent discs and end plates are removed. The patient is then placed prone and the posterior element and remainder of the pedicle is excised. Fixation by either screws or hooks can close the space created. The results have been recently reported by Bollini *et al.*[10]

■ Resection by a posterior approach and fusion

This technique is performed via a standard posterior approach. The posterior elements of the hemivertebra are removed and the pedicle resected and the posterior and posterolateral aspects of the vertebra are visualized. The bone of the hemivertebra is removed and the adjacent end plates and discs excised as much as can be done safely. Posterior instrumentation is then used to close the space created. This technique and results were described by Ruf and Harms.[11]

■ Simultaneous anterior and posterior resection and fusion

In this technique the patient lies in a lateral position and a 'T' incision is made along the spine posterior and transversely across the trunk. The dissection involves division of the erector spinae and psoas on one side. This approach does give an excellent view of the bone to be removed but it is quite a destructive approach and is mentioned here for completeness and not for promotion.

Instrumentation and fusion

Where possible, instrumentation of the affected area should be done; this will add some certainty to the outcome. Growth of these anomalous vertebrae is unpredictable and hence fusion or epiphyseodesis is also unpredictable. In any procedure that may make the spine unstable, stabilization by instrumentation should be initially established.

Distraction techniques

When there are multiple hemivertebrae, distraction techniques may be used to try to gain spinal length. Distraction can also reduce the secondary effects of the congenital deformity on adjacent vertebrae. While it has been assumed in the past that anomalous vertebrae cannot grow, more recent experience has shown that spinal growth of these vertebrae can be enhanced by these distraction techniques. Whether this is simply revealing the potential growth of the anomalous vertebra or actually producing growth by a callotasis effect is unknown.[12]

However, all distraction techniques are fraught with complications which include failure of fixation and risk of infection from repeated procedures.

■ Vertical expanding prosthetic titanium rib

This device was developed for chest expansion for asphyxiating thoracic dystrophies. It has been shown to be of particular value where the chest wall deformity is due to rib fusions. A secondary benefit has been the correction of the associated spinal deformity.

■ Spinal distraction using dual growing rods

The technique is the same as that used for juvenile idiopathic scoliosis.

Osteotomy or resection and instrumentation

Deformity due to failure of segmentation could be treated by fusion *in situ* if the deformity is acceptable. This is safer when compared with the risk of performing an osteotomy of the spine.

If the deformity is unacceptable it can be addressed by spinal osteotomy and instrumentation or, alternatively, by vertebral resection and instrumentation.

Factors to be taken into consideration while planning treatment

Recommended treatment

- Progression of the deformity
- Site and number of vertebrae in the deformity
- Maturity of the patient
- Neurological compromise
- Chest wall involvement.

The treatment recommended for dealing with hemivertebrae is shown in Table 21.5.

Table 21.5 ● Outline of treatment of congenital scoliosis due to hemivertebrae

INDICATIONS		
Single hemivertebra + Curve progression present + Hemivertebra situated mainly posteriorly + Kyphotic spine ⇩	Single hemivertebra + Curve progression present + Hemivertebra situated mainly anteriorly + Lordotic spine ⇩	Multiple hemivertebrae + Early curve progression present + No neurological compromise ⇩
Hemivertebra excision and fusion through a posterior approach	Hemivertebra excision and fusion through anterior AND posterior two-stage approach	Distraction technique (Vertebral expanding prosthetic titanium rib if there is chest wall deformity OR growing rods if chest wall is normal) as a stop gap measure + Definitive fusion at a later date
TREATMENT		

Iliac hypoplasia

Within this group of patients there are some in whom spinal imbalance is a significant deformity. These patients were described by Millis and Hall[13] as having 'postural imbalance in the transverse plane'. Some of these patients have a pelvic obliquity due to a deficiency of the S1 segment and/or the ilium and this is often accompanied by a modest leg length discrepancy.

In patients with a significant lumbar curve in whom correction is anticipated it becomes apparent that unless the pelvic obliquity is corrected there is a real risk of leaving the patient unbalanced or with an acute lumbosacral scoliosis.

The obliquity can be addressed relatively simply by employing the technique of transiliac lengthening as described by Millis and Hall[13] (Figure 21.13). This is particularly useful where there

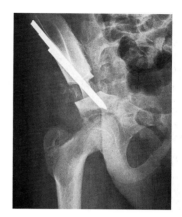

Figure 21.13 ● Iliac hypoplasia treated by transiliac lengthening by the technique of Millis and Hall.[13]

is associated acetabular dysplasia. The use of a carbon fibre wedge implant with the bone graft provides structural support and prevents graft collapse and loss of height.

An alternative procedure is to lengthen the shorter limb although this will leave the acetabulae at differing heights which may not be appropriate if there is any degree of acetabular dysplasia.

References

1. Mehta MH. Growth as a corrective force in the early treatment of progressive infantile scoliosis. *J Bone Joint Surg Br* 2005; **87**: 1237–47.
2. Riseborough E, Wynne-Davies R. A genetic survey of idiopathic scoliosis in Boston, Massachusetts. *J Bone Joint Surg Am* 1973; **55**: 974–82.
3. Mehta MH. The rib-vertebra angle in the early diagnosis between resolving and progressive infantile scoliosis. *J Bone Joint Surg Br* 1972; **54**: 230–43.
4. Akbarnia BA, Breakwell LM, Marks DS *et al*. Dual growing rod technique followed for three to eleven years until final fusion: the effect of frequency of lengthening. *Spine* 2008; **33**: 984–90.
5. Cambell RM Jr, Smith MD, Mayes TC *et al*. The effect of opening wedge thoracostomy on thoracic insufficiency syndrome associated with fused ribs and congenital scoliosis. *J Bone Joint Surg Am* 2004; **85**: 1659–74.
6. Lenke LG, Betz RR, Harms J *et al*. Adolescent idiopathic scoliosis: a new classification to determine the extent of spinal arthrodesis. *J Bone Joint Surg Am* 2001; **83**: 1169–81.
7. Smith BG. *Management of Neurogenic Scoliosis. Orthopedic Management of Cerebral Palsy*. Salt Lake City, UT: Pediatric Orthopaedic Society of North America, 2002.
8. Alman BA, Raza SN, Bigger WD. Steroid treatment and the development of scoliosis in males with Duchenne muscular dystrophy. *J Bone Joint Surg Am* 2004; **86**: 519–24.
9. McMaster MJ. Congenital scoliosis. In: Weinstein SL (ed.). *The Pediatric Spine*. Philadelphia, PA: Lippincott Williams and Wilkins, 2001.
10. Bollini G, Docquier PL, Viehweger E, Launay F, Jouve JL. Lumbar hemivertebra resection. *J Bone Joint Surg Am* 2006; **88**: 1043–52.
11. Ruf M, Harms J. Hemivertebra resection by a posterior approach: innovative operative technique and first results. *Spine* 2002; **27**: 1116–23.
12. Campbell RM Jr, Hell-Volke AK. Growth of the thoracic spine in congenital scoliosis after expansion thoracoplasty. *J Bone Joint Surg Am* 2003; **85**: 409–20.
13. Millis MB, Hall JE. Transiliac lengthening of the lower extremity. *J Bone Joint Surg Am* 1979; **61**: 1181–94.

Kyphotic deformities of the spine

Ian Torode

22

Introduction

Kyphosis is defined as a deformity of the spine in the sagittal plane. Pure kyphotic deformities are not complicated by rotation as opposed to kyphoscoliosis. Historically, many idiopathic scoliosis curves were described as kyphoscoliotic because the rib hump gave the patients a kyphotic appearance; however, the true deformity in scoliosis is actually lordotic in most instances and kyphoscoliosis is an uncommon deformity. This chapter will cover what are essentially pure kyphotic deformities that include postural and structural kyphosis.

The normal kyphosis of the thoracic spine ranges from 20 to 50° and when the kyphosis exceeds this range it may be considered as being pathological.

Postural kyphosis (synonym: postural round back)

Children with this deformity stand with a slouch; they are not unwell and pain is not an issue. Their parents have usually been telling them to 'stand up straight' for some time with little success. The children are usually in their second decade.

Problems of management

Cosmetic problem
Postural kyphosis is essentially a cosmetic problem.

Progression from a postural deformity to a structural deformity
If neglected, some deformities may become fixed or structural.

Treatment itself is often cosmetically unsatisfactory
Treatment with a brace is far from cosmetically pleasing.

Psychological issues
This deformity is not uncommon in girls attempting to disguise breast development. Sensitivity is required by the physician when dealing with these children.

Aims of treatment

- Improve posture in the growing child
  An effort must be made to provide the patient with an insight into the relationship between habitual posture and fixed deformity.
- Avoid a fixed or structural deformity before the end of growth
  Treatment should be instituted before the deformity becomes structural.

Treatment options

Education
Education regarding appearance and development will suffice for a large proportion of children who have what is, essentially, a normal variation or physiological deformity.

Physiotherapy with extension exercises
Moderately severe deformities detected in the growing child can be addressed by extension exercises. Most children will respond to treatment with extension exercises although compliance may be an issue.

Milwaukee brace
Deformities which are becoming stiffer with time can be improved with the use of a Milwaukee brace.

Fixed deformities treated by the use of a Milwaukee brace usually resolve quickly if compliance is reasonable. The problem of brace treatment is that it is profoundly non-cosmetic and the underlying issue is largely a cosmetic problem.[1]

Factors to be taken into consideration while planning treatment

- The degree of deformity
- The age of the child
- The flexibility of the deformity.

Recommended treatment

An outline of treatment of postural kyphosis is shown in Table 22.1.

Table 22.1 ● Outline of treatment of postural kyphosis

INDICATIONS		
Early teens + Mild kyphosis + Flexible deformity	Mid-teens + Moderate kyphosis + Flexible deformity ⇩	Any age + Any degree of severity + Deformity becoming rigid ⇩
⇩	Education regarding adopting a normal posture and risk of progression to a structural deformity if posture is not corrected + Extension exercises	Milwaukee brace to be worn constantly until correction of deformity has been obtained
Education regarding adopting a normal posture and risk of progression to a structural deformity if posture is not corrected		
TREATMENT		

Structural kyphosis

Structural kyphosis is defined as a kyphotic deformity of the spine associated with deformity of the vertebrae that may be either developmental or congenital in origin.

Introduction

Structural deformities may be due to congenital vertebral anomalies or developmental disorders of the spinal column such as Scheuermann's disease, deformities secondary to bone dysplasias or deformity arising from soft tissue laxity. Sepsis in the growing child may damage the vertebral growth plates leading to a progressive deformity that has some similarities to congenital kyphosis.

Scheuermann's disease

This disorder is usually seen in children over the age of ten years. Both pain and deformity usually accompany the thoracic kyphosis, which is the site of deformity of true Scheuermann's disease, although the lumbar spine may also be affected.[2] This disease may be more appropriately described as an osteochondritis. In the early stages of the disease mild wedging of the vertebrae or loss of signal in the anterior portion of the growing vertebrae and intervertebral discs may be evident on magnetic resonance imaging. There is often associated end plate irregularity and loss of disc height. Progressive notching of the anterior margins of the vertebrae and further wedging of the vertebral bodies occur (Figure 22.1). In the lumbar spine, pain rather than deformity is usually the presenting complaint although a modest kyphosis at the thoracolumbar junction can occur. The disease itself is self-limiting and resolves by the end of spinal growth, but the deformity may be permanent.

Problems of management

Minimal long-term disability

Management can be controversial because the long-term disability is mild in most instances and the treatment unattractive to teenage children.

Development of structural changes

Treatment needs to begin before major structural changes in the vertebrae have developed.

Delay in presentation and treatment

Often the deformity is thought to be postural and thus presentation may be late, particularly if pain is not an issue.

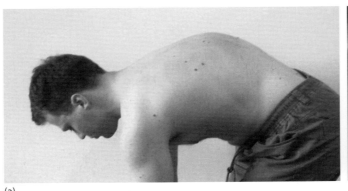
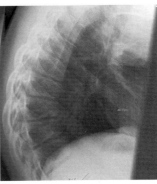

(a) (b)

Figure 22.1 ● Kyphosis due to Sheuermann's disease is seen in this adolescent **(a)**; the radiograph shows wedging of the vertebrae and end-plate irregularities **(b)**.

Neurological damage

Frank neurological impairment is rare but can occur. Spinal cord irritation as evidenced by hamstring tightness and or clonus is not uncommon.

Pain

Pain is a common feature in this condition.

Aims of treatment

- Early correction of deformity
  The deformity must be corrected early in the course of the disease while there is significant growth left to allow for remodelling of the vertebrae.
- Prevent neurological impairment
  If signs of irritation are evident early intervention is mandatory.
- Relieve pain

Treatment options

Extension exercises

Children with a mild thoracic kyphosis (<60°) can be managed with extension exercises and close observation and serial radiographs.

Brace treatment

A moderate thoracic kyphosis (>60°) can be managed by a Milwaukee brace.[3] In osteochondritis of the thoracolumbar spine where the apex of the deformity is below T10 a TLSO or Boston brace is effective.

Instrumentation and fusion of the spine

More severe deformities (>75°) may require surgical intervention, particularly if there is evidence of cord involvement.[4] In severe and rigid deformities towards the end of growth an anterior discectomy and posterior spinal fusion is necessary. If there is a more diffuse pattern of deformity, particularly if there is growth remaining, then a pure posterior approach will gain good correction. Pedicle screws may be more effective than hooks in these patients[5] (Figure 22.2).

Factors to be taken into consideration while planning treatment

- The skeletal maturity of the child
- The degree of deformity of the spine
- The level of vertebral deformity and the extent of the disease throughout the spine
- The presence of neurological involvement.

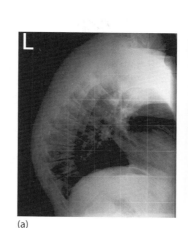

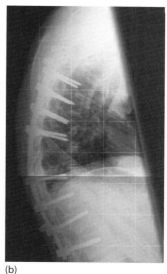

Figure 22.2 ● Kyphosis due to Scheuermann's disease **(a)** treated by posterior instrumentation with pedicular screw fixation **(b)**.

(a) (b)

Recommended treatment

An outline of treatment of Scheuermann's kyphosis is shown in Table 22.2.

Table 22.2 ● Outline of treatment of Scheuermann's kyphosis

INDICATIONS					
<60° kyphosis + No neurological deficit	60–75° kyphosis + No neurological deficit + Apex of kyphosis above T10 vertebra	60–75° kyphosis + No neurological deficit + Apex of kyphosis below T10 vertebra	>75° kyphosis + No neurological deficit + Diffuse pattern of involvement + Growth remaining	>75° kyphosis + No neurological deficit + More localized rigid deformity + Approaching end of skeletal growth	Any degree + Neurological deficit
⇩	⇩	⇩	⇩	⇩	⇩
Extension exercises	Milwaukee brace	TLSO or Boston brace	Posterior spinal fusion alone (preferably with pedicular screws)	Anterior discectomy + Posterior spinal fusion	Anterior discectomy + Posterior spinal fusion
TREATMENT					

Rationale of treatment suggested

While in most cases the deformity is a cosmetic issue, a worsening thoracic and thoracolumbar kyphosis is associated with an increased lumbar lordosis and back pain in later life. Correction of the deformity can effectively treat the pain and neurological impairment and produce a pleasing improvement in the cosmetic appearance.

Kyphosis due to bone dysplasias

Introduction

A progressive kyphotic deformity of the thoracolumbar junction spine is commonly seen in achondroplasia. An outwardly similar deformity is also seen in storage disorders such as Morquio or Hurler's disease.[6] In achondroplasia the deformity is often associated with significant spinal stenosis whereas the latter group often has proximal cervical spine instability and cerebral impairment from the underlying disease process. In both groups there is deformity of the vertebrae with a kyphotic deformity that is often present early in life. The common feature of these groups of children is that the kyphosis is usually localized to a couple of vertebral segments despite generalized disease and widespread changes elsewhere in the spine (Figure 22.3). The spinal problems may be aggravated by weakness of the trunk extensors, ligamentous laxity and the weight from a relatively large head. Impaired cerebral function can make history-taking difficult and hence regular reviews involving careful neurological examination and radiological studies are essential.

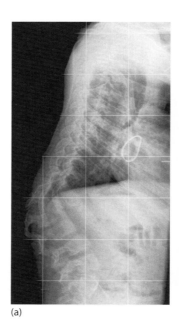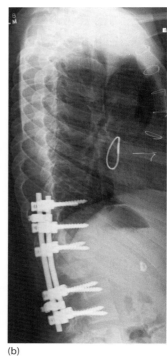

Figure 22.3 ● Severe kyphosis in a child with skeletal dysplasia **(a)** treated by posterior instrumentation **(b)**.

(a)   (b)

Problems of management

Neurological impairment

Worsening kyphosis in the thoracolumbar region can cause neurological compromise and it also results in an increase in lumbar lordosis which may, in turn, worsen any pre-existing spinal stenosis.

Factors affecting bracing

Brace management may be compromised by the short stature and mental impairment or behavioural issues.

Problems related to surgical intervention

Laminectomy may be necessary in order to deal with neurological compromise. However, laminectomy in the growing child, particularly in an area of kyphosis, can of itself lead to an increase in that deformity. Stabilization of the spine prior to laminectomy or in conjunction with the laminectomy should be considered for this reason. Surgical intervention may sometimes become necessary in early childhood but, in general, it is not a good option during the first five years. Furthermore, at this time, the family is still coming to grips with the complexities of the conditions.

Aims of treatment

It is important to emphasize that a cure of the disease is not possible and the aims of treatment are:
- Control of deformity and prevention of neurological impairment
  The aim of treatment early in life is to control the deformity and prevent neurological deterioration at an age when surgical intervention is not a good option.
- Correct deformity
  Correction of the deformity may be indicated as a measure to prevent neurological damage from occurring or it may be as an adjunct to decompression of the cord once neurological deficit has developed.
- Prevent deterioration of neurological status once neurological signs are evident
  Once there is evidence of neurological impairment it is imperative that further progression of the neurological damage is prevented.

Treatment options

- TLSO or similar underarm brace
- Posterior spinal fusion with continued anterior growth
- Combined anterior and posterior spinal fusion
- Posterior vertebrectomy and spinal fusion with instrumentation.

Factors to be taken into consideration while planning treatment

- The age of the patient
- The site and localization of the deformity within a widespread disease
- The presence of neurological impairment
- The associated clinical features and disabilities of the underlying condition.

Recommended treatment and rationale of treatment

Under two years of age the management is by observation and education of the families as to the natural history of the particular condition. Beyond two years of age an underarm brace may be employed if the associated clinical issues permit. After five years of age a posterior-only fusion may gain stability and allow for the anterior vertebrae to grow out the deformity. This is more useful where the secondary changes from growth are greater than the deformity of the vertebra due to the disease. By the end of the first decade the vertebrae may be of a size to permit a definitive fusion, which may be a combined anterior discectomy and posterior instrumentation. If the deformity is due to focal disease a posterior-only approach with vertebrectomy and posterior instrumentation and fusion is employed.

An outline of treatment of kyphotic deformity in skeletal dysplasia is shown in Table 22.3.

Table 22.3 ● Outline of treatment of kyphosis in skeletal dysplasia

INDICATIONS				
<2 years of age	2–5 years of age	5–10 years of age	>10 years of age[a] + Deformity involves several vertebral segments	>10 years of age[a] + Deformity localized to one or two segments
			⇩	⇩
		⇩	Anterior discectomy of affected segments + Posterior spinal instrumentation and fusion	Vertebrectomy + Posterior spinal instrumentation and fusion (both procedures performed through posterior approach)
⇩	⇩	Posterior spinal fusion		
Observation and education of family	TLSO			
TREATMENT				

[a] If neurological deficit appears, definitive surgery may be needed at an earlier age.

Congenital kyphosis

Kyphosis of congenital origin can arise because of failure of formation of vertebrae, failure of segmentation or due to congenital dislocation of the spine. The deformity in congenital kyphosis is often far more dramatic than congenital scoliosis. The major issue is the high risk of neurological involvement, particularly for deformities at or above the thoracolumbar junction.

Failure of formation

Dubousset[7] has described three types of failure of formation leading to kyphosis:

- Partial failure of formation with a well-aligned canal: Symmetrical deficiency is typically seen with a butterfly hemivertebra (Figure 22.4). An asymmetrical deficiency will lead to a kyphoscoliotic deformity.
- Partial failure of formation with a dislocated canal: This was described in 1973 as a 'congenital dislocation of the spine'. The risk to the cord, which is frequently dysraphic, is great and progression of the deformity can be rapid.

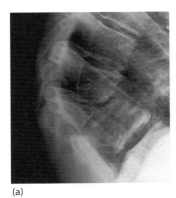
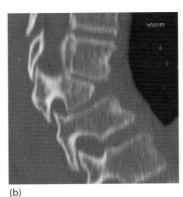
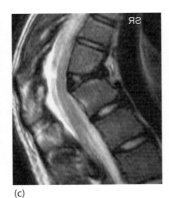
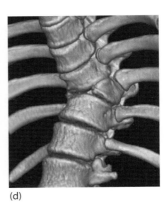

(a)　　　　　　　　　　　(b)　　　　　　　　　　　(c)　　　　　　　　　　　(d)

Figure 22.4 ● Congenital kyphosis due to agenesis of vertebral elements seen on the plain lateral radiograph **(a)**, computed tomography (CT) scan **(b)**, magnetic resonance imaging **(c)** and 3-D reconstruction of CT images **(d)**.

● Total failure of formation of vertebral bodies: Total failure of formation of one or more vertebrae is usually associated with congenital paralysis. This syndrome blends in with sacral agenesis.

Failure of segmentation

Failure of segmentation of the anterior elements and continued growth posteriorly results in a smooth kyphosis. The fusion anteriorly may not be apparent early in life and the appearance may be similar to Scheuermann's disease. There may be multiple vertebrae involved and severe deformity may develop.

Problems in management

Growth imbalance

Growth imbalance, on account of failure of growth of the anterior part of the vertebral column with growth of the posterior elements, will lead to progressive deformity. Once progression is documented surgical treatment should follow.

Mechanical factors

If the posterior elements are intact the spine may be stable but progression of the deformity will be rapid. If there are deficiencies in the posterior elements as well the resultant instability may lead to sudden neurological injury.

Neurological factors

Cord compromise may be antenatal in origin, secondary to malformation of the cord itself or develop in childhood secondary to the progressive deformity of the spine. Only cord compromise due to the latter can be expected to recover. Lesions of gradual onset, incomplete cord lesions and young age are better prognostic factors. The more long-standing and more severe the neurological deficit, the less likely are the chances of recovery.

Aims of treatment

- Prevent neurological impairment
  This may entail correction of deformity, preventing the progression of existing deformity or stabilizing an inherently unstable spine.
- Correct deformity
  Ideally, the deformity needs to be corrected before it becomes severe enough to put the cord in jeopardy.
- Prevent deterioration of neurological status once neurological signs of recent onset are evident
  The same measures considered for prevention of neurological deficit may need to be applied.
- Improve function
  If there is no likelihood of neurological improvement as in children with established long-standing neural damage, attention needs to be directed towards improving other functions. If spinal surgery can facilitate improvement of function (e.g. improving sitting balance in a child with spina bifida) it should be considered.

Treatment options for kyphosis without neurological deficit

Traction or distraction casting

If the kyphosis is flexible, traction or distraction casting can be utilized to lessen the deformity. Dubousset[7] recommends a period in a distraction cast. However, the author is more familiar with traction.

Excision of hemivertebra, posterior fusion and posterior instrumentation (posterior approach)

In the young child with a posterolateral hemivertebra, resection of the hemivertebra via a posterior approach and a short segment fusion with internal fixation is the treatment of choice[8,9] (Figure 22.5).

Anterior disc excision and posterior fusion and instrumentation (anterior and posterior approach)

In the older child coming to the end of growth with an established or worsening deformity, the flexibility of the apex may dictate treatment. Anterior excision of discs and soft tissue followed by posterior fusion with internal fixation will be necessary if the deformity is becoming rigid.

Anterior disc excision, anterior strut grafting, anterior instrumentation and fusion (anterior approach)

If the deformity is moderate and the patient is symptom free without neurological compromise, an anterior approach with excision of discs and anterior instrumentation around a strut may be the less risky approach in regard to the spinal cord.

Anterior strut grafting and fusion *in situ* without correcting the deformity (anterior approach)

In severe deformities anterior struts may be used. If the apex is rigid then it may be preferable to accept the deformity and fuse *in situ* rather than risk neurological injury by exploration of the cord.

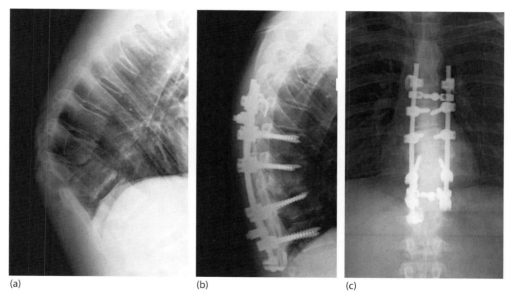

(a)   (b)   (c)

Figure 22.5 ● Surgical correction of a patient with congenital kyphosis **(a)** by excision of the hemivertebra, posterior instrumentation and fusion **(b,c)**.

Treatment options for kyphosis associated with neurological deficit

Indirect decompression by traction

Traction may be used as a method of indirect decompression of the spinal cord in children with early recent onset neurological impairment. If the cord recovers by this indirect decompression then stabilization by fusion is necessary but can be performed in the position gained by the traction. Careful neurological monitoring is required while the child is in traction to ensure that there is no deterioration of the neurological deficit.

Indirect decompression by distraction casting

Distraction casting works in much the same way as traction and the same precautions need to be taken while this is being attempted.

Direct spinal decompression

Cord or nerve compression of recent duration that does not resolve by conservative means will require direct decompression. This is usually accomplished via a posterior approach as it is the posterior aspect of the vertebral body that must be resected. Care must be taken to get above and below the apex of the offending lesion and surgical plans must incorporate stabilization as resection of anterior and posterior elements will render the spine more unstable. The decompression may then be followed by an anterior strut graft or posterior instrumentation. Posterior osteotomies or bone resection should be preceded by implant insertion and stabilization of the vertebral column to control any instability induced.

Spinal stabilization without spinal decompression

If there is a long-standing deficit or an incomplete lesion from birth then the surgical plan should be directed to stabilization rather than decompression.

Congenital kyphosis with spina bifida is virtually always associated with a complete high lumbar or thoracic cord lesion which is permanent. In these children the indications for surgery include recurrent skin breakdown, sitting imbalance and the need to use hands for support instead of for activities of daily living. The treatment of choice is vertebral column resection and internal fixation. Intramedullary fixation of the lumbar spine with thoracic sublaminar wires is simple, cost-effective and readily available.

Factors to be taken into consideration while planning treatment

- Age of the child
- Flexibility of the deformity
- Severity of the deformity
- Duration of neurological deficit, if present.

Recommended treatment

An outline of treatment is presented in Table 22.4.

Rarer causes of kyphosis

Kyphosis at the lumbosacral junction

The two principal abnormalities that cause a kyphotic deformity at the lumbosacral junction are congenital abnormalities and dysplastic spondylolisthesis (Figure 22.6). Both groups have a structural basis of congenital origin.

In the former group the issue is usually one of neurological impairment rather than the kyphotic deformity. Treatment in this group is usually directed towards surgical decompression rather than correction of the kyphosis.

In the latter group the problems may be a combination of pain, deformity and neurological compromise. If the clinical problem is one of pain and deformity the treatment is directed towards correction of the sagittal alignment and fusion. Note, however, that correction of the spinal alignment may be through the L4/L5 interspace with fusion to the sacrum from L4. Alternatively, in some patients correction of the kyphosis and listhesis is possible at the L5/S1 level. This requires instrumentation and fusion with an interbody graft.

If there is objective neurological loss, then decompression via reduction is necessary with fusion to the sacrum from either L4 or L5.

Kyphosis at the sacroiliac level

Kyphotic deformities are seen in two groups of patients and may also be considered as iatrogenic problems. Spina bifida patients who have undergone vertebral resection early in life with a fusion to the sacrum from the thoracic spine can subluxate through the sacroiliac joints. This presumably arises from excessive loads on immature joints. Correction is very difficult. The implication is that spine bifida patients with a congenital kyphosis should not undergo correction until the skeleton has matured significantly.

The second group are those patients who are normally active but who have had a long fusion to the pelvis at a time when there is still significant growth to come. In both groups the option of

Table 22.4 ● Outline of treatment of congenital kyphosis

INDICATIONS						
No neurological deficit + Young child + Posterolateral hemivertebra	No neurological deficit + Older child + Flexible deformity of moderate degree	No neurological deficit + Older child + Rigid deformity of moderate degree	No neurological deficit + Older child + Rigid deformity of severe degree	Neurological deficit present + Neurological impairment of recent onset + Flexible deformity + No neurological recovery noted with traction or distraction cast	Neurological deficit present + Neurological impairment of recent onset + Flexible deformity + Neurological recovery noted with traction or distraction cast	Neurological deficit present + Long-standing neurological impairment
⇩ Resection of hemi-vertebra + Posterior fusion (short segment) + Posterior instrumentation (posterior approach)	⇩ Traction or distraction cast + Anterior disc excision + Posterior fusion + Posterior instrumentation (anterior and posterior approach)	⇩ Anterior disc excision + Anterior fusion with strut graft + Anterior instrumentation (anterior approach)	⇩ Accept deformity + Anterior fusion *in situ* with strut graft (anterior approach)	⇩ Indirect decompression of spinal canal by traction or distraction cast + Fusion in position gained by traction or cast	⇩ Direct decompression of spinal canal + Fusion + Instrumentation	⇩ Fusion + Instrumentation (NO decompression of spinal canal)
TREATMENT						

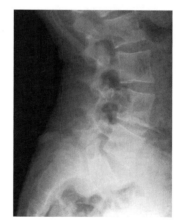

Figure 22.6 ● Lateral radiograph of the lumbosacral spine showing dysplastic spondylolisthesis in an adolescent.

delaying treatment of the primary deformity is not always possible. However, the parents and sometimes the patients need to be aware of this possible outcome.

Iatrogenic kyphosis following laminectomy

Conditions such as spinal cord tumours may demand multiple laminectomies and often at an early age. Kyphosis often results in this setting. Laminoplasty procedures may provide a protective barrier to the spinal cord but unfortunately do not protect against the development of a kyphosis over time.

Consideration for the use of long-term brace wear should be given to prevent the deformity arising during the period when the natural history of the tumour is becoming apparent. Consideration should be given to internal fixation and spinal fusion where progression of the deformity is documented. Age can be a barrier to early intervention.

Summary

Kyphotic deformities of the spine are a common feature of many disease processes. While the deformity may be viewed as purely cosmetic in neurologically intact patients, the possibility of developing neurological impairment is real. Patients presenting with a recent neurological loss may require early stabilization and fusion, and possibly spinal cord decompression. Patients with long-standing paraplegia may warrant stabilization but the spinal cord cannot be expected to recover, and thus decompressive procedures are not indicated.

References

1. Gutowski WT, Renshaw TS. Orthotic results in adolescent kyphosis. *Spine* 1988; **13**: 485–9.
2. Scheuermann HW. Kyphosis dorsalis juvenilis. *Orthop Chir* 1921; **41**: 305.
3. Sachs B, Bradford D, Winter R *et al*. Scheuermann kyphosis. Follow-up of Milwaukee-brace treatment. *J Bone Joint Surg Am* 1987; **69**: 50–7.
4. Ryan MD, Taylor TKF. Acute spinal cord compression in Scheuermann's disease. *J Bone Joint Surg Br* 1982; **64**: 409–12.
5. Lee SS, Lenke LG, Kukio TR *et al*. Comparison of Scheuermann kyphosis correction by posterior-only thoracic pedicle screw fixation versus combined anterior/posterior fusion. *Spine* 2006; **31**: 2316–21.
6. Levin TL, Berdon WE, Lachman RS *et al*. Lumbar gibbus deformity in storage diseases and bone dysplasias. *Pediatr Radiol* 1997; **27**: 289–94.
7. Dubousset J. Congenital kyphosis and lordosis. In: Weinstein SL (ed.). *The Pediatric Spine*. Philadelphia, PA: Lippincott Williams and Wilkins, 2001.
8. Ruf M, Harms J. Posterior hemivertebra resection with transpedicular instrumentation: early correction in children aged 1 to 6 years. *Spine* 2003; **28**: 2132–8.
9. Ruf M, Harms J. Hemivertebra resection by a posterior approach: innovative operative technique and first results. *Spine* 2002; **27**: 1116–23.

Torticollis

Ian Torode

23

Introduction

Torticollis or wry neck is a combined deformity of the neck with tilt of the head to one side and rotation of the chin to the opposite side (Figure 23.1). There are numerous causes of torticollis, of which congenital muscular torticollis is the one that will concern orthopaedic surgeons. However, making the appropriate diagnosis when confronted with other causes of torticollis is highly important. While we exist in an era of multiple investigations the appropriate diagnosis is usually reached by attention to the history and examination.

The important points from the history are the age of onset, presence of precipitating factors, whether the deformity is constant or intermittent and whether the deformity is painful.

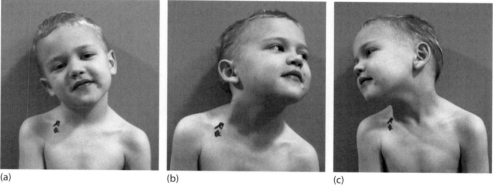

(a) (b) (c)

Figure 23.1 ● Classical appearance of muscular torticollis in a child. The deformity is evident when the child looks forwards **(a)** and the contracted sternocleidomastoid muscle can be identified when the child turns to either side **(b,c)**.

From the examination one should note:

- if the deformity is a tilt and rotation or tilt alone;
- if the sternocleidomastoid muscle is contracted on the side of the tilt;
- if there is facial asymmetry and/or plagiocephaly;
- if there are other features such as a short neck, low hairline or webbed neck;
- if eye movement and vision are normal;
- if there is an adduction contracture of the hip in the infant with torticollis;
- if the gait and balance are normal in the walking child.

Types of torticollis

Acute wry neck

This is a relatively common condition that may present in a previously well child with no history of deformity. It occurs after infancy, may occur spontaneously and is often seen after waking. Occasionally, it is seen after minimal trauma or associated with an upper respiratory tract infection. Clinically, there should not be plagiocephaly, there may be muscle spasm but this is diffuse and not confined to the sternocleidomastoid and there may be signs of lymphadenitis if a respiratory infection is at the root of the problem.

Treatment is directed towards resting the neck with a soft collar or traction and the use of simple analgesics or antispasmodic drugs. If the problem does not resolve readily then one should investigate to exclude atlantoaxial subluxation (see Chapter 34, Atlantoaxial instability).

Congenital anomalies

There are a wide variety of anomalies at the occipitocervical junction that can present with torticollis or head tilt. In these children there is usually no muscle spasm and there is usually a short neck with restricted motion in most directions. In some cases there will be webbing of the soft tissues and a low hairline. These deformities will usually have been present from birth although occasionally a hemivertebra may escape notice until the deformity worsens with growth. In other children the pattern of development may relate to a more widespread condition. Usually symptoms arise in later life. Very occasionally, there may be sternocleidomastoid spasm that warrants surgical intervention, although this will not cure the underlying condition.

Ocular torticollis

A child presenting with predominantly a head tilt but without pain and without contracture of the sternocleidomastoid and with a good range of motion in the cervical spine should alert the examiner to consider an ocular cause for the posture. One should look for strabismus (misalignment of the eyes) or nystagmus (rapid jerking movement of the eye). Weakness of the superior oblique muscle is a common cause of ocular torticollis in children. Duane syndrome is a rare ocular cause of torticollis due to a congenital disorder of eye movement.[1] Referral to an ophthalmologist is appropriate.

Neurogenic torticollis

The most important diagnosis in this group is that of a posterior fossa tumour or tumour of the lower cranial nerves. The presenting feature may be torticollis; however, there is commonly absence of a contracture of sternocleidomastoid. There may be signs of irritability or pain or stiffness.[2] Deviation of the tongue will point to a lesion of the XII cranial nerve.

Congenital anomalies of the cord such as a Chiari malformation can also cause torticollis.

Intermittent torticollis as opposed to a persistent deformity is a feature of cervical dystonia. This is the most common form of the focal dystonias. Usually the onset is in adult life but can present in children. It affects women more commonly and a small proportion of cases are familial. Botulinum toxin may be of benefit to some patients. Selective peripheral denervation is also employed.[3] Sandifer syndrome is a rare condition characterized by gastro-oesophageal reflux, spastic torticollis and dystonic body movements. The diagnosis may be difficult but possibly underreported.[4]

Hysterical or psychogenic torticollis

This is a particularly difficult situation to diagnose and treat. Usually the patient presents with a short history of a visible deformity but without any causative focus. The patient is likely to be adolescent rather than a younger child. There will not be facial asymmetry and no tightness of sternocleidomastoid initially. The deformity will readily correct in the early stages under anaesthetic although after some time a fixed deformity can develop. Clearly, all efforts are made to find an organic cause before making the diagnosis and this will involve a magnetic resonance scan to look for occult tumours as outlined above. Psychiatric assistance is mandatory.

Muscular torticollis

This could be termed a classical deformity in orthopaedics. In Jones's monograph on the subject the descriptions have been traced in writings from Hippocrates (500BC) to the present day. It is the most common form of torticollis in infants and children. The deformity is due to a contracture of sternocleidomastoid. The head is tilted to the involved side and the chin rotated to the opposite side.

■ Aetiology

The definitive cause is unknown. It is possible that birth trauma is a factor resulting in muscle trauma to the sternocleidomastoid. This was suggested by Van Rooenhyze (1670) and by André (1743) in *Orthopaedia*. A disproportionate number of children in some series have a history of being primiparous, breech or a difficult delivery. However there is no doubt that torticollis is seen after normal births or following caesarean section. Furthermore, specimens from autopsies of neonates have revealed mature fibrotic changes within the sternocleidomastoid muscle which clearly place the onset of the disease in the intrauterine period. Mikulicz (1895) and Volker (1902) proposed anoxia as the cause of fibrosis and suggested that these changes came on during the birth process. More recently, the fibrosis as a sequel of compartment syndrome due to intrauterine position has been suggested.[5] Neurological injury has also been proposed due to injury to the spinal accessory nerve and secondary fibrosis. There are occasional descriptions of a familial incidence; however, the vast majority of children are isolated cases. On the other hand, the large numbers in the series by Cheng *et al.*[6] implies that there is a racial difference in incidence.

■ Clinical findings

The clinical features will vary depending on the age of the child. If noted in the post-natal period a 'tumour' may be palpated in the neck. This mass is non-tender and soft to firm but not hard. The mass tends to resorb in the following weeks and the clinical picture is then one of a contracture of the sternocleidomastoid and the associated torticollis. As time passes and the age of presentation increases, the incidence and degree of facial asymmetry increases. Plagiocephaly is associated with the facial asymmetry. These changes can be expected to improve with time after correction of the deformity.

The presence of deformity without tightness of the sternocleidomastoid should encourage one to look for an underlying vertebral anomaly. Spasm of the sternocleidomastoid can occasionally occur in the presence of a vertebral anomaly and require treatment.[7] Fibrosis of both sternocleidomastoid muscles has been described, resulting in a restricted range of motion but not necessarily deformity.

■ Pathology

The fibrotic changes in the sternocleidomastoid muscle have often been described. These descriptions arise from necropsy specimens and from surgical specimens. The extent of fibrosis can vary from a relatively short segment to fibrosis of the entire length of the muscle. Histological studies have not clarified the aetiology of the deformity except to place the time frame in the intrauterine period prior to the onset of labour.

Problems of management

- Delay in presentation and, consequently, a less satisfactory outcome in regard to facial asymmetry and plagiocephaly.
- Recurrence of the deformity.
- Failure to recognize that the sternocleidomastoid is not the prime mover in some of these patients. Suspicion of an alternative diagnosis must always be considered if there is no demonstrable contracture of sternocleidomastoid.

Aims of treatment

- To correct the deformity and restore the range of motion of the cervical spine
- To achieve a satisfactory outcome in regard to facial asymmetry and plagiocephaly
- To avoid recurrence of the deformity
- To achieve the above without complications or unsightly scars

Treatment options

Manual stretching and active positioning

In a large series of patients >90 percent of success was achieved with a programme of manual stretching performed three times a week by a trained physiotherapist, coupled with a home programme of active positioning.[8] The stretch that has been applied to the sternocleidomastoid is documented by the report of rupture of that muscle during the stretching programme. This occurrence was not associated with any deleterious effect.[9] Lorenz, in 1891, attempted closed myorrhexis, but with complications including brachial plexus palsy this procedure was abandoned.[10]

Injection of Botulinum toxin

For recalcitrant congenital muscular torticollis satisfactory outcomes have been achieved by the use of Botulinum toxin type A in an attempt to avoid surgical release.[11] However, since the toxin blocks the neuromuscular junction it may only be effective in relieving spasm and have little effect on established contracture.

Surgical lengthening of the sternocleidomastoid musculotendinous unit

The surgical principle of correction of deformity due to a muscle contracture by lengthening that muscle has long been established. In relation to torticollis a percutaneous technique was described by Tulp (cited in Jones[10]) While this technique is no longer in vogue, the modern day equivalent is the use of endoscopy to achieve the lengthening and avoid noticeable scars.[12]

The alternative procedure is to surgically lengthen the muscle by an open procedure.[13] This can be achieved by open division in the mid-substance of the sternocleidomastoid[10] or by utilizing a bipolar approach (Figure 23.2). The latter entails the use of a transverse incision behind the ear to visualize and divide the origin of the sternocleidomastoid from the mastoid process. A second transverse incision just above the clavicle gives access to the heads of insertion of the sternocleidomastoid.

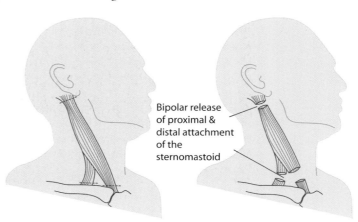

Bipolar release of proximal & distal attachment of the sternomastoid

Figure 23.2 ● Technique of releasing the sternocleidomastoid muscle.

Factors to be taken into consideration while planning treatment

- The correlation of the deformity with a treatable cause, i.e. sternocleidomastoid contracture.
- The presence of congenital vertebral anomalies.
- The age of the child.
- The degree of associated facial asymmetry and plagiocephaly.

Recommended treatment

The outline of treatment of torticollis is shown in Table 23.1.

Table 23.1 ● Outline of treatment of torticollis

INDICATIONS					
Torticollis + No contracture of the sternomastoid muscle + Weakness of external ocular muscles or nystagmus	Torticollis + No contracture of the sternomastoid muscle + No demonstrable ocular pathology	Torticollis + No contracture of the sternomastoid muscle + No demonstrable ocular or neurological pathology	Torticollis of recent onset + Spasm of the sternomastoid muscle + Pain	Torticollis + Contracture of the sternomastoid muscle + Infant	Torticollis + Contracture of the sternomastoid muscle + Older child + Facial asymmetry
					⇩
					Release of sternomastoid
		⇩	⇩	⇩	
	⇩	Refer to psychiatrist to exclude psychogenic cause	Investigate to exclude atlantoaxial instability	Regular stretching of the sternomastoid	
⇩	Refer to neurologist to exclude neurological cause				
Refer to ophthalmologist for treatment					
TREATMENT					

The author's favoured approach for surgical treatment of muscular torticollis is to make the distal incision and localize the offending tendons. A tape is passed around those tendons and the second proximal incision is made. By applying traction to the distal tape the proximal origin is readily identified and its release confirmed. The distal tenotomy is then performed and the wounds closed. An asymmetrical collar is then used in older children to encourage appropriate head posture. Supervised stretching via a physiotherapist is often helpful and a mirror can be used to assist in the re-education of the children as to what is an 'erect' posture. The proximal incision is not visible and the distal incision heals well and is not a cosmetic impairment (Figure 23.3).

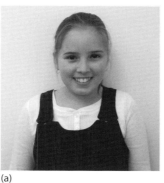 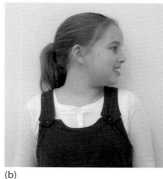 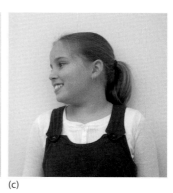

(a) (b) (c)

Figure 23.3 ● **(a–c)** Clinical result after release of the sternocleidomastoid. There is no residual tightness of the muscle and the scar is inconspicuous.

References

1. Williams CRP, O'Flynn E, Clarke NM, Morris RJ. Torticollis secondary to ocular pathology. *J Bone Joint Surg Br* 1996; **78**: 620–4.
2. Gupta AK, Roy DR, Conlan ES, Crawford AH. Torticollis secondary to posterior fossa tumors. *J Pediatr Othop* 1996; **16**: 505–7.
3. Factor SA, Lew MF, Trosch RM. Current and emerging treatments for cervical dystonia. *CNS Spectr* 2000; **5** (6 Suppl): S1–8.
4. Lehwald N, Krausch M, Franke C *et al.* Sandifer syndrome – a multidisciplinary and diagnostic challenge. *Eur J Pediatr Surg* 2007; **17**: 203–6.
5. Davids JR, Wenger DR, Mubarak SJ. Congenital muscular torticollis: sequela of intrauterine or perinatal compartment syndrome. *J Pediatr Orthop* 1993; **13**: 141–7.
6. Cheng JC, Tang SP, Chen TM, Wong MW, Wong EM. The clinical presentation and outcome of treatment of congenital muscular torticollis in infants – a study of 1,086 cases. *J Pediatr Surg* 2000; **35**: 1091–6.
7. Brougham DI, Cole WG, Dickens DR, Menelaus MB. Torticollis due to a combination of sternomastoid contracture and congenital anomalies. *J Bone Joint Surg Br* 1989; **71**: 404–7.
8. Cheng JCY, Wong MWN, Tang SP *et al.* Clinical determinants of the outcome of manual stretching in the treatment of congenital muscular torticollis in infants. *J Bone Joint Surg Am* 2001; **83**: 679–87.
9. Cheng JC, Chen TM, Tang SP *et al.* Snapping during manual stretching in congenital muscular torticollis. *Clin Orthop Relat Res* 2001; **384**: 239–44.
10. Jones PG. *Torticollis in Infancy and Childhood. Springfield, IL:* Charles C Thomas, 1968.
11. Joyce MB, de Chalain TM. Treatment of recalcitrant idiopathic muscular torticollis in infants with botulinum toxin type a. *J Craniofac Surg* 2005; **16**: 321–7.
12. Burstein RFD, Cohen SR. Endoscopic surgical treatment for congenital muscular torticollis. *Plast Reconstr Surg* 1998; **101**: 20–4.
13. Cheng JC, Tang SP. Outcome of surgical treatment of congenital muscular torticollis. *Clin Orthop Relat Res* 1999; **362**: 190–200.

SECTION 2

Dislocations

Developmental dysplasia of the hip

Randall Loder

24

Introduction

Developmental dysplasia of the hip (DDH) includes a wide spectrum of pathology ranging from mild acetabular dysplasia, which may not present until late adolescence or adulthood, to a fixed, total, irreducible dislocation of the hip diagnosed at birth. Management of this broad range of pathology requires considerable knowledge and thought on the part of the treating surgeon in diagnosis and treatment of the disorder as well as in communicating an honest prognosis to the parents.

In the past, DDH was known as congenital dislocation of the hip; however, there is now significant evidence that most hips are not dislocated at birth.[1] It is for this reason that the term DDH is now used. In this chapter we will not discuss the relatively rare teratologic hip dislocation which occurs early in fetal life, presents as a fixed, high-riding dislocation at birth, and is often associated with syndromes or other congenital malformations or genetic disorders (see Chapter 27, Teratologic hip dislocation in multiple congenital contractures).

Problems of management

Establishing a diagnosis and differentiating between neonatal hip instability, acetabular dysplasia, subluxation and complete dislocation

This is the key to management as the magnitude of involvement has a profound bearing on the necessary treatment. While complete dislocation may be easily diagnosed, neonatal hip instability or isolated acetabular dysplasia can be overlooked, unless an effort is made specifically to look for these forms of hip dysplasia.

Obtaining a reduction

Obtaining a reduction is relatively simple in cases of neonatal instability. However, once the hip dislocates and remains dislocated for some time, soft tissue impediments may develop and prevent reduction of the femoral head into the acetabulum. These include contracture of muscles crossing the hip – in particular, the iliopsoas and the adductor muscles, and contracture of the inferomedial part of the hip capsule (Figure 24.1).

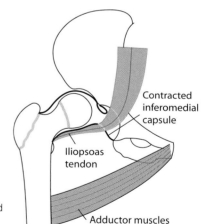

Contracted inferomedial capsule

Iliopsoas tendon

Adductor muscles

Figure 24.1 ● Structures that can impede reduction of a dislocated hip in a child with developmental dysplasia of the hip.

Obtaining a concentric reduction

Although simplistic in concept, this may be quite difficult in certain circumstances. Since the long-term goal is to have a perfect hip, a perfect concentric reduction is a prerequisite. In order for this to be achieved it is important to recognize impediments to a concentric reduction and to remove them.

In the young infant a concentric reduction is usually the rule as soft tissue changes only develop when the hip remains dislocated for some time. When the hip remains dislocated, the ligamentum teres becomes thicker and longer; the acetabular labrum with the capsule attached to it (the limbus) gets inverted into the acetabulum, the fibro-fatty tissue in the non-articular area of the floor of the acetabulum (the pulvinar) hypertrophies and the transverse acetabular ligament gets contracted. Each of these structures can prevent concentric reduction of the femoral head into the acetabulum (Figure 24.2).

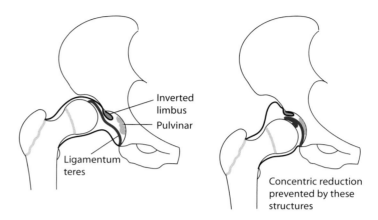

Figure 24.2 ● Factors that can contribute to failure to achieve a concentric reduction.

Maintaining a stable reduction

The concept appears quite simple, but subluxation or dislocation may recur even after seemingly satisfactory reduction of the hip. It is important to be aware of the factors that contribute to persistent instability of the hip. These factors include laxity of the superolateral capsule of the hip, coxa valga, femoral anteversion, acetabular dysplasia and abnormal acetabular version (Figure 24.3).

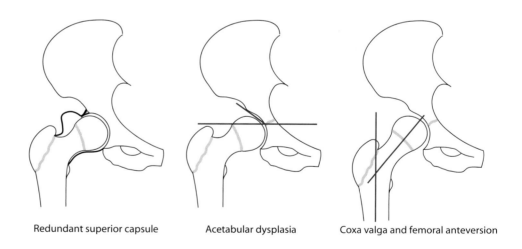

Redundant superior capsule   Acetabular dysplasia   Coxa valga and femoral anteversion

Figure 24.3 ● Factors that contribute to persistent instability after reduction of the hip in developmental dysplasia of the hip.

Avoiding complications

The complications of DDH are usually those of treatment and they include proximal femoral growth disturbances and avascular necrosis of the femoral capital epiphysis. Proximal femoral growth disturbance may result in shortening of the limb or deformities such as coxa vara or coxa valga; the latter deformity can lead to progressive subluxation during growth.[2] Avascular necrosis can lead to an incongruous joint and secondary degenerative arthritis.[3,4]

Allowing for normal growth and development of the hip

Early concentric reduction favours resumption of normal acetabular growth and this may enable correction of acetabular dysplasia in many instances, thus reducing the need for later pelvic osteotomy. Normal growth of the femoral ossific nucleus indicates that proximal femoral growth disturbance or avascular necrosis has not occurred.

Aims of treatment

- Obtain a concentric reduction
  It is imperative that the reduction that is obtained is concentric if the hip is to function normally in the long term. The quality of reduction must be documented to ensure that it is, in fact, a concentric reduction.
- Maintain stability of the hip
  The stability of the reduction needs to be maintained until growth is complete and the child needs to be followed up until skeletal maturity to ensure that the reduction remains stable.
- Stimulate normal growth and development of the hip
  Obtaining a concentric reduction with redirection of joint forces such that they become normal is key to the remodelling of the femoral head and acetabulum.
- Prevent complications
  In particular, avoid damage to the blood supply to the proximal femur.

Treatment options

Splinting of the hip

■ Rigid splints

Various rigid splints that hold the hips abducted were used in the past. Currently, they are not widely used.

■ Pavlik harness

In most children under four months of age, an initial trial with a Pavlik harness is recommended (Figure 24.4). It is the ideal treatment for a child with an Ortolani or Barlow positive hip instability. Circumstances in which it may not be indicated are in the older child (e.g. over six months) where a considerable time of immobilization is necessary. Once children begin to roll over and crawl it becomes very difficult to maintain reduction simply with a Pavlik harness.

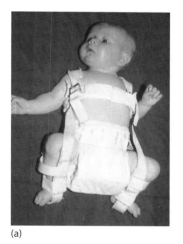
(a)

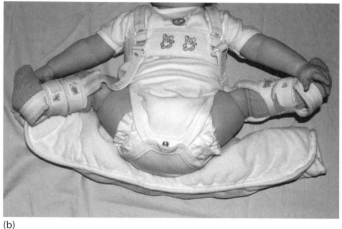
(b)

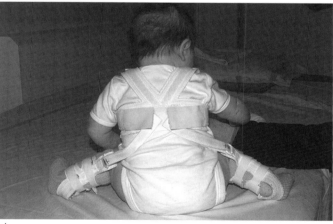
(c)

Figure 24.4 ● A Pavlik harness is used in infants under four months of age **(a)**. The position of the straps in front ensure that the hips are held flexed **(b)** while the straps at the back ensure that the hips remain abducted **(c)**. The harness is less effective in an older infant such as this who has begun to sit **(b,c)** or crawl.

In those children in whom the hip cannot be reduced on physical examination (Ortolani negative), the Pavlik harness can be tried but must be closely monitored. After application of the harness, the child must be re-examined within one to two weeks to document reduction both clinically and with imaging studies (e.g. hip ultrasound or radiographs). If a reduction cannot be obtained within two to four weeks, then the harness must be abandoned and a different treatment chosen.[5]

Pitfalls in Pavlik harness treatment include: inability to obtain and maintain reduction, which compounds the pathology by development of posterior acetabular insufficiency and instability; femoral nerve palsy; inferior or obturator dislocation; and avascular necrosis.[6,7] Posterior acetabular insufficiency occurs when the femoral head remains dislocated posteriorly over a prolonged time; the femoral head presses upon the posterior acetabular rim with resultant indentation and creation of a very shallow acetabulum (similar to a teacup saucer, rather than the teacup).[8] Femoral nerve palsy arises from hyperflexion. It is also for this reason that children in a Pavlik harness need to be re-examined on a frequent basis (every two to three weeks) to check the reduction, assess for appropriate fit of the harness and document active knee extension. Inferior obturator dislocation again may arise from hyperflexion, and is discovered on imaging studies during follow-up. Avascular necrosis usually arises from fixed hyperabduction, but will not be appreciated for many months after the harness has been stopped (failure or delay in ossification of the femoral head, irregular ossification of the femoral head, late physeal arrest resulting in either progressive valgus or varus deformity).

Closed reduction and spica cast application

When a Pavlik harness fails, or if the child is too large or mobile for a Pavlik harness, then an attempt at a gentle closed reduction under general anaesthesia with spica cast immobilization is the next option. The reduction should always be documented with an arthrogram to ensure that the reduction has truly occurred, and that there are no significant obstacles preventing complete reduction.[9]

Once the hip is reduced the stability of reduction is checked. While holding the hip in 90° of flexion the maximum abduction that is possible is noted. The hip is then slowly adducted and the point at which it redislocates is recorded. The arc of movement between maximum abduction and the point at which dislocation occurred is the 'safe zone'. The greater the arc of the safe zone, the more stable the hip. The arc of the safe zone is assessed with the hip in neutral rotation, internal rotation and external rotation to determine the most stable position of reduction.

If stable reduction is possible with less than 60° of abduction a spica cast is applied which extends from above the costal margin to the tips of the toes. The hips are held in at least 90° of flexion, approximately 45° of abduction and as near neutral rotation as possible. Documentation of the reduction in the spica cast must be performed. Imaging modalities that can be employed to document the reduction are a computed tomography (CT) scan, ultrasound or magnetic resonance imaging (MRI).

Adductor tenotomy and closed reduction

In some instances when a closed reduction is being attempted, tightness of the adductors may be noted that may prevent reduction. Percutaneous tenotomy of the adductors may then facilitate reduction. In most children between six and 18 months of age closed reduction, adductor tenotomy and spica cast immobilization are indicated.[10]

Once satisfactory reduction is achieved the treatment in a spica cast is as discussed above.

Open reduction

An open reduction is needed if: (1) closed reduction fails; (2) if after closed reduction the hip remains very unstable; (3) if stability after closed reduction can only be achieved by holding the hip in an extreme degree of abduction or internal rotation; or (4) if the reduction is not concentric.

Open reduction must address all the obstacles preventing a stable, concentric reduction. In a child less than one year of age open reduction can be performed via either a medial or anterior approach. If there is an inverted limbus, medial pulvinar or large ligamentum teres, then the medial approach is contraindicated, since these obstacles can not be adequately addressed from the medial approach. In a child older than one year the anterior approach is preferred.

Femoral osteotomy

Different forms of femoral osteotomy may be needed in order to achieve stable reduction. The femoral osteotomy can be either subtrochanteric or intertrochanteric if only shortening or rotation is desired; an intertrochanteric osteotomy is preferred if varus is desired. Fixation is achieved with dynamic compression types of plate for a subtrochanteric osteotomy and a blade plate or hip screws for an intertrochanteric varus osteotomy.

■ Varus osteotomy

If the hip remains stable only in wide abduction, a varus osteotomy is needed.

■ Derotation osteotomy

If after open reduction the anteversion requires significant internal rotation for the reduction to be stable, a derotation osteotomy is indicated. The derotation osteotomy corrects the associated femoral anteversion, reducing the need for extreme internal rotation in the post–operative cast position. This reduces the incidence of avascular necrosis.

■ Varus derotation osteotomy

If the hip remains stable only in abduction and internal rotation, a varus derotation osteotomy is necessary.

■ Femoral shortening

In older children, a femoral shortening osteotomy may be necessary to enable reduction of the hip. Shortening is also needed if the hip is so high riding that it is unstable following reduction due to increased tension from the longitudinal traction necessary to obtain reduction.[11]

A femoral shortening osteotomy reduces the tension on the femoral head and reduces the risk of avascular necrosis.[12–14]

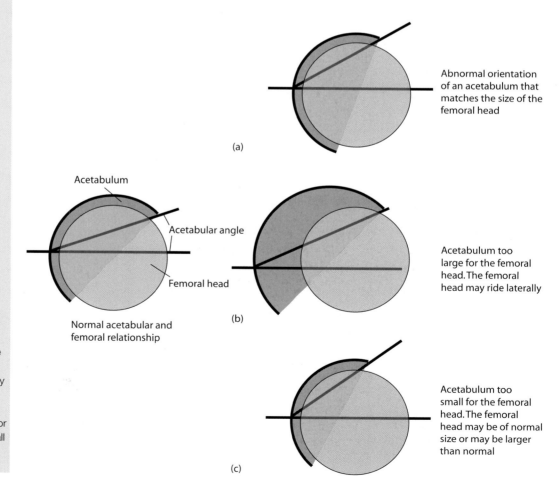

Figure 24.5 ● Acetabular dysplasia may be on account of three factors: the acetabular orientation may be such that the femoral head is not adequately covered **(a)**; the acetabulum may be too large and shallow permitting the femoral head to ride proximally and laterally **(b)**; or the acetabulum may be too small to adequately cover the femoral head **(c)**.

Abnormal orientation of an acetabulum that matches the size of the femoral head

(a)

Acetabulum

Acetabular angle

Femoral head

Normal acetabular and femoral relationship

Acetabulum too large for the femoral head. The femoral head may ride laterally

(b)

Acetabulum too small for the femoral head. The femoral head may be of normal size or may be larger than normal

(c)

Correction of acetabular dysplasia

Acetabular dysplasia or inadequate coverage of the femoral head by the acetabulum may be due to three reasons: (1) the acetabulum may be abnormally oriented although of adequate capacity; (2) the acetabulum may be too large so that the femoral head can ride laterally and become uncovered; or (3) the acetabulum may be too small relative to the size of the femoral head (Figure 24.5). Operations to remedy each of these problems have been devised.[15]

■ Redirectional osteotomies (volume neutral)

One essential prerequisite for all redirectional osteotomies is that concentric reduction must first be achieved.

Volume neutral redirectional osteotomies that can be used are the Salter innominate, Sutherland double innominate, triple innominate of Steel or Tönnis, dial (e.g. Eppright) and the Ganz periacetabular osteotomy.

As the child becomes older, less coverage is obtainable by the Salter osteotomy, as the hinge points (sciatic notch and symphysis pubis) are a considerable distance from the acetabulum. Osteotomies that hinge or rotate closer to the acetabulum give better coverage in older patients. As the point of rotation of the osteotomy becomes closer to the acetabulum, greater coverage is obtainable in more planes (Figure 24.6).

■ Salter osteotomy

An osteotomy from the sciatic notch to the anterior inferior iliac spine and which hinges on the pubic symphysis and the sciatic notch (Figure 24.6a).

■ Double innominate osteotomy

Osteotomies from the sciatic notch to the anterior inferior iliac spine, and the conjoined pubis, which hinge on the pubis and the sciatic notch (Figure 24.6b).

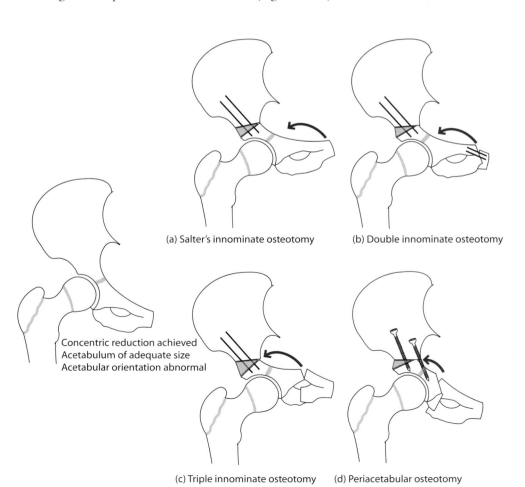

(a) Salter's innominate osteotomy

(b) Double innominate osteotomy

Concentric reduction achieved
Acetabulum of adequate size
Acetabular orientation abnormal

(c) Triple innominate osteotomy

(d) Periacetabular osteotomy

Figure 24.6 ● Examples of redirectional osteotomies of the pelvis used to treat acetabular dysplasia.

■ Triple innominate osteotomy

Osteotomies from the sciatic notch to the anterior inferior iliac spine, and the ischial and pubic rami, and which hinge on the pubis and the sciatic notch (Figure 24.6c).

■ Bernese periacetabular osteotomy of Ganz

Osteotomies performed in the pubis, ilium and ischium, which allow for extensive acetabular reorientation; they can only be performed when the triradiate cartilage has closed (Figure 24.6d).

■ Augmentation (volume increasing)

Operations that increase the volume of the acetabulum are various forms of shelf operations such as the Staheli acetabular augmentation and the Japanese tectoplasty. These operations improve coverage of the femoral head by adding bone graft over the uncovered part of the femoral head. The Chiari osteotomy improves femoral head coverage by displacing the acetabulum under a 'shelf' created by the innominate osteotomy. After all these operations the undersurface of the new shelf is not lined by articular cartilage, and a part of the capsule intervenes between the femoral head and the shelf.

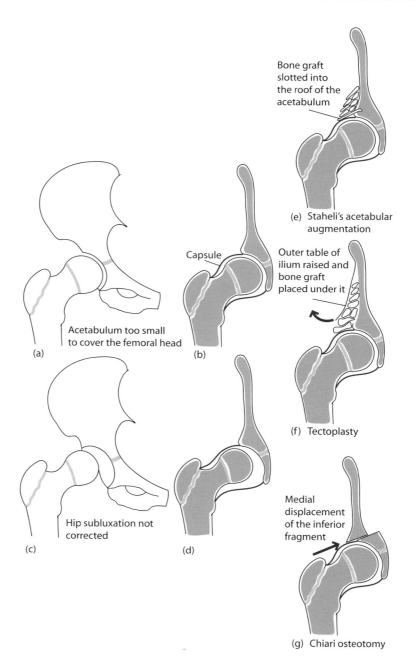

Figure 24.7 ● Examples of operations that attempt to increase the volume of the acetabulum that may be performed if the acetabulum is too small to cover the femoral head **(a,b)** or if hip subluxation cannot be adequately reduced **(c,d)** are shown. In these operations **(e–g)** the improved bony cover for the femoral head is lined by the hip capsule.

■ Staheli acetabular augmentation

An augmentation of the lateral acetabulum with placement of strips of corticocancellous bone graft between the hip capsule and the reflected head of the rectus femoris; it is a salvage osteotomy with no redirectional or hinge component (Figure 24.7e).

■ Tectoplasty

A proximally based flap of the outer cortex of the ilium that extends up to the margin of the joint capsule is raised and bone graft is packed under the flap to keep it elevated. This creates an extended acetabular roof. (Figure 24.7f).

■ Chiari osteotomy

A complete iliac osteotomy following the plane between the reflected head of the rectus femoris and the hip capsule, exiting posteriorly into the sciatic notch and anteriorly to the anterior inferior iliac spine; it is angled approximately 10–15° cranially. The distal fragment is then displaced medial relative to the proximal fragment (Figure 24.7g).

■ Reduction (volume reducing)

■ Pemberton osteotomy

An incomplete osteotomy with the lateral iliac cut starting equidistant between the anterior superior and anterior inferior iliac spines, parallel to the hip capsule and stopping at the ilioischial limb of the triradiate cartilage (Figure 24.8a). The amount of lateral coverage versus anterior coverage can be selected by the position of the medial cut relative to the lateral cut (equal gives anterior coverage, inferior gives more lateral coverage).

■ Dega osteotomy

An incomplete osteotomy of only the lateral ilium hinging on the triradiate cartilage (Figure 24.8b).

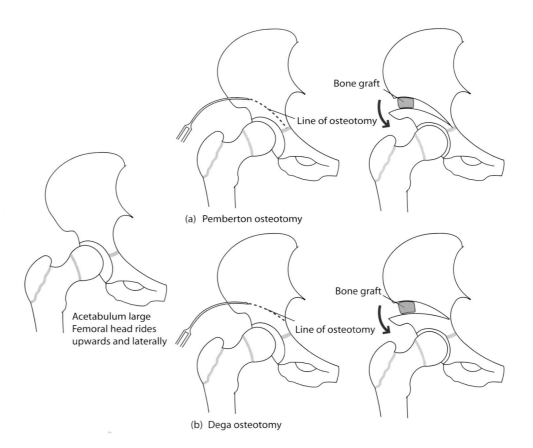

(a) Pemberton osteotomy

Acetabulum large
Femoral head rides
upwards and laterally

(b) Dega osteotomy

Figure 24.8 ● Examples of osteotomies that reduce the volume of the acetabulum.

The age of the child

This is very important when deciding if reduction or any treatment should even be attempted and, if reduction is to be performed, what the treatment options are. The treatment varies greatly as the age of the child advances.

Is the pathology instability, dysplasia, subluxation or dislocation?

This is very important to consider, along with the age of the child, as the treatment will vary with the nature of the underlying pathology.

Is there unilateral or bilateral dislocation?

Children with bilateral involvement are often diagnosed later than those with unilateral involvement. This is due to the fact that although the hip abduction is reduced in absolute magnitude it is not noticed since both sides are equally affected. A major hip reconstruction in the older child may require many months before adequate healing and rehabilitation permits treatment of the opposite hip. Thus there may be an insufficient amount of time necessary to treat both hips before the child passes the threshold age beyond which reduction hastens rather than forestalls degenerative hip disease. Many authors do not recommend reduction in children with bilateral dislocations after the age of six years, but will reduce a unilateral hip dislocation up to the age of eight years.

What are the obstacles preventing reduction?

This is important when deciding the type of treatment to be attempted and, if an open reduction is necessary, what approach to use (e.g. medial versus anterior). If an arthrogram shows minimal pulvinar and no other obstructions, then a simple closed reduction will probably suffice. In contrast, an inverted limbus or a constricting iliopsoas tendon or transverse acetabular ligament will require open reduction. A tight transverse acetabular ligament can be addressed through a medial approach, but an inverted limbus can only be addressed through an anterior approach.

Is the triradiate cartilage open or shut?

This is important when selecting the type of pelvic osteotomy – the Pemberton and Dega types can only be performed when the triradiate cartilage is still open. The Ganz periacetabular osteotomy can be performed only when the triradiate cartilage is closed.

Is the femoral head small, normal or large in size compared to the acetabulum?

This is very important when selecting a pelvic osteotomy – volume neutral, volume reducing or volume increasing.

What is the magnitude and location of acetabular dysplasia?

This is important when deciding the type of pelvic and femoral osteotomy needed. In the younger child (18 months to eight years), if the femoral head centres nicely on a simple abduction and internal rotation anterioposterior (AP) radiograph, then a femoral varus with or without a simpler redirectional osteotomy may be all that is required to obtain appropriate coverage. In older children, one must also ascertain whether the femoral head can be centred on the abduction internal rotation view; however, if the residual acetabular dysplasia is significant (>10° increase in acetabular index or Sharp's angle) compared to the opposite hip, then a more complex acetabular osteotomy will probably be needed (e.g. triple innominate, periacetabular).

In older adolescents and adults, there may be significant anterior uncoverage that will not necessarily be noted on standard AP radiographs. Here the false profile view, which demonstrates the anterior centre-edge (CE) angle of Lequense, will guide in the selection of the osteotomy and the extent of anterior coverage that is necessary.[16]

The outline of treatment of DDH in children is shown in Tables 24.1–24.4. and is briefly summarized below.

Table 24.1 ● Outline of treatment of developmental dysplasia of the hip in children under the age of four months

INDICATIONS		
Hip reducible by Ortolani manoeuvre	Hip not reducible by Ortolani manoeuvre	Unsatisfactory response to Pavlik harness (i.e. persistent instability, OR poor acetabular development, OR failure to achieve reduction) ⇩
⇩	⇩	Examine under anaesthesia and closed reduction and hip spica as outlined in Table 24.2
1 Pavlik harness for full-time use + 2 Monitor improvement of acetabular development (reduction in the β angle and an increase in the α angle of Graf) and Monitor for improved clinical stability of the hip + 3 Wean harness when hip has become stable + 4 Follow-up until skeletal maturity OR • If hip has not become stable in 6 weeks • Acetabular development not satisfactory after 6 weeks, follow steps of column 3	Pavlik harness for full-time use + Monitor at 1–2 weeks to ensure that reduction has occurred + IF reduction has been achieved, follow steps 2, 3, 4 of column 1 OR IF reduction not achieved in 2 weeks, follow steps of column 3	
TREATMENT		

Hip subluxation and dislocation

■ Age: Under four months

In the child with hip instability demonstrated by a positive Ortolani or Barlow sign, a Pavlik harness is recommended. After one to two weeks in the harness, both clinical examination and ultrasound examination[17] are performed to document improvement in both stability and acetabular development. The acetabular development can be quantified by ultrasound (Figure 24.9). On the ultrasound scan two angles are measured (the bony roof angle or α angle and the cartilage roof angle or β angle). An α angle greater than 60° and a β angle less than 55° suggests that the acetabular

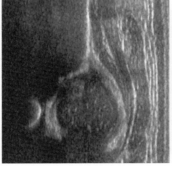
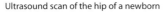
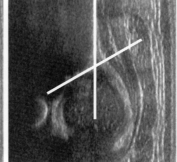
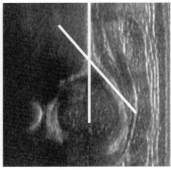

Figure 24.9 ● Ultraound images of a neonate's hip showing the angles measured to assess acetabular development.

Ultrasound scan of the hip of a newborn   The alpha angle   The beta angle

Table 24.2 ● Outline of treatment of developmental dysplasia of the hip in children between the age of 4 and 18 months

INDICATIONS			
Hip reducible when examined under anaesthesia + Reduction stable in neutral position	Hip reducible when examined under anaesthesia BUT Adductors are tight	Hip reducible when examined under anaesthesia BUT Very unstable (narrow safe zone) OR Hip stable only in extreme abduction or internal rotation OR Arthrogram following reduction shows non-concentric reduction ⇩	Hip NOT reducible by closed means when examined under anaesthesia even after adductor tenotomy ⇩
⇩	⇩	Open reduction + Hip spica x 6–12 weeks + Follow-up until skeletal maturity	Arthrogram to identify the impediments to reduction + Open reduction + Hip spica x 6–12 weeks + Follow-up until skeletal maturity
Confirm concentric reduction with arthrogram + Spica cast + Confirm concentric reduction in cast with CT/MRI + Sequential cast change at 6-week intervals until hip stable + Follow-up until skeletal maturity	Adductor tenotomy + Closed reduction + Confirm concentric reduction with arthrogram + Spica cast + Confirm concentric reduction in cast with CT/MRI + Sequential cast change at 6-week intervals until hip stable + Follow-up until skeletal maturity		
TREATMENT			

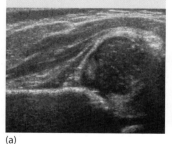
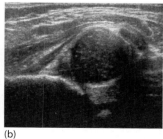
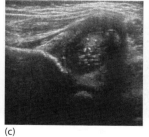
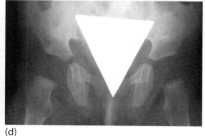

(a)   (b)   (c)   (d)

Figure 24.10 ● This six-week-old girl presented with an Ortolani positive right hip dislocation. The ultrasound obtained before reduction demonstrates the dislocation **(a)**. Immediately after harness application, even though the hip clinically felt reduced, an ultrasound documented incomplete reduction **(b)**; after two weeks in a Pavlik harness, the hip has become completely reduced **(c)** but still with residual acetabular dysplasia as noted by the shallow α Graf angle. An anteroposterior pelvis radiograph at five months of age documents reduction of both hips, early appearance of both ossific nuclei and equal acetabular indices **(d)**.

Table 24.3 ● Outline of treatment of developmental dysplasia of the hip in children between the ages of 18 months and 8 years

Open reduction is indicated in all cases + Femoral osteotomy as indicated below		
INDICATIONS FOR FEMORAL OSTEOTOMY		
Reduction stable in: Neutral position No undue tension (a rare situation) ⇩	Reduction stable only in: (a) Internal rotation OR (b) Abduction OR (c) Abduction and internal rotation ⇩	Considerable difficulty encountered in reducing the hip after release of all soft tissue impediments ⇩
Open reduction without femoral osteotomy	Open reduction to be combined with femoral osteotomy as indicated: Derotation if (a) Varus if (b) Varus derotation if (c)	Femoral shortening ± Varus or derotation femoral osteotomy if indicated, as shown in column 2
If there is radiological evidence of acetabular dysplasia treat as shown in Table 24.4		
TREATMENT		

Table 24.4 ● Treatment of acetabular dysplasia

INDICATIONS					
18 months–6 years		6 years–skeletal maturity		Skeletal maturity	
Concentric reduction achieved + Normal size acetabulum ⇩	Concentric reduction achieved + Large acetabulum ⇩	Concentric reduction achieved + Normal size acetabulum ⇩	Concentric reduction NOT possible OR Small acetabulum ⇩	Concentric reduction achieved ⇩	Concentric reduction NOT possible OR Small acetabulum ⇩
Salter osteotomy	Pemberton OR Dega osteotomy	Salter (until 8 years) OR Steel OR Tönnis osteotomy	Shelf procedure OR Chiari osteotomy	Steel OR Tönnis OR Ganz osteotomy	Chiari osteotomy
TREATMENT					

development is normal. If the reduction is satisfactory the harness is kept in place for six weeks, by which time the hip ought to have become stable and the acetabular development should have been restored to near normal (Figure 24.10).[18]

When a Pavlik harness fails or the child is too large or mobile for one, then a gentle closed reduction and spica cast immobilization is performed. If reduction requires significant abduction, an adductor tenotomy is performed.

If the reduction remains unstable, then open reduction and spica casting is needed (Figure 24.11). The author prefers the anterior approach for all open reductions. The author also routinely performs a capsulorraphy in all open reductions to improve stability, although some authors do not feel a capsulorraphy is as critical. After any reduction and spica cast application, documentation and maintenance of the reduction must be performed (Figure 24.11d).

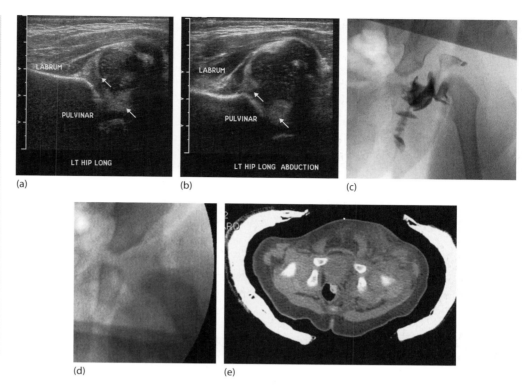

(a) (b) (c)

(d) (e)

Figure 24.11 ● This six-week-old girl presented with an apparent Ortolani positive hip dislocation, which was extremely unstable. The hip remains dislocated with interposed labrum and pulvinar **(a)**, even with a reduction manoeuvre in abduction **(b)**. An arthrogram at ten weeks of age demonstrates an inverted limbus **(c)** which required an open reduction **(d)**. Note the vague outline of the femoral head from retained arthrogram contrast after the open reduction. Computed tomography scan after the open reduction demonstrates maintenance of the reduction **(e)**.

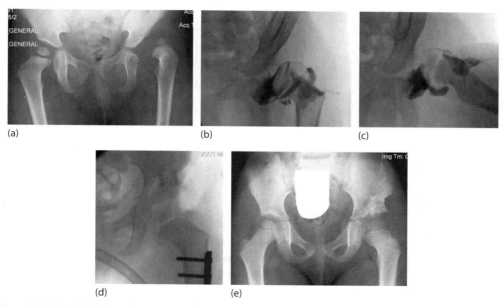

(a) (b) (c)

(d) (e)

Figure 24.12 ● A child aged one year and ten months with a newly diagnosed left developmental hip dislocation **(a)**. A closed reduction was not possible due to neolimbus which required open reduction **(b,c)**, femoral shortening and a Pemberton osteotomy **(d)**, using the femur removed from the shortening for the Pemberton osteotomy graft. Radiographs at three years and ten months demonstrate maintenance of the reduction with an intact Shenton's line and good acetabular remodelling **(e)**.

■ Age: four to 18 months

Initially an arthrogram, closed reduction, adductor tenotomy and spica cast immobilization is performed. If reduction cannot be obtained or is unstable, then an open reduction is performed. In rare cases femoral shortening with or without rotation is necessary. With either a closed or open reduction and spica cast immobilization, a post-reduction CT scan is performed to document reduction.

■ Age: 18 months to eight years

An open reduction, femoral and pelvic osteotomy, and spica cast immobilization is the treatment of choice.[12–14,19–22] Pre-operative traction is not used. In younger children (typically less than three years) a subtrochanteric femoral osteotomy is used (Figure 24.12). In older children, an intertrochanteric osteotomy with blade plate fixation is used so that a component of varus can be added.

■ Age: eight years to mid-adolescence

In these children, unless there are extenuating circumstances, simple observation without reduction of the hip is recommended.

■ Age: Mid-adolescence and adulthood

Again, in these patients observation without reduction of the hip is recommended.

Residual acetabular dysplasia alone (either primary or after previous reduction)

If the acetabulum is capacious, then a Pemberton pelvic osteotomy is selected.

If the joint can be made congruent and the acetabular volume is similar to that of the femoral head, then a redirectional pelvic osteotomy (most commonly the Salter osteotomy), with a possible femoral osteotomy, is recommended. In children less than four years of age with residual acetabular dysplasia and subluxation, a proximal femoral varus osteotomy alone may suffice.[23] Particular care and attention must be taken when a Salter osteotomy is performed along with a femoral rotational osteotomy. The Salter osteotomy gives anterior coverage at the expense of posterior coverage. If excessive femoral rotation is performed for correction of anteversion in concert with a Salter osteotomy, posterior dislocation, which is a very vexing condition, can occur.

In children over eight to ten years of age, a Salter osteotomy is not usually used, but rather the Steel osteotomy. If the triradiate cartilage is closed and there is significant dysplasia, then a Ganz periacetabular osteotomy is recommended. The periacetabular osteotomy must be performed by a surgeon who has the appropriate expertise and experience.

In the adolescent with asymptomatic mild dysplasia without subluxation (e.g. CE angle <20°, early sourcil sclerosis, etc.) and in whom reconstruction would require a large procedure, the author recommends that no intervention be undertaken until symptoms appear.

References

1. Ilfeld FW, Westin GW, Makin M. Missed or developmental dislocation of the hip. *Clin Orthop Relat Res* 1986; **203**: 276–81.
2. Campbell P, Tarlow SD. Lateral tethering of the proximal femoral physis complicating the treatment of congenital hip dysplasia. *J Pediatr Orthop* 1990; **10**: 6–8.
3. Malvitz TA, Weinstein SL. Closed reduction for congenital dysplasia of the hip. *J Bone Joint Surg Am* 1994; **76**: 1777–92.
4. Cooperman DR, Wallenstein R, Stulberg SD. Post-reduction avascular necrosis in congenital dislocation of the hip. *J Bone Joint Surg Am* 1980; **62**: 247–58.
5. Harding MGB, Harcke HT, Bowen JR, Guille JT, Glutting J. Management of dislocated hips with Pavlik harness treatment and ultrasound monitoring. *J Pediatr Orthop* 1997; **17**: 189–98.
6. Mubarak S, Garfin S, Vance R, McKinnon B, Sutherland D. Pitfalls in the use of the Pavlik harness for treatment of congenital dysplasia, subluxation, and dislocation of the hip. *J Bone Joint Surg Am* 1981; **63**: 1239–48.
7. Lerman JA, Emans JB, Millis MB *et al*. Early failure of Pavlik harness treatment for developmental hip dysplasia. *J Pediatr Orthop* 2001; **21**: 348–53.
8. Jones GT, Schoenecker PT, Dias LS. Developmental hip dysplasia potentiated by inappropriate use of the Pavlik harness. *J Pediatr Orthop* 1992; **12**: 722–6.

9. Forlin E, Choi IH, Guille JT, Bowen JR, Glutting J. Prognostic factors in congenital dislocation of the hip treated with closed reduction. *J Bone Joint Surg Am* 1992; **74**: 1140–52.

10. Vitale MG, Skaggs DL. Developmental dysplasia of the hip from six months to four years of age. *J Am Acad Orthop Surg* 2001; **9**: 401–11.

11. Zadeh HG, Catterall A, Nejad-Hashemi A, Perry RE. Test of stability as an aid to decide the need for osteotomy in association with open reduction in developmental dysplasia of the hip. *J Bone Joint Surg Br* 2000; **82**: 17–27.

12. Williamson DM, Glover SD, Benson MKDA. Congenital dislocation of the hip presenting after the age of three years. *J Bone Joint Surg Br* 1989; **71**: 745–51.

13. Ryan MG, Johnson LO, Quanbeck DS, Minkowitz B. One-stage treatment of congenital dislocation of the hip in children three to ten years old. *J Bone Joint Surg Am* 1998; **80**: 336–44.

14. Galpin RD, Roach JW, Wenger DR, Herring JA, Birch JG. One-stage treatment of congenital dislocation of the hip in older children, including femoral shortening. *J Bone Joint Surg Am* 1989; **71**: 734–41.

15. Gillingham BL, Sanchez AA, Wenger DR. Pelvic osteotomies for the treatment of hip dysplasia in children and young adults. *J Am Acad Orthop Surg* 1999; **7**: 325–37.

16. Clohisy JC, Barrett SE, Gordon JE, Delgago ED, Schoenecker PL. Periacetabular osteotomy for the treatment of severe acetabular dysplasia. *J Bone Joint Surg Am* 2005; **87**: 254–9.

17. Song KM, Lapinsky A. Determination of hip position in the Pavlik harness. *J Pediatr Orthop* 2000; **20**: 317–19.

18. Wientroub S, Grill F. Ultrasonography in developmental dysplasia of the hip. *J Bone Joint Surg Am* 2000; **82**: 1004–18.

19. Schoenecker PL, Strecker WB. Congenital dislocation of the hip in children. Comparison of the effects of femoral shortening and of skeletal traction in treatment. *J Bone Joint Surg Am* 1984; **66**: 21–7.

20. Salter RB. Innominate osteotomy in the treatment of congenital dislocation and subluxation of the hip. *J Bone Joint Surg Br* 1961; **43**: 518–39.

21. Lindstrom JR, Ponseti IV, Wenger DR. Acetabular response after reduction in congenital dislocation of the hip. *J Bone Joint Surg Am* 1979; **61**: 112–18.

22. Harris NH. Acetabular growth potential in congenital dislocation of the hip and some factors upon which it may depend. *Clin Orthop Relat Res* 1976; **119**: 99–106.

23. Schoenecker PL, Anderson DJ, Capelli AM. The acetabular response to proximal femoral varus rotational osteotomy. *J Bone Joint Surg Am* 1995; **77**: 990–97.

Paralytic hip dislocation: cerebral palsy

25

Benjamin Joseph

Introduction

Hip subluxation and dislocation are common in children with cerebral palsy. Ideally, the diagnosis of hip dysplasia should be made sufficiently early, so that the subluxated hip can be prevented from progressing on to a frank dislocation. This can only be achieved if children with cerebral palsy are regularly monitored for signs of impending hip dislocation.[1,2] Measurement of the migration percentage made on anteroposterior radiographs of the pelvis (Figure 25.1) will enable the surgeon to quantify the severity of hip subluxation.[3]

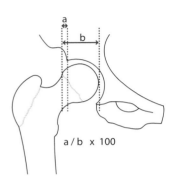

a / b x 100

Figure 25.1 ● Measurement of the Reimer's migration percentage can be used as a measure of the severity of hip subluxation.

The frequency of hip dysplasia varies with the topographic pattern of involvement. Dislocation of the hip is most frequent in children with total body involvement; it is significantly less frequent in diplegics and rare in hemiplegics.[4]

The implications of hip dislocation are also profoundly different in these groups. In diplegic children, hip dislocation can lead to losing their ability to walk. On the other hand, in children with total body involvement the consequences of hip dislocation include development of painful arthritis, problems in sitting and personal hygiene. There also seems to be an association between hip dislocation and the development of scoliosis, although a causative relationship has not been proven.

Problems of management

Spasticity of the adductor and flexors

The primary cause for hip dislocation in all types of cerebral palsy is spasticity of the hip flexors and adductors.

Muscle imbalance

The spasticity results in muscle imbalance between the flexors and extensors and between the adductors and the abductors. As a result the hip tends to lie in adduction and flexion.

Flexion and adduction contractures

Uncontrolled spasticity of the adductors and flexors leads to progressive limitation of passive abduction and extension of the hip and, eventually, adduction and flexion contractures develop.

Coxa valga and anteversion

Coxa valga and femoral anteversion develop and these contribute to the propensity for hip subluxation (Figure 25.2).

Globally deficient acetabulum

The acetabulum also fails to develop normally. Unlike in developmental dysplasia of the hip where the acetabulum is characteristically deficient anterolaterally, in cerebral palsy the acetabulum is globally deficient. As a result of this the hip can dislocate anteriorly, posteriorly or superiorly.[5]

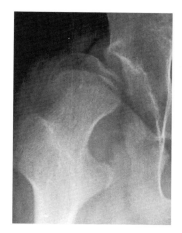

Figure 25.2 ● Radiograph of an ambulant child with diplegic cerebral palsy with severe subluxation of the right hip. Coxa valga, femoral anteversion and acetabular dysplasia are all present.

Articular cartilage erosion

Once the hip remains dislocated for some time, the articular cartilage may become eroded and the hip then becomes painful (Figure 25.3).

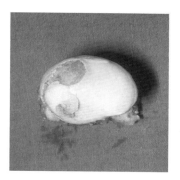

Figure 25.3 ● Articular cartilage is eroded over a large area of this femoral head that was excised from an adolescent with cerebral palsy and painful hip dislocation.

Aims of treatment

- Prevent hip subluxation and dislocation

  In the young child with early subluxation, prevention of hip dislocation is relatively simple as the adaptive bony changes in the femur and the acetabulum have not developed. Here the treatment is directed towards reducing the spasticity of the flexors and adductors of the hip and preventing these muscles from becoming contracted.

- Reduce the dislocated hip and prevent redislocation if the hip is not painful

  If the hip is severely subluxed or frankly dislocated, it is imperative to assess whether the hip has become painful or not. If the hip is not painful it may be assumed that the articular cartilage of the femoral head is not denuded. The hip needs to be concentrically reduced and redislocation must be prevented. This can be achieved by: release of soft tissue contractures, restoration of muscle balance, correction of coxa valga and femoral anteversion or correction of acetabular dysplasia.

  In order to reduce the hip the soft tissue contractures have to be released. To prevent redislocation, the muscle balance needs to be restored, the neck-shaft angle and the degree of femoral anteversion reduced and the acetabulum augmented.

- If the hip is painful, relieve pain

  If the hip has been dislocated for some time and is painful the main aim of treatment is to relieve pain. If the femoral articular cartilage is eroded, reduction of the hip will not relieve pain and thus should not be attempted.[6]

Treatment options

Options for reducing spasticity of adductors and flexors of the hip

■ Stretching exercises and appropriate posturing

Irrespective of whatever other form of treatment is instituted, stretching exercises and posturing are essential.

■ **Myoneural blocks**

Myoneural blocks will help only if there is no contracture of the muscles (see Chapter 61, General principles of management of upper motor neuron paralysis).

■ **Neurectomy of the obturator nerve**

Neurectomy of the obturator nerve, which was once popular, is best avoided as it runs the risk of producing an abduction deformity of the hip.[7]

Options for restoring muscle balance

Muscle imbalance can be improved by weakening the adductors and flexors and by augmenting the abductors and extensors of the hip. The adductors can be weakened by releasing the adductor muscles from their origin, transferring the origin of the adductor to the ischium or by performing an obturator neurectomy.

■ **Adductor release**

The origin of the adductor longus and the gracilis muscles are erased from the pubis. Occasionally in the more severely adducted hips some fibres of the adductor brevis may also need to be released.

■ **Adductor transfer**

The adductor muscles are released from the pubis and transferred more posteriorly to the ischium. The rationale of this operation is to reduce the strength of the adductors and at the same time to augment the hip extensor power.

■ **Obturator neurectomy**

Division of the anterior division of the obturator nerve may be justifiable if there is severe spasticity in the non-ambulant child. However, the risk of creating an abduction deformity by excessive weakening of the adductors should be kept in mind.

■ **Iliopsoas tenotomy at the lesser trochanter**

The flexors can be weakened by releasing the iliopsoas from the lesser trochanter. This option is reserved for the non-ambulant child and should be avoided in the ambulant child as it may weaken the hip flexor power too much.

■ **Intramuscular iliopsoas recession at the brim of the pelvis**

In the ambulant child the tendon of the psoas is released at the brim of the pelvis without division of the iliacus muscle fibres.

■ **Improving hip abductor power**

The strength of the hip abductors improves if adequate physiotherapy is given after the overactive adductors have been effectively weakened. The other option is to augment the abductors by performing an iliopsoas transfer.

Correction of coxa valga and femoral anteversion

Minor degrees of coxa valga and femoral anteversion may correct spontaneously once muscle balance is restored. A subtrochanteric femoral varus derotation osteotomy will be needed to correct the more severe degrees of these structural changes.

Correction of acetabular dysplasia

As mentioned earlier, the acetabulum is globally deficient and thus redirecting the acetabulum is risky. The improvement of acetabular coverage on one side results in worsening of the coverage in another region if a redirectional osteotomy is performed. Thus the options are restricted to procedures that can augment the acetabulum or procedures that reduce the capacity of the acetabulum (see Chapter 24, Developmental dysplasia of the hip). These procedures include Staheli's acetabular augmentation, shelf operations and Dega or Pemberton osteotomy.

Relieving pain

Once the hip is painful, it is necessary to ascertain whether the pain is due to articular cartilage destruction. The exact extent of cartilage damage will need to be confirmed at the time of surgery although appropriate imaging may help in giving the surgeon an approximate estimate pre-operatively.

If there has been extensive cartilage erosion, reduction of the hip will not relieve pain. The options available include the following.

■ Proximal femoral resection

The technique described by Castle and Schneider[8] involves extraperiosteal resection of the proximal femur from below the lesser trochanter. The capsule of the hip and the abductor muscles are sutured over the acetabulum. Post-operative traction is applied until the soft tissues have healed. The two main complications of this procedure are heterotopic ossification and proximal migration of the femoral shaft.

■ Valgus osteotomy with femoral head resection

Another option is to resect the femoral head and neck and to perform a valgus osteotomy of the femur at the subtrochanteric region with 45° angulation at the osteotomy.[9] The results of this procedure have been satisfactory in terms of pain relief; in addition, mobility of the hip is maintained. The frequency of heterotopic ossification appears to be less than that seen after proximal femoral resection.

■ Arthrodesis of the hip

Pain from the dislocated hip can also be effectively relieved by performing an arthrodesis.[10] This has the disadvantage of rendering the hip stiff and may make it difficult for the carer of a dependent child to move the child.

■ Total joint replacement

Total hip replacement has also been performed on a small number of patients with variable results.[11]

Recommended treatment

Weakening the overactive adductors

The recommended treatment for weakening the adductors is an open adductor release. This entails release of the adductor longus and the gracilis muscles close to their origins from the pubic bone. In more severe degrees of adductor contracture, the adductor brevis may also have to be released.

It is safer to avoid division of the obturator nerve or its branches unless it has been clearly demonstrated that the abductor power is very weak. If the hip abductor power is grade III (Medical Research Council) or more, obturator neurectomy must not be performed. If there is any doubt about the power of the abductors, avoid the neurectomy.

Weakening the overactive flexors of the hip

In the ambulant child avoid release of the iliopsoas completely from the lesser trochanter as this can weaken hip flexor power to an unacceptable degree.[3] The recommended option is to perform an intramuscular division of the psoas tendon at the pelvic brim, taking care not to divide the fibres of the iliacus muscle.

Correcting coxa valga and anteversion

In order to correct the coxa valga and the anteversion, an intertrochanteric or subtrochanteric osteotomy is performed. Although pre-operative measurement of the degree of coxa valga and the anteversion by appropriate imaging methods gives an insight into the magnitude of these deformities, often this may not be essential. In the operating theatre the hip is held in abduction and internal rotation and the best position that shows a concentric reduction is confirmed by radiography. The thigh is held in the chosen position of abduction and internal rotation and the femoral head is temporarily transfixed to the acetabulum with a stout K-wire. The femoral osteotomy is then performed and the distal fragment is adducted and externally rotated until the limb is in the neutral position. The fragments are fixed with a plate after which the K-wire is removed.

Correcting acetabular dysplasia

Staheli's acetabular augmentation operation and the shelf procedures have the advantage of allowing the freedom to place the grafts appropriately over the most deficient areas of the acetabulum (Figure 25.4).

The Dega or the Pemberton may not give as much global cover but may be preferred when the acetabulum is too shallow and large as they reduce the size of the acetabulum.

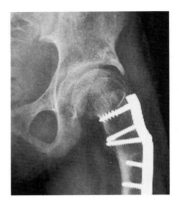

Figure 25.4 ● Acetabular dysplasia in a child with cerebral palsy treated by Staheli's acetabular augmentation. A femoral varus osteotomy was also performed to correct coxa valga.

Relieving pain

The recommended procedure for a painful hip in a non-ambulant child is excision of the femoral head and valgus subtrochanteric osteotomy as described by McHale *et al.*[9]

Very rarely, in an ambulant adolescent or young adult will there be justification in considering a total joint replacement.

Table 25.1 ● Outline of treatment of hip subluxation and dislocation in cerebral palsy

INDICATIONS					
Passive hip abduction <30°	Subluxation (Reimer's migration 20–40%) + No coxa valga OR femoral anteversion OR acetabular dysplasia	Subluxation (Reimer's migration 40–60%) ± Coxa valga + No acetabular dysplasia	Subluxation (Reimer's migration 40–60%) ± Coxa valga + Acetabular dysplasia	Subluxation severe (Reimer's migration >60%) OR Dislocation + Hip not painful	Severe subluxation or dislocation with articular cartilage damage OR Painful hip
	⇩	⇩	⇩	⇩	⇩
				Arthrotomy + Inspect the femoral articular surface + If articular cartilage healthy, open reduction + Femoral or acetabular procedure as in column 3 or 4	Excision of femoral head + Valgus subtrochanteric osteotomy + Muscle interposition (McHale's procedure)
⇩	Adductor release + Intramuscular release of psoas at pelvic brim	Adductor release + Iliopsoas release (intramuscular release of psoas at pelvic brim in ambulant child OR Release from lesser trochanter in non-ambulant child) + Varus derotation osteotomy	Adductor release + Iliopsoas release (intramuscular release of psoas at pelvic brim in ambulant child OR Release from lesser trochanter in non-ambulant child) + Varus derotation osteotomy + Acetabular augmentation if acetabulum is small OR Dega osteotomy if acetabulum is too large		
Adductor release + Physiotherapy					
TREATMENT					

Factors to be taken into consideration while planning treatment

The factors that need to be taken into consideration while planning treatment include:

- the ambulatory status of the child;
- the severity of neurological involvement;
- the general condition of the patient;
- the presence or absence of pain in the hip.

In the ambulant child all degrees of subluxation and dislocation of the hip need to be treated aggressively as hip dislocation may interfere with the ability to walk.

In the non-ambulant child subluxation of a mild or moderate degree may be left untreated in a child with severe neurological involvement who is bedridden. However, these children need to be followed up very closely to ensure that the subluxation is not progressing.

In a bedridden child with quadriplegic cerebral palsy, the decision to operate on a painless hip dislocation will depend on the general condition of the child. The potential benefits of operating on the hip in order to prevent the possible onset of pain must be weighed against the risks of subjecting the child to major surgery. Children with repeated respiratory infections and children who do not have good gag reflex are particularly prone to developing post-operative complications. However, in these children, pain from the dislocated hip that is severe enough to affect the quality of life may be an overriding indication to operate. In such instances, if a decision is made to operate, it must be with the fully informed consent of the parents who have been made aware of the potential risks of anaesthesia and surgery.

An outline of the overall management of hip subluxation and dislocation in cerebral palsy is presented in Tables 25.1 and 25.2.

Table 25.2 ● Overall outline of management of hip subluxation and dislocation in cerebral palsy

Ambulatory status	Status of the hip	General condition of the child	Presence of pain in the hip	Recommended treatment
Ambulant child	Subluxation or dislocation	Good	No pain	Treat as in Table 25.1
Non-ambulant child	Subluxation not progressing	Good	No pain	Observe for progression
	Progressive subluxation	Good	No pain	Treat as in columns 2, 3, 4 of Table 25.1
		Poor	No pain	Withhold surgery
	Dislocation	Good	No pain	Treat as in column 5 of Table 25.1
		Poor	No pain	Withhold surgery
		Good OR poor	Painful	Treat as in column 6 of Table 25.1 (McHale's procedure)

Rationale of treatment suggested

Why is McHale's procedure recommended for dislocated hips that are painful?
This procedure retains mobility at the hip which is why it is preferred to an arthrodesis. The frequency of heterotopic ossification after McHale's procedure appears to be less than that seen after proximal femoral resection by Castle and Schneider's technique.

References

1. Dobson F, Boyd RN, Parrott J, Nattrass GR, Graham HK. Hip surveillance in children with cerebral palsy: impact on the surgical management of spastic hip disease. *J Bone Joint Surg Br* 2005; **84**: 720–26.
2. Hagglund G, Andersson S, Duppe H *et al*. Prevention of dislocation of the hip in children with cerebral palsy: the first ten years of a population-based prevention programme. *J Bone Joint Surg Br* 2005; **87**: 95–101.

3. Reimers J. The stability of the hip in children: a radiological study of the results of muscle surgery in cerebral palsy. *Acta Orthop Scand Suppl* 1980; **184**: 1–100.
4. Bleck EE. The hip in cerebral palsy. *Orthop Clin North Am* 1980; **11**: 79–104.
5. Brunner R, Picard C, Robb J. Morphology of the acetabulum in hip dislocations caused by cerebral palsy. *J Pediatr Orthop B* 1997; **6**: 207–11.
6. Flynn JM, Miller F. Management of hip disorders in patients with cerebral palsy. *J Am Acad Orthop Surg* 2002; **10**: 198–209.
7. Spiegel DA, Flynn JM. Evaluation and treatment of hip dysplasia in cerebral palsy. *Orthop Clin North Am* 2006; **37**: 185–96.
8. Castle ME, Schneider C. Proximal femoral resection-interposition arthroplasty. *J Bone Joint Surg Am* 1978; **60**: 1051–4.
9. McHale KA, Bagg M, Nason SS. Treatment of the chronically dislocated hip in adolescents with cerebral palsy with femoral head resection and subtrochanteric valgus osteotomy. *J Pediatr Orthop* 1990; **10**: 504–9.
10. Root L, Goss JR, Mendes J. The treatment of the painful hip in cerebral palsy by total hip replacement or hip arthrodesis. *J Bone Joint Surg Am* 1986; **68**: 590–98.
11. Weber M, Cabanela ME. Total hip arthroplasty in patients with cerebral palsy. *Orthopaedics* 1999; **22**: 425–7.

Paralytic hip dislocation: spina bifida and polio

26

Benjamin Joseph

Introduction

Hip subluxation and dislocation are often seen in children with spina bifida and, less frequently, following polio.

In spina bifida the frequency of hip dislocation varies with the level of neurological deficit. The consequences of hip dislocation also differ in children with high level lesions and those with low level lesions. In the latter group, there is a good chance of children remaining community ambulators throughout life and hence a hip dislocation can impair their walking ability. In children with high level lesions who have a poor prognosis for long-term ambulation, unilateral hip dislocation may compromise sitting balance or predispose to ischial pressure sores. However, bilateral hip dislocation in children with high level lesions may not be disabling.

In polio, the vast majority of children will walk even when there is severe involvement of both lower limbs provided there are no severe deformities that preclude standing and provided an appropriate orthosis is fitted. Furthermore, despite their impairments, these children have a good chance of remaining community ambulators in adult life.

Problems of management

Muscle imbalance

As in other paralytic conditions where hip dislocation occurs, in both spina bifida and polio muscle imbalance is one factor that contributes to hip instability.[1] If the hip flexors and adductors are working while the abductors and extensors are weak or paralysed the hip tends to dislocate. However, muscle imbalance alone does not seem to account for all cases of hip dislocation in spina bifida as it has been noted that in a sizeable proportion of children with no demonstrable muscle imbalance hip dislocation can occur.[2] In polio, it is exceedingly rare to see hip instability in the absence of muscle imbalance.[3]

Deformities of the hip, pelvis and spine

Fixed deformities of the hip occur quite commonly in both spina bifida and polio and they too can contribute to hip instability (Figure 26.1). An adduction deformity or abduction deformity of the hip leads to obliquity of the pelvis which, in turn, predisposes to hip dislocation. Rigid lumbar scoliosis can also result in pelvic obliquity. In all these situations, the adducted hip is likely to dislocate.

Adaptive bony changes

In both spina bifida and polio, acetabular dysplasia, femoral anteversion and coxa valga add to the propensity for hip dislocation.

Aims of treatment

- Obtain a stable concentric reduction in children with good long-term potential for independent community ambulation
- Prevent loss of sitting balance in children with unilateral hip dislocation and poor walking ability
- Minimize the risk of development of ischial pressure sores if sensation is lost

Treatment options

Correcting muscle imbalance

■ Iliopsoas and adductor release

In spina bifida the easiest way to restore muscle balance is to weaken the stronger side by tenotomizing the iliopsoas and the adductor muscles. This is simpler than performing a tendon transfer and is particularly appropriate in spina bifida where the results of simple tenotomy have been shown to be comparable to transfer of the iliopsoas and adductor tendons.[4] In polio, the results of tendon transfers are more predictable and it seems a waste not to utilize the power of potentially useful muscles by performing a defunctioning tenotomy.

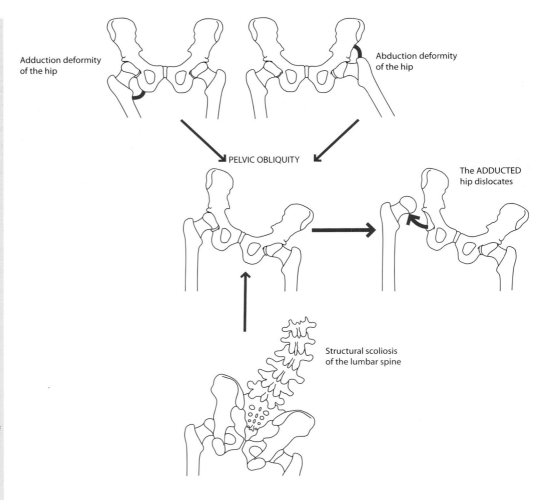

Figure 26.1 ● Diagram demonstrating how deformities of the hip and scoliosis can result in pelvic obliquity and tendency for the adducted hip to dislocate.

■ Adductor release and iliopsoas transfer

Release of the adductor muscles weakens one force that contributes to hip dislocation. Transfer of the iliopsoas augments hip abductor power, which helps to stabilize the hip.

■ External oblique, adductor and tensor fascia lata transfer

A combination of external oblique muscle transfer to the greater trochanter, adductor transfer to the ischium and posterior transfer of the origin of the tensor fascia lata has been advocated as a method of restoring muscle balance in paralytic hip dislocation.[5] These transfers aim to augment the hip abductor and extensor power and concomitantly weaken the hip adductor power.

Correcting adaptive bony changes in the femur and acetabulum

Coxa valga should be corrected if reduction of the dislocation is being undertaken. In a young child a simple open wedge osteotomy performed at the time of reduction and muscle rebalancing can be held in position in a plaster spica (Figure 26.2). In the older child a more formal fixation of the osteotomy with an appropriate plate and screws will be necessary. Acetabular dysplasia should be corrected if it is severe enough to compromise the stability of reduction. In paralytic dislocation, the deficiency of the acetabulum may not be in the anterolateral margin of the acetabulum as it is in developmental dysplasia but may involve the posterior margin. If this is so, a Salter type osteotomy is to be avoided as the posterior deficiency will become more severe following the operation, which increases the tendency for hip dislocation (Figure 26.3). For this reason, an acetabular augmentation is preferred as it can create a shelf at the region of the acetabulum that is most deficient.

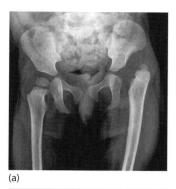

(a)

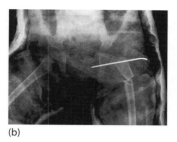

(b)

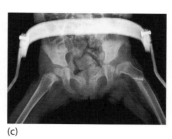

(c)

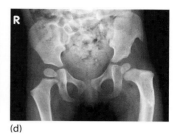

(d)

Figure 26.2 ● Radiograph of a dislocated left hip in a child with spina bifida **(a)**. Severe coxa valga is also evident. The hip has been reduced by performing an open reduction, varus osteotomy of the femur, release of the adductor muscles and an iliopsoas transfer to the greater trochanter **(b)** The Kirschner wire stabilizes the femoral head in the acetabulum; no internal fixation has been used for the femoral osteotomy and a spica cast has been applied. After removal of the spica cast and the Kirschner wire an abduction splint has been applied **(c)**. The follow-up radiograph after a year shows satisfactory reduction **(d)**.

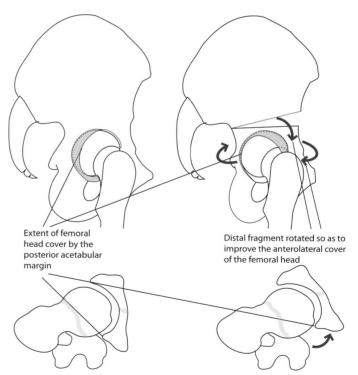

Extent of femoral head cover by the posterior acetabular margin

Distal fragment rotated so as to improve the anterolateral cover of the femoral head

Figure 26.3 ● Diagram demonstrating how a Salter osteotomy can make posterior deficiency of the acetabulum worse.

Correcting pelvic obliquity

■ Releasing contractures of the hip

Abduction and adduction contractures of the hip should be released if they are causing pelvic obliquity. In the young child release of the contracted muscles and fascia should suffice. In older children with severe deformity, a subtrochanteric or intertrochanteric osteotomy may be needed to correct residual deformity that may be present after soft tissue release.

Factors to be taken into consideration while planning treatment

■ Correcting lumbar scoliosis

A rigid lumbar scoliosis will need to be corrected if it is severe enough to produce pelvic obliquity.

Level and extent of neurological deficit

It has been clearly shown that children with spina bifida and functioning quadriceps muscles are likely to retain their ability to walk independently as community ambulators. Hence every effort must be made to reduce hips in children with a neurological level at or below L4. Children with high lesions tend to abandon walking and adopt wheel chair mobility by the time they reach adolescence. In these children reduction of dislocated hips are not indicated as a measure to improve their ability to walk. However, reduction may be undertaken for other indications.

Long-term walking potential

If the likelihood of retaining ambulatory ability is high, an attempt must be made to reduce hip dislocation.

Unilateral or bilateral dislocation

Reduction of both hips may be considered in children with low level lesions in spina bifida and in those with polio. However, bilateral hip dislocations may be ignored in children with high lesions in spina bifida. Reduction of unilateral dislocations should be considered irrespective of the level of neurological deficit in spina bifida[6] and should always be attempted in children with polio.

Presence of demonstrable muscle imbalance

If the hip flexors and adductors are clearly stronger than the abductors and the extensors the muscle imbalance should be corrected.

Presence of adaptive bony changes in the hip, acetabulum and pelvic obliquity

Deformities of the proximal femur, acetabulum or the pelvis that contribute to hip instability need to be addressed as indicated previously.

Recommended treatment

An outline of treatment of paralytic hip dislocation in spina bifida and polio is shown in Table 26.1.

Rationale of treatment suggested

Why is lateral transfer of the iliopsoas being recommended for both polio and spina bifida?
The results of tendon transfers in these conditions are fairly predictable and a strong hip flexor can be converted into a hip abductor in a proportion of cases. This is very valuable in improving gait and achieving dynamic hip stability. Even if active abduction does not occur and the transfer works only as a tenodesis, the tenodesis effect may help in improving the stability of the hip.
The risk of reattachment of the tendon back to the lesser trochanter and recurrence of muscle imbalance following simple tenotomy is also avoided when the lateral transfer is performed.
The lateral transfer is not very difficult to perform, unlike the posterior transfer suggested by Sharrard.[1]

In children with spina bifida, why is the lateral transfer of the iliopsoas being recommended only if the neurological level is below L4?
Children with low spina bifida (below L4) have a good chance of remaining community ambulators throughout their life and in these children any improvement in abductor power is worthwhile. However, in children with a poor long-term prognosis for community ambulation, increasing abductor power is not necessary and a simpler method of restoring hip stability by defunctioning the iliopsoas is preferred.

Table 26.1 ● Treatment of paralytic hip subluxation and dislocation in spina bifida and polio

INDICATIONS						
Spina bifida with neurological level at L3 or above + Bilateral dislocation	Spina bifida with neurological level at L3 or above + Unilateral dislocation	Polio OR Spina bifida with neurological level at L4 or below + Unilateral hip subluxation + Abduction deformity of the opposite hip with pelvic obliquity	Polio OR Spina bifida with neurological level at L4 or below + Unilateral hip subluxation + Lumbar scoliosis with pelvic obliquity	Polio OR Spina bifida with neurological level at L4 or below + Unilateral hip subluxation/ dislocation + Muscle imbalance (flexor and adductors stronger than extensors and abductors) + Flexion or adduction contracture	Polio OR Spina bifida with neurological level at L4 or below + Unilateral hip subluxation/ dislocation + Muscle imbalance (flexor and adductors stronger than extensors and abductors) + Coxa valga	Polio OR Spina bifida with neurological level at L4 or below + Unilateral hip subluxation/ dislocation + Muscle imbalance (flexor and adductors stronger than extensors and abductors) + Acetabular dysplasia
⇩	⇩	⇩	⇩	⇩	⇩	⇩
No intervention	Flexor adductor tenotomy + Femoral varus osteotomy	Release abduction contracture of opposite hip and see if hip remains stable (if unstable treat as in columns 5, 6, 7)	Correct scoliosis and fuse lumbar spine and see if hip remains stable (if unstable treat as in columns 5, 6, 7)	Release of adductors + Lateral transfer of the iliopsoas	Femoral varus osteotomy + Lateral transfer of the iliopsoas	Shelf acetabuloplasty + Lateral transfer of the iliopsoas
TREATMENT						

References

1. Sharrard WJW. Posterior iliopsoas transplantation in the treatment of paralytic dislocation of the hip. *J Bone Joint Surg Br* 1964; **46**: 426–44.
2. Broughton NS, Menelaus MB, Cole WG, Shurtleff DB. The natural history of hip deformity in myelomeningocele. *J Bone Joint Surg Br* 1993; **75**: 760–63.
3. Joseph B, Rajasekaran S. Poliomyelitis. In: Bulstrode C, Buckwalter J, Carr A *et al.* (eds). *Oxford Textbook of Orthopedics and Trauma*, Vol. 2. Oxford: Oxford University Press, 2002: 1511–32.
4. Weisl H, Fairclough JA, Jones DG. Stabilisation of the hip in myelomeningocele. Comparison of posterior iliopsoas transfer and varus-rotation osteotomy. *J Bone Joint Surg Br* 1988; **70**: 29–33.
5. Yngve DA, Lindseth RE. Effectiveness of muscle transfers in myelomeningocele hips measured by radiographic indices. *J Pediatr Orthop* 1982; **2**: 121–5.
6. Fraser RK, Bourke HM, Broughton NS, Menelaus MB. Unilateral dislocation of the hip in spina bifida – a long-term follow-up. *J Bone Joint Surg Br* 1995; **77**: 615–19.

Teratologic hip dislocation in multiple congenital contractures

27

Benjamin Joseph

Introduction

A teratologic hip dislocation is characterized by a stiff hip that is dislocated at birth, unlike developmental dysplasia where the hip dislocates in the neonatal period. Teratologic dislocations are associated with several conditions that manifest with multiple congenital contractures. Among these the most common is the classical arthrogryposis or amyoplasia.[1–4] Caudal regression syndrome or sacral agenesis and diastrophic dwarfism are less common causes for teratologic dislocation.[1]

In teratologic dislocation the Ortolani test will be negative, indicating that the hip is irreducible. In addition to the hip dislocation, congenital dislocation of the knee and rigid equinovarus or vertical talus are frequently seen in these children.

Problems of management

Irreducibility

Since the hip cannot be reduced by closed methods even when the child is anaesthetized, open reduction is mandatory. In a proportion of children with teratologic dislocations the femoral head may have ridden very proximally (Figure 27.1). Such high dislocations are difficult to reduce even at open reduction.

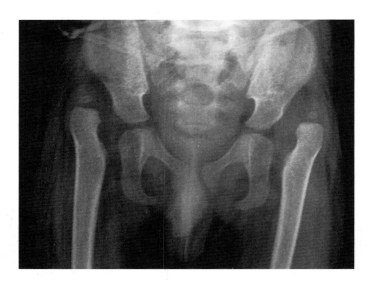

Figure 27.1 ● High teratological dislocation of the hips in a child with multiple congenital contractures.

Associated deformities of the lower limb

The associated deformities of the knee and foot may influence decisions regarding the timing and nature of surgery on the hip. Upper limb weakness and deformity may have a bearing on the long-term outcome since children with severe weakness of the lower limbs may require the use of walking aids.

Associated muscle weakness

Some children have significant weakness of muscles around the hip and knee. These children may not succeed in walking independently even if satisfactory reduction of the hips is achieved.

Aims of treatment

- Facilitate independent ambulation
  The prime aim is to facilitate independent ambulation and planning how to achieve this aim takes precedence over obtaining reduction of the hip. In addition to the hip dislocation, the children often have muscle weakness and limited motion of the hips and knees. All these factors may limit the ability to walk. A clear plan of appropriate bracing and deformity correction should be outlined before embarking on surgery to reduce the hip.

- If possible, obtain stable concentrically reduced hips
Since a dislocated hip does contribute to difficulty in walking in these children, it is ideal if the hip can be reduced. However, as previously mentioned, reduction is often difficult and attempts at reduction may be associated with a high complication rate.[2] The complications include avascular necrosis (close to 50 percent in some series), redislocation and persistent subluxation.

Treatment options

No intervention

In view of the difficulty in achieving satisfactory reduction of these hips some authors have suggested that bilateral dislocations be left untreated.[3,5] Others have suggested that reduction of the hip is unlikely to be of benefit in children who have severe muscle weakness.[4] In such children avoiding any intervention to reduce the hip may be justified.

Open reduction

A few authors have suggested that open reduction be attempted in all teratologic dislocations in an attempt to improve the mechanics of the hip and to prevent pain.[1,4,6,7]

Staheli *et al.*[6] prefer the medial approach while the anterolateral approach has been recommended by others.[1,4,7]

■ Open reduction by the medial approach

Through a Ludloff approach the adductor muscles and the iliopsoas are released. The medial capsule is opened and a reduction is attempted.

■ Three-stage procedure of adductor and iliopsoas release, followed by open reduction and varus derotation osteotomy of the femur

LeBel and Gallien[1] recommend preliminary open adductor and iliopsoas release followed by skin traction for two weeks. An open reduction is then performed and reduction is held in a spica with the hip abducted and internally rotated. Six weeks later a varus derotation osteotomy is performed.

■ Open reduction with circumferential capsulotomy

Akazawa *et al.*[7] also prefer the anterolateral approach but they perform an extensive soft tissue release with a circumferential capsulotomy.

■ Open reduction with femoral shortening

Gruel *et al.*[2] recommend femoral shortening as a means of reducing the risk of avascular necrosis and facilitating reduction.

Factors to be taken into consideration while planning treatment

Unilateral or bilateral involvement

It is generally accepted that unilateral dislocations should be treated and that an attempt must be made to reduce the dislocated hip.

Associated deformities of the knee

In a child with associated congenital dislocation of the knee, the reduction of the knee should precede surgery on the hip. This is for two reasons: first, reduction of the knee dislocation will relax the hamstrings and this, in turn, will facilitate reduction of the hip; second, it will be exceedingly difficult to apply a hip spica following hip surgery with the unreduced knee dislocation.

Extent of muscle weakness and severity of upper limb involvement

If there is profound muscle weakness and the upper limb function is poor, independent walking may never be achieved. In such children it would be appropriate to ignore the hip dislocation.

The age of the child

In the infant, the medial approach is preferred while in the older child a more extensive capsular release may be needed and this will require the anterolateral approach.

Recommended treatment

An outline of treatment of teratologic dislocation of the hip is shown in Table 27.1.

Table 27.1 ● Outline of treatment of teratologic dislocation of the hip

INDICATIONS					
Unilateral OR bilateral dislocation + Severe muscle weakness + Poor prognosis for walking	<1 year of age + Unilateral OR bilateral dislocation + Reasonably good prognosis for independent walking	1–2 years of age + Unilateral dislocation + Reasonably good prognosis for independent walking	1–2 years of age + Bilateral dislocation OR High unilateral dislocation + Reasonably good prognosis for independent walking	>2 years of age + Unilateral dislocation + Reasonably good prognosis for independent walking	>2 years of age + Bilateral dislocation
⇩	⇩	⇩	⇩	⇩	⇩
No intervention for the hip dislocation	Open reduction by medial approach	Open reduction by anterolateral approach ± Femoral osteotomy as indicated	Open reduction by anterolateral approach + Femoral shortening	Open reduction by anterolateral approach + Femoral shortening	No intervention for hip dislocation
TREATMENT					

Rationale of treatment suggested

Why is open reduction by the medial approach reserved for children under one year of age?
The chances of avascular necrosis are higher when the medial approach is used in the older child.

Why is femoral shortening routinely recommended for teratologic dislocation in a child over two years of age?
This is likely to reduce the risk of avascular necrosis and facilitate reduction.

Why is no intervention recommended for bilateral dislocation over the age of two years?
The chance of obtaining a concentric reduction of both hips decreases with increasing age of the child. Complications are also likely to be higher in the older child.

References

1. LeBel M-E, Gallien R. The surgical treatment of teratologic dislocation of the hip. *J Pediatr Orthop B* 2005; **14**: 331–6.
2. Gruel CR, Birch JG, Roach JW, Herring JA. Teratological dislocation of the hip. *J Pediatr Orthop* 1986; **6**: 693–702.
3. Friedlander HL, Westin GW, Wood WL Jr. Arthrogryposis multiplex congenita: a review of forty-five cases. *J Bone Joint Surg Am* 1968; **50**: 89–112.
4. Lloyd-Roberts GC, Lettin WF. Arthrogryposis multiplex congenita. *J Bone Joint Surg Br* 1970; **52**: 494–508.
5. Gibson PA, Urs NDK. Arthrogryposis multiplex congenita. *J Bone Joint Surg Br* 1970; **52**: 483–93.
6. Staheli LT, Chew DE, Elliot JS, Mosca VS. Management of hip dislocation in children with arthrogryposis. *J Pediatr Orthop* 1987; **7**: 681–5.
7. Akazawa H, Oda K, Mitani S *et al.* Surgical management of hip dislocation in children with arthrogryposis multiplex congenita. *J Bone Joint Surg Br* 1998; **80**: 636–40.

Post-infective hip dysplasia

Benjamin Joseph

28

Introduction

The nature and the severity of damage to the hip following septic arthritis depend to a large extent on the age at which the infection occurs. The long-term sequelae of septic arthritis of the hip are most profound when the infection occurs in infancy because the major part of the proximal femur is not ossified.[1–3] The unossified hyaline cartilage can be partly or totally destroyed during the infective episode. The extent, location and pattern of cartilage damage also determines the outcome.

Patterns of damage to the hip

The sequelae of septic arthritis of the hip in childhood can be very varied and elaborate classifications of these sequelae have appeared in the literature.[1,2] The pattern of damage varies depending on whether the ossific nucleus of the femoral epiphysis has appeared and whether the growth plate is well formed. Accordingly, the epiphyseal cartilage, the growth plate cartilage or the articular cartilage may be the primary region of damage.

In the infant before the ossific nucleus of the femoral head has appeared

In the young infant the femoral head and neck are completely formed of hyaline cartilage (articular cartilage and epiphyseal cartilage); the growth plate cartilage is yet to differentiate. Septic arthritis at this stage of development of the hip can result in partial or total destruction of the femoral head and neck (Figure 28.1a). If the damage is predominantly in the region of the neck, the neck alone may be destroyed and a pseudarthrosis may develop (Figure 28.1b). If the infection is controlled after partial dissolution of the cartilage has occurred the femoral head shape may become distorted.

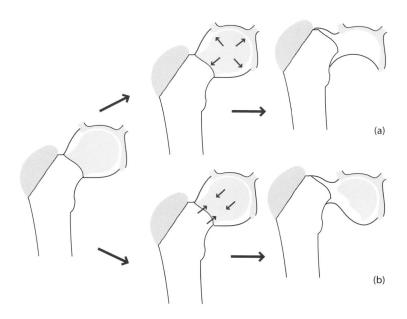

(a)

(b)

Figure 28.1 ● Diagram illustrating destruction of the femoral head and neck of the femur in septic arthritis in an infant.

In the child after the growth plate has formed

Once the growth plate has developed it may be damaged following septic arthritis. The consequence of the growth plate damage will depend on whether the growth plate is completely damaged or whether there is partial asymmetric damage. Asymmetric growth plate damage can result in coxa vara, coxa valga, femoral anteversion or femoral retroversion, depending on which part of the growth plate fuses prematurely (Figure 28.2). Complete damage to the growth plate will result in a foreshortened femoral neck. The greater trochanter will continue to grow normally and, in due course, outgrow the femoral neck, resulting in a Trendelenburg gait.

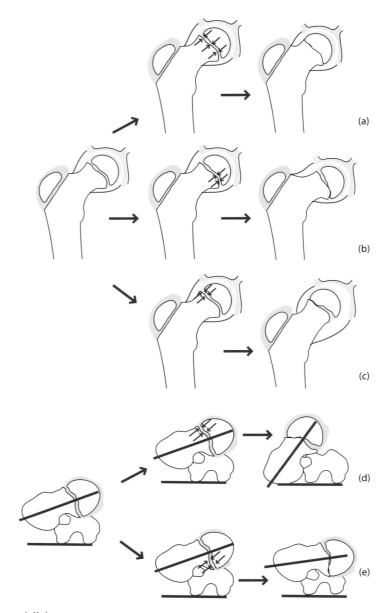

Figure 28.2 ● Diagram illustrating the various patterns of damage to the capital femoral growth plate that can lead to coxa brevis **(a)**, coxa vara **(b)**, coxa valga **(c)**, femoral anteversion **(d)** and femoral retroversion **(e)**.

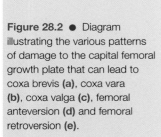

In the older child

In the older child damage to the triradiate cartilage can result in its premature fusion and this, in turn, can lead to acetabular dysplasia (Figure 28.3a). When the major part of the femoral capital epiphysis has already ossified cartilage damage may be predominantly limited to the articular cartilage, and if contiguous articular surfaces of the femoral head and acetabulum are destroyed bony ankylosis of the hip may follow (Figure 28.3b).

In addition to these complications of septic arthritis listed above, joint stiffness, varying degrees of joint incongruity due to distortion of the articular contours of the femur or acetabulum, joint subluxation or frank dislocation can occur.

Instability of the hip

Instability of the hip can develop in these children for various reasons and the strategies for dealing with each underlying cause will necessarily vary profoundly. If the femoral head is destroyed the fulcrum of the joint is non-existent and this is the most problematic cause of instability. If the neck of the femur is destroyed the lever arm of the femoral neck is broken and this results in instability of the hip. Coxa vara will also result in hip instability due to altered mechanics of the hip and lever arm dysfunction. Finally, if the hip is dislocated there will be instability.

Problems of management

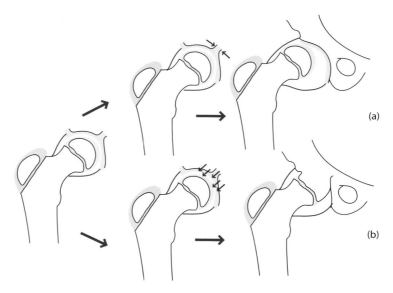

Figure 28.3 ● Diagram illustrating that damage to the triradiate cartilage can lead to acetabular dysplasia **(a)** and how articular cartilage destruction can lead to bony ankylosis **(b)**.

Deformity

Deformities of the proximal femur (angular and torsional deformities) or the acetabulum (acetabular dysplasia) can develop and these deformities may contribute to hip instability, limb length inequality or gait abnormalities.

Shortening

Shortening of the femur will be quite significant if the capital femoral growth plate is totally destroyed in infancy, while the degree of shortening will be less if premature fusion of the growth plate occurs later in childhood.

Altered mobility of the hip

When either the head or the neck of the femur is destroyed the range of movement of the hip usually becomes excessive. On the other hand, permanent residual stiffness can occur when the articular cartilage is partially damaged. Movement is totally abolished if bony ankylosis occurs.

Pain

Pain is more likely to occur in hips where the articular contour has become irregular and the joint is not congruent than when the head and neck have been resorbed.

Aims of treatment

- Restore stability of the hip
  It is important to restore stability of the hip as instability results in an awkward, energy consuming Trendelenburg gait.
- Correct deformities that may compromise hip function
  Any deformity that is progressive, compromises normal function of the hip or is likely to lead to early degenerative arthritis must be corrected. This includes coxa vara, coxa valga, excessive femoral anteversion and acetabular dysplasia.
- Correct shortening of the limb
  In order to avoid a limp, apart from restoring stability of the hip, the limb length inequality must be addressed.
- Retain mobility of the hip
  It is important to try to retain mobility of the hip. Restoring stability at the expense of mobility is not an acceptable approach in most instances as loss of hip movement can be quite disabling.
- Relieve pain if present and minimize the risk of pain developing later
  It is of paramount importance to ensure that pain is relieved if the hip is painful and also to ensure that any treatment option that is employed does not result in a painful hip. Despite the inherent disadvantages of walking with an unstable hip, it is preferable to have an unstable painless hip rather than a painful stable hip.

Treatment options

Restoring stability

■ **Improving stability by correcting deformities that compromise stability and improving the relationship between the femoral head and the acetabulum**

If coxa valga, acetabular dysplasia or femoral anteversion are causing the hip to subluxate, an appropriate osteotomy of the proximal femur or the acetabulum should be performed in order to correct the hip subluxation.[4]

■ **Creating a stable femoral–acetabular articulation in the absence of the femoral head**

■ Trochanteric arthroplasty

When the femoral head and neck have been destroyed, the trochanter can be placed into the acetabulum to function similarly to the femoral head.[5] The abductor muscles are transferred distally and the femur is angulated to create the semblance of a 'neck-shaft' angle (Figure 28.4). The operation is based on the assumption that the trochanteric apophysis that is covered by hyaline cartilage will remodel into a spherical shape. The operation, however, is limited by its unpredictable outcome, with unsatisfactory results in a third of patients under the age of six years and virtually all patients over the age of six years.[4] Among the problems following this operation listed in the literature are: development of avascular necrosis of the proximal femur, stiffness, abductor weakness, recurrent subluxation and degenerative arthritis.

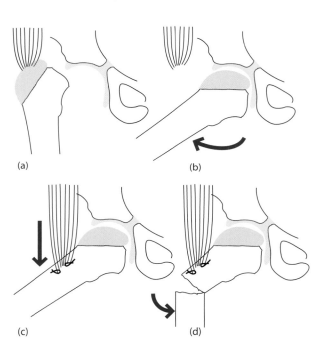

(a)　　　　(b)

(c)　　　　(d)

Figure 28.4 ● Diagram illustrating the steps of a trochanteric arthroplasty.

■ Harmon's procedure

If the femoral head is destroyed but there is a remnant of the femoral neck covered by unossified hyaline cartilage, the remnant of the neck can be placed in the acetabulum.[6] The upper end of the femur is split in the sagittal plane and the medial fragment is angulated in order to facilitate placement of the neck of the femur into the acetabulum. The split in the femur is held apart by a cartilage or bone graft from the iliac crest (Figure 28.5). Again, the results of this procedure are not predictable.

■ **Creating extra-articular stability in the absence of the femoral head (pelvic support osteotomy)**

The pelvic support osteotomy was advocated by Milch[7] and more recently by Ilizarov[8] for restoring hip stability in patients in whom the femoral head is destroyed. The femur is divided around the level of the ischial tuberosity and the distal fragment is angulated laterally. The degree of angulation is about 15° more than the range of passive adduction that is possible at the hip. This ensures

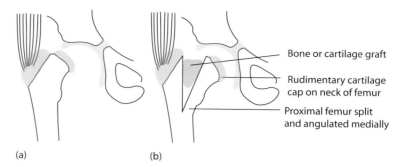

Bone or cartilage graft

Rudimentary cartilage cap on neck of femur

Proximal femur split and angulated medially

(a)   (b)

Figure 28.5 ● Diagram illustrating the Harmon operation for restoring hip stability if a cartilage covered remnant of the head is present.

that no free adduction of the limb will be possible following the surgery (Figure 28.6). Consequently, the Trendelenburg gait is eliminated. An additional advantage of the operation is that the abductor mechanism is improved by lateralizing the tip of the trochanter. A more distal osteotomy of the femur is performed in order to restore the mechanical axis of the limb and, at the same time, lengthening of the femur can be done through this osteotomy.

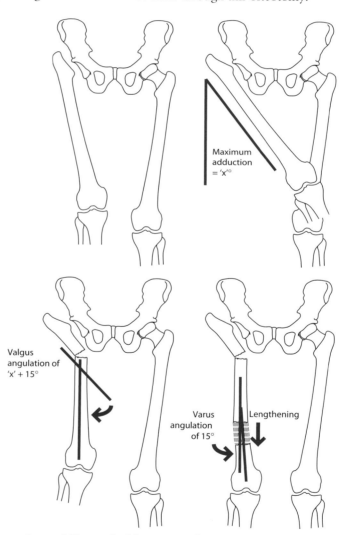

Maximum adduction = 'x'°

Valgus angulation of 'x' + 15°

Varus angulation of 15°

Lengthening

Figure 28.6 ● Diagram illustrating the technique of performing a pelvic support osteotomy to restore stability of the hip.

The operation retains mobility at the hip, restores hip stability and when combined with limb lengthening addresses the problem of limb length inequality. However, if done in children, the femur remodels and the effect of the pelvic support is lost. The options available to deal with this problem are either to defer surgery until after skeletal maturity or to perform the operation even in younger children but be ready to redo the angulation as and when the remodelling occurs. Choi *et al.*[4] advocate early operation as this will improve hip abductor muscle function sooner whereas in the adolescent the hip abductor may not function well after surgery since it has remained ineffective for so long.

Correcting deformities that compromise function

■ Coxa valga

Coxa valga can contribute to subluxation of the hip and in such a situation an intertrochanteric varus osteotomy may be performed.

■ Coxa vara

Coxa vara of a minor degree may not be of consequence; however, if it is severe enough to result in a Trendelenburg gait, a valgus osteotomy is indicated.

■ Femoral anteversion

If femoral anteversion is contributing to instability of the hip or if there is an unacceptable degree of in-toeing, a derotation osteotomy may be required.

■ Femoral retroversion

If femoral retroversion is contributing to posterior instability of the hip a derotation osteotomy is needed.

■ Acetabular dysplasia

Acetabular dysplasia should be corrected in order to improve hip stability if this is a contributing factor. If, however, the primary cause of hip instability is destruction of the femoral head or neck, correction of acetabular dysplasia will not in any way restore stability unless the primary problem is effectively remedied.

Correcting shortening of the limb

Limb length inequality needs to be addressed in the majority of children with sequelae of septic arthritis of the hip.

Retaining mobility of the hip

Whenever possible the mobility of the hip should be retained. This entails selecting options for restoring hip stability that have a low risk of resulting in hip stiffness.

Relieving pain

If the hip is painful when the child first presents, it is important to identify the possible cause of pain. If a near-normal relationship between the femoral head and the acetabulum cannot be restored and if movement of the hip produces pain, two options are available. The first is to abolish movement at the hip by an arthrodesis. The second option is to avoid any contact between the two damaged articular surfaces; this can be achieved by excising the deformed femoral head remnant.

Status of the femoral head

The first and foremost issue that needs to be considered is whether the femoral head is intact or resorbed. If the femoral head is intact it is necessary to know if it is distorted, if it is vascular and if it is capable of moving freely within the acetabulum.

Status of the femoral neck

Treatment depends on whether the femoral neck is intact or resorbed. If it is intact, the alignment of the neck to the shaft needs to be considered; coxa vara, coxa valga, anteversion and retroversion may need to be addressed. If the neck is short, the abductor mechanism is ineffective and the trochanter may need to be lateralized to overcome this problem.

Status of the acetabulum

The status of the acetabulum is only of relevance if it is considered appropriate to place the femoral head or the remnant of the head and neck or the trochanter into it. If the proximal femur is to articulate with the acetabulum, any acetabular dysplasia that may compromise stability needs to be corrected.

Factors to be taken into consideration while planning treatment

Recommended treatment

An outline of treatment of the sequelae of septic arthritis of the hip is shown in Table 28.1.

Table 28.1 ● Outline of treatment of post-infective dysplasia of the hip

INDICATIONS						
Femoral head and neck intact + Head spherical + Well-developed acetabulum + Hip subluxed OR dislocated	Femoral head and neck intact + Head spherical + Well-developed acetabulum + Premature fusion of the entire capital femoral growth plate	Femoral head and neck intact + Head spherical + Well-developed acetabulum + Coxa vara/Coxa valga/Femoral anteversion or femoral retroversion of unacceptable degree	Femoral head and neck intact + Head spherical + Acetabular dysplasia	Bony ankylosis	Femoral head intact + Femoral neck resorbed with pseudarthrosis + Head vascular + Head mobile in acetabulum	Femoral head resorbed OR Femoral head and neck resorbed OR Femoral neck resorbed but head avascular or not mobile in acetabulum
⇩	⇩	⇩	⇩	⇩	⇩	⇩
Open reduction and follow-up as for developmental dysplasia of the hip (DDH) (see Chapter 24)	Observe and follow up for development of coxa brevis and plan for: Trochanteric epiphyseodesis in childhood OR Trochanteric advancement at skeletal maturity	Corrective osteotomy of the femur at intertrochanteric or subtrochanteric level	Treat acetabular dysplasia as for DDH (see Chapter 24)	No intervention if position of ankylosis is acceptable OR Corrective osteotomy if position is unacceptable	Restore continuity of neck by bone grafting	Pelvic support osteotomy[a] + Distal realignment osteotomy of femur + Limb lengthening
TREATMENT						

[a]The pelvic support osteotomy of the femur will remodel in skeletally immature children. When this happens the Trendelenburg gait will recur and the osteotomy needs to be repeated in order to restore hip stability.

Rationale of treatment suggested

Why is pelvic support osteotomy preferred to either trochanteric arthroplasty or the Harmon procedure?
First, the long-term results of trochanteric arthroplasty are unpredictable.[1] Second, additional operations are often needed to restore stability of the hip after trochanteric arthroplasty and the Harmon operation. Finally, the most compelling reason for opting for the pelvic osteotomy is because the mobility of the hip is not compromised following this procedure, while a proportion of hips become stiff following trochanteric arthroplasty. The Harmon procedure does not result in a truly congruous hip and this is fraught with the risk of development of pain or early degenerative arthritis.

Why not wait until skeletal maturity before performing the pelvic support osteotomy in order to avoid the need for redoing the operation for remodelling of the osteotomy in skeletally immature children?

Following destruction of the femoral head the trochanter will migrate proximally and this shortens the gluteal muscles resulting in abductor weakness. The pelvic support osteotomy improves the strength and mechanical efficiency of the gluteal muscles by lateralizing the trochanter. If this is done in childhood, the muscles will begin to function efficiently at an early age. If the trochanter is left in the elevated position until skeletal maturity the gluteal muscles may never regain their power as they have remained ineffective for so long.

References

1. Choi IH, Pizzutillo PD, Bowen JR, Dragann R, Malhis T. Sequelae and reconstruction after septic arthritis of the hip in infants. *J Bone Joint Surg Am* 1990; **72**: 1150–65.
2. Hunka L, Said SE, MacKenzie DA *et al.* Classification and surgical management of the severe sequelae of septic hips in children. *Clin Orthop Relat Res* 1982; **171**: 30–36.
3. Choi IH, Shin YW, Chung CY *et al.* Surgical treatment of the severe sequelae of infantile septic arthritis of the hip. *Clin Orthop Relat Res* 2005; **434**: 102–9.
4. Choi IH, Yoo WJ, Cho T-J, Chung CY. Operative reconstruction for septic arthritis of the hip. *Orthop Clin North Am* 2006; **37**: 173–83.
5. Weissman SL. Transplantation of the trochanteric epiphysis into the acetabulum after septic arthritis of the hip: report of a case. *J Bone Joint Surg Am* 1967; **49**: 1647–51.
6. Harmon PH. Surgical treatment of the residual deformity from suppurative arthritis of the hip occurring in young children. *J Bone Joint Surg* 1942; **24**: 576–85.
7. Milch H. The pelvic support osteotomy. *J Bone Joint Surg* 1941; **23**: 581–95.
8. Ilizarov GA. Treatment of disorders of the hip. In: Green SA (ed.). *Transosseous Osteosynthesis*. Berlin: Springer Verlag, 1992: 668–96.

Congenital dislocation of the knee

Randall Loder

29

Introduction

Congenital dislocation of the knee may occur as an isolated deformity or more commonly in association with syndromes, such as Larsen syndrome or arthrogryposis.[1] The child frequently has other anomalies of the musculoskeletal system, typically hip dysplasia and foot deformities.[2] Children with an underlying syndrome may have other organ system issues that need to be addressed.

The characteristic hyperextension deformity can vary from a mild deformity which rapidly responds to simple stretching to a severe deformity that is associated with complete dislocation and proximal migration of the tibia relative to the distal femur (Figure 29.1).

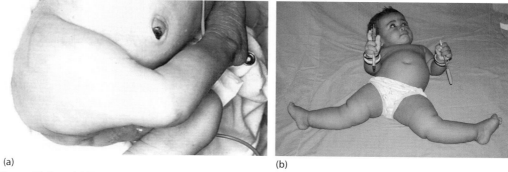

(a)   (b)

Figure 29.1 ● **(a)** The clinical appearance of a right congenital knee dislocation in a newborn child. Note the prominent posterior femoral condyles. **(b)** The appearance of an infant with congenital dislocation of both knees.

Problems of management

Contracture of the quadriceps muscle

Contracture of the quadriceps muscle appears to be the primary problem in this condition. The severity of contracture varies and, accordingly, the knee may be hyperextended, subluxated or dislocated (Figure 29.2).

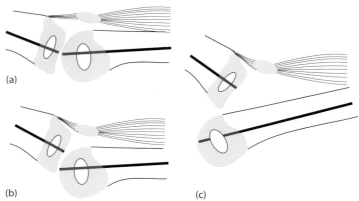

(a)

(b)   (c)

Figure 29.2 ● Three types of congenital hyperextension of the knee: **(a)** recurvatum, **(b)** subluxation and **(c)** dislocation.

Abnormalities of the cruciate ligaments

In a proportion of children with congenital dislocation of the knee the cruciate ligaments may be hypoplastic and stretched or totally absent. Although the ligament laxity may not manifest itself until later in life it is often quite symptomatic and disabling for the patient, and may also lead to late genu valgum or genu varum deformities (Figure 29.3).

(a)

Figure 29.3 ● The lateral radiographs of knees of a boy with hyperextension deformity of the right knee **(a)** and congenital dislocation of the left knee **(b)**. After successful open reduction of the left knee and closed reduction of the right knee, there was mild valgus instability of the left knee at age three years and two months **(c)**. This resolved without intervention; however, varus instability of the right knee developed at age 13 years 2 months **(d)**.

(b)

(c)

(d)

Associated hip dysplasia

It is very important to ascertain the status of the hip as soon as possible as hip dislocation imparts an even greater sense of urgency for obtaining reduction of the knee (Figure 29.4). It is essential that adequate knee flexion is obtained and the hamstrings are relaxed in order to facilitate reduction of hip dislocation.[2] Hence it is imperative that the hip dysplasia is recognized and the knee dislocation corrected promptly to enable early reduction of the hip.

Figure 29.4 ● The lateral radiographs of both knees of a one-day-old girl with bilateral congenital hyperextension deformities of the knees **(a)**. An ultrasound of the right hip **(b)** documents hip dysplasia, with no significant contact between the femoral head (star) and the acetabulum (arrow).

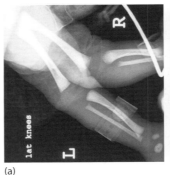

(a)

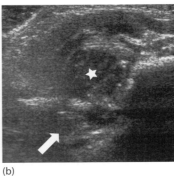

(b)

Aims of treatment

- Obtain tibiofemoral reduction
  Correction of the deformity and reduction of the dislocation is necessary to enable the child to walk.[3]
- Obtain an arc of motion necessary for daily activities
  The arc of knee motion generally regarded as necessary for adequate daily activities is 90° and the goal of treatment is to obtain this arc of motion.

- Obtain strong extensor function
  Good quadriceps strength is necessary for daily activities and ambulation and therefore it is important to avoid weakening the quadriceps by over-lengthening.
- Avoid instability and deformity
  An effort must be made to prevent or minimize anteroposterior laxity due to cruciate hypoplasia and avoid late valgus and varus deformity of the knee.[1,4]

Treatment options

Serial stretching and casting

Gentle longitudinal traction on the tibia with gentle gradual correction of the hyperextension deformity is attempted initially. After each session of stretching, a long leg cast is applied to maintain the correction obtained. The goal is to obtain at least 90° of flexion and reduction of the deformity over a course of several weeks. Care must be taken not to create 'pseudo-correction' through an iatrogenic fracture of the proximal tibial physis (Figure 29.5).

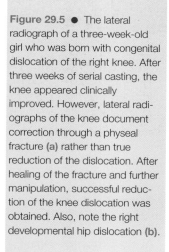
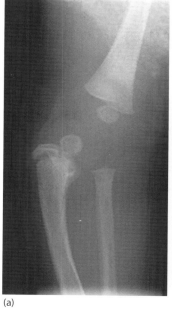
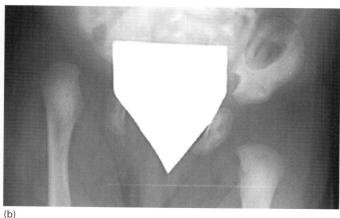

Figure 29.5 ● The lateral radiograph of a three-week-old girl who was born with congenital dislocation of the right knee. After three weeks of serial casting, the knee appeared clinically improved. However, lateral radiographs of the knee document correction through a physeal fracture **(a)** rather than true reduction of the dislocation. After healing of the fracture and further manipulation, successful reduction of the knee dislocation was obtained. Also, note the right developmental hip dislocation **(b)**.

(a)   (b)

Pavlik harness

Once 90° of flexion of the knee is obtained, further improvement in flexion can be achieved by using a Pavlik harness.[5] This will also assist in the treatment of any associated hip dysplasia.

Open reduction

This is reserved for those children who do not respond to a programme of stretching and cast immobilization.

Factors to be taken into consideration while planning treatment

Presence of other musculoskeletal anomalies

The hyperextension deformity places the hamstrings on stretch, which also stresses the hip and exacerbates any hip dysplasia. In order to treat hip dysplasia, the hamstrings must be relaxed.

Associated foot deformities, such as clubfoot, also need treatment. Serial casting for clubfoot deformity requires a flexed knee to relax the gastrocnemius muscle and the Achilles tendon to assist in correction of the equinus deformity. Thus, the coexistence of foot deformity similarly imparts a sense of urgency to obtain reduction of the knee in order to relax the triceps surae and allow correction of the clubfoot.

Magnitude of the extension deformity

If the deformity is just hyperextension, it is likely that simple stretching and casting will result in an acceptable result. If the deformity is a dislocation with proximal migration of the tibia anteriorly on the femur and foreshortened quadriceps mechanisms, then surgical intervention is required.[2] This differentiation can often be assisted by an arthrogram or ultrasound to image the position of the tibia relative to the femur (Figure 29.6).

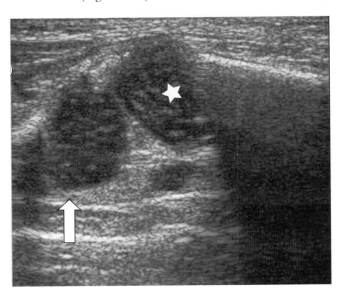

Figure 29.6 ● The lateral ultrasound of a three-week-old child after serial casting for congenital dislocation of the knee. Note that although there is still some residual hyperextension, there is complete contact between the tibia (arrow) and the femoral condyles (star), indicating that reduction has been achieved.

Recommended treatment

The outline of treatment is summarized in Table 29.1.

Table 29.1 ● The outline of treatment recommendations for congenital dislocation of the knee

INDICATIONS		
Congenital hyperextension OR Congenital subluxation OR Congenital dislocation of the knee without appreciable proximal overriding of the tibia	Congenital hyperextension OR Congenital subluxation OR Congenital dislocation of the knee without appreciable proximal overriding of the tibia + Passive knee flexion of up to 90° achieved by stretching and casting + Associated developmental dysplasia of the hip	Congenital dislocation of the knee without appreciable proximal overriding of the tibia + Inadequate response to serial stretching and splinting (i.e. 90° flexion not achieved) OR Congenital dislocation of the knee with proximal overriding of the tibia
⇩	⇩	⇩
Serial stretching and casting or splinting	Pavlik harness + Monitor for late instability and deformity	Open reduction and quadricepsplasty of Curtis and Fisher + Monitor for late instability and deformity
TREATMENT		

Serial stretching and casting

An initial trial of gradual stretching by gentle traction and flexion is performed. If there is a rapid response this can be continued. If there is minimal response, then further evaluation with an ultrasound (Figure 29.6) or plain radiographs to image the tibiofemoral relationship should be performed.[1] If 90° of flexion can be reached, then a Pavlik harness may be used. Night splinting is used for several months to maintain reduction.

Open reduction and quadriceps lengthening

Formal open reduction consists of quadriceps lengthening, anterior capsulotomy, reduction of the dislocation and long leg casting.[4,5] The technique used to lengthen the quadriceps is that of Curtis and Fisher[4] (Figure 29.7). In some instances the hamstrings need to be mobilized from their pathologic anterior position and placed into their normal position posterior to the knee. The cruciate ligaments should not be transected.[6] The correction must achieve at least 90° degrees of flexion. Although it may be possible to lengthen the quadriceps further, to obtain even more flexion of the knee, this may be at the risk of over-lengthening the muscle which results in permanent weakness of extension. The best results are obtained when surgery is performed before the age of six months.[7] An anteriorly placed incision runs the risk of poor wound healing due to tension on the wound once the knee is flexed. A lateral incision can avoid this problem (Figure 29.8).

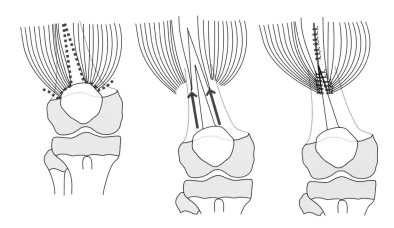

Figure 29.7 ● Technique of performing a V-Y plasty of the quadriceps tendon for congenital dislocation of the knee.

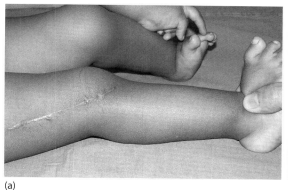 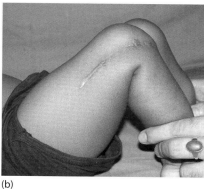

(a)   (b)

Figure 29.8 ● A laterally placed incision for reduction of congenital dislocation of the knee has healed well **(a)** and an excellent range of knee flexion has been restored **(b)** in this child.

Rationale of the choice of treatment

Why is the knee treated first when associated hip dislocation and clubfoot deformity are present?
Hyperextension of the knee results in stretching and increased tension on both the hamstrings and triceps surae. Stretching of these muscle groups exacerbates hip dysplasia and clubfoot deformity, respectively. Successful treatment of hip dysplasia and clubfoot first requires relaxed hamstrings and triceps surae. It is for this reason that the knee hyperextension deformity is addressed first.

Why is a Pavlik harness not used as the initial treatment since there is an increased incidence of hip dysplasia in children with congenital dislocation of the knee?
Placement of the Pavlik harness requires a minimum knee flexion of 90°. Since the knee is hyperextended, the child's lower extremity cannot be appropriately positioned in a Pavlik harness until this deformity is corrected.

References

1. Ko J-Y, Shih C-H, Wenger DR. Congenital dislocation of the knee. *J Pediatr Orthop* 1999; **19**: 252–9.
2. Ooishi T, Sugioka Y, Matsumoto S, Fujii T. Congenital dislocation of the knee. Its pathologic features and treatment. *Clin Orthop Relat Res* 1993; **287**: 187–92.
3. Ahmadi B, Shahriaree H, Silver CM. Severe congenital genu recurvatum. *J Bone Joint Surg Am* 1979; **61**: 622–4.
4. Curtis BH, Fisher RL. Congenital hyperextension with anterior subluxation of the knee. *J Bone Joint Surg Am* 1969; **51**: 255–69.
5. Nogi J, MacEwen GD. Congenital dislocation of the knee. *J Pediatr Orthop* 1982; **2**: 509–13.
6. Ferris B, Aichroth P. The treatment of congenital knee dislocation. A review of nineteen knees. *Clin Orthop Relat Res* 1987; **216**: 135–40.
7. Bensahel H, Dal Monte A, Hjelmstedt A *et al.* Congenital dislocation of the knee. *J Pediatr Orthop* 1989; **9**: 174–7.

Congenital dislocation of the patella

Randall Loder

30

Introduction

Congenital dislocation of the patella may occur as an isolated entity (Figure 30.1) or in concert with syndromes such as nail-patella syndrome (Figure 30.2), Down syndrome, Rubinstein–Taybi syndrome or in children with arthrogryposis.[1,2] If it is part of a more generalized syndrome, appropriate medical care may be needed for these children in addition to that for the patellar dislocation.

The patella may be dislocated at birth, or dislocate within the first year or two of life, due to hypoplasia of the patella, the femoral trochlear groove or both.[3–6] The hallmark features of congenital patellar dislocation are fixed flexion deformity of the knee, limited active knee extension, genu valgum and external tibial rotation. Secondary to external tibial rotation the position of the tibial tuberosity is abnormally lateral. Since the deformities do not interfere with crawling, congenital dislocation of the patella usually presents only in the second year of life as a delay or difficulty in walking. The knee flexion contracture, extensor weakness and external tibial rotation all contribute to the difficulty in walking.[7]

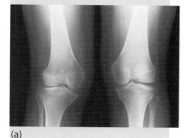
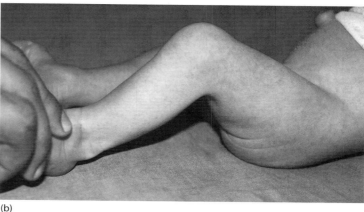

(a)   (b)

Figure 30.1 ● A new-born infant with a congenital dislocation of the patella of the left side. The characteristic external rotation of the tibia **(a)** and the fixed flexion deformity **(b)** are clearly seen.

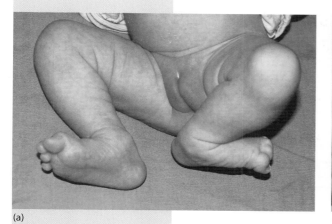
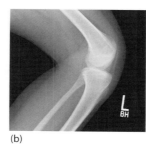
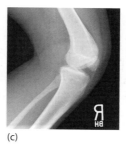
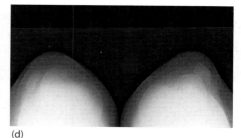

(a)   (b)   (c)   (d)

Figure 30.2 ● Anteroposterior **(a)**, lateral **(b,c)** and skyline **(d)** radiographs of a girl with nail-patella syndrome and bilateral congenital dislocation of the patellae.

Congenital dislocation of the patella must be differentiated from the much more common recurrent patellar dislocation which presents in late childhood or early adolescence and is due to simple patellar malalignment (see Chapter 31, Recurrent and habitual dislocation of the patella).[8]

Problems of management

Inability to actively extend the knee

Active contraction of the quadriceps does not produce any extension of the knee. This is not on account of actual weakness of the quadriceps but simply because the quadriceps mechanism lies posterior to the axis of movement of the knee. As a consequence of this, the child may be unable to stand on its feet and may begin to kneel-walk.

Knee deformity

The most severe component of knee deformity is flexion. While the major contribution to the deformity is the malaligned and contracted quadriceps mechanism which acts as a flexor of the knee, the hamstrings and the posterior joint capsule may also be contracted. Genu valgum is often present and the tibia is externally rotated.

Patellar and trochlear hypoplasia

The ability to maintain a normal patellar position after surgical realignment is influenced by the amount of patellar hypoplasia and size of the distal femoral trochlear groove. A markedly hypoplastic patella may not be palpable upon physical examination in a small child[5] and, since the patella does not ossify until three or four years of age, imaging using ultrasound, computed tomography or magnetic resonance imaging may be necessary to ascertain the presence or absence of the patella and quantify its size.

Aims of treatment

- Restore active knee extension
  This is the first and foremost goal. Successful ambulation requires strong knee extensors, which, in turn, requires normal patellofemoral anatomy and function.
- Correct the knee deformity
  Unless the flexion deformity of the knee is corrected the quadriceps cannot function effectively and therefore this deformity must be corrected. Correction of the genu valgum and the external rotation of the tibia are required to ensure stable reduction of the patella.
- Achieve stability of the patella with normal alignment of the quadriceps mechanism
  In order to maintain reduction of the patellofemoral joint, the malalignment of the quadriceps mechanism needs to be addressed. Structures on the lateral side of the knee that are contracted must be released and the lax medial structures need to be imbricated. Finally, any bony abnormality such as genu valgum and lateral rotation of the tibia must be corrected in order to ensure that all the destabilizing forces are removed.

Treatment options

Congenital dislocation of the patella requires surgical correction. The options that exist are only in the type and magnitude of realignment performed.

Restoring active knee extension

Realigning the quadriceps mechanism so that it lies anterior to the axis of movement of the knee will restore active knee extension. This requires complete release of the tight, fibrotic adhesions of the lateral retinaculum that may be adherent to the lateral intermuscular septum. The contracted vastus lateralis also needs to be released from the intermuscular septum as far proximal as is needed.

Correction of knee deformity

In most children lengthening of the contracted elements of the quadriceps muscle at the time of surgical reduction of the patella and realignment of the abnormal patellar tendon insertion usually solves knee flexion. In some instances release of the hamstrings and a posterior capsular release may be necessary when the capsule is also contracted.

Genu valgum also tends to become corrected once the contracted lateral soft tissue structures are adequately released.

Restoring patellar stability and realignment of the quadriceps mechanism

The strategies needed to achieve this aim include both dynamic and static stabilization of the patella. Plication of the vastus medialis is mandatory to improve the efficiency of the slack oblique fibres of the muscle. Lateral and distal advancement of the vastus medialis onto the surface of the patella provides a dynamic force that will counter any tendency for lateral displacement of the patella. The insertion of the patellar tendon is also moved medially to reduce the angle the quadriceps muscle makes with the patellar tendon. This further reduces the tendency for lateral subluxation of the patella. In young children with an open tibial physis this must be done without violating the proximal tibial apophysis (i.e. a bony procedure to shift the tibial tuberosity is contraindicated until physeal closure). It is important not to shift the insertion of the patellar tendon inferiorly as this may limit knee flexion. If, after performing these procedures, the patella still tends to subluxate laterally when the knee is passively flexed during the operation or if it has been clearly demonstrated that the femoral trochlear groove is very poorly developed, semitendinosus tenodesis is also performed.

Factors to be taken into consideration while planning treatment

In all cases of congenital dislocation of the patella, surgical release of the contracted structures is needed. The decision to release a specific structure depends upon the severity of deformity and the degree of patellar instability.

Severity of flexion deformity

If, after release of the contracted structures on the lateral aspect of the knee, flexion deformity persists, the hamstrings need to be released. Any residual flexion deformity after release of the hamstrings may be due to a posterior capsular contracture.

Degree of patellar instability

If, after adequate release of contractures, advancement of the vastus medialis and lateral shift of the patellar tendon, there is demonstrable instability, static stabilization by semitendinosus tenodesis is needed.

Size of patella and the trochlear groove

If the patella is very small and the trochlear groove is very shallow it may be more difficult to achieve stability of the patella. In such cases it is safer to perform a static tenodesis in addition to advancement of the vastus medialis.

Recommended treatment

The recommended treatment for congenital dislocation of the patella is shown in Table 30.1.

Table 30.1 ● Outline of the recommended management plan for treating congenital dislocation of the patella

INDICATION	
Following: Release of the lateral retinacular fibrosis + Release of the vastus lateralis from the intermuscular septum + Distal and lateral advancement of the vastus medialis onto the patella	
Flexion deformity of the knee persists ⇩	Patellar instability persists on passive knee flexion OR If the trochlear groove is shallow ⇩
Hamstring release Flexion deformity of the knee persists ⇩	Semitendinosus tenodesis
Release of posterior capsule of the knee	
TREATMENT	

Rationale of treatment choice

Why is the only option surgical realignment?

The pathoanatomy is such[4] that the very strong fibrotic lateral bands, lateral insertion of the patellar tendon and abnormal orientation of the vastus medialis can only be corrected surgically.

References

1. Mendez AA, Keret D, MacEwen GD. Treatment of patellofemoral instability in Down's syndrome. *Clin Orthop Relat Res* 1988; **234**: 148–58.
2. Stevens CA. Patellar dislocation in Rubinstein–Taybi syndrome. *Am J Med Genet* 1997; **72**: 188–90.
3. Ghanem I, Wattincourt L, Seringe R. Congenital dislocation of the patella. Part II: Orthopaedic management. *J Pediatr Orthop* 2000; **20**: 817–22.
4. Ghanem I, Wattincourt L, Seringe R. Congenital dislocation of the patella. Part I: Pathologic anatomy. *J Pediatr Orthop* 2000; **20**: 812–6.
5. Jones RDS, Fisher RL, Curtis BH. Congenital dislocation of the patella. *Clin Orthop Relat Res* 1976; **119**: 177–83.
6. Stanisavljevic S, Zemenick G, Miller D. Congenital, irreducible, permanent lateral dislocation of the patella. *Clin Orthop Relat Res* 1976; **116**: 190–99.
7. Langenskiöld A, Ritsilä V. Congenital dislocation of the patella and its operative treatment. *J Pediatr Orthop* 1992; **12**: 315–23.
8. Zeier FG, Dissanayake C. Congenital dislocation of the patella. *Clin Orthop Relat Res* 1980; **148**: 140–46.

Recurrent and habitual dislocation of the patella

31

Randall Loder

Introduction

In the normal individual, the patella has an inherent tendency to move laterally on account of the alignment of the quadriceps muscle and patellar tendon; the angle between the long axis of the muscle and the patella tendon (the Q-angle) creates a vector that pulls the patella laterally. Lateral subluxation of the patella is, however, prevented by the dynamic action of the distal fibres of the vastus medialis and by the static restraint offered by a sufficiently deep patellar groove on the femur, the larger lateral femoral condyle and the integrity of the medial capsule and retinaculum (Figure 31.1). Different pathological processes render these stabilizing mechanisms ineffective in congenital, recurrent and habitual dislocation of the patella (Table 31.1). A clear understanding of the factors that contribute to patellar dislocation will help in planning the requisite operative procedure.

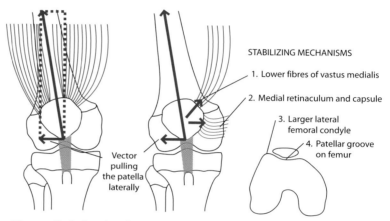

STABILIZING MECHANISMS

1. Lower fibres of vastus medialis

2. Medial retinaculum and capsule

3. Larger lateral femoral condyle

4. Patellar groove on femur

Vector pulling the patella laterally

Figure 31.1 ● Diagram illustrating the alignment of the normal quadriceps muscle and the patellar tendon. The laterally directed force vector tends to predispose to lateral displacement of the patella. The normal stabilizing factors that prevent patellar dislocation are shown.

Definitions

It is important to be clear about what recurrent, habitual and persistent dislocations of the patella are to avoid any confusion in the terminology. This differentiation is also necessary because treatment approaches are quite different for congenital, habitual and recurrent dislocation. Habitual dislocation always requires surgery proximal to the patella, while recurrent dislocation usually requires surgery at or distal to the patella.

Recurrent dislocation of the patella is an episodic, typically painful patellar dislocation, often due to an initial trauma. Its hallmark is capsular and retinacular laxity, in contrast to quadriceps contracture which is seen in congenital and habitual dislocation of the patella. Many children demonstrate a varying degree of underlying ligamentous laxity, upon which is superimposed an initial trauma that is often due to an athletic event.[1] In a smaller subset of patients there is an identifiable ligamentous laxity syndrome, such as Down syndrome,[2] Ehler-Danlos syndrome, etc. In the second subset the recurrent patellar dislocation can progress to persistent subluxation (Figure 31.2) and, finally, persistent dislocation.

Habitual, or obligatory, dislocation of the patella is a patellar dislocation that occurs every time the knee is flexed and is due primarily to a shortened but otherwise normally positioned quadriceps mechanism.[3,4] It is unlike congenital dislocation of the patella which is an irreducible dislocation that is present from birth and involves both a complete lateral displacement of the entire quadriceps mechanism as well as shortening. It also differs from recurrent dislocation of the patella in that the habitual dislocation is painless and without associated trauma, and demonstrates quadriceps contracture rather than capsular and retinacular laxity. In habitual dislocation the patella will reduce when the knee is in complete extension and full flexion of the knee is not possible while holding the patella firmly in the trochlear groove.

Table 31.1 ● Abnormalities that contribute to patellar instability in congenital, habitual and recurrent dislocation

Abnormality		Effect of this abnormality on normal stabilizing mechanisms	Role in particular type of patellar dislocation
Soft tissue	Ligament and capsular laxity	Stabilizing effect of medial capsule and medial retinaculum ineffective	Frequent in recurrent dislocation
Bony abnormalities	Shallow patellar groove	Ineffective static stability	May occur in recurrent, habitual and congenital dislocation
	Hypoplastic lateral femoral condyle	Ineffective static stability	May occur in recurrent, habitual and congenital dislocation (Figure 31.3)
	Genu valgum	Increases the Q-angle (this increases the vector that pulls the patella laterally)	Frequent in recurrent dislocation
	Torsional abnormalities of the femur and tibia (e.g. miserable malalignment syndrome)	Increases the Q-angle (this increases the vector that pulls the patella laterally)	May occur in recurrent dislocation (Figure 31.4)
	Abnormal size and shape of patella	More prone to ride out of the patellar groove of the femur	May occur in congenital, habitual and recurrent dislocation
Abnormalities of the quadriceps mechanism	Abnormal lateral insertion of patellar tendon	Increases the Q-angle	Often seen in recurrent dislocation
	Weak or abnormally inserted vastus medialis	Dynamic stability is lost	Often seen in recurrent dislocation
	Contracture of the vastus lateralis	The dynamic action of the vastus medialis cannot overcome the contracture of the vastus lateralis	Always seen in habitual and congenital dislocation
			May rarely be seen in long-standing recurrent dislocation
	Contracture of the rectus femoris and vastus intermedius	The dynamic action of the vastus medialis cannot overcome the contracture	Seen in habitual dislocation and congenital dislocation
			Not seen in recurrent dislocation
	Lateral displacement of the entire quadriceps mechanism	None of the stabilizing mechanisms can work since the quadriceps mechanism is displaced	Seen only in congenital dislocation

In *persistent dislocation of the patella*, as seen in congenital patellar dislocation and rarely following recurrent dislocation, the patella remains dislocated in both flexion and extension of the knee.

Aim of treatment

- Restore and maintain stability of the patella
  Irrespective of the type of dislocation the aim of treatment is to obtain a reduction and to prevent the patella from dislocating again.

Treatment options

Treatment of recurrent and habitual dislocation of the patella is directed to correcting the underlying abnormalities that are listed in Table 31.1. The specific strategies to address each of the abnormalities and the treatment options are shown in Table 31.2. It needs to be emphasized that several of these individual procedures may have to be combined in the operation in order to achieve satisfactory stability of reduction.

Factors to be taken into consideration while planning treatment

Is the child skeletally mature?

This is extremely important to determine since bony procedures that are standard in skeletally mature individuals cannot be used in skeletally immature children. A typical example is tibial tuberosity relocation; moving the tibial tuberosity in a child with significant remaining growth will result in an anterior growth arrest and secondary recurvatum deformity.

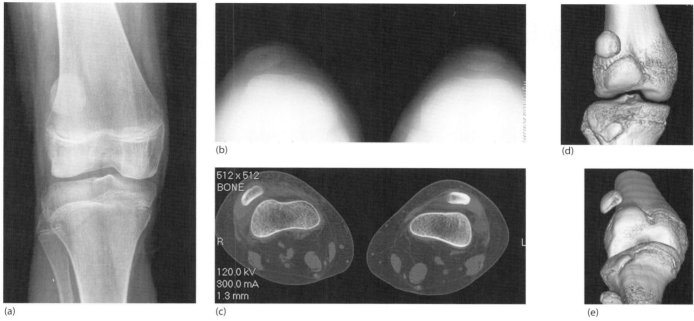

Figure 31.2 ● The anteroposterior **(a)** and Merchant's view **(b)** radiographs of a 13-year-old girl with recurrent right patellar dislocation. The axial computed tomography scan demonstrates lateral subluxation of the patella **(c)**, which is also nicely demonstrated on the 3-D reconstructions **(d,e)**.

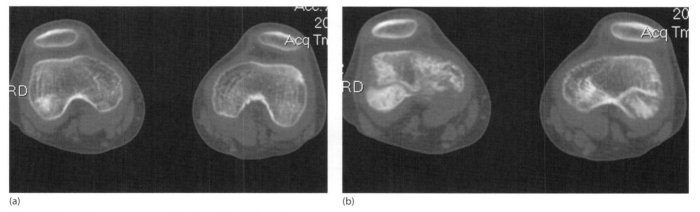

Figure 31.3 ● A seven-year-old girl with a habitual dislocation of the left patella. The computed tomography scan demonstrates a reasonably large patella with a hypoplastic patellofemoral groove, proximal to the physis **(a)** and at the level of the physis **(b)**.

What are the abnormalities of the soft tissue, bones and the quadriceps mechanism?

The specific abnormalities of the structures are listed in Table 31.1 and these will determine the nature of intervention.

Is there generalized ligament laxity?

The results of plication of the medial capsule may be poor on account of the inherent tendency for the soft tissue to stretch. In such situations it is safer to add other mechanisms to improve static or dynamic stability on the medial side (pes anserinus transfer or semitendinosus tenodesis).

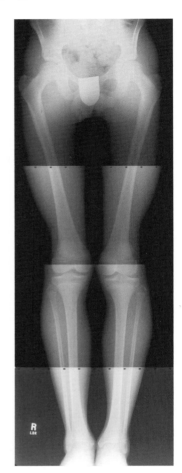

Figure 31.4 ● The standing anteroposterior radiograph of the lower extremities in a boy of 14 years and 5 months with recurrent dislocation of the patella that began five months earlier after a sporting injury. Note the lateral subluxation, as well as the slight rotational asymmetry of the femoral condyles indicating a mild femoral anteversion component.

Table 31.2 ● Treatment options for improving patellar stability

Strategy	Treatment options
Correction of medial capsular laxity	Medial capsular plication
Improving dynamic stability	Advance the insertion of vastus medialis distally and more medially and inferiorly onto the anterior surface of the patella (Figure 31.5b)
	Pes anserinus transfer (Figure 31.6b)
Improving static stability	Semitendinosus tenodesis (Figure 31.6c)
Reducing the Q-angle	Roux–Goldthwait transfer of lateral half of patellar tendon (Figure 31.7b)
	Medial transplantation of the tibial tuberosity (Figure 31.7c)
	Correction of genu valgum
	Correction of femoral and tibial torsion
Removing forces that favour dislocation	Release of the lateral capsule and retinaculum (Figure 31.5b)
	Release of the vastus lateralis
	Release of the rectus femoris and vastus intermedius

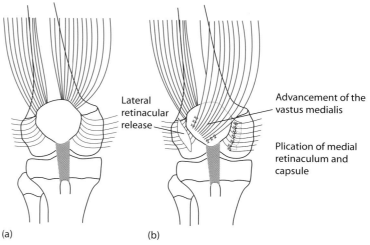

(a)   (b)

Figure 31.5 ● Diagram showing the technique of advancement of the vastus medialis to restore dynamic stability. Release of the lateral retinaculum and plication of the medial capsule and retinaculum are also shown.

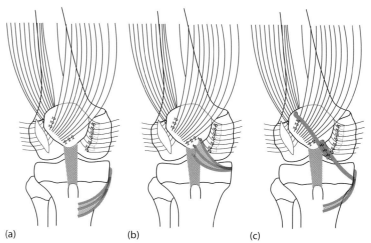

(a)   (b)   (c)

Figure 31.6 ● Diagram illustrating the technique of performing the pes anserinus transfer to augment the dynamic forces stabilizing the patella **(b)** and the technique of performing a semitendinosus tenodesis **(c)**.

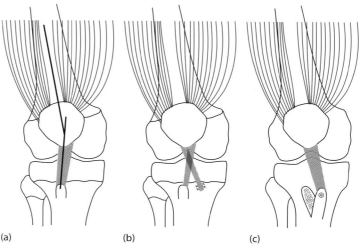

(a)   (b)   (c)

Figure 31.7 ● Diagram illustrating how an abnormally high Q-angle **(a)** can be effectively reduced by transferring the lateral half of the patellar tendon medially (the Roux–Goldthwait procedure) in a skeletally immature child **(b)** or by transplanting the tibial tuberosity laterally in the skeletally mature child **(c)**.

<table>
<tr><td>

Recommended treatment

</td><td>

Recurrent dislocation of the patella

■ Non-operative

If the problem appears to be simple subluxation rather than complete dislocation, then a rehabilitation programme designed to strengthen the vastus medialis and improve lateral retinacular flexibility should be prescribed.[1,5] Passive mobilization exercises of the lateral retinaculum along with progressive resistance short arc quadriceps exercises are initially prescribed, typically for eight weeks.

■ Operative

The outline of the surgical treatment is shown in Table 31.3 and summarized below.

</td></tr>
</table>

Table 31.3 ● Outline of operative treatment for recurrent dislocation of the patella

INDICATIONS		
In ALL cases perform: Release of the lateral retinaculum + Plication of the medial capsule + Advancement of the vastus medialis		
If the patella is still unstable after the above procedures + Normal Q-angle ⇩ Semitendinosus tenodesis	If the patella is still unstable after the above procedures + Abnormal Q-angle + No genu valgum or torsional abnormality + Skeletally immature ⇩ Roux–Goldthwait procedure	If the patella is still unstable after the above procedures + Abnormal Q-angle + No genu valgum or torsional abnormality + Skeletally mature ⇩ Tibial tuberosity transplantation
	If genu valgum or a torsional abnormality of the femur or tibia is contributing to the abnormal Q-angle, the bony deformity must be corrected prior to undertaking this operation	
TREATMENT		

If there is persistent recurrent instability after rehabilitation, or the patient has recurrent dislocation rather than subluxation, then operative treatment is strongly recommended. The very large number of described procedures indicates the difficulty in understanding the circumstances unique to any one patient and the inability to define the problem. This is aggravated in the paediatric condition, where the added dimension of growth must be considered. In general, reconstruction is designed in each case individually, and attempts to create a normal four quadrant balance,[5] both in static and dynamic conditions. Looking at the soft tissues first, it is important to consider both the peripatellar and infrapatellar structures. If a peripatellar lateral tether is present, then a lateral retinacular release is needed. This is often associated with concomitant medial capsular laxity, which is addressed by a medial plication and advancement of the vastus medialis to the lateral border of the patella and patellar tendon.[6] In the severe case a semitendinosus transfer through the patella to act as a check-rein tenodesis is also performed.[4,7] For the infrapatellar structures, the alignment of the patellar tendon and its insertion into the tibial tuberosity is evaluated. If the insertion is externally rotated or lateralized, then a transposition of the patellar tendon may be necessary.[8] In the skeletally immature patient, the procedure of choice is the Roux–Goldthwait transfer. If skeletally mature, then an actual translocation using an Elmslie–Trillat rotationplasty can be performed. Owing to the multiple soft tissue pathologies that must be addressed, these reconstructions need to be performed open rather than arthroscopically. In the extremely severe case, where there is significant malalignment of the femur and tibia (miserable malalignment syndrome – see Chapter 18, Femoral anteversion), concomitant femoral and tibial rotational osteotomies may be necessary. This is, however, an extremely unusual circumstance.

Habitual dislocation of the patella

Surgical realignment is always necessary. The two-incision approach, as described by Baksi,[4] is used. From the lateral incision, the tight lateral bands including the vastus lateralis are released from the patella. If patellar reduction can now be achieved in full flexion, then the vastus lateralis is reattached to the rectus femoris at the appropriate higher level. If reduction cannot be achieved, then a musculotendinous lengthening of the rectus femoris is performed; occasionally, the vastus intermedius also needs to be lengthened or released. Then the vastus lateralis, rectus femoris and vastus intermedius are reattached to each other at their appropriate new levels. Medial stabilization is next performed if lateral dislocation is still present during passive flexion. This involves medial plication of the vastus medialis, and often a pes anserinus transposition or semitendinosus tenodesis.

Rationale of treatment suggested

Why is short arc quadriceps exercise used in non-operative treatment of recurrent dislocation of the patella?
The patella rapidly dislocates with flexion, which makes long arc exercises contraindicated. Similarly, in flexion there is increased force across the patellofemoral joint which increases articular stress and the potential for cartilage degeneration.

Why perform the Roux–Goldthwait partial patellar tendon transfer in skeletally immature children?
This transfer does not violate the tibial tuberosity apophysis; a complete bony transfer will damage the anterior portion of the tibial physis and result in a recurvatum deformity due to anterior growth arrest.

Why is an isolated lateral retinacular release not indicated for recurrent dislocation of the patella?
This is reserved for those children in whom there is only lateral patellar tilt without any lateral translation. In the child with recurrent dislocation, there is lateral translation, by definition, and this recurrent dislocation leads to medial capsular ligamentous laxity which must also be corrected.

References

1. Hinton RY, Sharma KM. Acute and recurrent patellar instability in the young athlete. *Orthop Clin North Am* 2003; **34**: 385–96.
2. Mendez AA, Keret D, MacEwen GD. Treatment of patellofemoral instability in Down's syndrome. *Clin Orthop Relat Res* 1988; **234**: 148–58.
3. Bergman NR, Williams PF. Habitual dislocation of the patella in flexion. *J Bone Joint Surg Br* 1988; **70**: 415–19.
4. Baksi DP. Pes anserinus transposition for patellar dislocations. Long-term follow-up results. *J Bone Joint Surg Br* 1993; **75**: 305–10.
5. Stanitski CL. Patellar instability in the school age athlete. *Instr Course Lect* 1998; **47**: 345–50.
6. Vähäsarja V, Kinnunen P, Lanning P, Serlo W. Operative realignment of patellar malalignment in children. *J Pediatr Orthop* 1995; **15**: 281–5.
7. Deie M, Ochi M, Sumen Y *et al*. Reconstruction of the medial patellofemoral ligament for the treatment of habitual or recurrent dislocation of the patella in children. *J Bone Joint Surg Br* 2003; **85**: 887–90.
8. Bensahel H, Souchet P, Pennecot GF, Mazda K. The unstable patella in children. *J Pediatr Orthop* 2000; **9**: 265–70.

Recurrent and voluntary dislocation of the shoulder

32

Randall Loder

Introduction

Shoulder dislocation in children must be approached from a completely different perspective than in adults.

In children, dislocation of the shoulder may be paralytic (brachial plexus palsy, muscular dystrophy), associated with ligamentous laxity syndromes (e.g. Ehlers-Danlos), atraumatic (voluntary) or traumatic.

The foremost consideration is the underlying aetiology, since treatment, outcome and prognosis are closely linked to this. Prognosis entails both degenerative joint disease[1] as well as recurrence of dislocation or subluxation.[2–6]

Once the aetiology has been determined, then the shoulder dislocation should be classified according to three different criteria: subluxation or dislocation, severity of precipitating trauma (macro-trauma, repetitive micro-trauma or atraumatic) and mode of dislocation (involuntary, voluntary or habitual).

Types of dislocation

Types of dislocation are as follows:

- Acute traumatic anterior dislocation usually occurs following forced external rotation with abduction of the shoulder. The overall prognosis after the first acute, traumatic, anterior dislocation of the shoulder in children and adolescents is controversial, but most authors believe that many if not all children will eventually need surgical treatment.[2–5]
- Recurrent traumatic anterior dislocation.
- Multidirectional instability is instability in all three directions: anterior, posterior and inferior; it is relatively rare in children. Children with this instability tend to have their initial episode around ten years of age, while those with anterior or posterior instability tend to have their first episode around 14 years of age.[6]
- Voluntary subluxation or dislocation typically develops in school-age children for no obvious reason and without any history of trauma. The literature is clear that voluntary subluxation or dislocation should nearly always be treated non-operatively.[7]
- Dislocation associated with soft tissue disorders can, in a way, be viewed as the most severe type of multidirectional instability, since the underlying soft tissue disorder imparts significant global laxity to all of the capsular structures.
- Dislocation associated with obstetric brachial plexus palsy is now known to occur much earlier than thought, and should be aggressively searched for.[8–10] The most important clinical feature is loss of passive external rotation; other associated signs are asymmetric axillary skin folds and an apparent humeral shortening. If physical examination suggests that there may be posterior subluxation or dislocation, ultrasonography can be used, much as in developmental dislocation of the hip, to aid in diagnosis.

Problems of management

What is the aetiology and type of the dislocation?

This is the most important issue to decide as certain types do poorly with surgical intervention (e.g. voluntary),[6] yet with other types surgery is probably the best choice (e.g. obstetric brachial plexus palsy, traumatic dislocation). The treating physician, on the basis of history and physical examination, must determine the underlying aetiology.

In what direction is the dislocation?

It is important to know the direction of instability to guide both non-operative and operative treatment. The typical traumatic dislocation is anterior, yet the dislocation associated with obstetric brachial plexus palsy is posterior. Voluntary dislocation is usually multidirectional. Repair of instability in just one direction will clearly fail if the instability is multidirectional.

Muscle imbalance and capsular abnormalities

In paralytic dislocation there is underlying muscle imbalance that should be addressed while treating the dislocation. In obstetric brachial plexus palsy, internal rotation contracture, which may involve the internal rotators and the anterior capsule of the joint, predisposes to posterior dislocation. In recurrent dislocation there is usually varying degrees of capsular laxity. Capsular contracture or excessive laxity of the capsule needs to be corrected.

Adaptive bony changes

In children with paralytic dislocations there may be adaptive bony changes of the glenoid that include altered glenoid version and dysplasia.[8,9,11]

Aims of treatment

- Reduction and maintenance of dislocation
  Achieving reduction in the acute or recurrent involuntary dislocation is generally simple and performed by closed means. In long-standing neuromuscular or traumatic dislocations open reduction may be indicated. Maintaining reduction is especially problematic with traumatic and voluntary dislocations. Post-reduction rehabilitation is crucial.
- Rebalancing or realignment of muscle and capsular soft tissue structures
  This is important in neuromuscular dislocations as well as in multidirectional or unidirectional involuntary recurrent dislocation.
- Correction of associated bony adaptive changes
  If paralytic dislocation is reduced early, mild degrees of associated glenoid version or dysplasia may improve spontaneously.

Treatment options

Closed reduction and immobilization

Acute dislocations must be reduced as soon as possible followed by a period of immobilization. The type and time of immobilization (prolonged sling and swathe to minimal immobilization) appears to have no significant influence on the risk of recurrent dislocation, including time of immobilization.[2] With these considerations in mind, non–operative treatment involves immediate reduction, type of and time of immobilization determined by the treating physician and progressive rehabilitation.

Rehabilitation

The rehabilitation programme must attempt to optimize the dynamic stabilizers of the shoulder.

■ Anterior dislocation

The first issue to address is the dynamic stabilizer compression muscles (subscapularis, infraspinatus, teres minor, inferior rotator cuff, anterior deltoid). Next, attention is paid to the rehabilitation of dynamic tension, i.e. the rotator cuff tendons and muscles. The third component involves neuromuscular control by exercising the unstable shoulder in positions that maximally challenge the dynamic stabilizers. Finally, scapular stabilization must be addressed by strengthening the trapezius and serratus anterior muscles.

■ Posterior dislocation

For posterior dislocations, the strengthening focuses on the posterior deltoid, external rotators and scapular stabilizing muscles.

■ Multidirectional instability

Initially, a graduated rehabilitation programme is tried.[12]

■ Dislocation associated with soft tissue disorders

Intensive rehabilitation is initially instituted before considering any surgical intervention.

Surgical stabilization

■ Acute traumatic anterior dislocation

Immediate, initial operative care for an acute traumatic anterior dislocation is typically reserved for extenuating examples, such as a locked dislocation in an athlete who is desirous of returning to collision sports immediately. Surgery is typically considered only if symptoms persist despite a rehabilitation programme. If selected as the initial care, the surgery can be performed arthroscopically if the dislocation can be reduced under a general anaesthetic, otherwise open techniques will be necessary. The acute capsular stretch seen in the first-time dislocation may recover if the labral detachment is repaired and normal kinematics resume. This is the probable explanation for the much improved success rate of arthroscopic repair for the first-time dislocation patient compared to the recurrent dislocation patient. Whether open or closed, the avulsion of the labral attachment must be repaired.[13]

■ Recurrent traumatic anterior dislocation

The surgery involves capsular and ligamentous repair and plication along with reattachment of the labral avulsion (Bankart lesion).[14,15] If the instability has a component of multidirectional instability, then a capsular shift must also be performed.[16] These procedures can often be performed either arthroscopically or open; the superiority of one method over another is controversial,[17] but the data tend to show better outcomes with open repairs,[18] especially in those under 18 years of age.[19] Thermal capsulorraphy should not be used because of significant complications, such as axillary nerve injury and chondrolysis, that can arise from that method,[20] as well as many unsatisfactory results even at two to five year follow-up.[21]

■ Multidirectional instability

The inferior capsular shift procedure is the workhorse for multidirectional instability. This consists of a superolateral shift of the redundant inferior capsule followed by an inferior shift of the superior capsule. Bony disruption or avulsion, such as with an avulsion of the labrum from the inferior glenoid, is also repaired if present. The approach may be either anterior or posterior, based upon the predominant direction of the instability. Post-operative immobilization for six weeks, followed by gradual and specific rehabilitation is paramount. Sports activities should be restricted for at least one year.

■ Dislocation associated with soft tissue disorders

These should be approached surgically as any other multidirectional instability using an inferior capsular shift procedure. The prognosis is guarded due to the genetic nature of the underlying soft tissue problem (e.g. Ehlers-Danlos) and this must be seriously discussed with the patient prior to surgery.

Capsulorraphy and correction of glenoid version

True recurrent posterior dislocation is typically associated with glenoid version abnormalities. Thus a posterior glenoplasty along with the posterior capsular imbrication is often necessary.[22]

Muscle release and tendon transfer

Dislocations in children with obstetric palsy are typically seen in Erb's (upper plexus) palsy. There are two major issues that must be addressed: the first is the dislocation and the second is the muscle imbalance. Either closed reduction[23] or open reduction[24] along with soft tissue balancing is typically needed.[11] A release of the pectoralis major insertion, latissimus dorsi and teres major is first performed, and this permits reduction of the dislocation. The latissimus dorsi and teres major are then transferred to the rotator cuff to balance the musculature (see Chapter 58, The paralysed shoulder in the child).[23]

No active intervention

As previously noted, surgical intervention should not be undertaken in children who dislocate the shoulder voluntarily. Most of these children can be managed by 'skilful neglect', that is no restriction of activities or physiotherapy. Psychological counselling may be needed.

Factors to be taken into consideration while planning treatment

Type of dislocation

It is vital to consider the type of dislocation as the outcome and prognosis of either non-operative or operative treatment can then be discussed with the child and family. For a young child who has sustained the first traumatic anterior dislocation, the risk of recurrence is high, along with the relatively high chance of needing surgical repair, but with a very good prognosis afterwards. For the child with multidirectional instability, graduated rehabilitation programmes often succeed; if not, then a capsular shift procedure has a good chance of success. For a child with voluntary dislocation, surgery should not be proposed since recurrence is almost inevitable.

Direction of dislocation

In addition to the aetiological type, the direction of dislocation must also be considered. If the dislocation is posterior, then a computed tomography scan might be indicated to search for abnormal glenoid version or glenoid hypoplasia, as these may need to be addressed if surgery is being considered.

Recommended treatment

The outline of treatment of shoulder dislocation in children is shown in Table 32.1 and summarized below:

- For acute traumatic anterior dislocation treatment is with initial closed reduction, followed by immobilization until comfortable and then aggressive rehabilitation is undertaken.
- In the case of recurrent traumatic anterior dislocation a trial of good rehabilitation can be prescribed.[12] If this fails, then open anterior Bankart repair with or without capsular shift is performed. Arthroscopic repair can also be performed, but is not the author's recommended treatment. Thermal capsulorraphy should not be done.
- In posterior subluxation or dislocation the initial event is treated with a closed reduction followed by rehabilitation. In the rare child with persistent instability, posterior capsulorraphy with or without posterior glenoplasty is recommended.
- In multidirectional instability a graduated rehabilitation programme is first begun.[12] If this fails, then an inferior capsular shift procedure is performed.
- For voluntary subluxation or dislocation, only non-operative care is recommended, either benign neglect or at the most a muscle strengthening programme.
- Dislocation associated with soft tissue disorders is approached as a multidirectional instability, but with a more guarded prognosis for operative care due to the underlying systemic soft tissue disorder.
- In dislocation associated with obstetric brachial plexus birth palsy operative care is the primary treatment of choice due to the underlying muscle imbalance along with the associated soft tissue contractures which arise from the underlying muscle imbalance. This consists of the transfer of the teres major and latissimus dorsi to the rotator cuff along with release of the pectoralis major and closed or open reduction of the dislocation. The intervention should be done early before any deformation of the humeral head occurs. Glenoid retroversion and hypoplasia may also need to be corrected.

Table 32.1 ● Outline of treatment of shoulder instability in children

INDICATIONS					
Recurrent anterior dislocation OR Recurrent posterior dislocation OR Multidirectional instability OR Dislocation associated with soft tissue abnormality	Recurrent anterior dislocation + Rehabilitation unsuccessful	Recurrent posterior dislocation + Rehabilitation unsuccessful	Multidirectional instability OR Dislocation associated with soft tissue abnormality + Rehabilitation unsuccessful	Posterior subluxation or dislocation in child with brachial plexus palsy	Voluntary dislocation
⇩	⇩	⇩	⇩	⇩	⇩
Aggressive, graduated rehabilitation programme	Anterior open reduction, capsulorraphy and Bankart repair	Posterior open reduction, capsulorraphy ± Glenoplasty	Capsular shift procedure	Internal rotator release and transfer of latissimus dorsi and teres major to the infraspinatus	No active orthopaedic intervention + Counselling
TREATMENT					

Rationale of treatment suggested

Why is arthroscopic repair for the recurrent anterior dislocation not recommended?
The capsular ligamentous structures have been markedly stretched, and imbrication, capsulorraphy or capsular shift is needed. Most series favour improved outcomes with open procedures compared to arthroscopic repair in the very young.

Why is thermal capsulorraphy not recommended?
Although the results in adolescents and young adults are initially promising, it has been shown that there is significant recurrence along with the potential for other soft tissue complications and articular chondrolysis.

Why is operative care not recommended for the voluntary subluxation/dislocation patient?
Operative results are abysmal and there is often associated psychopathology that cannot be surgically remedied.

Why is non-operative care not recommended for the dislocation associated with brachial plexus palsy?
Owing to the underlying muscle imbalance, muscle balancing procedures must be performed. The weakness due to the palsy cannot be improved by simple muscle strengthening.

References

1. Hovelius L. The natural history of primary anterior dislocation of the shoulder in the young. *J Orthop Sci* 1999; **4**: 307–17.
2. Marans HJ, Angel KR, Schemitsch EH, Wedge JH. The fate of traumatic anterior dislocation of the shoulder in children. *J Bone Joint Surg Am* 1992; **74**: 1242– 4.
3. Deitch J, Mehlman CT, Foad SL, Obbehat A, Mallory M. Traumatic anterior shoulder dislocation in adolescents. *Am J Sports Med* 2003; **31**: 758–63.
4. Walton J, Paxinos A, Tzannes A *et al*. The unstable shoulder in the adolescent athlete. *Am J Sports Med* 2002; **30**: 758–67.
5. Te Slaa RL, Wijffels MPJM, Brand R, Marti RK. The prognosis following acute primary glenohumeral dislocation. *J Bone Joint Surg Br* 2004; **86**: 58–64.
6. Lawton RL, Choudhury S, Mansat P, Cofield RH, Stans AA. Pediatric shoulder instability: presentation, findings, treatment, and outcomes. *J Pediatr Orthop* 2002; **22**: 52–61.
7. Huber H, Gerber C. Voluntary subluxation of the shoulder in children. A long-term follow-up study of 36 shoulders. *J Bone Joint Surg Br* 1994; **76**: 118–22.
8. Beischer AD, Simmons TD, Torode IP. Glenoid version in children with obstetric brachial plexus palsy. *J Pediatr Orthop* 1999; **19**: 359–61.
9. Pearl MT, Edgerton BW. Glenoid deformity secondary to brachial plexus birth palsy. *J Bone Joint Surg Am* 1998; **80**: 659–67.
10. Moukoko D, Ezaki M, Wilkes D, Carter P. Posterior shoulder dislocation in infants with neonatal brachial plexus palsy. *J Bone Joint Surg Am* 2004; **86**: 787–93.
11. Waters PM, Jaramillo D. Glenohumeral deformity secondary to brachial plexus birth palsy. *J Bone Joint Surg Am* 1998; **80**: 668–77.
12. Burkhead Jr. WZ, Rockwood Jr. CA. Treatment of instability of the shoulder with an exercise program. *J Bone Joint Surg Am* 1992; **74**: 890–96.
13. Postacchini F, Gumina S, Cinotti G. Anterior shoulder dislocation in adolescents. *J Shoulder Elbow Surg* 2000; **9**: 470–74.
14. Rowe CR, Patel D, Southmayd WW. The Bankart procedure. A long-term end-result study. *J Bone Joint Surg Am* 1978; **60**: 1–16.
15. Wirth MA, Blatter G, Rockwood Jr CA. The capsular imbrication procedure for recurrent anterior instability of the shoulder. *J Bone Joint Surg Am* 1996; **78**: 246–59.
16. Pollock RG, Owens JM, Flatow EL, Bigliani LU. Operative results of the inferior capsular shift procedure for multidirectional instability of the shoulder. *J Bone Joint Surg Am* 2000; **82**: 919–28.
17. Cole BJ, L'Insalata J, Irrgang J, Warner JJP. Comparison of arthroscopic and open anterior shoulder stabilization. *J Bone Joint Surg Am* 2000; **82**: 1108–14.
18. Steinbeck J, Jerosch J. Arthroscopic transglenoid stabilization versus open anchor suturing in traumatic anterior instability of the shoulder. *Am J Sports Med* 1998; **26**: 373–8.

19. Savoie III FH, Miller CD, Field LD. Arthroscopic reconstruction of traumatic anterior instability of the shoulder: the Caspari technique. *Arthroscopy* 1997; **13**: 201–9.
20. Levine WN, Clark Jr AM, D'Alessandro DF, Yamaguchi K. Chondrolysis following thermal capsulorraphy to treat shoulder instability. *J Bone Joint Surg Am* 2005; **87**: 616–21.
21. D'Alessandro DF, Bradley JP, Fleischli JE, Connor PM. Prospective evaluation of thermal capsulorraphy for shoulder instability. Indications and results, two- to five-year follow-up. *Am J Sports Med* 2004; **32**: 21–33.
22. Kawam M, Sinclair J, Letts M. Recurrent posterior shoulder dislocation in children: the results of surgical management. *J Pediatr Orthop* 1997; **17**: 533–8.
23. Hoffer MM, Phipps GJ. Closed reduction and tendon transfer for treatment of dislocation of the glenohumeral joint secondary to brachial plexus birth palsy. *J Bone Joint Surg Am* 1998; **80**: 997–1001.
24. Torode I, Donnan L. Posterior dislocation of the humeral head in association with obstetric paralysis. *J Pediatr Orthop* 1998; **18**: 611–5.

Radial head dislocation

Benjamin Joseph

33

Introduction

Of the various causes of radial head dislocation in children, congenital dislocation is the most common; developmental dislocation, traumatic dislocation and paralytic dislocations are less frequently seen. Congenital radial head dislocation, which is the most common congenital anomaly in the region of the elbow, may occur as an isolated entity or in association with several generalized skeletal malformation syndromes.[1] Familial aggregations of radial head dislocation have also been reported.

Developmental dislocation of the radial head may occur in children with hereditary multiple osteochondromatosis or diaphyseal aclasis. The radial head subluxates as a consequence of retarded growth of the ulna. If the relative lengths of the radius and ulna are not restored, the radial head will dislocate. In paralytic dislocation, muscle imbalance between the pronators and the supinators can result in radial head dislocation. Although traumatic isolated radial head dislocation has been described, most often, subtle injury to the ulna is also present.

The radial head can dislocate anteriorly, posteriorly or laterally, and the consequences of the dislocation vary accordingly.

Consequences of radial head dislocation and the problems of management

No disability

Often the dislocated radial head produces virtually no appreciable disability in childhood, especially if the dislocation is of congenital origin.

Limitation of elbow movement

Anterior dislocations tend to limit terminal flexion of the elbow, while posterior dislocations may limit terminal extension.

Limitation of pronation and supination

Some restriction of pronation and supination is common with all forms of radial head dislocation.

Deformity

Lateral dislocation of the radial head tends to cause cubitus valgus. The dislocated radial head may produce an ugly prominence even if a deformity is not apparent (Figure 33.1).

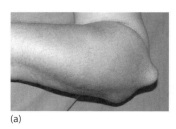
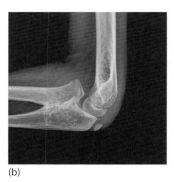

(a)　　　　　　　　　　　(b)

Figure 33.1 ● **(a)** Appearance of the elbow of an adolescent with radial head dislocation who had no symptoms and good elbow function. The prominence on the lateral aspect of the elbow is evident. **(b)** The limitation of flexion was quite significant in this young boy with a dislocated radial head associated with radio-ulnar synostosis.

Pain

Pain may develop in adolescence or adult life, particularly if the radial head is subluxated. Pain is less frequently seen in patients with complete dislocation of the radial head.

Aims of treatment

- Relieve pain
  The prime reason for treating radial head dislocation is to relieve pain.
- Improve the range of motion of the elbow and forearm if possible
  If restriction of movement is severe enough to impair function of the limb, an effort must be made to restore movement. However, it is seldom possible to restore full range of motion in these children.
- Improve the appearance of the limb
  If the child is concerned about the prominence of the dislocated radial head, surgery may be justified even if there is no functional disability. However, it needs to be clearly explained to the child and the parents that any surgery to improve the appearance will leave a visible scar in the region.

Treatment options

No intervention

If there are no symptoms related to the radial head dislocation and if the function of the limb is satisfactory, no intervention is required. This is the approach to adopt in the majority of instances of congenital dislocations, particularly if the dislocation has been detected accidentally in the older child.

Reduction of the radial head with reconstruction of the annular ligament

Traumatic radial head dislocation of recent onset may be successfully reduced. The annular ligament that has been torn should either be repaired or a new ligament must be fashioned from tissue in the vicinity of the elbow. A popular technique entails creating a ligament from a strip of fascia raised from the triceps aponeurosis (Figure 33.2).[2]

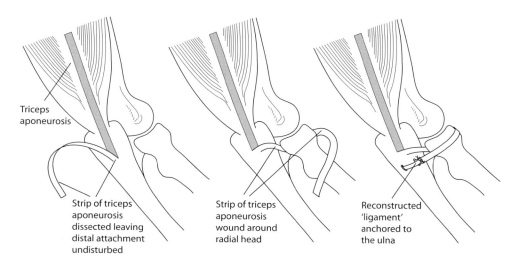

Triceps aponeurosis

Strip of triceps aponeurosis dissected leaving distal attachment undisturbed

Strip of triceps aponeurosis wound around radial head

Reconstructed 'ligament' anchored to the ulna

Figure 33.2 ● Technique of reconstruction of the annular ligament after reduction of the dislocated radial head.

Reduction of the radial head with lengthening of the ulna

Radial head subluxation and dislocation seen in children with hereditary multiple osteochondromatosis can been treated by gradual lengthening of the ulna.[3–5] The radial head falls back into position as the lengthening of the ulna progresses (Figure 33.3).

Reduction of the radial head with shortening of the radius

Reduction of the chronically dislocated radial head can be facilitated by shortening of the radius; this may be done at the time of open reduction of the radial head.[6] Acute shortening of the radius is preferred to gradual lengthening of the ulna when there is no true growth retardation of the ulna.

Excision of the radial head

In the skeletally mature adolescent with symptoms, the radial head may be excised. Excision of the radial head is not advisable in the young child as proximal migration of the radius and inferior radioulnar subluxation can develop as normal growth of the ulna progresses. Although the range of movement may not always increase following radial head excision, some improvement may occur.[7]

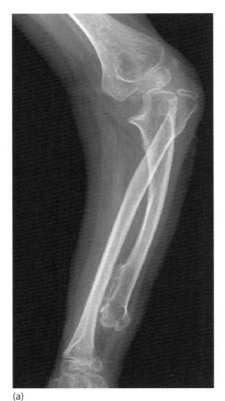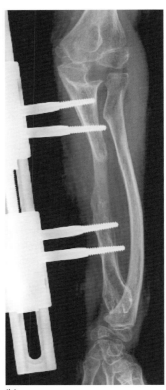

(a)   (b)

Figure 33.3 ● Dislocation of the radial head in a child with hereditary multiple osteochondromatosis treated by gradual lengthening of the ulna. Reduction of the radial head occurred spontaneously once the length of the ulna was restored.

Factors to be taken into consideration while planning treatment

Age of the child

In children under the age of three years, reduction of a congenital dislocation of the radial head may have a good outcome.[6] In the older child the capitellum will have become hypoplastic and the radial head may also be deformed and reduction may result in an incongruous joint.

Symptoms and disability

If the child is totally asymptomatic, surgical intervention is not justified. On the other hand, if there is pain or significant functional impairment, treatment is warranted.

Underlying primary cause of the dislocation and the duration since dislocation

A long-standing congenital radial head dislocation and paralytic radial head dislocations are difficult to reduce. In contrast, reduction of a traumatic dislocation of recent onset or a developmental dislocation is more simple.

Shape of the capitellum of the humerus and the radial head

Irrespective of the cause of radial head dislocation, if the radial head remains dislocated, both the capitellum and the radial head will become distorted. Reduction of the dislocation after these structural changes in the bones have occurred is likely to have a poor outcome.

Presence of muscle imbalance

Since muscle imbalance is the underlying cause of paralytic radial head dislocation, the muscle imbalance needs to be corrected if the radial head is to remain reduced. In several instances it may just not be possible to restore muscle balance.

Relative lengths of the radius and the ulna

A relatively long radius or a short ulna predisposes to radial head dislocation. It is important to restore the normal relative length of the radius and the ulna in order to achieve stable reduction. This may entail lengthening of the ulna or shortening of the radius.

Recommended treatment

The recommended treatment of radial head dislocation is outlined in Table 33.1.

Table 33.1 ● Outline of treatment of radial head dislocation

INDICATION						
Congenital dislocation + Child under 3 years + No syndromic association + Parents keen to get radial head reduced	Congenital dislocation + Child over 3 years + No symptoms + No functional deficit	Congenital dislocation + Child over 3 years + Functional limitation involving the dominant hand + No gross deformation of the femoral head or capitellum	Developmental dislocation or subluxation + Short ulna (e.g. as in diaphyseal aclasis)	Unreduced traumatic dislocation ± Ulnar bowing	Paralytic subluxation or dislocation + No symptoms	Radial head dislocation of any cause + Adolescent + Pain OR Limitation of elbow movement causing functional disability ⇩ Radial head excision
⇩ Open reduction of radial head + Reconstruction of annular ligament	⇩ No intervention	⇩ Radial shortening + Open reduction + Reconstruction of annular ligament	⇩ Gradual lengthening of ulna and indirect reduction of radial head	⇩ Ulnar osteotomy if ulnar bowing present + Open reduction + Reconstruction of annular ligament	⇩ Attempt to restore muscle balance if feasible (If not feasible, no intervention for radial head subluxation)	
TREATMENT						

References

1. Joseph B. Elbow problems in children. In: Gupta A, Kay SPJ, Scheker LR (eds). *The Growing Hand*. London: Harcourt, 2000: 769–82.
2. Bell Tawse AJS. The treatment of malunited anterior Monteggia fractures in children. *J Bone Joint Surg Br* 1965; **47**: 718–23.
3. Masada K, Tsuyuguchi Y, Kawai H *et al*. Operations for forearm deformity caused by multiple osteochondromas. *J Bone Joint Surg Br* 1989; **71**: 24–9.
4. Fogel GRT, McElfresh EC, Peterson HA, Wicklund PT. Management of deformities of the forearm in multiple hereditary osteochondromatas. *J Bone Joint Surg Am* 1984; **66**: 670–80.
5. Pritchett JW. Lengthening of the ulna in patients with hereditary multiple exostosis. *J Bone Joint Surg Br* 1986; **68**: 561–5.
6. Tachdjian MO (ed). *Pediatric Orthopedics*, 2nd edn. Philadephia: WB Saunders, 1990: 184–7.
7. Campbell CC, Waters PM, Emans JB. Excision of the radial head for congenital dislocation. *J Bone Joint Surg Am* 1992; **74**: 726–33.

Atlantoaxial instability

Ian Torode

34

Ian Torode

Introduction

Instability of the proximal cervical spine may arise from trauma or from developmental abnormalities in the skeleton or in the ligamentous structures. The relatively large head in infancy, coupled with ligamentous laxity and the horizontal plane of the facet joints in this region, all contribute to the increased risk of instability in the upper cervical spine.

Instability at the atlantoaxial level can occur in both the axial or horizontal plane and in the sagittal plane at the atlantoaxial level. At the occipitospinal junction transient instability in the long axis of the spine occurs in distraction injuries in children. Despite the fact that the occipitoatlas joint usually returns to a stable position with removal of the distraction force, these injuries are often fatal.

Children can present with instability and cord compromise because of unrecognized structural deficiencies in the upper cervical region. One should be aware of the potential for instability in conditions such as Down syndrome, mucopolysaccharidoses and congenital anomalies of the occipitocervical junction.

Instability in the transverse plane

Rotatory displacement at the atlantoaxial segment

This condition has a number of aetiological factors. Most involve minor trauma, falls, inflammation or unprotected positioning of the head and neck when the child is under general anaesthetic. The condition was possibly first described by Sir Charles Bell in 1830. Later, in 1930, a similar condition was reported by Grisel.[1,2] Others have reported the condition as Maladie de Grisel. It is important to recognize that there are different types of rotatory displacement since the treatment and potential complications differ (Figure 34.1).

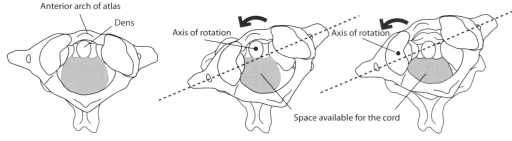

Figure 34.1 ● Diagram showing the normal atlantoaxial relationship and the space available for the spinal cord **(a)**. Two types of rotatory instability are shown **(b,c)**. There is gross reduction of the space available for the cord when the atlas pivots around the atlantoaxial joint.

(a) Normal atlantoaxial relationship

(b) Rotary instability: Atlas pivots around the dens

(c) Rotary instability in Grisel syndrome: Atlas pivots around the atlantoaxial joint

■ Acute and transient rotatory displacement

In children this deformity can occur without recognized cause or following minor trauma, upper respiratory infections or after general anaesthetic. The child has a cocked robin torticollis and resists attempts to correct the deformity. There is often pain and muscle spasm.

■ Fixed rotatory displacement

Some of the first group may fail to resolve and other children may present with a more chronic deformity that is not necessarily painful. Occasionally, this variety is associated with more severe trauma.

The investigation of choice is a computed tomography (CT) scan with the head turned maximally to both sides. The radiographic feature is subluxation or dislocation anteriorly of one of the facets of the axis that does not change with rotation of the head to the opposite side. Frequently, this displacement does not reduce with simple measures such as traction.

■ Chronic rotatory displacement with destruction of the atlantoaxial joint (Grisel's syndrome)

The term Grisel's syndrome should be reserved for the situation of fixed displacement of the atlantoaxial joint on one side associated with a long history of middle ear infection or adjacent sepsis. In these children the axis of rotation shifts to the more normal atlantoaxial joint and this results in a pincer effect with the risk of spinal cord compression (Figure 34.1c and 34.2). This is a far more dangerous clinical setting than the previous forms of atlantoaxial displacement described. A careful review of the literature reveals cases of sudden death with atlantoaxial dislocation. In many of these cases the underlying sepsis has been documented, although at presentation the signs of infection may have resolved with treatment of an ear infection for example.

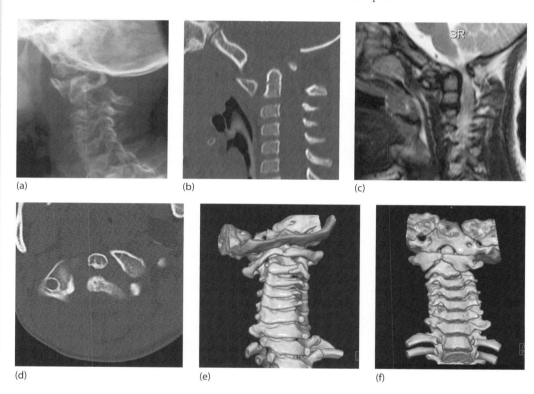

Figure 34.2 ● A lateral radiograph **(a)**, computed tomography (CT) scan and magnetic resonance scan images **(b–d)** and 3-D reconstruction of the CT images **(e,f)** show the displacement of the atlas in a child with Grisel syndrome.

Instability in the sagittal plane

Anomalies of the odontoid

■ Congenital hypoplasia or aplasia of the odontoid

Hypoplasia or aplasia of the odontoid may result in incompetence of the cruciate ligament complex. In marked hypoplasia of the dens the cruciate and alar ligaments may be unable to contribute to stability as they subluxate over the rudimentary structure in flexion. This may result in clinical atlantoaxial instability, though not all children with odontoid hypoplasia have demonstrable instability at the atlantoaxial junction. However, there is a significant incidence of rapid onset quadriparesis and/or sudden death in these children. Therefore, while prophylactic fusion of C1 to C2 may not be indicated, one should be aware and the parents educated of the need to recognize myelopathic symptoms and signs.

■ Os odontoideum

This term refers to a small separate bone seen cranially to the axis and first used by Giacomini in 1886.[3] There is evidence that many of these lesions are post-traumatic in origin; however, in others the os odontoideum is part of a hypoplastic dens syndrome. It is also seen in association with laxity syndromes such as Down or Morquio syndromes.[4,5] These children may present with neurological symptoms or signs that demand stabilization. If the anomaly is detected coincidentally then careful examination of flexion-extension is necessary. In some the os will move with the clivus with resultant compression of the cord. These children are at risk and stabilization is recommended. In others the os will move with the atlas and axis which implies a competent ligamentous complex.

Assimilation of the atlas

Occipitalization of the atlas or failure of segmentation of the occiput and C1 results in fusion of the occipitocervical junction. This may occur as an isolated finding but is often associated with other congenital anomalies such as fusions of the mid-cervical spine. In some series there is a common finding of basilar invagination and Chiari malformation.[4] The association of a fused occiput–C1 and fusions involving C2 obviously puts great strain on the C1–C2 junction. Stabilization may be necessary to avoid a neurological catastrophe but obliteration of most or all of the cervical motion is a significant compromise in a child who is asymptomatic.

Down syndrome

Instability in the sagittal plane in Down syndrome is well recognized (Figure 34.3). Problems can occur at both the atlanto-occipital level and at the atlantoaxial level. The underlying pathology is one of collagen defects and ligamentous laxity. However, developmental anomalies are not uncommon in Down syndrome.[6] The incidence of instability varies from 9 to 22 percent although symptomatic instability is much less common.

Symptoms of instability may be local with pain, head tilt or torticollis. However, generalized disturbances in gait, hyperreflexia or quadriparesis may also be due to cervical instability.

Screening programmes have not been shown to be effective in reducing injury and the relationship to organized sports is, at best, unclear. There may be difficulties in obtaining a clear history and the physical signs may vary depending on the dynamic nature of compression of the spinal cord which may be positional in nature.

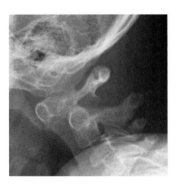

Figure 34.3 ● Lateral radiograph of the cervical spine of a child with Down syndrome showing atlantoaxial instability.

Mucopolysaccharidoses

Mucopolysaccharidoses (MPS) is a family of recessively inherited diseases that have in common a defect in lysosomal storage. Owing to the lack of specific degradative enzymes, mucopolysaccharides accumulate causing a broad spectrum of clinical findings. In Hurler's (type 1 MPS) and in Morquio's (type 4 MPS) there is an increased incidence of odontoid hypoplasia and also an increase in the presence of abnormal excessive soft tissue adjacent to the odontoid.[7,8]

Diagnostic difficulties arise in these children when instability is not readily apparent and stenosis of the spinal column is not clear-cut. These children can accumulate the metabolic products within the spinal cord which can in itself cause myelopathy and perhaps also make the children more susceptible to cord malfunction in the face of less obvious instability or stenosis. Myelopathy in MPS should not be ascribed to either instability or stenosis without clear radiographic evidence. If instability is evident then posterior fusion is appropriate.[9] However, surgical decompression or fusion is not without risk and may not be appropriate in all cases.

Problems of establishing a diagnosis

● Mentally retarded children with poorly developed communication skills may be unable to provide an adequate history.
● As instability may be a dynamic malfunction of the spinal column, demonstration and documentation may be difficult.

Aims of treatment

● Correct malalignment of the spine
● Stabilize a demonstrably unstable spine
● Prevent or relieve neurological compromise

Treatment options

Observation

Asymptomatic instability in Down syndrome without myelopathy may be best managed by observation rather than either restriction of activities or surgical intervention.

Halter traction

In children with acute transient rotatory instability, muscle relaxants such as diazepam and halter traction usually result in spontaneous realignment of the spine and relief of pain.

Halo vest

Most fixed rotatory subluxations in children will reduce with the application of a halo and longitudinal traction. Occasionally, while applying the halo under general anaesthetic, a click is felt and the child awakes with the head in a normal position. If reduction is achieved, a period in a halothoracic vest follows. Reduction must be documented with a CT scan.

Halo vest followed by fusion

If reduction of a fixed rotatory subluxation is not achieved by halo traction then it is necessary to proceed to an open reduction and posterior fusion. The halo vest is retained for post-operative support.

Open reduction and fusion

Children with a Grisel's syndrome should be treated as an emergency with stabilization using a halo and traction under close observation. The definitive treatment is a posterior fusion of C1 and C2. If there is an accompanying myelopathy careful documentation is required followed by an attempted reduction. The best decompression is by reduction of the subluxation or dislocation. It may be necessary to perform an open reduction by a lateral approach to the atlantoaxial joint.[10] An alternative approach is by anterior transoral release of the dislocated and fixed atlantoaxial joint followed by posterior fixation and fusion of C1 and C2.[11]

C1-C2 fusion

The only definitive treatment for atlantoaxial instability in the sagittal plane is fusion. However, there is a significant failure rate in obtaining a fusion in Down syndrome children. Surgical stabilization in Down syndrome should be reserved for those children with symptoms of cord irritation or signs of cervical myelopathy. The occiput-C1 level should also be carefully examined as instability at that level may warrant stabilization. Abnormalities of C1, such as a deficient posterior arch, may also result in inclusion of the occiput-C1 level in the fusion.

■ Wiring and bone grafting by the posterior approach

The Gallie technique and the Brooks and Jenkins technique are the most well known (Figure 34.4). These techniques are inexpensive and readily available. They are relatively easy to perform and reasonably safe. They involve exposure of the posterior elements but mostly in the midline and thus under vision. These techniques do not expose the vertebral arteries or nerve roots to injury. However, they are less effective at controlling rotation and anterior translation. In osteoporotic bone the fixation may be less secure and without halo vest external support the risk of non-union is significant. Furthermore, they may not be possible in the face of cord compression requiring laminectomy.

■ Transarticular screw fixation

The transarticular screws are inserted from the posterior aspect of the lateral mass of C2 and pass proximally across the C1-C2 joint to enter the anterior aspect of C1 (Figure 34.5).

This technique can be used where the posterior elements have been compromised. The fixation is biomechanically superior to wiring, with a higher union rate. The technique does require a larger exposure for the inferior approach to C2 and the positioning of the patient is more demanding.[12] Furthermore, it is necessary to check the anatomy of the C1 and C2 levels to ascertain whether it is possible to insert the screw safely past the vertebral artery. The screw fixation can be supplemented with posterior wiring.

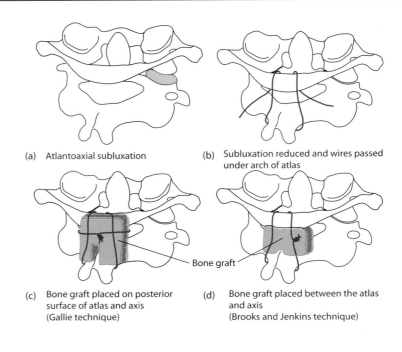

(a) Atlantoaxial subluxation

(b) Subluxation reduced and wires passed under arch of atlas

Bone graft

(c) Bone graft placed on posterior surface of atlas and axis (Gallie technique)

(d) Bone graft placed between the atlas and axis (Brooks and Jenkins technique)

Figure 34.4 ● Techniques of atlantoaxial fusion using wiring and bone graft.

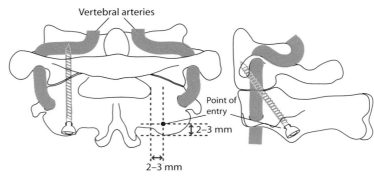

Vertebral arteries

Point of entry

2–3 mm

2–3 mm

Figure 34.5 ● Technique of transarticular screw fixation for atlantoaxial fusion.

■ Segmental screw fixation

This technique involves insertion of screws individually into the lateral mass and pedicles of C1 and C2. This permits the reduction using the screws as a second procedure and then stabilization with rods inserted into the screws. The exposure is less extensive than for transarticular screw fixation. The technique of screw insertion in C1 can be either the lateral mass technique or the posterior arch technique.[13–15] The pedicle screw technique, the subarticular, pars or laminar techniques can be used for screw insertion into C2.[16] Exposure of the entry point for the C1 screws can demand control of venous bleeding. The C2 nerve root may be irritated by the exposure and the screw.

Occipitocervical fusion

Fixation to the skull may be via wires through burr holes or around screws. Fixation can also be achieved with plates and screws. Distal fixation may be through sublaminar wires or cables, or screws inserted into the lateral masses or into pedicles, depending on the level (Figure 34.6). These devices can be fixed or placed around rods, plates or bone segments.

- The type of displacement.
- Reducibility of the displacement with traction.
- Integrity of the posterior arch of the atlas.
- Presence of associated instability at the occipitoatlas joint.
- Presence of neurological deficit.

Factors to be taken into consideration while planning treatment

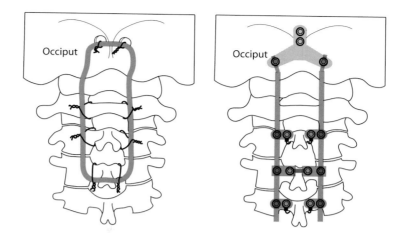

Figure 34.6 ● Methods of fixation used for occipitocervical fusion.

Recommended treatment

Rationale of treatment

An outline of treatment of rotatory subluxation of the atlantoaxial joint is shown in Table 34.1 and an outline of treatment for sagittal plane instability of the atlantoaxial joint is shown in Table 34.2.

In children the rate of fusion is usually better than in adult patients and hence simple techniques are often safer, less expensive and more user friendly. Thus, in most instances, C1-C2 stabilization with wires is often employed. If a posterior defect in the ring of C1 or occasionally C2 is evident then screw techniques can be utilized providing the anatomy permits. Where fusion to the skull is necessary, plate and screw fixation to the skull produces the most stable fixation. External support with a halo is well tolerated by children and should be used if there is any doubt concerning the stability of internal fixation.

Table 34.1 ● Outline of treatment of rotatory displacement of C1-C2 joint

INDICATIONS				
Acute rotatory displacement	Fixed rotatory displacement	Fixed rotatory displacement + Not reduced by halo traction	Grisel's syndrome	Grisel's syndrome + Not reduced by halo traction OR Myelopathy present ⇩
⇩	⇩	⇩	⇩	Urgent open reduction by lateral approach + C1-C2 fusion Halo vest for 6 weeks
Halter traction + Muscle relaxants	Halo application under general anaesthesia + Traction through halo vest + Retain halo for 6 weeks if reduction obtained (confirmed by CT scan) + Mobilization in halo vest If reduction not obtained treat as in column 3	Open reduction by posterior approach + C1-C2 fusion Halo vest for 6 weeks	Urgent halo traction + C1-C2 fusion if reduction achieved + Halo vest for 6 weeks If reduction not obtained treat as in column 5	
TREATMENT				

Table 34.2 ● Outline of treatment of sagittal plane instability of C1-C2 joint

INDICATIONS			
Asymptomatic C1-C2 instability in Down syndrome + No neurological impairment	C1-C2 instability + Early neurological signs + Posterior arch of atlas intact	C1-C2 instability + Early neurological signs + Posterior arch of atlas deficient ⇩	C1-C2 instability + Early neurological signs + Associated instability at occipitoatlas joint ⇩ Occipitocervical fusion
⇩ Observation	⇩ Fusion by either wiring or screw techniques.	Screw stabilization of C1-C2 joint from a posterior approach + Bone grafting	
TREATMENT			

References

1. Grisel P. Enucleation de l'atlas et torticollis nasopharyngien. *La Presse Medicale* 1930; **38**: 50–53.
2. Grisel P, Bourgois H. Un nouveau cas de torticollis naso-pharyngien. *Ann d'otolaryngol* 1931; **7**: 725.
3. Giacomini C. Sull' esistenza dell "os Odontoideum" nel' momo. *G Acad Med Torino* 1886; **49**: 24–8.
4. Menezes AH. Os Odontoideum – pathogenesis, dynamics and management. *Concepts Pediatr Neurosurg* 1988; **8**: 133–45.
5. Menezes AH, Ryken TC. Craniovertebral abnormalities in Down's syndrome. *Pediatr Neurosurg* 1992; **18**: 24–33.
6. Crockard HA, Stevens JM. Craniovertebral junction anomalies in inherited disorders: part of the syndrome or caused by the disorder? *Eur J Pediatr* 1995; **154**: 504–12.
7. Thomas SL, Childress MH, Quinton B. Hypoplasia of the odontoid with atlanto-axial subluxation in Hurler's syndrome. *Pediatr Radiol* 1985; **15**: 353–4.
8. Lipson SJ. Dysplasia of the odontoid process in Morquio's syndrome causing quadriparesis. *J Bone Joint Surg Am* 1977; **59**: 340–4.
9. Ransford AO, Crockard HA, Stevens JM, Modaqheh S. Atlanto-axial fusion in Morquio-Brailsford syndrome – a 10 year experience. *J Bone Joint Surg Br* 1996; **78**: 307–13.
10. Crockard HA, Rogers MA. Open reduction traumatic atlanto-axial rotary dislocation with use of an extreme lateral approach. A report of 2 cases. *J Bone Joint Surg Am* 1996; **78**: 431–6.
11. Wang C, Yan M, Zhou HT, Wang SL, Dang GT. Open reduction of irreducible atlantoaxial dislocation by transoral anterior atlantoaxial release and posterior internal fixation. *Spine* 2006; **15**: 306–13.
12. Magerl F, Seeman PS. Stable posterior fusion of the atlas and axis by transarticular screw fixation. In: Kehr P, Weidner A (eds). *Cervical Spine,* vol 1. New York, NY : Springer-Verlag; 1987: 322–7.
13. Harms J, Melcher RP. Posterior C1-C2 fusion with polyaxial screw and rod fixation. *Spine* 2001; **26**: 2467–71.
14. Goel A. Double insurance atlantoaxial fixation. *Surg Neurol* 2007; **67**: 135–9.
15. Tan M, Wang H, Wang Y *et al*. Morphometric evaluation of screw fixation in atlas via posterior arch and lateral mass. *Spine* 2003; **28**: 888–95.
16. Wright NM. Posterior C2 fixation using bilateral, crossing C2 laminar screws: case series and technical note. *J Spinal Disord Tech* 2004; **17**: 158–62.

SECTION 3

Deficiencies

Fibular hemimelia

Ian Torode

35

Introduction

Fibular hemimelia is a relatively common deficiency of the lower extremity. The incidence rate is about one or two per 100 000 live births. As noted in Chapter 37, Congenital short femur and proximal focal femoral deficiency, fibular hemimelia is associated with femoral deficiency in 50 percent of cases (Figure 35.1). Although fibular hemimelia can occur as an 'isolated' deficiency, it is the author's belief that one should treat all children with fibular deficiency as having whole limb involvement to a greater or lesser extent. Fibular hemimelia can be classified into types I and II: type I is mere fibular hypoplasia or partial absence of the fibula and type II is complete absence of the fibula.[1] While it is traditional to name the deficiency by the major bone absence, in fibular hemimelia, the extent of involvement of the other bones of the limb often dictates management.

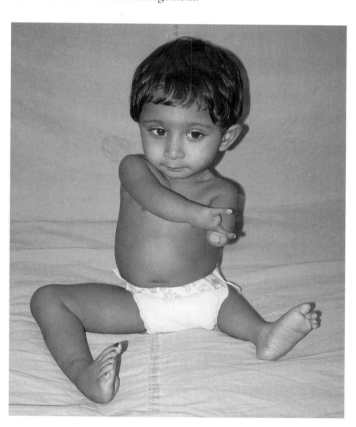

Figure 35.1 ● This child has fibular hemimelia and proximal focal femoral deficiency of the left lower limb in addition to reduction defects of the upper limbs and clubfoot on the right side.

The classical presentation is a newborn noted to have a foot lying in a valgus attitude at the ankle with absence of one or more of the lateral rays or toes and varying degrees of syndactyly (Figure 35.2). Usually some degree of equinus is also evident. There will always be limb length inequality depending on the amount of femoral and tibial involvement.

Problems of management

Deformities

Static deformities of the ankle, subtalar and midtarsal joints prevent the normal weight-bearing sole from resting on the ground (the foot is no longer plantigrade). The deformities of the foot and ankle are often compounded by deformities of the leg and knee. Ability to bear weight may also be compromised by an associated leg length discrepancy.

■ Knee

At the knee a valgus deformity is usually present and this arises from a deficiency in development of the lateral femoral condyle. It is important to address this deformity irrespective of whether the foot

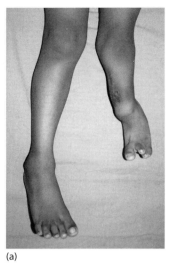
(a)

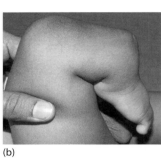
(b)

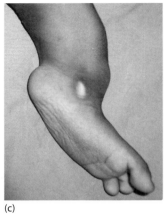
(c)

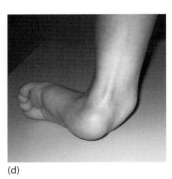
(d)

Figure 35.2 ● The appearance of the limbs of children with fibular hemimelia. The shortening and absence of lateral rays of the foot **(a)** anterior bowing of the leg **(b)**, the equinus **(c)** and valgus deformity of the foot **(d)** are all clearly seen.

is retained or ablated. In both groups the mechanical loads on the knee are inappropriate and may also lead to patellar subluxation or dislocation even if a patellar tendon supracondylar prosthesis is employed. If the valgus is left untreated in children using a prosthesis following ablation of the foot, it can make alignment of the prosthetic foot difficult. The prosthetist will need to shift the foot medially to get the foot close to the mechanical axis of the limb. This will be increasingly difficult as the child grows and the prosthesis will have an unsightly bump on its lateral aspect.

■ Leg

In more severe cases of fibular hemimelia the tibia is often significantly deficient in length and may have a kyphotic deformity. A skin dimple or a longitudinal crease overlies the apex of the deformity. The tibia will usually have a valgus angulation at that level. Often this component of valgus is initially overlooked until the deformity becomes more obvious with the passage of time.

■ Ankle

Valgus deformity of the ankle joint is often present in complete fibular hemimelia. This may be due to lack of lateral support as the lateral malleolus is missing. In addition to this, the distal tibial physeal growth may be asymmetrical and the distal epiphysis may be wedge shaped.[2] Where the distal fibula is present, fibular hemimelia is often associated with a ball and socket ankle joint; however, that finding should not be of concern. A ball and socket ankle is far more stable than an ankle with a complete absence of the fibula and dysplasia of the distal tibia.

■ Foot

Deformities within the foot are common in fibular hemimelia. Simple anomalies of the toes are rarely an issue. Tarsal coalitions often occur and a common coalition is between the talus and calcaneus. The coalesced bone usually has a significant valgus deformity. Another group of children have a joint between the talus and calcaneus, yet the joint is not normal, and with growth, weight bearing and probably a contribution from increased loads with limb lengthening, the calcaneus drifts laterally.

Not all feet in fibular hemimelia lie in valgus; while uncommon, an equinovarus deformity may occur in association with fibular hemimelia (Figure 35.3). It can trap the unwary into thinking that the underlying condition is metatarsus adductus or clubfoot. The presence of ligament laxity of the knee in a child with an equinovarus deformity points to limb deficiency.[3]

Instability of joints

■ Ankle

Instability of the ankle joint may result in progressive deformity particularly during tibial lengthening.

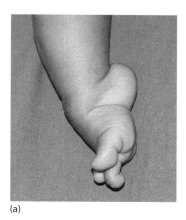
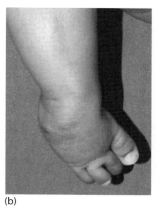
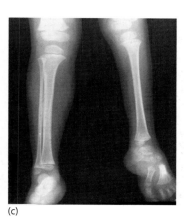

(a)   (b)   (c)

Figure 35.3 ● Foot of an infant with fibular hemimelia and an equinovarus deformity **(a,b)** and the radiograph of the leg of an older child with complete fibular hemimelia and an equinovarus deformity **(c)**.

■ Patella

The patella is often small and high riding in these children. The genu valgum, hypoplasia of the lateral femoral condyle and the underdeveloped patella all predispose to patellar subluxation and dislocation.

Shortening of the limb

All segments of the limb contribute, to varying degrees, to the overall shortening. The limb proportions that are present at birth will remain unchanged until skeletal maturity and hence a fairly accurate estimate of the final limb length discrepancy can be made at the initial presentation.

■ Femur

The femur very rarely may be totally absent (Figure 35.4); more frequently the proximal femur may be deficient or there may be a mild degree of shortening. The shortening of the limb depends on the extent of femoral deficiency.

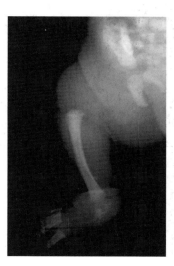

Figure 35.4 ● Radiograph of a child with complete fibular hemimelia and total agenesis of the femur.

■ Tibia

The tibia is short and the shortening may be as much as 40 percent of the normal tibial length.[4]

■ Foot

Although the major component of the shortening occurs in the femur and tibia, the foot also contributes to the limb length deficiency and this needs to be taken into consideration when planning procedures to equalize limb lengths.

Absence of rays of the foot

Deficiencies of the lateral rays and the leg length inequality will add to the weight-bearing difficulties. There have been suggestions that the number of rays can help predict the likelihood of retaining the foot; the chances of retaining the foot appear poor if less than three rays are present.[4]

Aims of treatment

- Obtain a plantigrade foot with a stable ankle if the foot can be retained
  Once a decision has been made to try to retain the foot, it is imperative that the foot is made plantigrade. If ankle instability persists after making the foot plantigrade the ankle must be stabilized.
- Restore limb length equality by skeletal maturity
  Again, in children in whom the foot is being retained, strategies need to be worked out to ensure that the limb lengths are equalized by skeletal maturity.
- Correct the associated valgus deformities of the knee, tibia and ankle
  Deformities of the knee and the tibia need to be addressed in all children irrespective of the fate of the foot. In children in whom the foot is retained, in addition to dealing with deformities of the knee and leg, any ankle deformity should be corrected.
- Facilitate optimal prosthetic fitting if the foot is ablated
  Once the foot is ablated, all deformities of the limb that interfere with optimal prosthetic fitting should be corrected.

Treatment options

Foot ablation and prosthetic fitting

■ Timing

The best age for this procedure is between 12 and 18 months. Although delay is not crucial the procedure should be completed before three years of age as the child will then have 'ownership' of the limb and psychological loss may be an issue. Earlier surgery is not necessary as the foot will not inhibit crawling. Prosthetic fitting at that age is a waste. The concept held by some parents that they want their child to share in the decision-making is invalid and cruel when the foot is clearly useless.

■ The procedure

While commonly referred to as a Syme or Boyd amputation this is not strictly correct. The author's preferred procedure is as follows.

A longitudinal incision is made posteriorly approximately at the junction of the proximal two-thirds and distal one-third of the calf. Through that incision the Achilles tendon is completely divided and the foot firmly dorsiflexed. A second incision is made on the dorsal aspect of the foot from a point one finger breadth anterior to the medial malleolus to a similar point laterally. The medial and lateral extent of the dorsal incision is then connected across the sole of the foot. The dissection then continues close to the talus and calcaneus, which may be separate entities although they are commonly coalesced into one bony mass. Care must be taken to stay close to the bone so as not to injure the vascular bundle posteromedially and to maintain integrity of the skin. Once the removal of the bones is complete the tourniquet is then deflated and the skin flaps inspected. The wound is closed over a drain. A pin may be used to hold the heel pad in the desired position. Prior to closure the tibial deformity may need to be addressed.

Where there is a significant kyphotic and valgus deformity of the tibia there will be a longitudinal crease in the skin at the apex of this deformity. An incision that excises that skin crease will expose the tibia. A trapezoidal segment of bone is removed that will allow both correction and relaxation of the tissues. The osteotomy is then fixed by inserting a stout pin through the heel pad, which is then passed into the tibia and across the osteotomy. The skin is then closed over a drain and a plaster splint applied that is fashioned in a loop around the stump and across the top of the knee.

■ Prosthetic fitting

The post-operative care when foot ablation has been performed is to wrap the leg in a plaster splint for four weeks, or six weeks if a tibial osteotomy has also been performed. After four weeks the stump should be non-tender and able to be handled for limb fitting. In the tibial osteotomy group the plaster splint and pin are removed at six weeks. If there is some residual swelling then stump shrinkers can be employed for a short time until the prosthetist is comfortable to proceed.

In this age group minimal gait training is needed and most of the education is directed towards parents. These children grow rapidly in the first few years of life and with maturation of the stump the second prosthesis is usually required in six to nine months.

Stabilization of the ankle

Different operations have been attempted to obtain stability of the ankle. However, only a few cases have been included in reports.[5–7] The first three of the four operations listed below attempt to restore stability while retaining ankle motion.

■ Gruca operation

The Gruca operation creates a lateral support by bifurcating the distal tibial articular surface (Figure 35.5b). Since the operation transgresses the growth plate, growth arrest can occur and this may further increase the limb length inequality.

■ Bending osteotomy through the distal tibial physis

The operation attempts to improve the stability of the ankle by deepening the tibial articular surface in a manner similar to a Pemberton or Dega osteotomy for developmental dysplasia of the hip (Figure 35.5c).

■ Reconstruction of the malleolus with iliac graft

An attempt has been made in a child to construct the lateral malleolus with a composite graft from the ilium (Figure 35.5d).

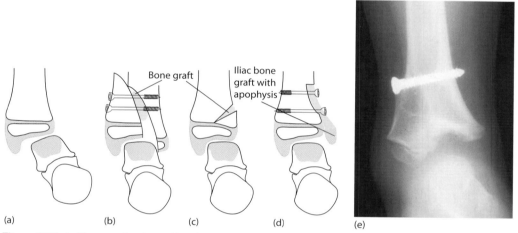

Figure 35.5 ● Diagram showing ankle valgus in fibular hemimelia **(a)** and the techniques of performing operations to correct this valgus instability. The Gruca operation **(b)**, the bending osteotomy of Exner **(c)** and reconstruction of the lateral malleolus with iliac graft along with a piece of the iliac apophysis **(d)** are shown. Radiograph of the ankle of a child who has undergone a Gruca operation shows satisfactory alignment of the ankle **(e)**.

■ Tibiotalar arthrodesis

Arthrodesis of the ankle can stabilize the joint although the foot will become very stiff especially if there is talocalcaneal coalition.

Limb length equalization

For the first few years of life there may be no need for any assistance as the child will compensate for a modest deficiency. Some children will be assisted by the use of a shoe raise; however, a raise of greater than 4 cm will probably produce instability in gait.

■ Limb lengthening

Limb lengthening is employed in some children and frequently this entails sequential lengthening in at least two sittings. The technique is described in Chapter 44, Length discrepancy of the tibia. In children with a congenital deficiency and a ligamentous deficiency of the knee, care has to be taken during the lengthening to prevent a knee flexion contracture developing which may herald the onset of subluxation. Fixation across the joint is not absolutely necessary as an extension orthosis fixed to the frame and to the thigh during the distraction phase to protect the knee is important. The tendency to develop an equinus deformity with lengthening must be addressed and fixation across the ankle to a pin in the calcaneus is frequently employed to prevent proximal migration of the heel.

■ Contralateral epiphyseodesis

Contralateral epiphyseodesis is employed in some children. These children are usually in the category of minor dysplasias of the limb. The more severely involved children will have either a foot ablation or a limb lengthening. However, this is a good tool for relatively minor adjustments to length when employed at the appropriate age (see Chapter 44, Length discrepancy of the tibia).

Correction of genu valgum, tibial, ankle and subtalar deformity

■ Correction of genu valgum

Irrespective of whether the foot is ablated or not, all children with genu valgum will be helped significantly by an appropriately timed screw hemiepiphyseodesis. This technique avoids having a staple under the skin where the prosthesis may be loading (Figure 35.6). Alternatively, a distal femoral osteotomy can be performed; however, this is considerably more surgery with a concomitantly greater time of disability for the child.

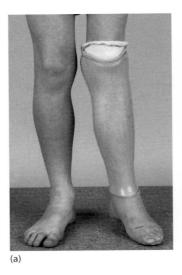
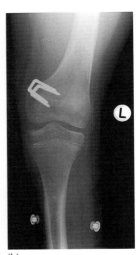

Figure 35.6 ● Genu valgum is evident in a child who has undergone a Syme amputation **(a)** treated by stapling **(b)**.

(a)   (b)

■ Correction of tibial bowing

Bowing of the tibia may be corrected at the time of limb lengthening in children in whom the foot is being retained. In children undergoing foot ablation, it is more appropriate to address the tibial deformity at the time of foot ablation rather than subject the child to a tibial osteotomy later in life or compel the child to wear a cosmetically unattractive limb which also mechanically loads the knee inappropriately.

■ Correction of ankle valgus

Minor deformities at the ankle level in the minimally deficient limb are usually managed by a hemiepiphyseodesis by a screw inserted through the medial malleolus. This is particularly the case if the distal aspect of the fibula is preserved. More significant degrees of valgus require a distal tibial osteotomy.

■ Correction of subtalar valgus

Subtalar valgus can be corrected by a subtalar fusion. However, this will stiffen an already stiff foot. Where there is a talocalcaneal coalition, an osteotomy through the coalition mass can allow a medial shift on the heel. However, one cannot expect the midfoot and hindfoot to be mobile and adjust to this shift as is expected when a heel shift is performed in other circumstances.

■ Correction of the equinovalgus in infancy

In cases where there is a relatively normal foot lying in an equinovalgus position, it may be reasonable to consider a posterolateral release to make the foot plantigrade. However, before committing the child to that procedure it is necessary to be reasonably certain that the ankle is stable and the limb length discrepancy not so great as to make ablation of the foot a consideration. Once parents have emotionally committed to the foot being kept it will be difficult to change the surgical plans. The release entails division of the Achilles tendon, lengthening of the peronei and complete excision of the fibrous or cartilaginous fibular anlage.[8]

Table 35.1 ● Outline of treatment of fibular hemimelia

INDICATIONS							
Shortening of limb too great to consider limb length equalization (e.g. in children with associated proximal femoral deficiency (PFFD))	No associated PFFD + <3 rays present + Gross valgus deformity of foot + Unstable ankle	Shortening of the limb within limits of safe limb lengthening + 3 or more rays present + Foot plantigrade + Ankle stable	Shortening of the limb within limits of safe limb lengthening + 3 or more rays present + Valgus deformity of foot + Child <4 years of age	Projected shortening at skeletal maturity <5 cm + 3 or more rays present + Valgus deformity of foot	Projected shortening at skeletal maturity >5 cm + 3 or more rays present + Valgus deformity of foot + Child over 4 years	Projected shortening at skeletal maturity >5 cm + 3 or more rays present + Unstable ankle + Child over 4 years	Older child with residual shortening following earlier correction of knee, ankle and foot deformities and first-stage limb lengthening
⇩	⇩	⇩	⇩	⇩	⇩	⇩	⇩
TREATMENT							
Foot ablation + Prosthetic fitting (manage as for PFFD)	Foot ablation + Simultaneous correction of genu valgum and tibial bowing + Below knee prosthesis	Retain foot + Correct genu valgum + Staged limb lengthening procedures	Retain foot + Posterolateral soft tissue release + Orthosis with shoe raise until old enough for limb lengthening	Retain foot + Correct deformities of the knee, tibia and ankle in early childhood + Contralateral femoral or tibial epiphyseodesis at optimal time	Retain foot + First-stage limb lengthening + Simultaneous correction of genu valgum, tibial bowing and ankle deformity	Retain foot + First-stage limb lengthening + Simultaneous correction of genu valgum, tibial bowing + Tibiotalar fusion	Fine-tune the limb length inequality by second lengthening OR Contralateral epiphyseodesis

Factors to be taken into consideration while planning treatment

Extent of limb length inequality

If the extent of shortening is massive on account of an associated proximal focal femoral deficiency, lengthening of the tibia should not be considered. Since the recommended approach is to ablate the foot and fit a prosthesis, deformities of the ankle and foot are also of no consequence. Only when it is considered possible to achieve limb length equalization by skeletal maturity should limb lengthening be considered.

Stability of the ankle

A foot with a stable ankle is more likely to be retained. However, if other criteria dictate retaining the foot an unstable ankle can be stabilized.

Presence of deformities of the knee, leg, ankle and foot

The severity of deformity of the foot often dictates the need for ablation. However, the deformities of the knee and leg need to be addressed in all children with fibular deficiency.

Bilateral deficiencies

Treatment for children with bilateral deficiencies needs to be individualized. Often patients with bilateral lower limb deficiencies have upper limb involvement and this may necessitate a different approach. If a child does not have two good hands to manipulate prostheses, it may be necessary to keep feet that would otherwise be less than useful. Furthermore, in bilateral deficiencies, length is adjusted to the longer limb and not to 'normality'.

Parental choice and social factors

In certain societies amputation is not readily accepted and the cost and availability of prosthetic services may justify retaining the foot even if it is not an ideal choice.

Recommended treatment

The outline of treatment is shown in Table 35.1.

References

1. Acherman CA, Kalamchi A. Congenital deficiency of the fibula. *J Bone Joint Surg Br* 1979; **61**: 133–7.
2. Choi IH, Lipton GE, Mackenzie W, Bowen JR, Kumar SJ. Wedge-shaped distal tibial epiphysis in the pathogenesis of equinovalgus deformity of the foot and ankle in tibial lengthening for fibular hemimelia. *J Pediatr Orthop* 2000; **20**: 428–36.
3. Torode IP, Gillespie R. Anteroposterior instability of the knee: a sign of congenital limb deficiency. *J Pediatr Orthop* 1983; **3**: 467–70.
4. Stanitski DF, Stanitski CL. Fibular hemimelia: A new classification system. *J Pediatr Orthop* 2003; **23**: 30–4.
5. Exner GU. Bending osteotomy through the distal tibial physis in fibular hemimelia for stable reduction of the hindfoot. *J Pediatr Orthop B* 2003; **12**: 27–32.
6. Thomas IH, Williams PF. The Gruca operation for congenital absence of the fibula. *J Bone Joint Surg Br* 1987; **69**: 587–92.
7. Weber M, Siebert CH, Goost H, Johannisson R, Wirtz D. Malleolus externus plasty for joint reconstruction in fibular aplasia: preliminary report of a new technique. *J Pediatr Orthop B* 2002; **11**: 265–73.
8. McCarthy JJ, Glancy GL, Chang FM, Eilert RE. Fibular hemimelia: comparison of outcome measurements after amputation and lengthening. *J Bone Joint Surg Am* 2000; **82**: 1732–5.

Tibial hemimelia

Ian Torode

36

Ian Torode

Introduction

Tibial hemimelia is a less common deficiency of the lower extremity in comparison to fibular hemimelia or femoral deficiencies. The occurrence rate quoted in the United States is about one per million live births.[1] In the author's experience the incidence is far more common, affecting approximately one child per 100 000 live births. However, tibial deficiencies occur more frequently than fibular deficiencies in syndromic children. The deficiency may be bilateral and where part of a 'syndromic' presentation, other abnormalities may be readily apparent. It can occur both as an isolated deficiency and as an inherited condition.

The knee, leg and foot in tibial hemimelia

Kalamchi and Dawe classified these patients into three groups[1] (Figure 36.1).

■ Type I: Complete absence of the tibia

The entire tibia is absent; the fibular head is proximally situated. These children have a grossly unstable knee and ankle.

■ Type II: Absence of the distal portion of the tibia

These children will have a grossly unstable ankle. The foot itself may appear normal. The spike of the distal tibia is commonly palpable and visible and often has a skin dimple nearby.

■ Type III: Distal tibiofibular diastasis

In these children the foot will resemble a resistant congenital talipes equinovarus but with significant midfoot adductus and varus at the ankle.

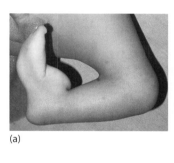
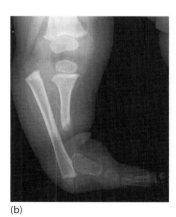
(a)

(b)

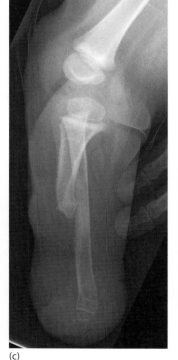
(c)

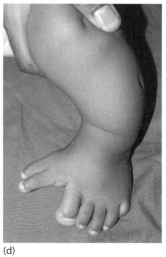
(d)

Figure 36.1 ● The entire tibia may be absent (type I) and this is associated with flexion deformity of the knee and equinovarus deformity of the foot **(a)**. In partial tibial hemimelia (type II) there is either mild flexion or no deformity of the knee **(b,c)**. In tibial hemimelia there may loss of rays of the foot **(b)** or duplication of toes **(d)**.

Associated anomalies of the limbs

The hip, femur and the upper limbs may have associated anomalies that may require treatment. These associated anomalies may also have a bearing on the treatment of the tibial defect.

■ The hip in tibial hemimelia

The hip in tibial hemimelia may be dislocated from birth. This is uncommon but does raise treatment difficulties as the usual orthoses such as the Pavlik harness may not be appropriate for treating the hip dislocation in the presence of an unstable knee and ankle in type I patients. It may be necessary to use a hip spica if a closed reduction is possible. If the hip is irreducible then an open reduction via a medial approach is advised for typical dislocations. However, some children have a grossly deficient acetabulum and then prolonged cast treatment may be necessary.

■ The femur in tibial hemimelia

The femur may be duplicated to a varying degree. This may be seen as simply a broad distal end of the femur or as a complete divarication with two separate femoral condyles.

■ The upper limb in tibial hemimelia

Deformities along the pre-axial aspect of the limb are not uncommon. These may be in the form of pre-axial polydactyly or alternatively pre-axial deficiencies. They may be seen as a floating thumb or extend to radial deficiencies.

Problems of management

Shortening of the limb

In all forms of tibial hemimelia there is some degree of shortening of the affected limb.

Poor quadriceps function

The quadriceps may not be able to extend the knee at all in many instances of type I deficiency because of the lack of distal skeletal insertion of the quadriceps tendon. However, in some instances of type I deficiency there is demonstrable active extension of the knee (Figure 36.2).

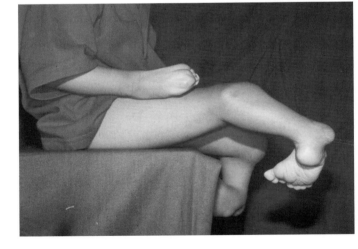

Figure 36.2 ● Quadriceps function may be present in some children with complete tibial hemimelia as seen in this child. Note that the child also has mirror polydactyly of the foot and complex syndactyly of the hands.

Instability of the knee

If the proximal tibia has not developed the knee will be unstable.

Knee deformity

Flexion deformity of the knee is often seen in children with types I and II tibial hemimelia. A lack of a quadriceps mechanism results in a flexion contracture and the inability to extend the 'knee'.

Ankle instability

The ankle is invariably unstable in all forms of tibial hemimelia.

Foot deformity

Equinovarus deformity is usually seen in these children.

The frequency and severity of these problems vary with the type of tibial hemimelia (Table 36.1). The options for treatment and issues that need to be considered while planning treatment are influenced by the severity of these problems.

Table 36.1 ● Severity of problems associated with different types of tibial hemimelia

Type	Shortening	Quadriceps function	Knee instability	Knee deformity	Ankle instability	Foot deformity
I	Severe	Often absent	Severe	Flexion deformity >45° common (especially if no quadriceps function)	Severe	Equinovarus
		Occasionally present				
II	Moderate	Usually present	Stable	Flexion deformity <45° may be present	Severe	Equinovarus
III	Mild or moderate	Present	Stable	Nil	Present	Equinovarus

Aims of treatment

- Provide a stable knee
- Make the foot plantigrade
- Equalize limb lengths

Treatment options

Type I deficiency

■ The Brown procedure and foot stabilization

A degree of joint stability can be attained by the Brown procedure which involves centralization of the fibula to the intercondylar region of the femur.[2–5] The prerequisite for the Brown procedure is adequate quadriceps function, which is not common in type I patients. However, the absence of collateral ligaments demands external support for stability. The foot can be stabilized by performing a talofibular fusion.

While early success may be attainable, the combination of knee instability and length deficiency coupled with the need for lifelong brace wear has led patients to request amputation in their teen years; this is far from a satisfactory outcome.

■ Fusion of the fibula to the femur, ablation of the foot and prosthetic fitting

This may be considered if there is significant shortening of the femur in association with tibial hemimelia. Since fusions at both knee and ankle severely impede function this option is not recommended if the foot is being retained and stabilized by talofibular fusion.

■ Disarticulation

The treatment of choice in most type I patients is knee disarticulation. The knee disarticulation needs to be personalized to the needs and anatomy of each patient as partial duplication of the femur is not uncommon. Usually a simple disarticulation is performed without any attempt to change the condylar anatomy. This broad end of the femur is utilized for prosthetic suspension and rotational control, and the option of removing a condyle later is still available.

Type II deficiency

■ Proximal tibiofibular synostosis, talofibular fusion and limb lengthening

Reconstruction of the distal deficiency involves creating stability at the ankle usually by fusing the distal fibular to the talus. Proximal stability is achieved by creating a synostosis between the proximal tibia and fibula. The syndesmosis creation requires mobilization of the biceps tendon which can be transferred to the proximal tibia. The proximal fibula is then resected and the fragment used as a bone graft at the syndesmosis. The fusion of the fibula to the tibia also requires mobilization of the soft tissues of the anterior compartment of the leg. It may be difficult to avoid division of the vessels traversing this compartment. Usually two or three screws can pass from fibula to tibia to create stability. It is advisable to protect the limb in a cast.

In taking this route it will later be necessary to perform a leg lengthening procedure, on one or more occasions. Before embarking on this plan it is vital to be certain that the quadriceps mechanism is functional.

■ Proximal tibiofibular synostosis, ablation of the foot and prosthetic fitting

As retention of the foot necessitates creating stability proximally and distally and adding length, the alternative plan of foot ablation followed by tibiofibular synostosis is not unreasonable (Figure 36.3). This avoids the need for lengthening procedures, and the function of a child in a well-fitted prosthesis and modern prosthetic foot is as good as or perhaps better than that following ankle fusion and multiple leg lengthening operations.

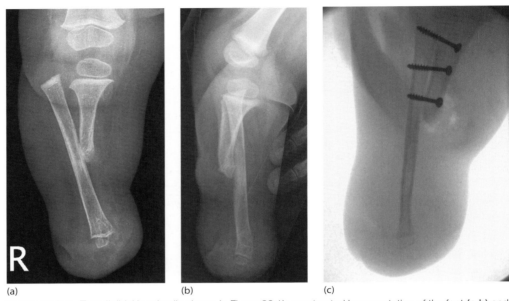

(a)   (b)   (c)

Figure 36.3 ● Type II tibial hemimelia shown in Figure 36.1b was treated by amputation of the foot **(a,b)** and creation of a synostosis between the proximal tibia and the fibula **(c)**.

Type III deficiency

■ Correction of foot deformity, ankle stabilization and limb lengthening

Treatment involves correction of the foot deformity with soft tissue releases in the early stages and then later correction of the bone deficiency within the tarsus. The ankle will require stabilization with a syndesmosis screw and, if needed, a tibial osteotomy. The ankle may be stabilized by talofibular fusion if this fails.

■ Ablation of the foot and prosthetic fitting

There is a tendency for relapse of the foot and ankle deformity with growth and then foot ablation may not be unreasonable.

The factors to be taken into consideration while planning treatment are:

● function of the quadriceps;
● severity of limb length inequality.

Factors to be taken into consideration while planning treatment

Recommended treatment

The outline of treatment of tibial hemimelia is shown in Table 36.2.

Table 36.2 ● Outline of treatment tibial hemimelia

INDICATIONS						
Type I tibial hemimelia + Functioning quadriceps + Flexion deformity of knee not severe	Type I tibial hemimelia + Quadriceps NOT functioning + Flexion deformity of knee severe	Type I tibial hemimelia + Congenitally very short femur	Type II tibial hemimelia + Moderate shortening of the leg	Type II tibial hemimelia + Severe shortening of the leg	Type III tibial hemimelia	Type III tibial hemimelia + Recurrent foot deformity
⇩	⇩	⇩	⇩	⇩	⇩	⇩
Brown's procedure + Talofibular fusion + Orthotic support for knee	Disarticulate knee + Prosthetic fitting (knee disarticulation prosthesis)	Fuse femur to fibula + Ablate foot + Prosthetic fitting (knee disarticulation prosthesis)	Proximal tibiofibular synostosis + Talofibular fusion + Limb lengthening	Proximal tibiofibular synostosis + Ablate foot + Prosthetic fitting (below-knee prosthesis)	Talofibular fusion + Limb lengthening	Ablate foot and prosthetic fitting (Syme's prosthesis)
TREATMENT						

References

1. Kalamchi A, Dawe RV. Congenital deficiencies of the tibia. *J Bone Joint Surg Br* 1985: **67**: 581–4.
2. Brown FW. The Brown operation for total hemimelia tibia. In: Aitken GT (ed.) *Selected Lower-limb Anomalies; Surgical and Prosthetic Management*. Washington, DC: National Academy of Sciences, 1971: 21–8.
3. Loder RT, Herring JA. Fibular transfer for congenital absence of the tibia: a reassessment. *J Pediatr Orthop* 1987; **7**: 8–13.
4. Wada A, Fujii T, Takamura K *et al*. Limb salvage treatment for congenital deficiency of the tibia. *J Pediatr Orthop* 2006; **26**: 226–32.
5. Epp Ch Jr, Tooms RE, Edholm CD, Kruger LM, Bryant DD 3rd. Failure of centralization of the fibula for congenital longitudinal deficiency of the tibia. *J Bone Joint Surg Am* 1991; **73**: 858–67.

Congenital short femur and proximal focal femoral deficiency

37

Ian Torode

Introduction

Congenital deficiencies of the femur represent one component of congenital limb deficiencies.[1] A deficiency of the femur should not be viewed in isolation as almost every affected child will have deficiencies, to a greater or lesser extent, in other components of the affected limb. However, for clarity, deficiencies of different segments of the lower limb will be discussed separately.

Classification

From a radiological standpoint, the subgroups of congenital femoral deficiencies may be many and are only limited by the number of cases witnessed by the author. Gillespie and Torode[2] attempted to correlate the clinical features with the radiological picture to restrict the subcategorization to only two groups to assist in the management of the patient.

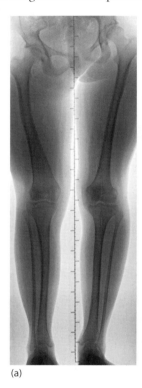 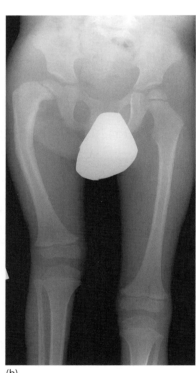

Figure 37.1 ● Radiograph of the lower limbs of a child with a congenital short femur **(a)**. The proximal femur is normally developed. Radiographs of another child with a congenital short femur **(b)** show that apart from coxa vara and a degree of acetabular dysplasia the proximal femur is well developed.

(a) (b)

For simplicity, the term congenital short femur (CSF) is used to categorize those children with significant leg length discrepancy but who have an intact femur (Figure 37.1). In contradistinction, the term proximal focal femoral deficiency (PFFD) is used for those children with a severe leg length discrepancy and a radiologically demonstrable defect in the proximal femur (Figure 37.2).

At one end of the spectrum of congenital femoral deficiencies is the modest leg length discrepancy that will require limb length equalization and at the other end is a gross limb deficiency and the clear need for prosthetic assistance. Therefore it is necessary for any surgeon to draw their line along this spectrum to separate those limbs that might be reconstructed from those that may be treated by limb ablation and prosthetic fitting. Where that line is placed will also be affected by social mores of any individual society, by the facilities available, by the skill and experience of the surgeon and by the wishes of the parents.

The advent of antenatal ultrasound has resulted in antenatal diagnoses being made which then demands of the doctor knowledge of the natural history of the problem. Furthermore, such a diagnosis is likely to be accompanied by anxiety and guilt in the future parents. This demands that the consulted doctor develops skills in passing on accurate information regarding the expected infant's clinical picture while, at the same time, providing some optimism regarding the child's future ability

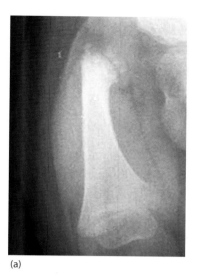
(a)

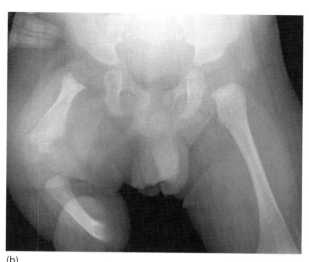
(b)

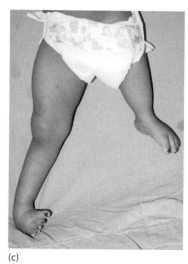
(c)

Figure 37.2 ● Proximal focal femoral deficiency is characterized by failure of development of proximal femur **(a)**. The shortening of the limb is severe in all these cases **(b,c)**.

to be mobile, functional and happy. The possibility of speaking to other parents of similar children may be invaluable.

Problems of management

Shortening

The most obvious problem confronting the surgeon is the shortening of the limb.

Associated deficiencies of the leg

Femoral deficiencies are associated with a significant deficiency below the knee in approximately 50 percent of cases. The severity of the below-knee deficiency will clearly have an impact on the treatment course applied to the femoral deficiency. The presence of a fibular deficiency is common to both CSF and PFFD but may alter the treatment protocol. For example, a patient with CSF with a marked femoral hypoplasia and a severe fibular hemimelia may be best treated as a PFFD patient, whereas the same degree of femoral deficiency with a relatively normal leg, ankle and foot may be treated by leg length equalization.

The specifics of management of fibular hemimelia are discussed in Chapter 35, Fibular hemimelia.

Dysplasia of the hip and pelvis

In children with PFFD there may be a defect in ossification of the neck of the femur, coxa vara or absence of the femoral head and neck. Varying degrees of pelvic involvement is commonly seen, which may present as abductor weakness or acetabular dysplasia.

Flexion deformities of the hip and knee

In both PFFD and CSF there are flexion deformities of the hip and knee, although they are less rigid and less severe in the group with CSF.

Genu valgum

Hypoplasia of the lateral femoral condyle will manifest itself as a valgus deformity of the knee in patients with CSF whereas in children with PFFD the issue may not be clinically relevant.

Knee instability

Instability of the knee due to cruciate ligament deficiency occurs both in CSF and PFFD; however, the contracture of the PFFD knee may disguise this feature.

Aims of treatment

- To provide reassurance and education for the family
  It must be remembered that the first visit to a doctor by parents, whether it be an antenatal consultation, in a maternity unit or in a clinic in the first few weeks of life, will be a meeting

involving people who expected that their child would be born complete and normal. The parents will be in emotional turmoil from a mixture of guilt and anxiety. Fears regarding walking ability, sporting capabilities, coupled with questions regarding aetiology will come to the fore.

If the first consultation does not take place for some months after delivery the best efforts by the surgeon to have a rational discussion will almost certainly have been compromised by 'helpful' advice from a relative, neighbour, taxi driver or checkout girl at the supermarket. It will make the doctor/parent/patient relationship substantially more straightforward if there is an antenatal consultation or a consultation in the first few days after delivery.

Other allies in this process will be the parents of other patients. It can be quite useful to have expectant parents sit outside a clinic so they may witness other children playing wearing prostheses and being normal children. Even when it is clear that there is no genetic input into the cause of the child's deficiency, a consultation with a geneticist may help quell the concerns that this problem has come from one family stream or another.

- To enable the child to walk and to optimize the gait pattern
  Children with even the most severe form of PFFD do walk even if they have had no treatment, although the gait pattern is far from optimal. With treatment, in the milder forms of CSF it should be possible to achieve a normal gait. In children with PFFD the aim would be to attempt to get the gait to as near normal a pattern as possible.
- Making the best use of the available components of the limb
  A decision must be taken whether to utilize the foot for normal weight-bearing function, weight-bearing function through an extension prosthesis or as a stump for prosthetic fitting.
- Eliminating deformities of the hip and knee
  The deformities that interfere with prosthetic fitting or normal walking must be corrected.
- Achieving limb length equality by adult life
  Actual limb length equalization may be feasible in CSF but in PFFD the limb length would have to be 'equalized' with the help of a prosthesis.

The first 12 months of life

During the first year of life no treatment is needed either for CSF or PFFD. The child will play and partake in the usual activities of a baby. The femoral shortness will not prevent the child crawling or sitting. This is a period of investment for the surgeon when a treatment plan that extends through skeletal maturity can be outlined with the family. The parents will develop an understanding of the condition and will remember the plans made. After the age of one year the treatment of CSF and PFFD differs and the treatment for CSF patients is discussed first.

Treatment of congenital short femur

Among children with CSF there are two subgroups, i.e. children with a good foot and ankle and children with a fibular hemimelia and a severely deficient foot and ankle.

Age: one to three years

■ Enabling gait

■ Shoe lift if the foot and ankle are normal

Children with a satisfactory foot and ankle will not require any assistance to walk at their appropriate age. A deficiency of even several centimetres will not require a shoe lift in the first instance. The child will adopt an equinus posture on the affected side and bend the opposite knee as needed. As the years pass and the length discrepancy increases a shoe lift may be helpful. It does not need to be equal to the actual discrepancy and, indeed, once the lift exceeds 4 cm it will engender a degree of instability.

■ Syme's amputation and prosthetic fitting if the foot is grossly deficient

Children with a grossly deficient foot and ankle are best treated by Syme's amputation[3,4] in the second year of life followed by fitting of a patellar-bearing prosthesis with a supracondylar strap.

Age: three to six years

■ Correction of deformities of the hip and knee

Children with CSF have a modest flexion deformity of the hip and knee in infancy. These deformities will spontaneously correct and so no surgical intervention is required.

The valgus attitude of the knee arises from a deficiency in the lateral femoral condyle. The degree of deformity varies and does not seem to equate to the shortness of the femur. The deformity may cause instability in gait. A distal femoral osteotomy can be used to correct the deformity. Since this deformity arises from an inherent growth deficiency it will recur and further treatment at an older age is needed.

Age: Six to twelve years

If the genu valgum has recurred, hemiepiphyseodesis with one or two screws across the medial side of the growth plate is performed (Figure 37.3).

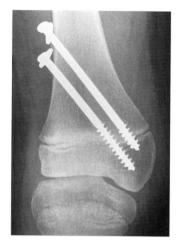

Figure 37.3 ● Genu valgum may be corrected by performing a screw epiphyseodesis.

■ Limb length equalization

In children with a relatively good foot and ankle there is a need to aim for leg length equality by skeletal maturity. The total amount of length needing to be addressed can be reasonably estimated early in life simply by using the known fact that the relative proportions of the skeleton will remain constant throughout life unless surgically altered. In other words, a 20 percent discrepancy in an infant will be a 20 percent discrepancy at maturity.

■ Transiliac lengthening

If hip dysplasia is present it is foolhardy to attempt a femoral lengthening. A pelvic osteotomy to correct the acetabular deficiency can be accompanied by pelvic lengthening to also gain 1.5–2 cm at around seven to ten years of age (Figure 37.4).[5]

■ Tibial lengthening

Even with a good foot and ankle it is common that the tibia may be slightly short. A tibial lengthening can be performed at an early age. It is helpful to gain 4–5 cm of length and to overlengthen the tibia. This avoids the need for a shoe lift for some years and also reduces the amount of future femoral lengthening. A slightly long below-knee segment or having knees at different heights does not inhibit childhood activity.

■ Femoral and tibial epiphyseodesis

Femoral and tibial epiphyseodesis of the longer limb has a low morbidity and disability compared with 3–4 cm of femoral lengthening.

■ Femoral lengthening

Femoral lengthening over a nail can markedly reduce the time for which the fixator needs to be retained. However the nail requires a femoral canal diameter of approximately 9 mm and hence a child needs, on average, to be more than ten years old.

- Attempt to obtain a stable hip if possible
  If the femoral head and neck or the acetabulum are not developed, hip stability cannot be restored. However, in children with a reasonably well-formed acetabulum with coxa vara, restoring the neck-shaft angle will improve the stability and consequently the gait.
- Ensure that the 'thigh' segment functions as a strong lever to propel the limb while walking and ensure that the knee is stable

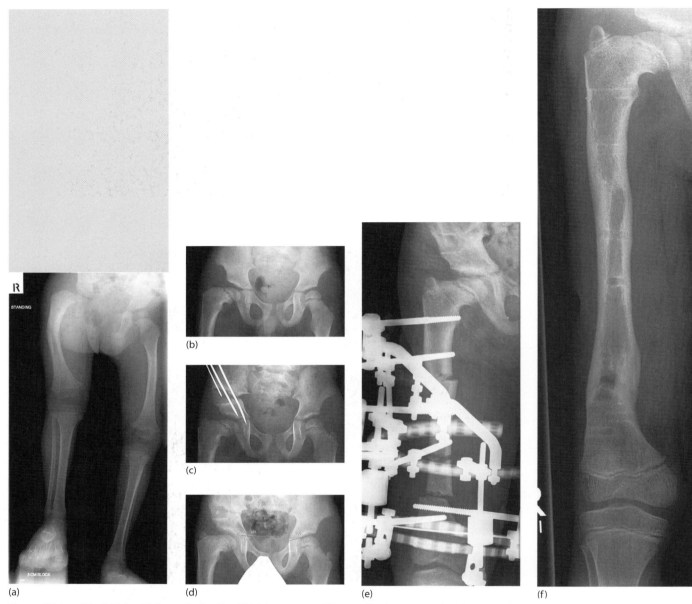

Figure 37.4 ● The limb-length inequality in this child **(a)** was treated by transiliac lengthening **(b–d)** followed by femoral lengthening **(e,f)**.

In children with PFFD, the short femur and the tibia *together* need to function as the 'thigh' segment. The presence of a mobile knee joint in the middle of the 'thigh' renders the segment weak. Fusion of the knee (Figure 37.5) and converting the child's femur and tibia into a single bone will provide a strong lever arm of virtually the same length as the normal femur. Fusion will also correct the knee instability.

- Provide an efficient and cosmetically appealing prosthesis

  It is well recognized that a below-knee amputation is superior to an above-knee amputation in terms of energy consumption and the efficiency of gait. If the ankle joint can be made to function like the knee by performing a rotationplasty, it is possible to make the limb similar to a below-'knee' amputation (Figure 37.6).[6] If this is not possible on account of poor function of the ankle and foot, a more appealing prosthesis can be made if the foot is amputated. However, in some societies parents may not agree to any form of ablative surgery. Children with PFFD and major deficiencies of the upper limbs with poor upper limb function may then develop prehensile function in the feet (Figure 37.7). In these two situations an extension prosthesis which accommodates the foot needs to be provided.

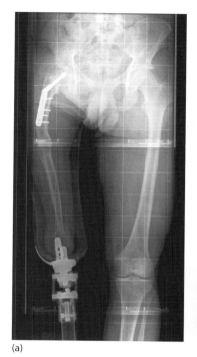 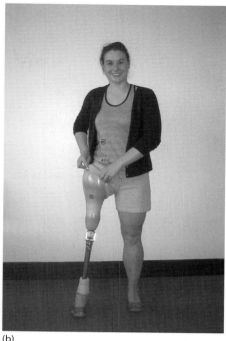

(a)   (b)

Figure 37.5 ● Fusion of the knee provides a stable thigh segment and facilitates the fitting of the prosthesis after the foot has been ablated.

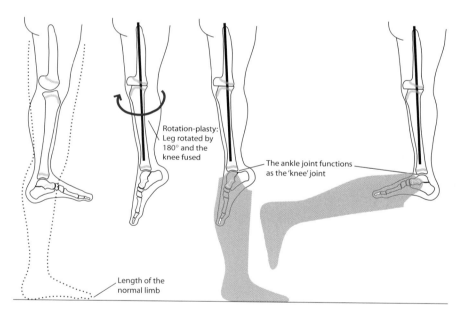

Rotation-plasty: Leg rotated by 180° and the knee fused

The ankle joint functions as the 'knee' joint

Length of the normal limb

Figure 37.6 ● Diagram showing how the ankle joint functions as the 'knee' joint facilitating the fitting of a below-knee prosthesis.

Treatment options for proximal focal femoral deficiency

Hip

■ Subtrochanteric valgus osteotomy

A subtrochanteric valgus osteotomy is needed if there is coxa vara.

■ Obtaining union at the neck

If there is an ossification defect that persists beyond the age of five to six years, a screw may be passed across this defect.

■ No intervention

No intervention is feasible when the femoral head and neck are not developed.

Knee

■ Arthrodesis

If the foot and ankle are not functional an arthrodesis of the knee is performed.

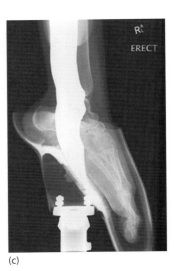

Figure 37.7 ● This child has bilateral proximal focal deficiency and major reduction defects of the upper limb. The feet need to be retained as they may have to assume a prehensile function. Apart from correction of the clubfoot deformity on the left to make the foot plantigrade (which is about to be undertaken) no other surgery on the feet are justified.

■ Van Nes rotationplasty

If the foot and ankle are normal a rotationplasty should be considered (Figure 37.8).

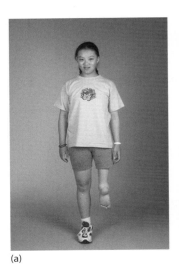

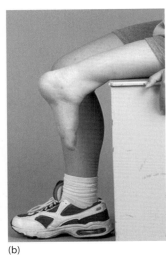

(a)   (b)   (c)

Figure 37.8 ● A Van Nes rotationplasty has been performed on this girl **(a)**. The ankle now functions as the "knee" **(b)**. The position of the foot in the prosthetic socket is seen in this radiograph **(c)**.

■ No intervention

If the femoral segment is very small, surgery at the knee may not be feasible or necessary.

Foot and ankle

■ Syme's amputation

If the foot is functionless and severely deformed, a Syme's amputation is the treatment of choice. If the foot is functional and the parents reject a rotationplasty, a Syme's amputation is offered.

■ Retain the foot

If the foot is performing prehensile functions or if the parents refuse any ablative surgery the foot is retained in the normal position. If a rotationplasty is performed the foot is retained but gets rotated backwards 180°.

Prosthesis

■ Below-knee prosthesis

A below-knee prosthesis is fitted after a Van Nes rotationplasty.

■ Above-knee prosthesis

An above-knee prosthesis that incorporates a prosthetic knee joint is needed after a Syme's amputation in children with PFFD.

Factors to be taken into consideration while planning treatment of proximal focal femoral deficiency

■ Extension prosthesis

An extension prosthesis is provided when the foot is retained without performing a rotationplasty.

Status of the foot

If the foot and ankle are functioning normally the foot can be used to function as the 'below-knee' segment after a Van Nes rotationplasty. If the foot and ankle are not functional the Van Nes rotationplasty cannot be considered.

Status of the knee

Fusion of the knee should be considered in most instances to improve stability, but if the knee is situated very proximally due to extreme shortness of the femur, surgery on the knee may not be necessary.

Status of the hip

The severity of the anomaly at the hip will determine the options for surgery on the hip.

Extent of shortening

The degree of shortening in PFFD is usually far too great to consider limb lengthening procedures.

Bilateral or unilateral involvement

A small proportion of children have bilateral PFFD and such a situation may influence the choice of treatment.

Presence of major congenital anomalies of the upper limb

Very occasionally a child may have major anomalies of the upper limb with little or no useful upper limb function. In this situation the treatment plan may have to be totally different as the foot may adapt and perform prehensile functions. It is vital that these functions are retained and in such a child surgery on the foot should be avoided at all costs.

The outline of treatment of PFFD is shown in Tables 37.1 and 37.2.

Recommended treatment of proximal focal femoral deficiency

Table 37.1 ● Outline of treatment of the foot and knee in children with proximal focal femoral deficiency

INDICATIONS				
Well-formed foot + Foot being used for prehensile function (e.g. in children with major upper limb deficiency with no useful hand function)	Well-formed foot + Foot not performing prehensile function + Parents willing for rotationplasty	Well-formed foot + Foot not performing prehensile function + Parents not willing for rotationplasty + Parents not willing for amputation	Well-formed foot + Foot not performing prehensile function + Parents not willing for rotationplasty + Parents willing for foot amputation	Deformed and non-functional foot
⇩	⇩	⇩	⇩	⇩
Retain foot + No knee fusion + Correction of knee deformities interfering with prosthetic fitting + Extension prosthesis accommodating the foot	Retain foot + Van Nes rotationplasty + Below-'knee' prosthesis	Retain foot + Knee fusion + Extension prosthesis accommodating the foot	Syme's amputation + Knee fusion + Above-knee prosthesis	Syme's amputation + Knee fusion + Above-knee prosthesis
TREATMENT				

Table 37.2 ● Outline of management of the hip in children with proximal focal femoral deficiency

INDICATIONS		
Acetabulum and femoral head and neck not formed	Acetabulum and femoral head and neck formed + No ossification defect in neck of femur + Coxa vara ⇩	Acetabulum and femoral head and neck formed + Ossification defect in neck of femur + Coxa vara ⇩ Subtrochanteric valgus osteotomy + Screw across neck
⇩ No intervention	Subtrochanteric valgus osteotomy	
TREATMENT		

References

1. Hamanishi C. Congenital short femur: clinical, genetic and epidemiological comparison of naturally occurring condition with that caused by thalidomide. *J Bone Joint Surg Br* 1980; **62**: 307–20.
2. Gillespie R, Torode IP. Classification and management of congenital abnormalities of the femur. *J Bone Joint Surg Br* 1983; **65**: 557–68.
3. Syme J. Amputation at the ankle joint. *London and Edinburgh Monthly J Med Sci* 1843; **3**: 93.
4. Birch JG, Walsh SJ, Small JM *et al.* Syme amputation for the treatment of fibular deficiency. An evaluation of long term physical and psychological functional status. *J Bone Joint Surg Am* 1999; **81**: 1511–18.
5. Millis MB, Hall JE. Transiliac lengthening of the lower extremity. A modified innominate osteotomy for the treatment of postural imbalance. *J Bone Joint Surg Am* 1979; **61**: 1182–94.
6. Torode IP, Gillespie R. Rotationplasty of the lower limb for congenital defects of the femur. *J Bone Joint Surg Br* 1983; **65**: 569–73.

Distal focal femoral deficiency

Benjamin Joseph

38

Introduction

Distal focal femoral deficiency is a very rare congenital anomaly characterized by failure of development of the distal part of the femur.[1,2] Apart from this intercalary deficiency there is no significant abnormality of the proximal part of the femur (Figure 38.1).

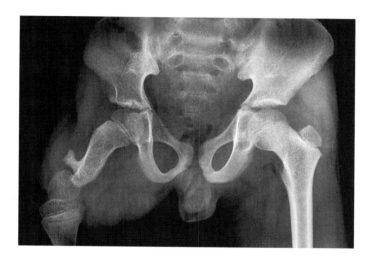

Figure 38.1 ● Radiograph of a child with distal focal femoral deficiency. The distal part of the femoral shaft has not developed. The distal femoral condyle is present but there is no continuity between the femoral shaft and the condyle.

Problems of management

Instability of the knee

Since the lower half of the femur has not developed there is no knee joint and there is no stable articulation between the distal end of the femoral shaft and the tibia. This makes bearing weight on the limb very difficult.

Shortening of the limb

The shortening of the limb is profound and the foot may be at the level of the opposite normal knee.

Aims of treatment

- Restore stability between the femur and tibia
  It is imperative that stability is restored between the distal end of the femur and the tibia.
- Manage the limb length inequality
  Since the shortening of the limb usually exceeds the limit for safe lengthening, the inequality in length must be compensated with an appropriate prosthesis.
- Optimize prosthetic fitting
  The most energy efficient design of prosthesis that can be provided in the situation must be chosen.

Treatment options

Restoring stability of the 'knee'

■ Control the knee instability by the prosthesis

Since a prosthesis is required, the instability at the articulation between the distal femur and the tibia may be controlled, to some extent, by the prosthesis when it is worn. The efficacy of the prosthesis in providing this stability is limited by the short femur and the fact that the prosthesis can only extend up to the trochanter. The child will find it difficult to raise the limb while recumbent without the prosthesis.

■ Fusion of the distal femur to the tibia

The best way to restore stability is to obtain bony continuity between the distal femur and the tibia (Figure 38.2). Care should be taken to avoid damage to the proximal tibial growth plate during the surgery.

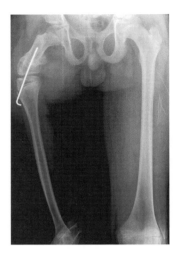

Figure 38.2 ● Radiograph of the same boy shown in Figure 38.1 after union between the femoral shaft and the condyle has been achieved. Some cartilage covering the femoral condyle and the tibial articular surface was removed and the wire transfixes the joint. A formal arthrodesis may be needed later if the knee remains unstable.

Managing limb length inequality

■ Limb lengthening

Limb lengthening may only be considered if the shortening is not severe. Since the shortening of the femur in this condition usually exceeds 50 percent of the normal femoral length, lengthening may not be a feasible option.

■ Prosthetic fitting

The limb length inequality can be compensated by the prosthesis.

Optimizing prosthetic fitting

■ Extension prosthesis

The foot is retained and accommodated in the extension prosthesis. This option has the advantage of retaining the foot which may be what children and parents in some communities prefer.

■ Syme's amputation followed by prosthesis fitting

After the foot is ablated formal prosthetic fitting can be done. The length of the stump will be comparable to that obtained by disarticulation of the knee in a normal limb. The prosthesis will have to incorporate an external knee joint.

■ Van Nes rotationplasty followed by below-knee prosthesis

A rotationplasty can be performed at the time of the arthrodesis. The tibia is rotated through 180° so that the foot faces backwards. The foot serves as a 'below-knee stump'; when the ankle is plantarflexed the 'knee' remains extended and when the ankle is dorsiflexed the 'knee' flexes.

Table 38.1 ● Outline of treatment of distal focal femoral deficiency

INDICATIONS		
Parents willing to accept Van Nes rotationplasty	Parents unwilling to accept Van Nes rotationplasty but will accept ablation of the foot	Parents unwilling to accept Van Nes rotationplasty OR Syme's amputation
⇩	⇩	⇩
'Arthrodesis' of distal femoral shaft to tibia + Van Nes rotationplasty + Below-knee prosthesis	'Arthrodesis' of distal femoral shaft to tibia + Syme's amputation + Above-knee prosthesis	'Arthrodesis' of distal femoral shaft to tibia + Extension prosthesis
TREATMENT		

This option has the advantage of avoiding the need to incorporate a knee joint into the prosthesis and this reduces the energy requirements for the child. However, the child and the parents must be willing to accept the bizarre appearance of the foot facing backwards when the prosthesis is removed. This may be unacceptable in societies where it is the norm to remove footwear inside the house and in places of worship.

Factors to be taken into consideration while planning treatment

The main factor that needs to be taken into consideration is the view of the parents regarding the treatment.

Recommended treatment

The outline of treatment of distal focal femoral deficiency is shown in Table 38.1.

References

1. Gilsanz V. Distal focal femoral deficiency. *Radiology* 1983; **147**: 105–7.
2. Tsou PM. Congenital distal femoral focal deficiency: report of a unique case. *Clin Orthop Relat Res* 1982; **162**: 99–102.

Radial club hand

Benjamin Joseph

39

Introduction

Radial club hand is a complex congenital anomaly involving failure of formation of structures on the pre-axial border of the upper limb (Figure 39.1). The deficiency involves the skeleton, muscles and tendons, nerves and vessels and other soft tissues of the entire upper limb to a greater or lesser extent.

The severity of the skeletal deficiency varies from a mildly hypoplastic radius to total absence of the radius, thumb, first metacarpal, scaphoid and trapezium.

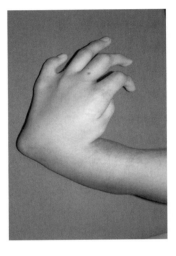

Figure 39.1 ● Clinical appearance of the forearm of a child with radial club hand.

Radial club hand may be an isolated anomaly or may be associated with one of a host of complex syndromes.[1] Unilateral radial club hand is often an isolated anomaly, while the bilateral form is more frequently associated with syndromes.[1] Several non-syndromic associated skeletal anomalies may be encountered in children with radial club hand and they include radio-ulnar synostosis, syndactyly, congenital elevation of the scapula, scoliosis, clubfoot and developmental dysplasia of the hip.

Anomalies of the cardiovascular system, the haemopoietic system, the gastrointestinal tract and the genitourinary tract may be present in these children and it is important to identify and treat these anomalies, if warranted, before embarking on treatment of the upper limb.

The severity of the deficiency varies (Figure 39.2) and is classified according to whether the radius is slightly short (type I), clearly hypoplastic (type II), partially absent (type III) or totally absent (type IV).[2]

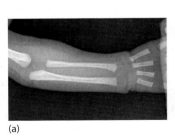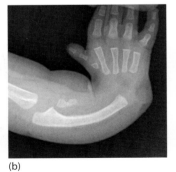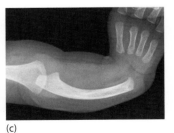

(a) (b) (c)

Figure 39.2 ● Radiographs of varying severity of radial club hand. In the mildest form or type I radial club hand the radius is slightly short, while in type II the radius is clearly hypoplastic **(a)**; in type III there is partial absence of the radius **(b)** and in type IV the entire radius is absent **(c)**.

Problems of management

Impaired hand function

Prehensile function and efficient grasp are both impaired in children with radial club hand and the reasons for the impairment of function may be attributed to the failure of normal development of the thumb, abnormality of the fingers and altered muscle function.

■ The thumb

In some cases the thumb is totally absent while in others the thumb may be present but be totally non-functional. In these situations prehensile function is lost. When the thumb is present, the range of movement of the thumb may be considerably reduced and a true pulp-to-pulp pinch is often not possible. In a small proportion of children with radial club hand the thumb is normal and these children tend to have thrombocytopenia.

■ The fingers

The index finger is often stiff; in general, the little finger is the most mobile. When the thumb is absent, the index or little finger substitutes for the thumb. The range of movement of the inter-phalangeal joints is reduced and this is one factor responsible for poor grip strength.

■ Muscles

The abnormally oriented muscles pull the hand into radial deviation and flexion. The finger flexors are ineffective in generating sufficient flexion of the fingers.

Instability of the wrist

The wrist is unstable and this contributes significantly to the poor hand function. The grip strength is markedly reduced because the wrist cannot remain in dorsiflexion while the child attempts to grasp an object.

Shortening of the forearm

The short forearm *per se* may not cause any functional limitation but it adds to the unsightly appearance of the limb. However, a short radius in a child with type II radial club hand contributes to instability at the wrist. In type I radial club hand the short radius contributes to the radial deviation deformity of the wrist.

Stiffness of the elbow

Stiffness of the elbow may occasionally be present and unless this can be overcome surgical correction of the hand deformity is contraindicated.

Aims of treatment

- Improve overall hand function
  Although it is desirable to improve the function of the hand, in certain situations this may not be possible. It is essential that these situations where hand function cannot be improved are clearly recognized as any attempt at surgical interference may actually compromise function further.
  In children who are considered as candidates for surgical intervention, an attempt must be made to restore prehensile function and to improve grasp.
- Improve the appearance of the limb
  The radial deviation and flexion at the wrist, the bowing of the ulna, the short forearm and the associated thumb deficiency may all have to be addressed in order to make the limb look better. However, it must be emphasized to the parents that the forearm and hand can never be made to look completely normal.

Treatment options

No intervention

No intervention is the preferred option if either the function of the hand is so near normal that surgery is unlikely to make a difference or when surgery may actually jeopardize existing function.[3]

Manipulation and splintage

In type I radial club hand with mild radial deviation of the wrist, serial manipulation and casting in early infancy is effective in correcting the deformity. Subsequent maintenance of correction by splints throughout the growing years can prevent recurrence of deformity. The splints are initially used throughout the day but later on night splinting should suffice.

Surgery to correct the wrist deformity and to stabilize the wrist

■ Radial lengthening

In type I and mild forms of type II radial club hand, wrist instability may be largely due to insufficient radial support on account of the short radius. Restoring the normal length of the radius relative to the distal end of the ulna can improve stability at the wrist.

■ Centralization

For over 30 years centralization has been a popular operation for severe degrees of types II, III and IV radial club hand.[4] It entails placing the distal end of the ulna into a slot in the carpus in line with the third metacarpal after releasing the contractures on the radial side of the wrist (Figure 39.3a–e). The more recent modifications of the operation try to ensure that the distal ulnar physis is not damaged and make an attempt to rebalance the muscles.

■ Radialization

Radialization was introduced more recently in an attempt to overcome some of the shortcomings of centralization.[5] The operation entails release of the contracted soft tissue on the medial side of the wrist and forearm, corrective osteotomy of the bowed ulna (if required), transfer of the flexor carpi radialis and the extensor carpi radialis to the extensor carpi ulnaris and realignment of the carpus onto the ulna. The ulna is transfixed with a stout wire to the second metacarpal with the wrist in some degree of ulnar deviation (Figure 39.3f). The operation avoids excision of any carpal bones and redistributes the muscle forces around the wrist in a manner that favours active ulnar deviation and retains mobility of the wrist. This operation appears to be a better procedure than centralization in young children, and for this reason it is recommended that this operation is performed in infants between the age of six months and one year.[1]

■ Wrist fusion

Wrist fusion can achieve stability and this alone can help in improving hand function. However, if done in a skeletally immature child, damage to the distal growth plate of the ulna can make an already short forearm even shorter. For this reason, this option should be reserved for the skeletally mature patient. In children with bilateral radial club hand it is not advisable to perform wrist fusion on both sides.

Surgery to correct bowing of the forearm

Corrective osteotomy of the bowed ulna may be performed in conjunction with either an operation to stabilize the wrist (radialization or centralization) or at the time of ulnar lengthening. When done at the time of the centralization or radialization, it may be necessary to shorten the ulna in order to reduce the soft tissue tension on the radial side. Concomitant gradual correction of the bowing can be performed while lengthening of the ulna is being done.

Surgery to lengthen the forearm

Lengthening of the forearm should be undertaken with caution as the procedure is fraught with the risk of several complications. Nevertheless, in the older child with unilateral radial club hand this option may be considered. This option has also been advocated in patients with a severe anomaly in whom previous attempts at centralization or radialization have failed.[1] While there is a possibility of increasing finger stiffness, due to increased tension on the tendons, improved overall function has been reported.[6]

Severity of the anomaly

In children with type I radial club hand, with a well-formed functional thumb and satisfactory function of the wrist and hand and no deformity, intervention is not necessary. On the other hand, if there is any functional limitation, the feasibility of improving function by surgery needs to be considered. In very severe cases where the neurovascular structures are severely contracted along with the surrounding soft tissues, correction of the deformity may jeopardize the blood supply.

Age of the patient

An adolescent or young adult who has had no prior treatment is usually not a candidate for intervention. By this age the patient will have adjusted to the disability and adapted quite remarkably

Factors to be taken into consideration while planning treatment

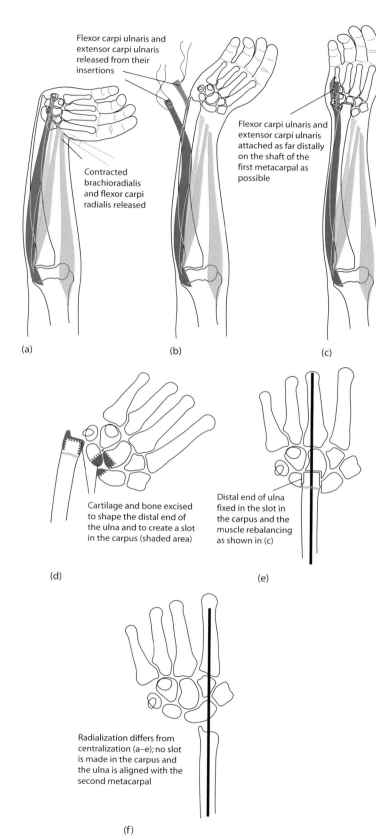

Figure 39.3 ● Diagrammatic representation of centralization **(a–e)** and radialization **(f)**.

by using the ulnar digits for activities of daily living (ADL). An infant with a severe degree of anomaly is likely to benefit far more from early surgery. Current data suggest that in the young child with radial club hand, the radialization operation works well. The results of centralization appear to be better in the older child.[1]

Severity and prognosis of associated anomalies

If the anticipated lifespan is short and the anomalies of other systems are not compatible with reasonable overall function, it may not be worthwhile to subject the child to a series of operations to improve hand function alone.

Range of movement of the elbow

In a child with less than 90° of elbow flexion, radial deviation of the wrist may be the only way the hand can reach the mouth. Correction of the wrist deformity in such a child would be counterproductive and should be avoided.

Hand function and independence in ADL

If the hand function is normal, as it is in some children with type I radial club hand, no intervention is needed. In the adolescent with a severe type of radial club hand who has adapted well to the deformity and is independent for ADL, surgery is better avoided as function may deteriorate following surgery.

Recommended treatment

An outline of recommended treatment is shown in Table 39.1. It is emphasized that when the thumb is absent or non-functional, pollicization may be required in order to improve hand function. The indications for pollicization are dealt with in Chapter 41, Thumb deficiencies.

Table 39.1 ● Outline of treatment of radial club hand

INDICATIONS								
Any type + Very poor prognosis for good quality of life and short anticipated life span due to associated systemic anomalies	Type I + Any age + Good hand function + Negligible deformity + Stable wrist	Type I + Infant + Good hand function + Mild radial deviation + Stable wrist	Type I or mild type II + Good hand function + Moderate radial deviation + Wrist unstable	Severe type II, type III or type IV + Poor hand function + Severe radial deviation + Unstable wrist + Stiff elbow	Severe type II, type III or type IV + Adolescent well adapted to ADL with ulnar digits + Severe radial deviation + Unstable wrist	Severe type II, type III or type IV + Infant (6–12 months of age) + Poor hand function + Severe radial deviation + Unstable wrist	Severe type II, type III or type IV + Older child + Poor hand function + Severe radial deviation + Unstable wrist	Severe type II, type III or type IV + Failed radialization or centralization procedure + Skeletally mature + Unilateral deficiency
⇩	⇩	⇩	⇩	⇩	⇩	⇩	⇩	⇩
No intervention	No intervention	Manipulation and casts followed by splint	Lengthening of the radius	No intervention	No intervention	Radialization	Centralization	Wrist fusion ± Ulnar lengthening
TREATMENT								

Acknowledgements

The author gratefully acknowledges the critical comments of Professor Bhaskaranand Kumar, Head of Hand and Microvascular Service, Kasturba Medical College, Manipal.

References

1. D'Arcangelo M, Gupta A, Scheker LR. Radial club hand. In: Gupta A, Kay SPJ, Scheker LR (ed). *The Growing Hand*. London: Harcourt Publishers Limited, 2000: 147–70.
2. Bayne LG, Klug MS. Long-term review of the surgical treatment of radial deficiencies. *J Hand Surg [Am]* 1987; **12**: 169–79.
3. Dobyns JH, Wood VE, Bayne LG. Congenital hand deformities. In: Green DP (ed.). *Operative Hand Surgery*, vol. 1, 3rd edn. New York: Churchill Livingstone, 1993: 288–303.
4. Lamb DW. Radial club hand. A continuing study of sixty-eight patients with one hundred and seventeen club hands. *J Bone Joint Surg [Am]* 1977; **59**: 1–13.
5. Buck-Gramcko D. Radialization as a new treatment for radial club hand. *J Hand Surg [Am]* 1985; **10**: 964–8.
6. Pickford MA, Scheker LR. Distraction lengthening of the ulna in radial club hand using the Ilizarov technique. *J Hand Surg [Br]* 1998; **23**: 186–91.

Ulnar club hand

Benjamin Joseph

40

Introduction

Ulnar club hand is a longitudinal deficiency of the postaxial border of the upper limb with abnormalities of the elbow, forearm, wrist and hand (Figure 40.1). Anomalies at each of these sites contribute to the overall disability. The condition is several times rarer than radial club hand. Three of four cases are unilateral although the contralateral upper limb may have some congenital anomaly in a large proportion of cases. Ulnar club hand is also frequently associated with other anomalies or syndromes.[1]

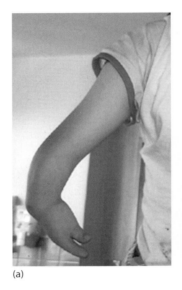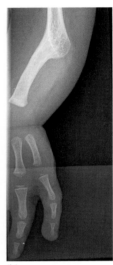

Figure 40.1 ● The appearance of the limb of a child with ulnar club hand **(a)** and radiograph of another child with ulnar club hand **(b)**.

(a)   (b)

Several classifications of ulnar club hand have been suggested; none of them is watertight and not every case falls into one of these classifications. One classification system that can be used to plan treatment is that suggested by Dobyns *et al.* (Table 40.1).[2]

Table 40.1 ● Classification of ulnar club hand and the various anomalies in the different types

Type	Ulna	Elbow	Radial head	Radius	Wrist and hand
I: Hypoplasia	Short but both proximal and distal ulnar epiphyses are present	Well formed	Dislocation ± No proximal migration	Mild bowing present but does not increase	Wrist not deviated Hand anomalies frequent and may be severe
II: Partial aplasia (commonest type)	Small ossified segment + Cartilage anlage in distal third	Humero-ulnar articulation formed	Dislocation + Proximal migration occurs	Short Bowing present which may progress	Wrist deviated Sloping distal radial epiphysis Hand anomalies frequent and may be severe
III: Total aplasia (very rare)	Absent No cartilage anlage	Fixed flexion deformity May be associated with cubital pterygium syndrome	No proximal radio-ulnar joint as ulna is totally absent	± Bowing	Hand anomalies severe
IV: Synostosis (very rare)	Small remnant present	Radiohumeral fusion OR Ulnohumeral fusion	No proximal radio-ulnar joint	± Bowing	Variable

Hand anomalies seen in ulnar club hand vary and they do not correlate to the severity of the forearm deformity. The hand anomalies include absent fingers (ectrodactyly) and syndactyly. Although the main deficiency is on the ulnar (post-axial) border, a significant proportion of children with ulnar club hand have thumb anomalies. On account of this it has been suggested that in addition to classifying the nature of the ulnar defect, it is probably as important to classify these cases on the basis of the severity of the thumb anomaly.[3]

About a third of the children with ulnar club have only two digits and another third have three digits. Thumb anomalies are seen in over a third of children; they include deficiency, duplication, syndactyly of the first web and adduction deformity.[1]

Problems of management

Progressive bowing of the radius

In type II ulnar club hand, progressive bowing of the radius tends to occur. Some authors attribute this to the presence of a fibrous tether between the cartilaginous anlage and the ulnar side of the distal radial epiphysis[4] and they recommend that the anlage and the fibrous tether be excised. Others disagree with this concept and feel that excision of the anlage is not warranted.[5,6]

Proximal migration of the dislocated radial head

Radial head dislocation is frequently seen in the different types of ulnar club hand. In type II there is a tendency for proximal migration of the dislocated radial head which contributes to the shortening of the forearm. Occasionally the proximally migrated radial head can limit elbow motion.[4]

Hand anomalies that compromise hand function

The various hand anomalies interfere with hand function; some of these anomalies are amenable to treatment that may improve hand function.

Loss of elbow motion

The elbow may be in severe flexion in children with a cubital pterygium syndrome or it may be stiff in extension in children with synostosis. In both these situations useful motion at the elbow cannot be restored.

Aims of treatment

- Improve hand function
  Specific anomalies of the hand such as syndactyly, hypoplasia or aplasia of the thumb and first web space contracture that may be seen in association with ulnar club hand should be corrected in order to improve hand function.
- Prevent progressive deformity of the forearm
  An attempt must be made to prevent the radius from bowing. If progression of bowing of the radius is observed, an effort must be made to prevent further progression.

Treatment options

Correction of specific hand anomalies

Standard techniques of syndactyly release, first web space release and surgery on the hypoplastic thumb (see Chapter 41, Thumb deficiencies) may be performed to improve function of the hand in children with any form of ulnar club hand.[1]

Splintage of the forearm to prevent bowing

In the infant and the young child, regular splinting of the forearm with thermoplastic splints may help to minimize the severity of radial bowing.[5,6]

Excision of the cartilaginous anlage of the distal ulna

Although there does not seem to be agreement on the efficacy of this procedure, excision of the cartilage anlage does appear to reduce the severity of radial bowing but has little effect on the proximal migration of the radial head.[4]

Radio-ulnar synostosis and creation of a single bone forearm

Function can be improved in children with type II ulnar club hand with significant proximal migration of the radial head by excision of the radial head and creation of a synostosis of the radius and ulna.[7] Simple techniques of fixation appear to be sufficient to obtain union between the two bones. The single bone forearm provides a more stable lever.

Amputation

If there is no potential for improving hand function in a child with no useful elbow movement, serious thought should be given to performing an above-elbow amputation. However, if the function of the opposite upper limb is also very poor, it may be difficult to put on the prosthesis.

Type of ulnar club hand

The severity of ulnar defect will influence the choice of options for intervention.

Function of the hand and potential for improving function

The function of the hand needs to be evaluated and corrective surgery should be considered if it is felt that function can be improved by operating on any anomaly of the hand.

The age of the child

Bracing of the forearm in an infant or young child may minimize the deformity of the radius. However, this is unlikely to be effective in the older child.

Factors to be taken into consideration while planning treatment

Table 40.2 ● Outline of treatment ulnar club hand

INDICATIONS						
Type I ulnar club hand	Type II ulnar club hand + Infant or young child	Type II ulnar club hand + Older child + Specific hand anomalies amenable to surgical correction + No progression of radial bow ± radial head dislocation (no proximal migration)	Type II ulnar club hand + Older child + Specific hand anomalies amenable to surgical correction + Progression of radial bow + Radial head dislocation with proximal migration	Type III ulnar club hand + Some useful motion at elbow + Specific hand anomalies amenable to surgical correction	Type IV ulnar club hand + Specific hand anomalies amenable to surgical correction	Type III ulnar club hand + Cubital pterygium syndrome + Very poor hand function
⇩	⇩	⇩	⇩	⇩	⇩	⇩
No intervention for forearm + Correct hand anomalies if present	Splint forearm to prevent bowing	Correct hand anomalies	Correct hand anomalies + Excise cartilage anlage of ulna + Excise radial head + Radio-ulnar synostosis and create single bone forearm	Correct hand anomalies	Correct hand anomalies	Above elbow amputation and prosthetic fitting
TREATMENT						

The status of the elbow

If the range of motion of the elbow is very limited and not in a functional arc (as in cubital pterygium with severe flexion deformity), then attempting to improve hand function may not be worthwhile.

Bowing of the radius and proximal migration of the radial head

Bowing of the radius and proximal migration of the radial head both contribute to shortening of the forearm and, hence, these problems need to be addressed.

The treatment of ulnar club hand is outlined in Table 40.2.

Recommended treatment

References

1. Sykes PJ, Eadie PA. Longitudinal ulnar deficiency in the hand. In: Gupta A, Kay SPJ, Scheker LR (eds). *The Growing Hand*. London: Harcourt Publishers Limited, 2000: 189–95.
2. Dobyns JH, Wood VE, Bayne LG. Congenital hand deformities. In: Green DP (ed.). *Operative Hand Surgery*, vol. 1. New York: Churchill Livingstone, 1993: 251–548.
3. Cole PJ, Manske PR. Classification of ulnar deficiency according to the thumb and first web. *J Hand Surg [Am]* 1997; **22**: 479–88.
4. Mulligan PJ. The elbow in ulnar club hand. In: Gupta A, Kay SPJ, Scheker LR (eds). *The Growing Hand*. London: Harcourt Publishers Limited, 2000: 197–202.
5. Marcus NA, Omer GE. Carpal deviation in congenital ulnar deficiency. *J Bone Joint Surg Am* 1984; **66**: 1003–7.
6. Broudy AS, Smith RJ. Deformities of the hand and wrist with ulnar deficiency. *J Hand Surg [Am]* 1979; **4**: 304–15.
7. Lloyd-Roberts GC. Treatment of defects of the ulna in children by establishing cross union with the radius. *J Bone Joint Surg Br* 1973; **55**: 327–30.

Thumb deficiencies

Benjamin Joseph

41

Introduction

Congenital deficiencies of the thumb include a spectrum of anomalies such as hypoplasia and aplasia, constriction band syndrome, brachydactyly and true transverse absence. The severity of the deficiency varies and in order to define an outline of treatment a practical classification was suggested by Blauth (Table 41.1).[1] It needs to be emphasized that every case may not fit into this classification system precisely and treatment may have to be tailored to the individual case. Nevertheless, the classification serves as a basic guideline for identifying specific problems of management and for planning treatment (Figure 41.1).

Table 41.1 ● Blauth classification of thumb deficiencies and the problems of management

Type	Characteristic features	Problems of management
Type I	Minor hypoplasia The thumb looks smaller than normal	Function of the thumb is normal
Type II	The thumb is smaller than normal The skeletal elements are all formed and the joints are developed Adduction contracture of the first web space is present The thenar muscles are absent The ulnar collateral ligament of the MCP joint is lax	Opposition is not possible MCP joint is unstable
Type III	The thumb is much smaller than normal The metacarpophalangeal (MCP) joint is unstable The carpometacarpal (CMC) joint is poorly developed The thenar muscles are absent The extrinsic muscles are abnormal or rudimentary	Opposition is not possible The MCP and CMC joints are unstable
Type IV	A floating thumb that is attached to the hand by a soft tissue stalk without any skeletal attachment	Totally non-functional thumb Unacceptable cosmetic appearance
Type V	Total absence of the thumb	

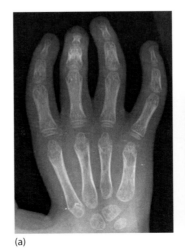
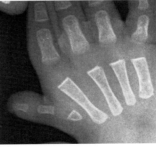

Figure 41.1 ● Examples of total **(a)** and partial thumb deficiency **(b)**.

(a)

(b)

Aims of treatment

- Provide a thumb that can oppose
  The prerequisites needed to enable opposition of the thumb are muscles to bring about the movement, mobile and stable carpometacarpal (CMC) and metacarpophalangeal (MCP) joints and a sufficiently wide web space. Treatment aimed at improving hand function must attempt to fulfil these prerequisites.
- Ensure that the thumb is stable
  Even if the thumb can perform the movement of opposition, a firm grip will not be possible unless the joints of the thumb remain stable when resistance is offered.
- Ensure that the appearance of the reconstructed thumb is cosmetically acceptable
  The hand is a part of the body that is visible whenever it is used and this makes it important to ensure acceptable appearance.

Treatment options for the partially functional deficient thumb

Restoration of power of opposition

■ Opponensplasty with flexor digitorum superficialis of the ring finger

The flexor digitorum superficialis (FDS) of the ring finger is transferred to the thumb metacarpal and proximal phalanx as is done for opponens paralysis (see Chapter 60, The paralysed hand and wrist).

■ Abductor digiti minimi transfer

The abductor digiti minimi transfer is a more demanding operation (Figure 41.2).[2] The appearance of the thenar eminence improves following this transfer. Occasionally, sufficient power of opposition may not be achieved by this transfer and then an FDS transfer may have to be added.

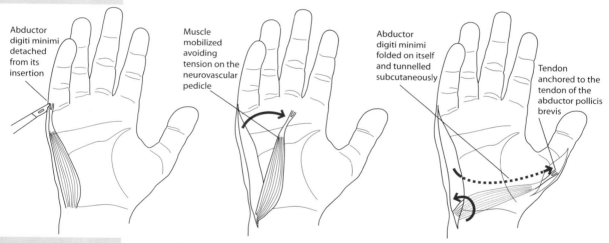

Figure 41.2 ● Diagram illustrating the technique of abductor digiti minimi transfer to facilitate thumb opposition.

■ Palmaris longus transfer

The palmaris longus can be transferred to the thumb with a free tendon graft.

Release of the contracted web space

A flap is usually needed to widen the web space.

Reconstruction of the ulnar collateral ligament

The ulnar collateral ligament can be reconstructed with the tendon of the FDS that is used for the opponensplasty (Figure 41.3).

Reconstruction of the CMC joint by metatarsophalangeal joint transfer

Shibata[3] performs an elaborate operation that entails a microvascular transfer of the metatarsophalangeal joint of the second toe to create a CMC joint in type III deficiency. This operation is combined with tendon transfers to enable the reconstructed thumb to function.

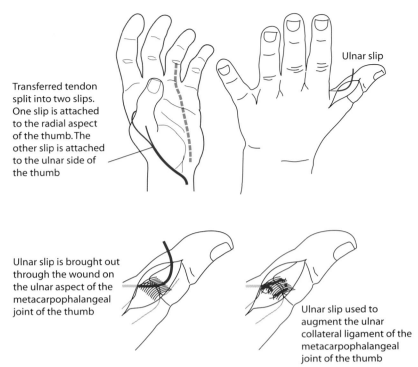

Transferred tendon split into two slips. One slip is attached to the radial aspect of the thumb. The other slip is attached to the ulnar side of the thumb

Ulnar slip

Ulnar slip is brought out through the wound on the ulnar aspect of the metacarpophalangeal joint of the thumb

Ulnar slip used to augment the ulnar collateral ligament of the metacarpophalangeal joint of the thumb

Figure 41.3 ● Diagram demonstrating how the flexor digitorum superficialis of the ring finger can be used to restore the power of opposition and to reconstruct the ulnar collateral ligament of the metacarpophalangeal joint of the thumb.

Treatment options for the non-functional or absent thumb

Pollicization

The operation was popularized by Buck–Gramcko[4] and consists of:

1. transposition of flaps to create a web space;
2. removal of the shaft of the second metacarpal to create a thumb consisting of three bones and of a length that is comparable to the length of a normal thumb (the head of the metacarpal is retained);
3. rotation of the index finger by 140–160° to achieve pulp to pulp opposition with the middle finger;
4. suturing of the head of the second metacarpal to the trapezoid (or the second metacarpal base) with a non-absorbable suture;
5. use of the first dorsal interosseous muscle to abduct the thumb and the first palmar interosseous muscle to adduct the thumb (Figure 41.4);
6. use of the extensor indicis to function as the new extensor pollicis.

Pollicization is recommended for all type IV and V deficiencies and quite gratifying functional and cosmetic results can be obtained by this intricate operation (Figure 41.5). There is disagreement regarding the preferred treatment for type III deficiency; most prefer to perform a pollicization while a few surgeons attempt reconstruction[3] as indicated earlier.

Microvascular toe transfer

In children in whom the index finger is also absent microvascular toe transfer is recommended.[5]

Factors to be taken into consideration while planning treatment

The type of deficiency

The severity of the deficiency will dictate the nature of reconstruction.

Presence of associated hand and forearm anomalies

Associated absence of the index finger precludes the option of index finger pollicization.

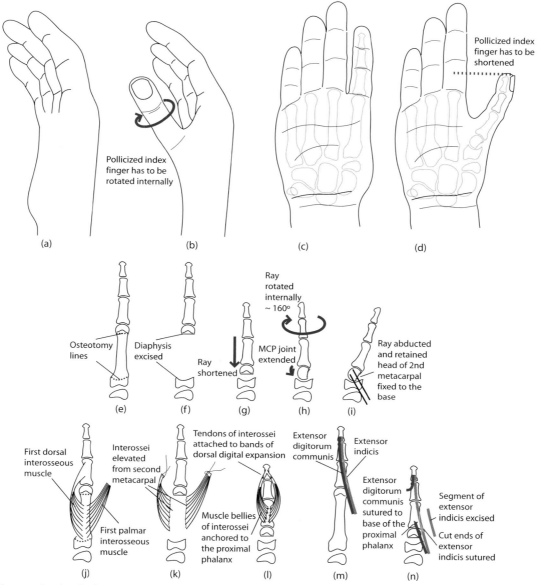

Figure 41.4 ● Diagram showing the important steps of pollicization of the index finger. The index finger has to be shortened, rotated internally and the muscles around the reconstructed 'thumb' have to be rebalanced. The appearance of the hand following pollicization is shown **(a–d)**. Details of how the metacarpal is shortened, rotated and fixed **(e–i)**, rebalancing of the intrinsic muscles **(j–l)** and the technique of rebalancing of the extrinsic muscles **(m,n)** are shown.

Recommended treatment

The outline of treatment of thumb deficiencies is shown in Table 41.2.

Rationale of recommended treatment

Why is the abductor digiti minimi transfer recommended for restoring opposition?
This transfer improves the appearance of the hand by increasing the bulk of the thenar eminence.

Why is pollicization preferred to reconstruction with metatarsophalangeal joint transfer for type III deficiencies?
Pollicization is a simpler operation than the microvascular joint transfer.

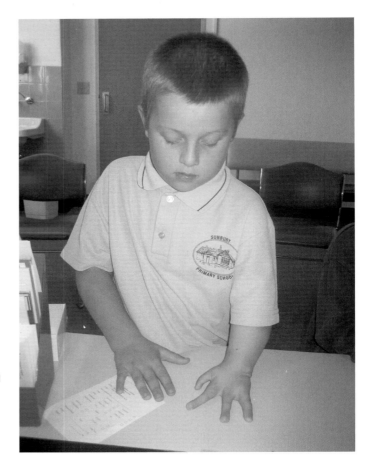

Figure 41.5 ● This boy had total agenesis of the left thumb. The appearance of the hand following pollicization of the index finger is good and the pollicized index finger is functioning as the thumb.

Table 41.2 ● Outline of treatment of thumb deficiencies

INDICATIONS			
Type I deficiency + Normal function	Type II deficiency + No active opposition + Unstable MCP joint	Type III/IV/V deficiency + Normal index finger	Type III/IV/V deficiency + Normal index finger not available for transfer
			⇩
⇩	⇩		Microvascular toe transfer
No intervention	Abductor digiti minimi transfer + Ulnar collateral ligament reconstruction	⇩ Pollicization of index finger (+ amputation of non-functional thumb in type III and type IV deficiencies)	
TREATMENT			

References

1. Scheker LR, Cendales LC. Correcting congenital thumb anomalies in children: Opponensplasty and pollicization. In: Gupta A, Kay SPJ, Scheker LR (eds). *The Growing Hand*. London: Harcourt Publishers Limited, 2000: 171–82.
2. Littler JW, Cooley SG. Opposition of the thumb and its restoration by abductor digiti quinti transfer. *J Bone Joint Surg Am* 1963; **45**: 1389–96.

3. Shibata M. Metatarsophalangeal joint transfer for Type III-B hypoplastic thumb. In: Gupta A, Kay SPJ, Scheker LR (eds). *The Growing Hand*. London: Harcourt Publishers Limited, 2000: 183–88.

4. Buck-Gramcko D. Pollicization of the index finger. Method and results in aplasia and hypoplasia of the thumb. *J Bone Joint Surg Am* 1971; **53**: 1605–17.

5. Kay SPJ. Microvascular toe transfer in children. Part A: The congenital defect. In: Gupta A, Kay SPJ, Scheker LR (eds). *The Growing Hand*. London: Harcourt Publishers Limited, 2000: 987–1000.

SECTION 4

Discrepancies of limb length

General principles of management of discrepancies of limb length in children

42

Selvadurai Nayagam

Introduction

Minor differences in limb length (of up to 15 mm) can exist as a normal variant. Larger discrepancies may not always be symptomatic; compensation mechanisms can be effective (especially with the upper limb) and hence treatment is not necessary. However, there are thresholds beyond which these compensatory mechanisms falter and, in the case of the lower limb, the individual displays a limp.

Altering the length of a bone in a child may be indicated in three situations:

- When there is a discrepancy of length between left and right sides (either upper or lower limb).
- In order to restore a normal length relationship between paired bones in the same limb segment (e.g. between the radius and ulna or between the tibia and fibula).
- To improve stature and body proportions in a child with disproportionate dwarfism.

This chapter focuses on the lower limb as this is where treatment is usually directed.

Surgery for limb length abnormalities include lengthening of the short bone, shortening of the long bone or a combination of the two. The treatment approach varies depending on the bone affected, the size of the discrepancy, the underlying cause and whether residual growth remains.

Problems of management

Limp

The limp from a shoulder dip is easy to pick out. However, the child may also display compensation manoeuvres: ankle equinus, vaulting (over the longer leg) or flexion and circumduction of the longer leg in swing-through. In mild discrepancies these compensations are able to reduce the vertical displacement of the centre of gravity but when length differences exceed 5.5 percent, toe-walking becomes clinically apparent.[1]

Fatigue tolerance

Efforts to reduce vertical oscillations of the centre of gravity induce an energy cost and ultimately affect walking tolerance. Simulations of leg length discrepancies appear to indicate an increased oxygen consumption and perceived exertion,[2] although this may be more noticeable in older adults than in young children.

Back symptoms

The association between leg length discrepancy and back pain is tenuous;[3-8] other possible aetiologies should be sought before leg length discrepancy is considered as a cause – so unusual is this association in children.

Uncovering the hip of the long leg – a prelude to early osteoarthritis?

When standing, the pelvis tilts lower on the side of the shorter leg, thereby 'uncovering' the hip of the longer side. This, coupled with the finding that the long leg is exposed to greater forces[9] in stance, has led some to associate leg length discrepancy with osteoarthritis.[8,10-12] As with back pain, the evidence is weak.

Aims of treatment

- Reduce limping
  This is a primary aim of treatment. In clinical conditions where other abnormalities (e.g. paralysis or coxa vara) are present in addition to shortening, limb length equalization will only partially reduce limping.
- Eradicate the need for footwear modification
- Increase a sense of well-being from improvement in body image

Assessment of limb length discrepancy

Measurement of the limb length discrepancy

■ Clinical techniques

The method of using blocks to level the pelvis (when assessed from behind the child and palpating the posterior iliac crests) is as accurate as computed tomography (CT) scan-derived measurements. The caveats are ensuring the child is able to cooperate with instruction and stand with both knees extended. This method is prone to error if the underlying cause is a hemihypertrophy or hemiatrophy as the hemipelvis may be unequal in size to the contralateral side. Tape measurements are useful in younger children but must be recognized as estimates and not 'measurements' as they are not accurately repeatable.

■ Imaging techniques

Standing radiographs using 1-metre film cassettes have been used as standard. CT-derived scanograms are often used but have the disadvantage of not being weight-bearing images; significant joint incongruity or laxity is unmasked in standing films. Newer digitally derived scanogram images are now available that are obtained using fluoroscopic image intensifiers linked to a computer – these are weight-bearing images from low radiation exposure.

Treatment options

- No treatment or footwear modification.
- Epiphyseodesis.
- Limb shortening.
- Limb lengthening.

Factors to be taken into consideration while planning treatment

Aetiology of leg length discrepancy

The underlying cause of the length discrepancy is relevant from several aspects:

- While most conditions cause a linear increase of limb length discrepancy with age, there are some that follow a curvilinear or even non-linear pattern (Figure 42.1). Awareness of this difference will prevent incorrect estimations of final leg length discrepancy to be made from tables or graphs that assume a linear increase.[13]
- Soft tissue-related complications are particularly difficult to resolve when lengthening in congenital longitudinal limb deficiencies.
- Soft tissue complications in limb lengthening are less marked in post-traumatic discrepancies. An exception is where multiple physeal damage occurs in neonatal septicaemia (purpura fulminans) – there are often large areas of soft tissue scarring associated with the thromboembolic infarcts produced in this condition.

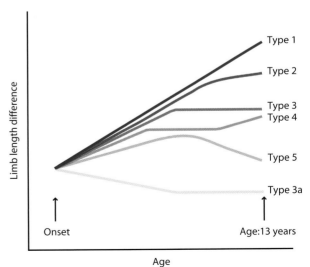

Figure 42.1 ● Patterns of changes in limb length discrepancy.
Type 1: Usually from physeal damage or in congenital longitudinal limb deficiency.
Type 2: Less common, seen in some congenital longitudinal limb deficiencies and in polio.
Type 3: Exemplified by femoral fractures where a difference may arise from stimulation (limb becomes longer and then stabilises) or has united shorter (type 3a) and grows faster to eventually reduce the difference.
Type 4: Perthes' disease and neonatal hip sepsis produce an initial shortening from loss of bone substance in the femoral head and neck, but the discrepancy then plateaus before increasing again when the capital physis closes prematurely.
Type 5: Chronic inflammatory disorders of the knee stimulate the distal femoral physis to greater growth. This effect is lost when the condition is medically treated. However, early physeal closure is not uncommon and the result is a curve that is typified by an upward slope-plateau-downward slope pattern. A similar pattern is seen when Perthes' disease occurs in early childhood; remodeling reduces the initial shortening from collapse of the femoral head.

Associated limb deformity

Many congenital and acquired causes of limb length discrepancy are associated with angular or rotational deformity; correction may be staged or simultaneous with that of length inequality (Figure 42.2).

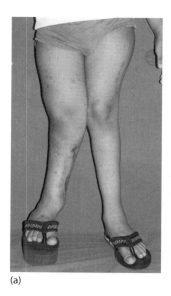
(a)

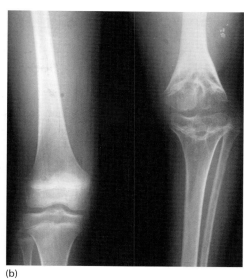
(b)

Figure 42.2 ● **(a)** Shortening of the right tibia is associated with an angular deformity in this boy with Ollier's disease. **(b)** Severe shortening due to physeal damage following osteomyelitis is associated with mild genu varum.

Estimating length discrepancy at maturity

This provides a yardstick for planning: there are many methods available for predicting this parameter.[14–17]

These methods fall into two groups: those based on the assumption that changes in length discrepancy are linear with respect to time (Moseley's straight line graph,[15] Paley's multiplier method[16]) and those (Eastwood[14]) which do not make this assumption and allow extrapolations to be made cognisant of the underlying aetiology and relevant shape of the graph (Shapiro[13]). Linear methods suffice most of the time but awareness of non-linear patterns is important lest the surgeon makes inappropriate estimations.

Predicted height at maturity

This is probably more relevant to the male population. Height predictions can be performed using bone age scores in a formula (the TW3 method[18]) or using a table of multipliers.[19] If a child has below average height potential, solving the leg length discrepancy by epiphyseodesis of the long leg may compromise this further. In such scenarios offering limb lengthening may produce a more acceptable result to the child and their family.

Limb reconstruction versus prosthetic management

Small to moderate final discrepancies (usually of less than 5 cm) are amenable to simple techniques such as epiphyseodesis. Larger differences may need to be addressed by limb lengthening or a combination of the two surgical techniques. In some children, there will be discrepancies so large that multiple attempts at limb lengthening will invariably result in:

● a childhood notable for hospitalizations and multiple surgeries;
● structural symmetry in length between the lower limbs but not functional parity; at times worse function than can be obtained through prosthetic management;
● extensive scarring (physical and psychological).

The surgeon's role in managing children with leg length discrepancies is to either eradicate or facilitate prosthetic and orthotic use. The decision to offer reconstruction or amputation is difficult in cases where the predicted final discrepancy is large; often pressure is generated by family members or cultural circumstances to avoid amputation at all costs. In the event reconstruction is decided upon, a useful rule of thumb is to limit each stage of lengthening to a 15–20 percent increase (especially in congenital deficiencies). In contrast, prosthetic management should be considered if the length discrepancy is greater than 30 percent or predicted to be greater than 25 cm at skeletal maturity and especially if associated foot anomalies cannot be reconstructed to provide a satisfactory platform for efficient walking (Figure 42.3).

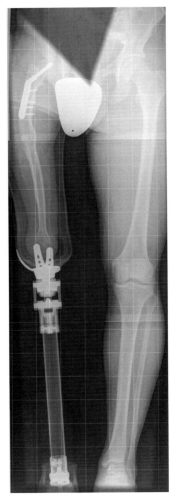

Figure 42.3 ● Prosthetic management may be more appropriate while dealing with severe shortening of the lower limb associated with major congenital limb deficiency.

Recommended treatment

The outline of treatment of lower limb length discrepancy is shown in Table 42.1.

Determine the cause of length discrepancy and estimate the final discrepancy as early as possible. This allows a strategy of management to be formulated. Small discrepancies (less than 5 cm) without deformity can be managed by epiphyseodesis unless stature considerations override. Significant deformity with similar magnitude of length discrepancy can be managed by osteotomy and lengthening. Large final discrepancies will either follow a route of lengthening coupled with contralateral epiphyseodesis or staged lengthening procedures. Keep any single stage of lengthening to less than a 15 percent increase over the starting length. These procedures may be linked to appropriate deformity corrections if needed. Finally, always consider prosthetic management for large discrepancies.

Table 42.1 ● Outline of treatment of lower limb length discrepancy

INDICATIONS					
Congenital or acquired cause + Final discrepancy <5 cm + No deformity + Predicted height at maturity not below average	Congenital or acquired cause + Final discrepancy <5 cm + Significant deformity	Acquired cause + Final discrepancy 5–15 cm + With or without significant deformity	Congenital cause + Final discrepancy 5–15 cm + With or without significant deformity	Congenital or acquired cause + Final discrepancy 15–25 cm + With or without significant deformity	Congenital or acquired cause + Final discrepancy >25 cm + With or without significant deformity
⇩	⇩	⇩	⇩	⇩	⇩
Contralateral epiphyseodesis	Corrective osteotomy + Lengthening (at the same site or different level within the same bone)	Corrective osteotomy (if deformity is present) + Lengthening (at the same site or different level within the same bone), repeated over two stages in childhood if necessary	Contralateral epiphyseodesis to reduce final discrepancy by 5 cm + Corrective osteotomy to improve axis alignment and joint stability + Lengthening (at the same site or different level within the same bone), repeated over two stages in childhood (*Divide total lengthening between the femur and tibia so as to reduce percentage of length increase on each bone. Stresses are reduced in soft tissues and across the joints, albeit with the disadvantage that the knee joints may end up at different levels.*)	Early amputation at around walking age + Prosthetic fitting OR Contralateral epiphyseodesis to reduce final discrepancy by 5 cm + Corrective osteotomy to improve axis alignment and joint stability + Lengthening (at the same site or different level within the same bone), repeated over three stages in childhood (*Divide total lengthening between the femur and tibia so as to reduce percentage of length increase on each bone. Stresses are reduced in soft tissues and across the joints, albeit with the disadvantage that the knee joints may end up at different levels.*)	Early amputation at around walking age + Prosthetic fitting
TREATMENT					

References

1. Song KM, Halliday SE, Little DG. The effect of limb-length discrepancy on gait. *J Bone Joint Surg Am* 1997; **79**: 1690–8.
2. Gurney B, Mermier C, Robergs R, Gibson A, Rivero D. Effects of limb-length discrepancy on gait economy and lower-extremity muscle activity in older adults. *J Bone Joint Surg Am* 2001; **83**: 907–15.
3. Grundy PF, Roberts CJ. Does unequal leg length cause back pain? A case-control study. *Lancet* 1984; **2**(8397): 256–8.

4. Hoikka V, Ylikoski M, Tallroth K. Leg-length inequality has poor correlation with lumbar scoliosis. A radiological study of 100 patients with chronic low-back pain. *Arch Orthop Trauma Surg* 1989; **108**: 173–5.

5. Soukka A, Alaranta H, Tallroth K, Heliovaara M. Leg-length inequality in people of working age. The association between mild inequality and low-back pain is questionable. *Spine* 1991; **16**: 429–31.

6. Kakushima M, Miyamoto K, Shimizu K. The effect of leg length discrepancy on spinal motion during gait – three-dimensional analysis in healthy volunteers. *Spine* 2003; **28**: 2472–6.

7. Tjernstrom B, Rehnberg L. Back pain and arthralgia before and after lengthening. 75 patients questioned after 6 (1–11) years. *Acta Orthop Scand* 1994; **65**: 328–32.

8. Friberg O. Clinical symptoms and biomechanics of lumbar spine and hip joint in leg length inequality. *Spine* 1983; **8**: 643–51.

9. Bhave A, Paley D, Herzenberg JE. Improvement in gait parameters after lengthening for the treatment of limb-length discrepancy. *J Bone Joint Surg Am* 1999; **81**: 529–34.

10. Gofton JP, Trueman GE. Studies in osteoarthritis of the hip. II. Osteoarthritis of the hip and leg-length disparity. *Can Med Assoc J* 1971; **104**: 791–9.

11. Bjerkreim I. Secondary dysplasia and osteoarthrosis of the hip joint in functional and in fixed obliquity of the pelvis. *Acta Orthop Scand* 1974; **45**: 873–82.

12. Nakagawa M, Iwata H, Sugiura S *et al.* The evaluation of intertrochanteric osteotomy in relation to osteotomized angle and leg-length discrepancy for osteoarthritis of the hip. *Clin Orthop Relat Res* 1980; **152**: 277–83.

13. Shapiro F. Developmental patterns in lower-extremity length discrepancies. *J Bone Joint Surg Am* 1982; **64**: 639–51.

14. Eastwood DM, Cole WG. A graphic method for timing the correction of leg-length discrepancy. *J Bone Joint Surg Br* 1995; **77**: 743–7.

15. Moseley CF. A straight-line graph for leg-length discrepancies. *J Bone Joint Surg Am* 1977; **59**: 174–9.

16. Paley D, Bhave A, Herzenberg JE, Bowen JR. Multiplier method for predicting limb-length discrepancy. *J Bone Joint Surg Am* 2000; **82**: 1432–46.

17. Menelaus MB. Correction of leg length discrepancy by epiphysial arrest. *J Bone Joint Surg Br* 1966; **48**: 336–9.

18. Tanner J, Healy M, Goldstein H, Cameron N. *Assessment of Skeletal Maturity and Prediction of Adult Height: TW3 Method*. London: WB Saunders, 2001.

19. Paley J, Talor J, Levin A, Bhave A, Paley D, Herzenberg JE. The multiplier method for prediction of adult height. *J Pediatr Orthop* 2004; **24**: 732–7.

Length discrepancy of the femur

Selvadurai Nayagam

43

Introduction

Large discrepancies of limb length are easy to identify early but attention may be drawn first by a concomitant limb deformity or absence of a limb part, as often occurs in congenital longitudinal deficiencies. In contrast, minor limb length discrepancies are usually brought to the attention of parents by health visitors, relatives or school teachers and the problem detected later in childhood. This chapter focuses on both congenital and acquired causes of a short femur but excludes proximal focal femoral deficiency (PFFD) which is covered in Chapter 37, Congenital short femur and proximal focal femoral deficiency.

Anterolateral bowing of the femur and varying degrees of longitudinal deficiency (previously termed congenital short femur or congenital femoral hypoplasia to distinguish it from true PFFD variants) account for most congenital cases. Longitudinal deficiencies not only present in the bone segment to which the deficiency is labelled but may affect adjoining segments as well – for instance in fibula hemimelia, a length discrepancy is often found in the fibula, tibia and femur. However, the type that finds its place in this chapter is one where the main length discrepancy is in the femur.

Acquired causes are mainly trauma and infection. There are major growth implications if the distal femoral physis is irrevocably damaged as this contributes to over a third (37 percent) of longitudinal growth of the lower limb. Early damage to the proximal femoral physis from neonatal sepsis also has far-reaching effects; the hip is poorly developed, instability is an issue and, to compound matters, the limb is short from absent growth at the capital physis – all leading to poor gait (see Chapter 28, Post-infective hip dysplasia). A similar but more severe scenario occurs in purpura fulminans, a complication of bacterial (usually meningococcal) septicaemia, where multiple areas of infarct in several physes lead to severe length discrepancies and deformity.

While attention is often focused on a shortened femur, a similar magnitude of gait anomaly arises if the femur is too long. This can be a consequence of overgrowth after fracture or the presence of a deep arteriovenous malformation.

The clinical and functional impact of length discrepancy is described in Chapter 42, General principles of management of discrepancies of limb length in children.

Problems of management

Length inequality in conjunction with deformity

Femoral length discrepancies are often seen with an associated deformity irrespective of the cause being congenital or acquired. Coxa vara, retroversion of the femoral neck[1] and knee valgus (from hypoplasia of the lateral femoral condyle) commonly coexist with shortening in the congenitally short femur. In addition, soft tissue anomalies and contractures at the hip are present, for example a fixed flexion deformity, adduction and external rotation.[2–4] Short femurs resulting from traumatic causes do not have these soft tissue associations.

In general, proximal femoral deformities need to be addressed early to improve hip congruence and stability. Distal deformities will need treatment depending on severity and the coincidental need for other surgical interventions; for example a corrective osteotomy for deformity is carried out at the same time as attempted excision of a bony tether in the distal femoral physis (Figure 43.1a–c). These procedures can also be combined with measures to address length discrepancy and so reduce the total number of interventions. Surgical techniques other than osteotomy are also applicable: with a congenitally hypoplastic lateral femoral condyle, hemiepiphyseodesis works well to correct the valgus deformity (Figure 43.1d). In contrast, some deformities may resolve with time and simply need monitoring in the first instance, for instance in anterolateral bowing.

Knee instability

Sagittal plane laxity from deficient cruciate ligaments is common with congenital femoral hypoplasia[5,6] (Figure 43.2). The severity varies from mild to moderate and correspondingly supportive measures are either none or bracing. However, the presence of such instability needs to be noted when limb lengthening is planned; soft tissue tension in muscles acting across the knee is increased by the process of lengthening and may induce subluxation.

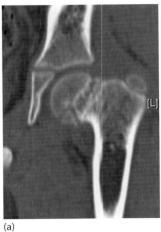
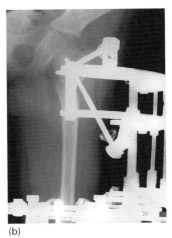
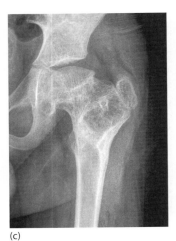
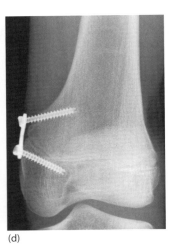

(a) (b) (c) (d)

Figure 43.1 ● Congenital longitudinal deficiencies of the femur are associated with deformity. Coxa vara and hypoplasia of the lateral femoral condyle are not uncommon, requiring correction by osteotomy **(a–c)** or hemiepiphyseodesis **(d)**.

Figure 43.2 ● Cruciate ligament deficiency is common in congenital causes of femoral shortening. It rarely produces symptoms of instability but is relevant if femoral lengthening is envisaged as knee subluxation may be induced during the process.

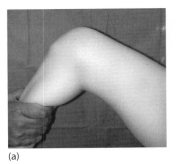
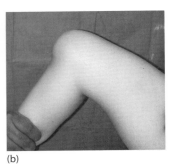

(a) (b)

Foot anomalies

In keeping with other varieties of longitudinal deficiency of the lower limb, foot anomalies may also be present in congenital femoral hypoplasia. This may take the form of missing rays, tarsal coalitions and soft tissue contractures.[3,4,7,8] Early restoration of a functional position is needed and is certainly a prerequisite to walking.

Estimating discrepancy at maturity

Caution is needed when using straight line and multiplier techniques for estimating the final length discrepancy.[9,10] These methods work well for many congenital causes but the shape of the discrepancy curve can vary (Chapter 42, General principles of management of discrepancies of limb length in children) and is significantly different for overgrowth from fracture, poliomyelitis, congenital arteriovenous malformations, sequelae of neonatal hip sepsis or multiple physeal arrest from infarcts in septicaemia.[11] An alternative method of estimation is the graphical method of Eastwood and Cole.[12]

Soft tissue resistance in congenital causes and its relevance

Despite advances in both techniques and devices for limb lengthening, soft tissue resistance (and the consequent problems) remains a major obstacle in the congenital case. While bone formation is reliable, the same is not true of muscle; soft tissue contractures can lead to loss of knee joint movement, joint subluxation and even dislocation.[13–17] Major length discrepancies in the femur due to congenital causes, in the event of being managed through limb lengthening, need to be addressed gradually through staged procedures that equalize a small percentage (less than 20 percent) of the discrepancy at a time. This reduces the onus on the soft tissues and minimizes the risk of unrecoverable complications.

Aims of treatment

Treatment options

Factors to be taken into consideration while planning treatment

Planning stages of treatment

Treatment can be planned to coincide with periods that have least impact on schooling or performance in statutory academic examinations. Earlier intervention may be warranted if deformity associated with length discrepancy prevents satisfactory ambulation, if the problem is unlikely to improve with time (cf. anterolateral bowing of the femur) or is associated with a joint instability (hip or knee). In the case of a timely epiphyseodesis, surgery needs to proceed regardless but in other instances of limb lengthening or deformity correction, surgery can be planned accordingly. Most major femoral limb length discrepancies (predicted final discrepancy up to 20 cm) will need three stages of lengthening, perhaps with the inclusion of a contralateral epiphyseodesis.

- To improve gait: pattern, energy cost and walking tolerance
- To eradicate dependence on orthotics or shoe modifications
- To improve psychological self-esteem

No intervention

Minor discrepancies do not need treatment. While many surgeons would consider a threshold of 20–25 mm as that beyond which some form of equalization is needed, it should be borne in mind that compensatory mechanisms are so effective in some children and adolescents that even 30 mm discrepancies are tolerated without clear evidence of gait problems or fatigue.

Non-surgical

Non-surgical treatment is mainly in the form of shoe raises (lifts) for minor discrepancies and extension prostheses in the more severe examples. It is usual to find poor compliance with shoe raises once the child is old enough to be aware of peer pressure. Forcing compliance only adds to the angst between the child, parents and the treating surgeon. It may be preferable to await surgical correction. By contrast, in major discrepancies the orthotic appliance is usually accepted as it represents the only way for the child to walk efficiently.

Epiphyseodesis

This is a good technique for equalization if predicted final discrepancies are less than 5 cm and especially when the abnormal femur is over-long as in the case of discrepancy from arteriovenous malformations. It can also be used as part of a strategy of equalization together with lengthening the short femur in cases of large discrepancies. Techniques include drill and curettage[18] or screws.[19]

Limb lengthening

Since the adoption of principles of the Ilizarov method, this option has enabled equalization to be achieved with reasonable preservation of limb function. However, it is still faced with the problems of soft tissue resistance described above.

Limb shortening

This is a reasonable option for the skeletally mature who is above average height or if there are local or patient factors that deem lengthening the short limb too risky (unstable joints, scarring, infection). This can be done with plate and screw or intramedullary nail stabilization, with the expected extensor lag in quadriceps function recovering with time.

Threshold for length equalization by surgery

An absolute threshold for intervention based on the single parameter of length difference is unwise. Some individuals with discrepancies of nearly 30 mm cope very well and display little difficulty in walking. Similarly, offering surgical equalization over prosthetic management to a child with a large length discrepancy may risk producing a childhood of multiple hospitalizations and a leg with poor function, albeit equal in length.

Predicted length discrepancy

This can be extrapolated by using charts or multipliers (see Chapter 42, General principles of management of discrepancies of limb length in children). It is an important basis in decision-making as it provides the surgeon with a measure by which the task ahead is estimated. The predicted length discrepancy allows provisional categorization into those individuals with realistic prospects of limb reconstruction as opposed to those in whom surgery is better focused on facilitating efficient prosthetic use.

Deformity and joint instability

Congenital and acquired causes of femoral shortening may be associated with either or both of the above. They cannot be isolated from the overall consideration as all will contribute to the functional outcome. Deformity can be addressed concomitantly with surgery for length equalization. Joint instability in the hip is dealt with early. Knee instability due to traumatic causes may benefit from ligament reconstruction but congenital causes rarely present such a need; in exceptional cases bracing may be appropriate.

Patient and family circumstances

The undertaking of limb lengthening in stages is not easy for the child or family. The treatment period is lengthy, onerous and repeated. In some domestic situations it may be preferable to offer equalization through a combination of epiphyseodesis and waiting. Circumstances may change in early adulthood which may then allow the surgeon to consider limb lengthening for any remaining discrepancy. The social and psychological impact of limb lengthening should not be underestimated.[20,21]

School curriculum

This may be a relatively minor factor to the surgeon but has an important impact on the child's education. Staged surgery should be scheduled to fit into school years that can best tolerate the intrusion.

Recommended treatment

The outline of treatment of femoral length discrepancy due to congenital and acquired causes is shown in Tables 43.1 and 43.2 and the details of the recommended treatment are discussed here.

Monitoring and providing support

At first presentation, which can be at any age from infancy to adolescence, it is preferable for the treating surgeon to obtain an overall view of the problem. The questions that need answering will be:

- What is the expected final discrepancy?
- Is there a deformity?
- How many years of growth are there remaining?
- Is this a congenital or acquired cause of femoral shortening?

The answers to the questions will enable a provisional plan of management to be outlined based on the size of the surgical undertaking.

Prescription of shoe raises

Children who present early require a minimum of intervention – usually in the form of shoe modifications and follow up of the increasing discrepancy, until such time that surgery is necessary. Forcing compliance with shoe modifications is unhelpful; the often-mentioned risk of 'back problems' unless complied with is unproven.

Advocating deformity correction

It should be undertaken in conjunction with surgery for lengthening or epiphyseodesis in order to reduce the number of in-hospital events. An exception is the presence of hip joint dysplasia or such similar deformity that will benefit from early intervention.

Timing the epiphyseodesis

The Australian (Menelaus) method of estimation is helpful – about 10 mm of annual growth occurs at the distal femoral physis and 6 mm at the proximal tibial.[22,23] Whether epiphyseodesis is used as the sole definitive treatment or as part of an overall strategy to reduce length discrepancy between the sides, the timing can be judged from the said estimation or from more formal charting techniques (Moseley straight line,[10] Eastwood and Cole[12]).

Table 43.1 ● Treatment of femoral length discrepancy from congenital causes

INDICATIONS						
Estimated final discrepancy at skeletal maturity ≤5 cm			Estimated final discrepancy at skeletal maturity >5 cm			
Anterolateral bowing of femur	Femoral hypoplasia + No proximal femoral deformity OR Femoral overgrowth (arteriovenous malformation or hemihypertrophy)	Femoral hypoplasia + Proximal femoral deformity + Poor hip congruence and stability	Femoral hypoplasia + No proximal femoral deformity + Estimated adult height is within normal limits	Femoral hypoplasia + No proximal femoral deformity + Estimated adult height below normal limits	Femoral hypoplasia + Proximal femoral deformity + Poor hip congruence and stability + Estimated adult height is within normal limits	Femoral hypoplasia + Proximal femoral deformity + Poor hip congruence and stability + Estimated adult height below normal limits
⇩	⇩	⇩	⇩	⇩	⇩	⇩
Epiphyseodesis of opposite femur (if estimated adult height is within normal limits) OR Lengthening of short femur (if estimated adult height is lower than normal)	Epiphyseodesis of opposite femur (if estimated adult height is within normal limits) OR Lengthening of short femur (if estimated adult height is lower than normal) + Corrective osteotomy of distal femur if needed for valgus deformity	Improve hip congruence and stability before schooling + As in column 2	Staged lengthening + Contralateral epiphyseodesis + Treat distal femoral valgus if needed by supracondylar osteotomy or hemiepiphyseodesis	Staged lengthening + Treat distal femoral valgus if needed by supracondylar osteotomy or hemiepiphyseodesis	Improve hip congruence and stability before schooling + As in column 4	Improve hip congruence and stability before schooling + As in column 5
			TREATMENT			

Staging limb lengthening episodes

The estimated final discrepancy will determine the number of stages (Figure 43.3). In any single stage of lengthening it is advisable to keep the length gained to less than 20 percent of the original limb length; this minimizes the potential for generating damaging forces across the various joints.[24,25] Most lengthening is performed using external fixators. In major reconstructions, some leg length can be restored through lengthening the tibia as well; while this results in the knee joints at different levels, it is arguably safer than restoring all length through the femur alone. There is no evidence to suggest the difference in knee joint levels (which will inevitably arise if the length inequality is addressed through both femoral and tibial lengthening) affects the final functional outcome.

Dealing with final discrepancy at maturity

The use of intramedullary lengthening devices or shortening of the contralateral longer femur are viable options for the skeletally mature. They may make the 'final hurdle' in a programme of staged equalization more surmountable and avoid yet another episode of external fixator-driven treatment. Contralateral femoral shortening is apt if the individual is tall.

Table 43.2 ● Treatment of femoral length discrepancy from acquired causes

INDICATIONS						
Estimated final discrepancy at skeletal maturity <5 cm			Estimated final discrepancy at skeletal maturity 5–15 cm		Estimated final discrepancy at skeletal maturity >15 cm	
Discrepancy in the absence of deformity	Discrepancy + Coexisting deformity not due to asymmetric physeal bar	Discrepancy + Coexisting deformity due to asymmetric physeal bar	Discrepancy in the absence of deformity	Discrepancy with coexisting deformity	Discrepancy in the absence of deformity	Discrepancy with coexisting deformity
⇩ Epiphyseodesis of opposite femur and or tibia (if estimated adult height is within normal limits) OR Lengthening of short femur (if estimated adult height is lower than normal)	⇩ Single-stage corrective osteotomy + Limb lengthening	⇩ Single-stage corrective osteotomy + Epiphyseodesis of viable part of physis + Limb lengthening (some over-lengthening needed to account for growth arrest following epiphyseodesis)	⇩ Single- or two-stage lengthening	⇩ Deformity correction + Epiphyseodesis of viable part of physis + Two-stage limb lengthening	⇩ Two-stage lengthening + Contralateral epiphyseodesis	⇩ Deformity correction + Epiphyseodesis of viable part of physis + Two- or three-stage limb lengthening + Contralateral epiphyseodesis
TREATMENT						

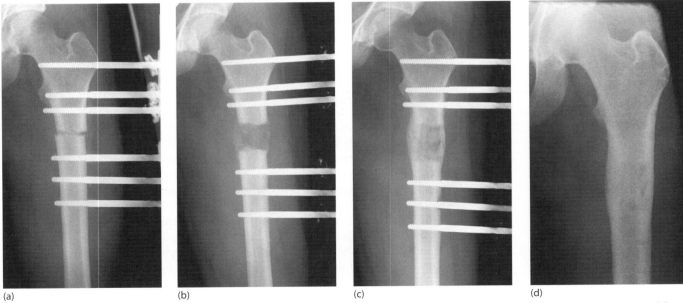

(a)　　　　　　(b)　　　　　　(c)　　　　　　(d)

Figure 43.3 ● Femoral lengthening is frequently performed through osteotomies in the subtrochanteric or supracondylar regions of the femur **(a)**. Stabilization with an external fixator facilitates controlled gradual elongation after an initial wait of five to ten days **(b)**; on reaching the desired length, a gradual strengthening of the regenerate column occurs. When sufficient consolidation is seen on radiograph (a homogeneous column with no defects and cortices beginning to form on both anteroposterior and lateral views) **(c)**, the external fixator can be removed **(d)**.

References

1. Stanitski DF, Kassab S. Rotational deformity in congenital hypoplasia of the femur. *J Pediatr Orthop* 1997; **17**: 525–7.
2. Pirani S, Beauchamp RD, Li D, Sawatzky B. Soft tissue anatomy of proximal femoral focal deficiency. *J Pediatr Orthop* 1991; **11**: 563–70.
3. Torode IP, Gillespie R. The classification and treatment of proximal femoral deficiencies. *Prosthet Orthot Int* 1991; **15**: 117–26.
4. Gillespie R, Torode IP. Classification and management of congenital abnormalities of the femur. *J Bone Joint Surg Br* 1983; **65**: 557–68.
5. Johansson E, Aparisi T. Missing cruciate ligament in congenital short femur. *J Bone Joint Surg Am* 1983; **65**: 1109–15.
6. Torode IP, Gillespie R. Anteroposterior instability of the knee: a sign of congenital limb deficiency. *J Pediatr Orthop* 1983; **3**: 467–70.
7. Pappas AM, Miller JT. Congenital ball-and-socket ankle joints and related lower-extremity malformations. *J Bone Joint Surg Am* 1982; **64**: 672–9.
8. Pappas AM. Congenital abnormalities of the femur and related lower extremity malformations: classification and treatment. *J Pediatr Orthop* 1983; **3**: 45–60.
9. Paley D, Bhave A, Herzenberg JE, Bowen JR. Multiplier method for predicting limb-length discrepancy. *J Bone Joint Surg Am* 2000; **82**: 1432–46.
10. Moseley CF. A straight-line graph for leg-length discrepancies. *J Bone Joint Surg Am* 1977; **59**: 174–9.
11. Shapiro F. Developmental patterns in lower-extremity length discrepancies. *J Bone Joint Surg Am* 1982; **64**: 639–51.
12. Eastwood DM, Cole WG. A graphic method for timing the correction of leg-length discrepancy. *J Bone Joint Surg Br* 1995; **77**: 743–7.
13. Glorion C, Pouliquen JC, Langlais J, Ceolin JL, Kassis B. Femoral lengthening using the callotasis method: study of the complications in a series of 70 cases in children and adolescents. *J Pediatr Orthop* 1996; **16**: 161–7.
14. Barker KL, Simpson AH, Lamb SE. Loss of knee range of motion in leg lengthening. *J Orthop Sports Phys Ther* 2001; **31**: 238–44; discussion 245–6.
15. Hosalkar HS, Jones S, Chowdhury M, Hartley J, Hill RA. Quadricepsplasty for knee stiffness after femoral lengthening in congenital short femur. *J Bone Joint Surg Br* 2003; **85**: 261–4.
16. Acharya A, Guichet J-M. Effect on knee motion of gradual intramedullary femoral lengthening. *Acta Orthop Belg* 2006; **72**: 569–77.
17. Barker KL, Shortt NL, Simpson HR. Predicting the loss of knee flexion during limb lengthening using inherent muscle length. *J Pediatr Orthop B* 2006; **15**: 404–7.
18. Canale ST, Christian CA. Techniques for epiphysiodesis about the knee. *Clin Orthop Relat Res* 1990: **255**: 81–5.
19. Metaizeau J-P, Wong-Chung J, Bertrand H, Pasquier P. Percutaneous epiphysiodesis using transphyseal screws (PETS). *J Pediatr Orthop* 1998; **18**: 363–9.
20. Ghoneem HF, Wright JG, Cole WG, Rang M. The Ilizarov method for correction of complex deformities. Psychological and functional outcomes. *J Bone Joint Surg Am* 1996; **78**: 1480–5.
21. Ramaker RR, Lagro SW, van Roermund PM *et al*. The psychological and social functioning of 14 children and 12 adolescents after Ilizarov leg lengthening. *Acta Orthop Scand* 2000; **71**: 55–9.
22. Menelaus MB. Correction of leg length discrepancy by epiphysial arrest. *J Bone Joint Surg Br* 1966; **48**: 336–9.
23. Westh RN, Menelaus MB. A simple calculation for the timing of epiphysial arrest: a further report. *J Bone Joint Surg Br* 1981; **63**: 117–19.
24. Stanitski DF. The effect of limb lengthening on articular cartilage. An experimental study. *Clin Orthop Relat Res* 1994: **301**: 68–72.
25. Stanitski DF, Rossman K, Torosian M. The effect of femoral lengthening on knee articular cartilage: the role of apparatus extension across the joint. *J Pediatr Orthop* 1996; **16**: 151–4.

Length discrepancy of the tibia

Selvadurai Nayagam

44

Introduction

Fibular hemimelia (see Chapter 35, Fibular hemimelia) is probably the most common congenital cause of a short tibia but it is a variant of a longitudinal deficiency. As such the femur is likely to be short and there may also be knee and foot anomalies. In contrast, leg length discrepancy arising only from the tibia should prompt the surgeon to look for specific diagnoses that typically produce this sign. When the condition presents in infancy, nearly all children have an associated deformity or radiological abnormality that heralds the diagnosis. These are:

- anterolateral bowing with or without concomitant tibial pseudarthrosis;
- posteromedial bowing;
- tibial hemimelia.

When the discrepancy is detected in later childhood, the cause can be one of many and some are present without deformity (Figure 44.1). They can be divided into those which are growth plate related, a result of bone dysplasia, neurological problems or a focal gigantism.

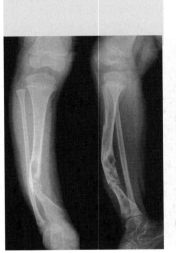

(a)

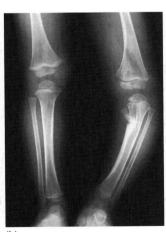

(b)

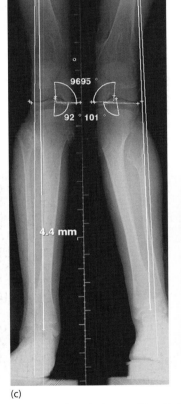

(c)

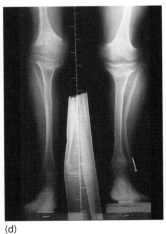

(d)

Figure 44.1 ● Bone, fibrous or cartilage dysplasias are conditions which produce tibial length abnormalities. Osteofibrous dysplasia, when extensive **(a)**, can produce deformity and length anomalies, as can enchondromas in Ollier's disease **(b)** and osteochondromas in the multiple hereditary form of the condition **(c)**. Growth plate damage from trauma or infection is the other major group; it is most marked when multiple physes are affected as can occur after meningococcal septicaemia **(d)**.

Growth plate disorders

Deformity is almost always present. Trauma and infection rank highest as causes, but physeal growth can be affected through the nearby presence of osteochondromas[1] and enchondromas.[2,3] Also included is infantile and adolescent Blount's disease.

Bone dysplasia

These include fibrous and osteofibrous dysplasia,[4,5] and focal fibrocartilaginous dysplasia.[6]

Neurological problems

Polio and cerebral palsy are principal causes. Occasionally, the idiopathic clubfoot deformity is accompanied by a significant tibial length discrepancy.[7]

Local gigantism

Neurofibromatosis can be a subtle cause, with café au lait spots appearing only later in childhood. In these cases anterolateral bowing may be absent but the ankle is in valgus owing to a wedged appearance to the epiphysis on the anteroposterior radiograph.

Problems of management

Predicting the final discrepancy

The techniques described in Chapter 42, General principles of management of discrepancies of limb length in children apply. One should be aware that not all will follow a type 1 Shapiro pattern and as such are not suitable for 'straight line' methods or multiplier techniques.

Addressing the length inequality – temporarily and definitively

Shoe raises can accommodate discrepancies of 3–4 cm and may be accepted by the child initially. Definitive treatment will depend on the final discrepancy, adult height potential, coexisting deformity and the presence of bone dysplasia. It may involve tibial lengthening or contralateral epiphyseodesis, and this may be done with surgical treatment for other features of the condition.

Addressing coexisting deformity

In many situations this will be the reason for surgery in the first instance. Small physeal bars may be successfully removed and restore balanced growth at the physis. When this is not possible, corrective osteotomies can be performed (simultaneously with lengthening if need be) and the procedure repeated when recurrence is significant. Where deformity arises because of bone 'disease', for example in congenital pseudarthrosis or osteofibrous dysplasia, segmental excision of the affected area may be needed and the limb then straightened; it follows that the resulting defect will need reconstruction. In general, restoring a normal mechanical axis to the limb is prioritized as deformity is usually the main cause of significant problems in walking; length discrepancy can be dealt with later.

Addressing the cause of discrepancy

This is possible in a few instances only; of note are small, accessible physeal tethers or benign tumours (osteochondromata) near the physis which can be excised. To a lesser extent, successful segmental resection of areas of pseudarthrosis or osteofibrous dysplasia can achieve the same.

Aims of treatment

- Restoration of normal limb alignment
- Equalization of limb length
- Preservation of knee and ankle joint function

Treatment options

Observation, shoe wear modification and epiphyseodesis

This is applicable for minor length discrepancies that are not associated with significant deformity. Surgical treatment for estimated final discrepancies of 2–5 cm will entail a contralateral epiphyseodesis.

Excising the physeal bridge with interposition

This is an established technique and works well for small physeal bridges; a prerequisite is that the bridge is mapped out by computed tomography (CT) scan or magnetic resonance imaging (MRI) before surgery (Figure 44.2). Success is better with centrally located bridges which occupy less than 30 percent of the total area of the physis (see Chapter 70, Physeal bar).

Completing the physeal arrest

Large tethers cannot be successfully removed. In order to avoid repeated corrective osteotomies, a completion of the physeal arrest and dealing with the consequent length inequality may be a more 'controlled' approach to a difficult problem.

Corrective osteotomy

This is a necessary adjunct to correcting length discrepancy if deformity is part of the problem (Figure 44.3). It may need to be repeated for physis–related problems unless exercising the physeal bridge with interposition or completing the physeal arrest are incorporated.

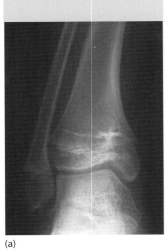
(a)
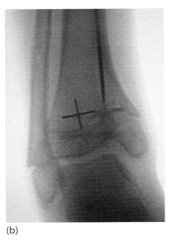
(b)
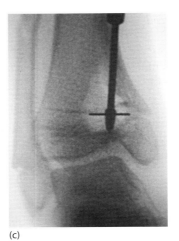
(c)
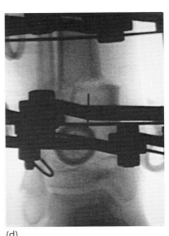
(d)

Figure 44.2 ● Physeal tethers produce anomalous growth leading to shortening and deformity **(a)**. In selected ones, usually determined by magnetic resonance imaging, epiphyseolyis accompanied by corrective osteotomy may resolve the problem **(b–d)**.

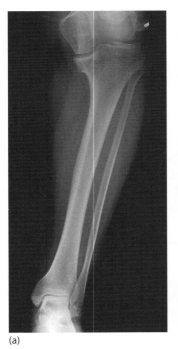
(a)
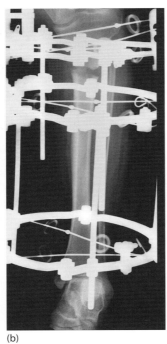
(b)
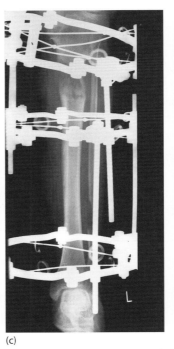
(c)
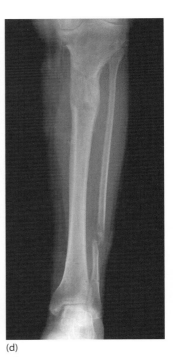
(d)

Figure 44.3 ● Simultaneous correction of deformity and length can be achieved using distraction osteogenesis **(a–d)**.

Limb lengthening

The need for lengthening will depend on the underlying cause of tibial shortening and the predicted final discrepancy. Some measure of lengthening is likely to be needed for early onset physeal tethers, particularly if these are located at both the proximal and distal tibia.

Major segmental tibial resection and reconstruction with bone transport or free vascularized fibula transfer

This technique is more likely to be needed for congenital pseudarthrosis due to neurofibromatosis or extensive osteofibrous dysplasia.

Several of the aetiologies listed above are dealt with separately and the relevant chapters should be consulted.

Spontaneous resolution

Limited tibial involvement by osteofibrous dysplasia is noted to offer the possibility of resolution by puberty.[5] In more extensive or progressive lesions the possibilities of fracture and pseudoarthrosis or the presence of an adamantinoma have prompted a more radical approach in the form of an extraperiosteal resection followed by reconstruction of the defect.[4]

In focal fibrocartilaginous dysplasia the infantile and early childhood tibia vara can spontaneously improve if the degree of varus is less than 30° but a length discrepancy may still need treatment.[6]

Deformity – degree, progression and recurrence

This may prompt correction even before the length discrepancy is significant. Correction is appropriate if the size of deformity predisposes to a fracture or interferes with activity.

In the case of partial physeal arrest, the size and site of the tether (whether produced through infection or trauma) acts as an indicator of the likely success should an attempt at removal be undertaken. CT scan or MRI mapping is helpful. A successful excision of a physeal bridge removes the problem and terminates the process of deformity and length discrepancy.

With other diagnoses, the cause may not be removable and repeated corrections should be anticipated.

Final length discrepancy

This influences the choice of strategy for equalization, as does the height potential and the presence of other features (e.g. deformity) that necessitate surgery. An approach is provided in the chapter on general principles (Chapter 42, General principles of management of discrepancies of limb length in children).

Factors to be taken into consideration while planning treatment

Recommended treatment

This is outlined in Table 44.1 and refers only to conditions where the discrepancy is solely in the tibia; consequently, fibula hemimelia is excluded and dealt with in Chapter 35, Fibular hemimelia.

Tibial length discrepancies not associated with deformity are treated along the lines described in Chapter 42, General principles of management of discrepancies of limb length in children. Tibial hemimelia (Chapter 36, Tibial hemimelia), anterolateral and posteromedial tibial bowing (Chapters 10, Anterolateral bowing of the tibia and congenital pseudarthrosis of the tibia and 11, Posteromedial bowing of the tibia) are also dealt with in separate chapters.

Table 44.1 ● Treatment of tibial length discrepancy

INDICATIONS					
Tibial shortening <5 cm + No deformity + Anticipated adult height normal	Tibial shortening <5 cm + No deformity + Anticipated adult height below normal OR Tibial shortening >5 cm	Tibial shortening <5 cm + Deformity with tendency for spontaneous correction (e.g. in posteromedial bowing, focal fibrocartilaginous dysplasia)	Tibial shortening + Deformity secondary to localized removable cause (e.g. physeal bar or juxta-physeal osteochondrom a)	Tibial shortening + Deformity secondary to progressive bone dysplasia (e.g. osteofibrous dysplasia)	Tibial shortening + Deformity due to extensive physeal arrest
⇩	⇩	⇩	⇩	⇩	⇩
Contralateral epiphyseodesis of tibia and fibula	Lengthening of short tibia	Monitor for improvement of angular alignment + Deal with shortening as in column 1 or 2	Corrective osteotomy + Excision of offending lesion (physeal bar or osteochondroma) + Deal with shortening as in column 1 or 2	Excise affected segment with simultaneous corrective osteotomy + Reconstruction of defect and concurrent limb lengthening + Deal with shortening as in column 1 or 2 should further discrepancy develop	Corrective osteotomy (repeated as necessary in early childhood) + Completion of physeal arrest (to prevent recurrence of deformity) + Epiphyseodesis of fibula + Limb lengthening in one or two stages (depending on severity of discrepancy)
TREATMENT					

References

1. Schmale GA, Conrad EU, Raskind WH. The natural history of hereditary multiple exostoses. *J Bone Joint Surg Am* 1994; **76**: 986–92.
2. Baumgart R, Burklein D, Hinterwimmer S, Thaller P, Mutschler W. The management of leg-length discrepancy in Ollier's disease with a fully implantable lengthening nail. *J Bone Joint Surg Br* 2005; **87**: 1000–4.
3. D'Angelo G, Petas N, Donzelli O. Lengthening of the lower limbs in Ollier's disease: problems related to surgery. *Chir Organi Mov* 1996; **81**: 279–85.
4. Lee RS, Weitzel S, Eastwood DM *et al*. Osteofibrous dysplasia of the tibia. Is there a need for a radical surgical approach? *J Bone Joint Surg Br* 2006; **88**: 658–64.
5. Campanacci M, Laus M. Osteofibrous dysplasia of the tibia and fibula. *J Bone Joint Surg Am* 1981; **63**: 367–75.
6. Dusabe J-P, Docquier P-L, Mousny M, Rombouts J-J. Focal fibrocartilaginous dysplasia of the tibia: long-term evolution. *Acta Orthop Belg* 2006; **72**: 77–82.
7. Shimode K, Miyagi N, Majima T, Yasuda K, Minami A. Limb length and girth discrepancy of unilateral congenital clubfeet. *J Pediatr Orthop B* 2005; **14**: 280–4.

Discrepancies of length in the fibula

Selvadurai Nayagam

45

Introduction

The fibula does not grow at the same rate as the tibia; neither is the growth rate equal at its proximal and distal physes. This means that proximal and distal tibiofibular relationships change with growth. At birth there is a relative shortening of the fibula at the ankle and a consequent valgus tilt of the mortise (Figure 45.1) – this reduces to 6° at the age of five years and eventually becomes neutral (about 90° to the long axis of the tibia) by the age of ten. This natural change of relationship at the ankle mortise is a consequence of:

- greater growth at the proximal fibula compared with the proximal tibia;[1]
- greater growth at the distal tibial physis compared with the distal fibula but not overcoming the length increase from the proximal fibula physis, thus leading to a gradual overall 'descent' of the lateral malleolus.[2]

Problems of disproportionate length relationships between tibia and fibula can manifest as deformity of the knee or ankle joint (Figure 45.2). The causes are:

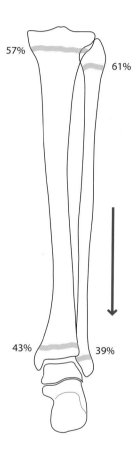

Figure 45.1 ● The proximal fibula physis grows faster than the distal. It also grows faster than the proximal tibial physis; both factors lead to a gradual descent of the distal fibula in the ankle mortise.

- Events (e.g. fracture, infection) which produce either a physeal arrest of the tibia or fibula; depending on which end of the leg is affected, the consequences may be either varus or valgus at the ankle or problems at the proximal tibiofibular joint.
- Bone dysplasias which include:
  - Achondroplasia (usually a varus ankle): Relative overgrowth of the fibula in achondroplasia has been linked to genu varum and a varus ankle alignment. The proximal tibiofibular joint is either subluxed or dislocated but, fortunately, seldom symptomatic. However, varus limb alignment at the knee and ankle are the usual presenting features.
  - Hereditary multiple osteochondromata (usually a valgus ankle).[3]
- Congenital hypoplasia, e.g. fibula hemimelia (usually a valgus ankle).
- Clubfoot (sometimes ankle valgus despite a varus inclination of the calcaneum at the subtalar joint).[4]
- Myelodysplasia or paralytic disorders (usually a valgus ankle).[5]
- Surgical resection of the shaft of the fibula, especially in the distal third, producing a valgus ankle.[6–8]
- Fibular pseudarthrosis from neurofibromatosis,[9] also leading to a valgus ankle.

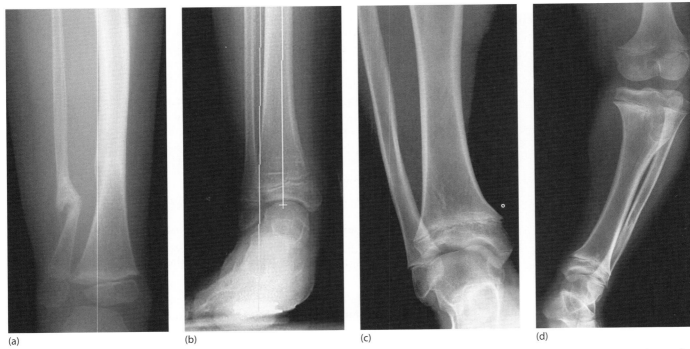

(a)   (b)   (c)   (d)

Figure 45.2 ● Disproportion between fibula and tibial lengths produce ankle or knee deformities. When the fibula is short at the ankle as the result of a pseudarthrosis **(a)** or congenital hemimelia **(b)**, a valgus deformity follows. Conversely, when overlong as in achondroplasia **(c,d)**, the resultant deformity at the knee and ankle is in varus.

Problems of management

Abnormal ankle alignment (varus or valgus) and consequent problems of stability

A change in the talocrural angle (Figure 45.3) will occur if the fibula (lateral malleolus) is too long or short at the ankle. This produces a tilt which, if minor, can be compensated for by a mobile subtalar joint.

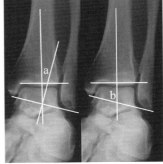

Figure 45.3 ● The talocrural angle describes the inclination of the tibial plafond in relation to a transmalleolar axis in a mortise view of the ankle. It can be measured in two ways: **(a)** the angle subtended by the two lines which varies between 8 and 15° (shown here as the angle between two perpendiculars drawn to the reference lines); **(b)** the angle between the perpendicular to the ankle plafond and the transmalleolar axis which ranges between 75 and 87°. Comparisons to the contralateral normal side should reveal less than 5° of variation.

However, if the deformity is moderate or cannot be compensated for by the subtalar joint, it can lead to fibula impingement, recurrent medial (valgus) or lateral ligament (varus) sprains. Clinical instability must be demonstrated and treatment not simply directed at radiograph measurements – note it is normal to have some degree of valgus at the ankle prior to the age of ten.

Subluxation of the proximal tibiofibular joint

The greater longitudinal growth of the fibula (as compared with the tibia) is exaggerated if either the proximal or distal tibial physis is damaged. Bowing of the fibula and eventual subluxation of the proximal tibiofibular joint may occur in order to accommodate the greater fibular length. The patient notices a prominent lump on the outer side of the knee which may or may not be painful.

Aims of treatment

- Restore ankle alignment and stability
- Stop development of a progressive deformity
- Improve local symptoms from a subluxed or dislocated proximal tibiofibular joint

Treatment options

Epiphyseodesis of the relevant physis

This will address a length imbalance only if the corresponding adjacent physis is growing normally.

Fibula lengthening or shortening

This applies to the ankle and is sometimes combined with corrective osteotomies of the distal tibia.

Distal tibial/fibula osteotomies

This can be dome or wedge osteotomies.

Restoring the structural integrity of the distal fibula

This applies to congenital pseudarthrosis or a non-union of the fibula which develops after a segment of the shaft is used as a source of strut graft.

Factors to be taken into consideration while planning treatment

Aetiology

While the underlying aetiology producing length disproportion between fibula and tibia may differ, the strategies described above are generally applicable. The exception to the rule is congenital pseudarthrosis of the fibula (often in association with neurofibromatosis) where a change of approach is needed in recognition of the poor results from standard surgical strategies.

Age and growth remaining

The simplest strategies lie with epiphyseodesis of the relevant physis. If this is performed with at least two years of growth remaining, a substantial correction can be anticipated and, with the exception of the most severe deformities, without recourse to any further surgery. This is helped further in that new techniques of hemiepiphyseodesis are available which are reversible on removal of implant.[10,11]

Mobility of the subtalar joint

Correction of the tilt of the ankle mortise should be considered in conjunction with the range of movement in the subtalar joint. A mobile subtalar joint tolerates alterations of ankle tilt and the forefoot can be placed flat on the ground after surgery. Conversely, a stiff subtalar joint has a fixed relationship between hindfoot and forefoot (midfoot movements are significantly diminished by a stiff subtalar joint) and therefore surgery to alter the position of the hindfoot must take into account the corresponding changes in position to the forefoot.

Recommended treatment

Ankle valgus from distal fibula shortening

For more details the reader is directed to Chapter 8, Valgus deformity of the ankle and subtalar joint.

■ Medial hemiepiphyseodesis of the distal tibia

It is not uncommon for relative shortening of the fibula at the ankle to be associated with a wedge-shaped distal tibial epiphysis.[3,12–14] If the distal fibula physis is growing normally, hemiepiphyseal arrest on the medial side of the distal tibial physis will gradually restore the talocrural angle. This can be accomplished by an oblique screw, staples or an 8-plate.[3,11,13,15] The technique is suitable if sufficient growth remains in the child (at least two years) and the cause of fibula shortening was not an arrest of the distal fibula physis.

■ Fibula lengthening

Step-cut lengthening was the usual technique before distraction osteogenesis, according to the principles of Ilizarov, became widely known.[3,16] Limitations in acute lengthening arise from resistance of the interosseous membrane – this needs to be divided and released along a segment of the distal fibula before 6–7 mm of lengthening can be accomplished. This restriction is overcome if a gradual lengthening technique is used.[17]

Fibula lengthening should be considered if:

- the distal fibula physis is closed;
- the valgus malalignment thereby arises principally from lack of lateral support from a short lateral malleolus;
- alignment of the tibial plafond to the tibial axis in the coronal plane is near normal (i.e. without a valgus tilt arising from a wedge-shaped epiphysis).

Traumatic or post-septic arrest of the distal fibula physis falls in this category. If the distal tibial physis is open and the child skeletally immature, a distal tibial epiphyseodesis may need to be done after fibula lengthening to avoid recurrence of deformity.

■ Supramalleolar osteotomy

If the fibula and tibial physes are closed and there is a valgus tilt to the tibial plafond, correction by a dome or wedge osteotomy will address the ankle malalignment.

Ankle valgus from fibula pseudarthrosis

■ Bone grafting and internal fixation

When fibula shaft resections (for use as autogenous strut grafts) lead to the development of a pseudarthrosis and proximal migration of the lateral malleolus, bone graft and internal fixation across the defect can resolve both problems simultaneously. Restoration of the structural integrity of the fibula permits the contribution of longitudinal growth from the proximal fibula physis to effect a gradual descent of the lateral malleolus and reduction of valgus tilt.[18]

■ Tibia-pro-fibula synostosis

Unlike the clinical scenario above, congenital pseudarthrosis of the fibula shares the same dismal outcome with the tibia if bone grafting attempts are made to bridge the defect. Ankle stability and cessation of increasing ankle valgus can be resolved by creating a cross-union between tibia and fibula proximal to the syndesmosis.[9]

A ball and socket type of ankle joint

This clinically valgus alignment of the ankle arises from both a short fibula and abnormal shape of the tibial plafond. It is associated with a congenital tarsal coalition which abolishes subtalar movement.

■ Orthotic use

A valgus heel support is sufficient for those who have mild symptoms.

■ Surgery

A hemiepiphyseodesis of the medial side of the distal tibial physis is simplest (Figure 45.4a). This can be accomplished using a transphyseal screw or 8-plate,[11,19] both of which produce less local irritation or prominence than staples.

Ankle varus from excessive distal fibula length

■ Distal fibula epiphyseodesis

Two screws across the distal fibula physis will arrest longitudinal growth (Figure 45.4e). Contribution from the proximal fibula physis to continued descent of the lateral malleolus must not be underestimated – it will take at least two years before the distal tibia is able to grow and restore an appropriate talocrural angle. Once this is obtained, it is then necessary to carry out an epiphyseodesis of the distal tibia lest a valgus deformity ensues. Any significant leg length discrepancies in the tibia can then be attended to by a timely contralateral proximal tibial epiphyseodesis (note the distal tibia contributes approximately 3 mm to leg length annually compared with 6 mm from the proximal tibia).

■ Distal tibial lengthening

The tibia can be lengthened independently of the fibula; this is indicated when the tibial plafond is neutral in alignment but the heel tilted into varus from an overlong fibula. Gradual descent of the distal tibia can be titrated until the talocrural angle is restored.

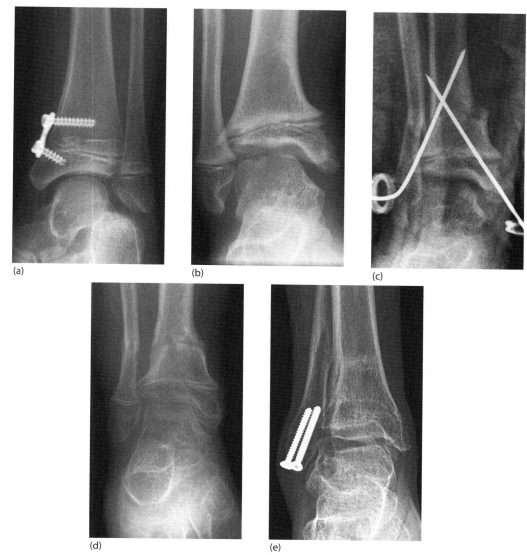

(a)   (b)   (c)

(d)   (e)

Figure 45.4 ● A short fibula in fibula hemimelia produces a valgus alignment of a ball-and-socket ankle joint. Hemiepiphyseodesis of the medial tibial physis helps to restore the length proportions **(a)**. An overlong fibula in achondroplasia produces a varus ankle. A supramalleolar osteotomy realigns the joint **(b–d)**. If the fibula is relatively too long as in achondroplasia or a consequence of distal tibial growth arrest **(e)**, a screw epiphyseodesis may help.

■ Supramalleolar osteotomy

A dome or wedge osteotomy is indicated if the tibial plafond is itself tilted in varus. An opening wedge osteotomy of the distal tibia can be combined with fibula shortening, thereby simultaneously addressing both length relationships and ankle alignment (Figure 45.4b–d).[20]

Subluxation of the proximal tibiofibular joint

This occurs with excessive fibula length. It is usually seen in achondroplasia in which laxity of the lateral collateral ligament of the knee is associated. Fortunately, proximal tibiofibular joint subluxation that develops gradually as a consequence of altered length relationships between tibia and fibula is not usually symptomatic – sometimes the patient notices the prominent fibula head laterally. If detected early and before skeletal maturity, a proximal fibular epiphyseodesis is helpful in resolving, or at least arresting, progression of lateral prominence of the fibula head. If laxity of the lateral collateral ligament is the main issue and the patient is skeletally mature, a proximal tibial lengthening can be performed with gradual distal transport of the fibula head.[21]

Rationale of treatment suggested

A length disproportion between fibula and tibia usually causes problems at the ankle joint. Small degrees of ankle varus are less well tolerated than equivalent degrees of valgus. Epiphyseodesis is a simple surgical technique which, if employed with sufficient growth remaining, can resolve many of these deformities. Even in premature physeal closure of the distal fibula, some distal migration of the lateral malleolus is possible due to the contribution of the proximal fibula physis – as long as the distal tibial physis is surgically closed early enough. The other strategies of treatment are described to provide solutions when epiphyseodesis is not feasible, when one or other physis is closed or for an adolescent near or after skeletal maturity (Table 45.1).

Table 45.1 ● Treatment of ankle deformity as a result of abnormalities of fibula length

INDICATIONS					
Valgus ankle from short fibula			Varus ankle from long fibula		
Congenital ball and socket ankle joint + Wedge-shaped distal tibial physis + 2 years growth remaining	Normal plafond alignment + Closed distal fibula physis + Skeletally immature OR Normal plafond alignment + Skeletally mature	Valgus plafond alignment + Skeletally mature	Open distal tibial physis + 2 years growth remaining	Normal plafond alignment + Closed distal tibial physis + Skeletally immature OR Normal plafond alignment + Skeletally mature ⇩ Distal tibial lengthening + Distal fibula epiphyseodesis on restoration of talocrural angle (if skeletally immature)	Varus plafond alignment + Skeletally mature ⇩ Supramalleolar osteotomy
⇩ Medial hemiepiphyseodesis of distal tibia	⇩ Fibula lengthening + Distal tibial epiphyseodesis on restoration of talocrural angle (if skeletally immature)	⇩ Supramalleolar osteotomy	⇩ Distal fibular epiphyseodesis		
TREATMENT					

References

1. Pritchett JW. Growth and growth prediction of the fibula. *Clin Orthop Relat Res* 1997; **334**: 251–6.
2. Karrholm J, Hansson LI, Selvik G. Changes in tibiofibular relationships due to growth disturbances after ankle fractures in children. *J Bone Joint Surg Am* 1984; **66**: 1198–210.
3. Snearly WN, Peterson HA. Management of ankle deformities in multiple hereditary osteochondromata. *J Pediatr Orthop* 1989; **9**: 427–32.
4. Stevens PM, Otis S. Ankle valgus and clubfeet. *J Pediatr Orthop* 1999; **19**: 515–17.
5. Dias LS. Valgus deformity of the ankle joint: pathogenesis of fibular shortening. *J Pediatr Orthop* 1985; **5**: 176–80.
6. Hsu LC, Yau AC, O'Brien JP, Hodgson AR. Valgus deformity of the ankle resulting from fibular resection for a graft in subtalar fusion in children. *J Bone Joint Surg Am* 1972; **54**: 585–94.
7. Frick SL. Valgus deformity after fibular resection in children. *J Pediatr Orthop* 2004; **24**: 345; author reply 345–6.
8. Frick SL, Shoemaker S, Mubarak SJ. Altered fibular growth patterns after tibiofibular synostosis in children. *J Bone Joint Surg Am* 2001; **83**: 247–54.
9. Langenskiold A. Pseudoarthrosis of the fibula and progressive valgus deformity of the ankle in children: treatment by fusion of the distal tibial and fibular metaphyses. Review of three cases. *J Bone Joint Surg Am* 1967; **49**: 463–70.

10. Khoury J, Tavares J, McConnell S, Zeiders G, Sanders J. Results of screw epiphysiodesis for the treatment of limb length discrepancy and angular deformity. *J Pediatr Orthop* 2007; **27**: 623–8.

11. Stevens PM. Guided growth for angular correction: a preliminary series using a tension band plate. *J Pediatr Orthop* 2007; **27**: 243–59.

12. Wiltse LL. Valgus deformity of the ankle – a sequel to acquired or congenital abnormalities of the fibula. *J Bone Joint Surg Am* 1972; **54**: 595–606.

13. Burkus JK, Moore DW, Raycroft JF. Valgus deformity of the ankle in myelodysplastic patients. Correction by stapling of the medial part of the distal tibial physis. *J Bone Joint Surg Am* 1983; **65**: 1157–62.

14. Stevens PM. Relative hypoplasia of the fibula and associated ankle valgus. *J Pediatr Orthop* 1987; **7**: 605.

15. Stevens PM, Belle RM. Screw epiphysiodesis for ankle valgus. *J Pediatr Orthop* 1997; **17**: 9–12.

16. Weber D, Friederich NF, Muller W. Lengthening osteotomy of the fibula for post-traumatic malunion. Indications, technique and results. *Int Orthop* 1998; **22**: 149–52.

17. Rozbruch SR, DiPaola M, Blyakher A. Fibula lengthening using a modified Ilizarov method. *Orthopedics* 2002; **25**: 1241–4.

18. Hsu LC, O'Brien JP, Yau AC, Hodgson AR. Valgus deformity of the ankle in children with fibular pseudarthrosis. Results of treatment by bone-grafting of the fibula. *J Bone Joint Surg Am* 1974; **56**: 503–10.

19. Stevens PM, Aoki S, Olson P. Ball-and-socket ankle. *J Pediatr Orthop* 2006; **26**: 427–31.

20. Beals RK, Stanley G. Surgical correction of bowlegs in achondroplasia. *J Pediatr Orthop B* 2005; **14**: 245–9.

21. Paley D, Bhatnagar J, Herzenberg JE, Bhave A. New procedures for tightening knee collateral ligaments in conjunction with knee realignment osteotomy. *Orthop Clin North Am* 1994; **25**: 533–55.

Length discrepancy in metatarsals

Selvadurai Nayagam

46

Introduction

In a paediatric setting, congenital causes of length discrepancy in metatarsals (brachymetatarsia) are more likely than acquired causes. Two common scenarios that present to the surgeon are: the adolescent female who has a short fourth metatarsal and as a consequence an unsightly fourth toe or the young child with a short first metatarsal (sometimes associated with duplication of the great toe) which presents as transfer metatarsalgia. Occasionally, length discrepancy of metatarsals is seen in Down or Apert syndrome. Acquired causes of short metatarsals in children are uncommon, with trauma[1] or infective complications to the growth plate being principal reasons.

Another condition where length discrepancy of the rays can be encountered is macrodactyly. Brachymetatarsia and macrodactyly are considered separately as the approach to treatment differs profoundly.

Brachymetatarsia

Problems of management

Decision to intervene in asymptomatic children

Many children with a length discrepancy of the metatarsals are asymptomatic. Problems usually arise in adolescence when perceptions of body image take precedence.

Problems with shoe wear

Occasionally, there are pressure-related problems caused by the associated toe deformities (the toe of a short fourth ray is usually elevated and rubs against the upper leather of the shoe; a short first ray can be associated with hallux valgus or varus) or there is reluctance on the part of the teenager to use adapted shoes.

Transfer metatarsalgia

A short metatarsal may lead to excessive loading of adjacent metatarsal heads and metatarsalgia.

Associated deformity of toes

The deformity of the toe may be the first presenting complaint (Figure 46.1) and the short metatarsal then identified on radiograph. Both problems are related and should not be addressed in isolation.

Aims of treatment

- Facilitate comfort and fitting in normal shoes
- Reduce transfer metatarsalgia
- Improve an unsightly deformity

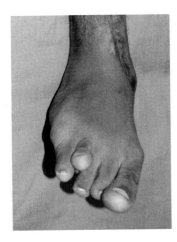

Figure 46.1 ● A short metatarsal may present as a toe deformity in this example of brachymetatarsia involving the fourth ray.

Treatment options

Observation and shoe wear modification

Observation is all that is needed if presentation is in early childhood. Symptoms may not manifest until later when the child is older and more conscious of their body image. Metatarsalgia can be relieved by insole modifications. Toe deformities can be accommodated by footwear alterations. Poor relief from these shoe adjustments (or reluctance to accept a continued need for them) added to the visual impact of the deformity usually prompts a review of the surgical options.

Surgical options

There are three surgical strategies for addressing length inequality: lengthening the short ray, shortening neighbouring long rays or a combination of both. With lengthening, both acute and gradual techniques are used – acute if the target lengthening is under 15 mm and gradual if greater.[2] Choice may be dictated by the surgeon's familiarity with a particular technique and other individual patient factors.

■ Metatarsal shortening strategy

This is performed in neighbouring rays – and includes metatarsals and proximal phalanges (see Bilateral brachymetatarsia). As much as 8 mm is possible although local soft tissue conditions may restrict the final quantity. This technique is usually employed when dealing with a short fourth ray, where reducing the length of second and third rays may either obviate the need of fourth ray lengthening or reduce the target length needed from lengthening.

■ Metatarsal lengthening strategy

Acute lengthening is performed by the application of a distractor in an osteotomy and slowly expanding the gap while the patient remains under anaesthesia. As much as 15 mm can be achieved, and the space then filled with bone graft. Gradual lengthening is accomplished with an external fixator applied in accordance with the principles of callotasis; bone graft is not usually needed.

■ Combined surgical strategies

In severe brachymetatarsia, shortening neighbouring rays can partially restore normal length relationships of the metatarsals, leaving the remaining difference to be obtained from lengthening of the short ray. This combined approach is important in cases with a >50 percent length discrepancy; addressing this magnitude of discrepancy purely by gradual lengthening techniques is associated with a high risk of complications.

Factors to be taken into consideration while planning treatment

The parabolic curve defined by the metatarsal heads

The metatarsal heads of a normal foot outline a parabolic arch. The normal first metatarsal can hold one of three relationships with the second ray[3]: (a) shorter (40 percent), (b) equal (22 percent) or (c) longer (38 percent) (Figure 46.2). However, these differences, when present, are in the order of a few millimetres. In contrast, the shortening in brachymetatarsia is many millimetres and can be less than half the length of neighbouring metatarsals. The parabolic arch of the normal contralateral foot can be used as a guide to the degree of shortening for the affected side. This is important if transfer metatarsalgia is present as a consequence of shortening of the first ray.

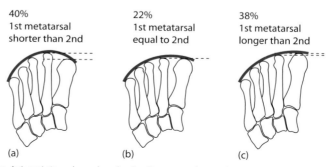

40%
1st metatarsal shorter than 2nd

22%
1st metatarsal equal to 2nd

38%
1st metatarsal longer than 2nd

(a)   (b)   (c)

Figure 46.2 ● The 1st metatarsal can be shorter than, equal to or longer than the second. The differences in length are usually small, a few millimetres at most. The metatarsal heads and tips of the toes subtend parabolic curves and surgery to adjust length discrepancies between metatarsals should recreate the curve defined on the normal contralateral side.

The presence of a plantarflexion deformity of the first ray

In some congenital short first rays the first metatarsal is plantarflexed. Lengthening this ray along the axis of the metatarsal may produce excessive loading of the first metatarsal head; the antero-posterior radiograph of the foot which allows the parabolic curve to be defined will mislead the surgeon to over-lengthening unless this sagittal plane deformity is identified in a weight bearing lateral radiograph of the foot. This enables an adjustment to the quantity of first ray lengthening to be made or a dorsiflexion osteotomy to correct the deformity prior to lengthening.

The length of the phalanges

The tips of the distal phalanges also outline a parabolic arch. Similarly, as with the arch defined by the metatarsal heads, the normal side can serve as a reference for surgical planning. When the purpose of surgery is to improve an unsightly deformity of the toes, matching the parabolic curve as defined by the tips of the distal phalanges is probably a more useful guide than that of the metatarsal heads.

The number of rays affected

When multiple rays are affected, a combination of shortening and lengthening strategies to restore the parabolic curve is usually necessary. Bone harvested from metatarsal shortening can conveniently be used as a graft for acute lengthening of short rays.[4]

Bilateral brachymetatarsia

When the same ray is affected in both feet, the template from a normal contralateral foot is obviously absent. Using the second ray as an index (the second ray is rarely affected), the ratio of the length of the first metatarsal to the second is 0.9 and that of the fourth metatarsal 1.0 in the feet of a random group of normal subjects. In brachymetatarsia, the ratios are reduced to 0.7 and 0.8 for the first and fourth metatarsals, respectively. Thus, the length of the second metatarsal serves as a guide for correction. A similar scenario is found with ratios of the lengths of proximal phalanges; again, using the second ray as the index, the ratios are 1.0 and 0.9 for the first and fourth proximal phalanges in normal feet. In those with brachymetatarsia, the ratios are altered to 0.8 and 0.7. This implies brachymetatarsia is a shortening of the ray and not just of the metatarsal. It emphasizes the need to recognize shortening of the proximal phalanx as part of the problem and, where significant, the inequality in length not addressed by lengthening of the metatarsal alone. In such situations, consideration should be given to shortening of neighbouring proximal phalanges.

Local soft tissue conditions

This may influence the choice between acute or gradual techniques, with the latter being more suited when poor soft tissue conditions render large incisions and acute changes of length risky.

Familiarity with technique

Both acute and gradual techniques of metatarsal lengthening can be fraught with complications,[2,5,6] which the surgeon will need to anticipate (Figure 46.3). In general, excessive brachymetatarsia of any single ray should be managed with a combination of techniques: shortening of neighbouring rays combined with a less ambitious lengthening of the affected ray.

Recommended treatment

The overall objective is to restore the parabolic arches of the metatarsal heads and toe tips using the simplest techniques or combination thereof. The percentage shortening and the affected ray will guide the surgeon as to which strategies are most useful. First ray shortening is usually addressed by lengthening; fourth ray shortening can be addressed by any of the techniques depending on the size of the discrepancy. In general, if callotasis is used, it is wise to reduce the target length (by shortening of neighbouring rays) to less than 40 percent as fewer complications are likely.

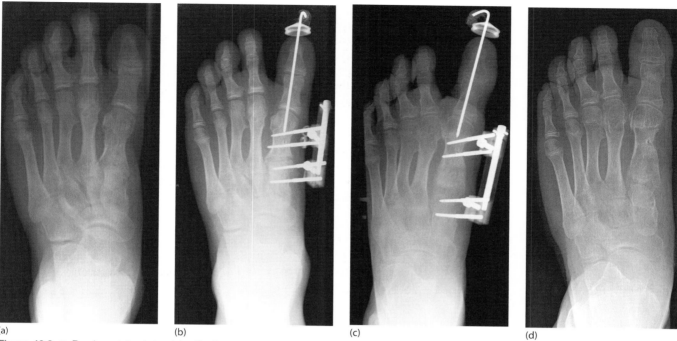

(a) (b) (c) (d)

Figure 46.3 ● Brachymetatarsia involving the first metatarsal **(a)** treated by gradual lengthening with an external fixator **(b–d)**. Metatarsal lengthening is based on the principles of distraction osteogenesis. A low energy osteotomy is made in the metaphyseal region and gradual distraction (usually 0.5 mm a day) is commenced after an interval delay of seven days. External fixator removal is after sufficient regenerate consolidation is visualized on the radiograph.

The outline of treatment is shown in Table 46.1.

Table 46.1 ● Outline of treatment of brachymetatarsia

INDICATIONS			
Symptomatic 1st or 4th ray shortening + Discrepancy 15 mm or less	Symptomatic 1st ray shortening + Discrepancy >15 mm + Overall target length <40% of original length of metatarsal ⇩	Symptomatic 4th ray shortening + Discrepancy >15 mm + Overall target length <40% of original length of metatarsal ⇩	Symptomatic 1st ray shortening + Discrepancy >40% of original length of metatarsal ⇩
⇩ Acute lengthening with bone graft	Gradual lengthening by callotasis	Shorten 2nd and 3rd metatarsals OR Gradual lengthening of 4th metatarsal by callotasis + Shortening of proximal phalanges of 2nd and 3rd rays if necessary to restore toe-tip parabolic arch	Shorten 2nd to 4th rays + Gradual lengthening of 1st ray by callotasis
TREATMENT			

Macrodactyly

Macrodactyly, which may affect one or more rays, is characterized by an abnormal increase in the girth and length of both the skeletal and soft tissue components of the affected ray (Figure 46.4). Macrodactyly can occur in a variety of conditions that include Klippel–Trenaunay–Weber syndrome, neurofibromatosis, Milroy disease and Proteus syndrome.[7,8] There appears to be two types of macrodactyly. In the first type, the toe is large from birth but the growth of the affected ray is proportionate to the growth of the rest of the foot. In the second type, there is rapid and disproportionate growth of the affected ray that far exceeds the normal growth of the rest of the skeleton.[8]

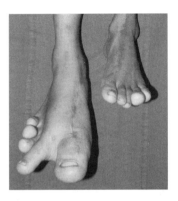

Figure 46.4 ● Macrodactyly affecting the first and second rays of the right foot in a child. There is a minor degree of macrodactyly of the fourth toe of the left foot.

An attempt must be made to reduce the girth and length of the foot and to try to restore the size of the foot to near normal by skeletal maturity. Strategies for reducing the girth include soft tissue debulking and ray amputation while the options for reducing the length include epiphyseodesis of the phalanges and the metatarsals, shortening of the metatarsal and excision of a phalanx. In the type of macrodactyly with rapid and excessive growth, early epiphyseodesis should be done while in the other type epiphyseodesis can be deferred until the length of the ray is close to the anticipated adult length.

References

1. Marcinko DE, Rappaport MJ, Gordon S. Post-traumatic brachymetatarsia. *J Foot Surg* 1984; **23**: 451–3.
2. Kim HT, Lee SH, Yoo CI, Kang JH, Suh JT. The management of brachymetatarsia. *J Bone Joint Surg Br* 2003; **85**: 683–90.
3. Harris RI, Beath T. The short first metatarsal: its incidence and clinical significance. *J Bone Joint Surg Am* 1949; **31**: 553–65.
4. Kim JS, Baek GH, Chung MS, Yoon PW. Multiple congenital brachymetatarsia. A one-stage combined shortening and lengthening procedure without iliac bone graft. *J Bone Joint Surg Br* 2004; **86**: 1013–15.
5. Choi IH, Chung MS, Baek GH, Cho TJ, Chung CY. Metatarsal lengthening in congenital brachymetatarsia: one-stage lengthening versus lengthening by callotasis. *J Pediatr Orthop* 1999; **19**: 660–4.
6. Oh CW, Satish BRJ, Lee S-T, Song H-R. Complications of distraction osteogenesis in short first metatarsals. *J Pediatr Orthop* 2004; **24**: 711–15.
7. Chang LH, Kumar SJ, Riddle EC, Glutting J. Macrodactyly of the foot. *J Bone Joint Surg Am* 2002; **84**: 1189–94.
8. Dennyson WG, Bear JN, Bhoola JD. Macrodactyly of the foot. *J Bone Joint Surg Br* 1977; **59**: 355–9.

Length discrepancy of the humerus

Selvadurai Nayagam

47

Introduction

Children tolerate minor and moderate length discrepancy in the upper limb well. Significant differences usually arise when the proximal humeral physis is damaged early in childhood, due to neonatal sepsis (Figure 47.1) or if the limb is congenitally hypoplastic. Less frequent causes are trauma or bone cysts, both of which can damage the proximal physis. Indications for undertaking limb equalization lie with the anticipated need for equality in length – sometimes this is brought upon by parental or patient pressure as a means to improve self-esteem and body image. At other times the need for equality in humeral length is seen as important for undertaking certain activities which involve coordinated movements between the arms – examples are playing the piano, typing, field sports which use sticks (hockey, golf), bats (cricket, baseball) or similar items. Even in these circumstances only large differences in humeral length are likely to have an impact on function.

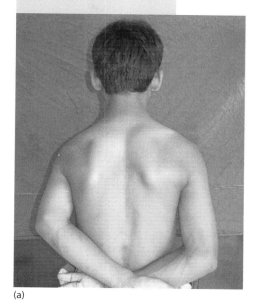

(a)

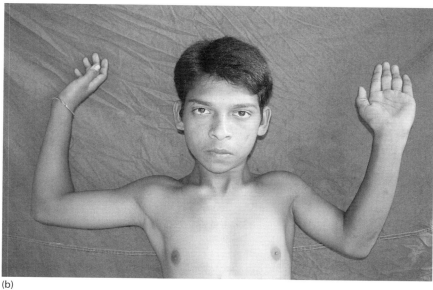

(b)

Figure 47.1 ● Appearance of an adolescent who had osteomyelitis of the humerus in early childhood. The proximal growth plate of the left humerus was damaged resulting in shortening of the arm **(a)** and limitation of abduction of the shoulder **(b)**.

Problems of management

Deciding to whom to offer surgery

The speed and quality of regenerate formation in the humerus is probably as good as the femur.[1] Even so, the temptation to offer surgical lengthening as a panacea to ills arising from length inequality needs to be resisted. As with other aspects of surgery, appropriate patient selection is important. It is difficult to quantify a threshold above which surgical intervention is indicated as the functional disability produced from differences in arm length is largely dependent on the anticipated use of both arms. In the activities cited in the text above, arm length inequality may hinder performance; otherwise differences of as much as 5–6 cm can be tolerated without too much difficulty.

Infrequently, children who have disproportionate short stature (e.g. achondroplasia) may present for humeral lengthening. This is a scenario quite different from arm length inequality and is an issue of body image and psychological well-being. A number of these children will undergo lower limb lengthening in stages in order to increase stature – from which there are functional gains to be had. However, the number resorting to bilateral humeral lengthening after having undergone staged lower limb surgery is fortunately small.[2]

Stability of the shoulder joint

Neonatal sepsis, causing destruction of the proximal humeral physis, is a leading cause of humeral length discrepancy. It often leads to a misshaped humeral head and inferior subluxation.[3] However, if the shoulder girdle muscles display good function, the shoulder joint should have sufficient stability to withstand moderate amounts of lengthening. Muscle weakness or paralysis around the shoulder should trigger caution against lengthening.

Aims of treatment

- Reduction of discrepancy in length
  Unlike the lower limb where length equality is a surgical objective, this is only necessary in certain circumstances for the humerus and approximate parity is sufficient to produce the necessary improvement in function.
- Improvement in function
  In the occasional instance where bimanual dexterity is impaired on account of shortening of the humerus, the aim would be to improve function.
- Improvement in psychological sense of well-being

Treatment options

Observation and advice

An initial period of observation is always wise; it allows the surgeon time to get to know the child and family in order to assess the impact of the arm length discrepancy on function. As the child grows the parents may realize that little (if any) function is lost from length inequality alone and may change their initial persuasive requests for surgical equalization. This period also allows selection of those cases that will benefit, either functionally or psychologically, from arm length equalisation.

Shortening of the longer humerus

This is rarely undertaken as it leads to disproportion of the upper limbs with respect to the rest of the body. An unusual scenario is when length inequality is due to overgrowth or hypertrophy, but here equalization is undertaken rarely as the length differences are usually minor.

Humeral lengthening

This is the commonest strategy for humeral length equalization (Figure 47.2). Potential complications include neurapraxia, joint stiffness and fracture after fixator removal.[4,5] A single osteotomy level can produce 6–8 cm of regenerate bone reliably; double level osteotomies achieve greater length at the risk of increasing soft tissue problems including joint stiffness and neurapraxia. In the event a 10–16 cm lengthening is needed, it may be preferable to divide this into two events of lengthening in childhood separated by a few years in between.

Factors to be taken into consideration while planning treatment

The predicted length discrepancy at skeletal maturity

The proximal humeral physis contributes to 80 percent of humeral length.[6] Proximal physeal closure occurs around 12–14 years in girls and 14–16 years in boys. From the age of seven, the humerus lengthens at approximately 1.2–1.3 cm per year, with almost 1 cm a year arising from the proximal physis.[7] These figures allow an estimate of final length discrepancy at skeletal maturity.

Threshold for intervention

Some authors recommend a threshold of intervention at 6 cm.[8,9] An absolute threshold is unwise and much depends on the effect of the length inequality on function, psychological well-being and the coordinated use of both arms for leisure or anticipated career activities. In the event that functional use is unimpaired and the cosmetic asymmetry tolerated, no intervention is wisest irrespective of the measured difference in length.

Patient circumstances with regard to extended use of an external fixator

The bone healing index for humeral lengthening is between 26 and 29 days/cm (in a mixed group of aetiologies[2,9]). If an average lengthening is in excess of 5 cm, then the period a fixator is left

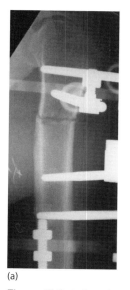
(a)

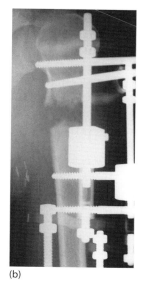
(b)

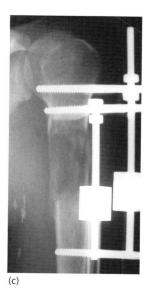
(c)

Figure 47.2 ● An osteotomy just distal to the surgical neck of humerus allows for sufficient room for placement of pins into the proximal humeral segment safely without risk to the radial nerve which runs further distal **(a)**. Distraction proceeds fractionally to gain approximately 1 mm a day. Regenerate formation and quality is akin to lengthening in the femur **(b)**. Removal of the fixator should not occur before a homogeneous appearance of the regenerate is observed with no lucencies visible. The striated appearance here, despite some evidence of corticalization, should prompt further waiting **(c)**.

in situ will be in excess of 5–6 months at a minimum. Careful pre-operative selection is therefore necessary to ensure the treatment is tolerated to completion. Family circumstances will need investigation to determine whether an adequate support structure exists for this type of treatment. Lack of compliance in any lengthening surgery produces poor results.

Concomitant deformity

Conditions which damage the proximal humeral physis (in particular, neonatal septic arthritis, juxtaphyseal bone cysts or trauma) lead to humeral shortening; in severe examples, there can be inferior subluxation at the shoulder and humerus varus (Figure 47.3).[3,10,11] Despite the radiological appearance, the functional range of shoulder abduction may be minimally impaired and corrective osteotomy unnecessary.[11] In those significantly affected, a closing wedge osteotomy with tension band fixation is effective.[12]

Figure 47.3 ● Humerus varus and shortening of the humerus due to physeal damage in early childhood.

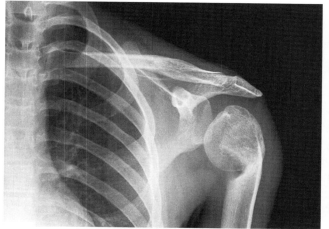
(a)

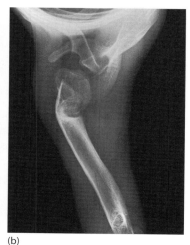
(b)

Recommended treatment

The recommended treatment of humeral length inequality is outlined in Table 47.1. It is based on several important precepts:

- Length inequality in the upper limb is well tolerated except for certain activities.
- Observation as an initial course of management is wise.
- Lengthening surgery can be offered to those whose family circumstances allow and whose expectations are realistic.
- Correction of humerus varus should be considered if the limitation of function is a result of compromised shoulder movement and length inequality.

Table 47.1 ● Outline of treatment of humeral length inequality

INDICATIONS			
Length inequality with no functional impairment even for activities which require coordinated action between arms	Length inequality producing impairment of leisure or anticipated career interests + Estimated final discrepancy <8 cm	Length inequality producing impairment of leisure or anticipated career interests + Estimated final discrepancy >8 cm ⇩ Double-stage lengthening with interval between events of surgery	Length inequality producing impairment of leisure or anticipated career interests + Restriction of shoulder movement from humerus vara ⇩ Corrective osteotomy of proximal humerus + Second-stage lengthening with interval between events of surgery
⇩ Observe, reassure and reassess at skeletal maturity	⇩ Single-stage lengthening with osteotomy proximal to deltoid insertion		
TREATMENT			

References

1. Tanaka K, Nakamura K, Matsushita T *et al.* Callus formation in the humerus compared with the femur and tibia during limb lengthening. *Arch Orthop Trauma Surg* 1998; **117**: 262–4.
2. Aldegheri R, Dall'Oca C. Limb lengthening in short stature patients. *J Pediatr Orthop B* 2001; **10**: 238–47.
3. Saisu T, Kawashima A, Kamegaya M *et al.* Humeral shortening and inferior subluxation as sequelae of septic arthritis of the shoulder in neonates and infants. *J Bone Joint Surg Am* 2007; **89**: 1784–93.
4. Lee FY-I, Schoeb JS, Yu J, Christiansen BD, Dick HM. Operative lengthening of the humerus: indications, benefits, and complications. *J Pediatr Orthop* 2005; **25**: 613–16.
5. Cattaneo R, Catagni MA, Guerreschi F. Applications of the Ilizarov method in the humerus. Lengthenings and nonunions. *Hand Clin* 1993; **9**: 729–39.
6. Pritchett JW. Growth plate activity in the upper extremity. *Clin Orthop Relat Res* 1991; **268**: 235–42.
7. Pritchett JW. Growth and predictions of growth in the upper extremity. *J Bone Joint Surg Am* 1988; **70**: 520–5.
8. Prevot J, Lascombes P, Gagneux E, Ramborum D. Arm lengthening in children. Report of 4 cases. *Chirurgie* 1990; **116**: 184–9.
9. Cattaneo R, Villa A, Catagni MA, Bell D. Lengthening of the humerus using the Ilizarov technique. Description of the method and report of 43 cases. *Clin Orthop Relat Res* 1990; **250**: 117–24.
10. Ogden JA, Weil UH, Hempton RF. Developmental humerus varus. *Clin Orthop Relat Res* 1976; **116**: 158–65.
11. Ellefsen BK, Frierson MA, Raney EM, Ogden JA. Humerus varus: a complication of neonatal, infantile, and childhood injury and infection. *J Pediatr Orthop* 1994; **14**: 479–86.
12. Ugwonali OF, Bae DS, Waters PM. Corrective osteotomy for humerus varus. *J Pediatr Orthop* 2007; **27**: 529–32.

Discrepancies of length in the forearm

Selvadurai Nayagam

48

Introduction

The functional impact of mild to moderate forearm shortening is minimal; examples are seen in bony and chondrodysplasias where a symmetrical limb shortening is often present and is compensated for with little effort (Figure 48.1). This ability to annul the effect of shortening also applies in asymmetrical discrepancies in length of the forearm as long as elbow and hand function are well preserved; the individual is usually able to adjust body position in activities that require simultaneous and coordinated bilateral hand function such as in driving or lifting heavy objects. In contrast, an altered length relationship of the radius and ulna in the same forearm produces deformity and limitation of movement as the close relationship of the two bones, linked proximally and distally in two mobile joints, is disrupted.

Such abnormality of length between the radius and the ulna may be congenital (as in radial or ulnar dysgenesis), developmental (as in hereditary multiple osteochondromatosis or Madelung deformity) or acquired (following physeal damage from trauma or infection). The common causes are listed below.

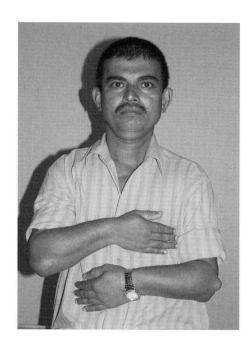

Figure 48.1 ● Short forearm of an adult with hereditary multiple osteochondromatosis. He is a stone mason and has no functional limitations at all.

Radial shortening

■ Congenital

Congenital radial hypoplasia can be present in varying degrees, from no detectable difference in length but deficient carpal bones on the radial side, through varying degrees of radial shortening to complete absence[1] (see Chapter 39, Radial club hand).

■ Distal radial physeal arrest

This may arise as a consequence of trauma or infection, or even occur insidiously as in Madelung deformity.

■ Developmental

Osteochondromas on the radius and ulna in children with hereditary multiple osteochondromatosis can variably affect forearm growth. While it is more common for ulnar shortening to occur with juxtaphyseal osteochondromas on that bone, radial shortening can occur with similarly located lesions.[2,3]

Ulna shortening

■ Congenital

Ulna dysplasia is rare and can vary from mild shortening through varying degrees of hypoplasia to complete absence, which if present may be associated with radiohumeral synostosis[4] (see Chapter 40, Ulnar club hand).

■ Physeal arrest

Physeal arrest at the distal ulna physis from trauma or infection can lead to an ulnar club hand deformity. The radial bow may become exaggerated and in severe cases dislocation of the radial head occurs.

■ Developmental

Growth retardation of the distal ulnar physis frequently occurs when an osteochondroma is situated in the distal ulna and changes in the radius similar to that seen with physeal arrest occur.

Problems of management

Malalignment of the hand and the forearm

The wrist is deviated either radially or ulnar-wards depending on which bone is shorter and there is a tendency for the longer bone to become bowed.

Instability of the wrist and loss of grip

The wrist can become unstable and grip is affected as finger flexor strength is dissipated from an inability to hold an efficient position of the wrist.

Progression of the deformity and shortening

Most developmental and acquired causes of shortening of the ulna or radius are due to physeal involvement and hence can progress as the child grows.

Psychological impact of the appearance

Moderate and severe degrees of shortening of the forearm bones result in very obvious deformity which can be distressing for the child.

Aims of treatment

- Correct alignment and length proportion
- Arrest progression of deformity
- Augment joint stability
- Improve cosmesis

Treatment options

Ignore

Minor degrees of inequality in lengths of the radius and ulna may not be discernable and also cause no deformity of the wrist or forearm; these may be ignored.

Physeal bar excision

Mapping of the size and location of the physeal tether is made by magnetic resonance imaging.[5,6] Lesions greater than 50 percent of the entire physis in children with less than two years of growth are unsuitable for attempted physeal bar resections (see Chapter 70, Physeal bar). Success is better with lesions involving less than 30 percent of the area of the physis.[7] These recommendations are usually quoted for physes of the lower limb, e.g. distal femur and proximal tibia. Surgery to remove a physeal tether in the distal radius is technically more difficult and only relatively small and easily accessible tethers should be attempted. In a Madelung deformity, the procedure proposed by Vickers and Nielsen describes resection of the tether on the ulnar side of the physis with fat interposition and division of an anomalous short radiolunate ligament[8] (see Chapter 20, Varus and valgus deformity of the wrist). Physeal bar excisions from the distal ulna are impractical owing to the small size of the physis.

Shortening the longer bone

If the overall forearm shortening is not excessive, a short ulna but with normal physes may be treated by growth arrest of the distal radius. This technique is applicable if the ulna physis is damaged but the effect then would be cessation of a further increase in length discrepancy, not an equalization to normal proportions.

Lengthening the shorter bone

In cases of acquired or developmental ulna shortening, a progressive increase in length discrepancy between the radius and the ulna produces an exaggeration of the radial curvature. It is important to monitor this radial deformity; the radial curvature and the ulnar deviation at the wrist increase with time and the radial head may dislocate. Early intervention is needed before this occurs. Gradual ulnar lengthening with correction of the radial bowing will restore alignment of the forearm and correct deviation at the wrist (see Chapter 20, Varus and valgus deformity of the wrist). A dislocated radial head can also be reduced by lengthening the ulna using Ilizarov techniques (as long as it has not been long-standing). This seldom improves the arc of supination–pronation; however, it may eliminate an extension block to the elbow that is present from the dislocation (see Chapter 33, Radial head dislocation).

Most examples of radial physeal damage present with significant radial shortening and it is necessary to employ gradual lengthening techniques. An ulnar physeal epiphyseodesis prevents recurrence if done on completion of radial lengthening (Figure 48.2).

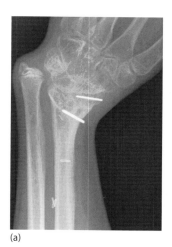
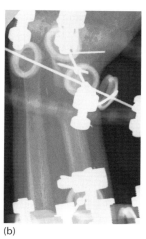
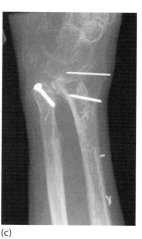

(a)   (b)   (c)

Figure 48.2 ● Acquired length discrepancies of the radius produce wrist deviations **(a)**. Correction of alignment and length inequality **(b)** will restore wrist and hand position; grip becomes more efficient. A distal ulna epiphyseodesis at the end of the procedure will prevent recurrence **(c).**

If the upper limb is so short as to interfere with reach, it is easier and safer to lengthen the humerus rather than attempt to lengthen the radius and ulna. Lengthening of forearm bones to achieve body proportions in achondroplasia and mesomelic dysplasia is discouraged; the potential for loss of wrist and elbow function coupled with a long period of external fixator use (forearm bones, when lengthened, need a longer time to consolidate compared with the lower limb or humerus) produce an inappropriate risk to benefit ratio.

Age at presentation

Both distal radial and ulnar physes account for 80 percent of the longitudinal growth of the respective bones and a major part of growth occurs by the age of 12 years. If there is evidence of a distal radial physeal tether in the young child, an attempt may be made to resect the tether to minimize the shortening of the bone. A minimum of two years of growth is needed for physeal bar resection to return an appreciable effect; attempts to resect physeal tethers of the distal radius after the age of 12 are questionable.

Degree of and unilateral or bilateral involvement

Mild deformities due to shortening of the radius or ulna, if not progressive, may be observed as the functional loss is slight and compensated for by good elbow and shoulder movement. Moderate and severe deformities may often require lengthening along with corrective osteotomies.

Overall length of the limb

Lengthening of both bones of the forearm to improve reach is rarely needed as compensatory adjustments by the body and arm enable very effective positioning.

Elbow stability and movement

Gradual lengthening of the radius or ulna in an external fixator, particularly if the cause is congenital dysplasia, needs to proceed with some caution as the elbow joint may be unstable; the fixator can be extended across the elbow to prevent iatrogenic subluxation.

Recommended treatment

An outline of treatment of a short radius or ulna is shown in Tables 48.1 and 48.2.

Table 48.1 ● Outline of treatment of a short radius

INDICATIONS			
Congenital radial hypoplasia (radial club hand type I or II)	Short radius + Osteochondroma on distal radius	Short radius + Distal physeal damage (amenable to physeal bar resection)	Short radius + Distal physeal damage (not amenable to physeal bar resection) ⇩
⇩	⇩	⇩	Gradual lengthening of the radius + Epiphyseodesis of the distal ulna
Gradual lengthening of the radius	Excision of osteochondroma + Radial lengthening (only if discrepancy is unlikely to correct with growth)	Excision of physeal bar + Radial lengthening (only if discrepancy is unlikely to correct with growth)	
	Concurrent correction of deformity of the radius if present		
TREATMENT			

Rationale of treatment suggested

Disproportionate shortening of one forearm bone produces deformity and loss of function. Either the radius or ulna may be responsible and treatment is offered to address those components which produce greatest disability. Lengthening of the short bone is a component of surgical strategy; treatment often includes corrective osteotomies, physeal bar excisions, wrist centralization and tendon transfers depending on the underlying problem. Significant improvement in hand and wrist function is achievable notwithstanding the benefits in appearance and body image.

In contrast, corrective surgery for a short forearm when the bones are proportionate should not be undertaken lightly. Forearm lengthening is complex and fraught with potential complications which affect wrist and elbow function. Compensatory manoeuvres for a short forearm are excellent if shoulder, elbow and wrist function are intact – in the event of a stiff elbow and wrist, lengthening the forearm will only increase the distance of the hand from the mouth and produce greater disability and as such should only be considered in exceptional circumstances.

Table 48.2 ● Outline of treatment of a short ulna

INDICATIONS		
Short ulna + Distal ulnar osteochondroma	Short ulna + Distal physeal damage + Approaching skeletal maturity + Mild discrepancy in length between radius and ulna	Short ulna + Distal physeal damage + Young child OR Severe discrepancy OR Radial head dislocated
	⇩	⇩
⇩	Radial epiphyseodesis	Gradual lengthening of the ulna
Excision of osteochondroma + Ulnar lengthening (if discrepancy is unlikely to correct with growth)		
	Concurrent correction of deformity of the radius if present	
TREATMENT		

References

1. Manske PR. Longitudinal failure of upper-limb formation. *J Bone Joint Surg Am* 1996; **78**: 1600–23.
2. Masada K, Tsuyuguchi Y, Kawai H *et al.* Operations for forearm deformity caused by multiple osteochondromas. *J Bone Joint Surg Br* 1989; **71**: 24–9.
3. Porter D, Emerton M, Villanueva-Lopez F, Simpson A. Clinical and radiographic analysis of osteochondromas and growth disturbance in hereditary multiple exostoses. *J Pediatr Orthop* 2000; **20**: 246–50.
4. Johnson J, Omer GJ. Congenital ulnar deficiency. Natural history and therapeutic implications. *Hand Clin* 1985; **1**: 499–510.
5. Ecklund K, Jaramillo D. Patterns of premature physeal arrest: MR imaging of 111 children. *AJR Am J Roentgenol* 2002; **178**: 967–72.
6. Borsa JJ, Peterson HA, Ehman RL. MR imaging of physeal bars. Radiology 1996; **199**: 683–7.
7. Williamson RV, Staheli LT. Partial physeal growth arrest: treatment by bridge resection and fat interposition. J Pediatr Orthop 1990; **10**: 769–76.
8. Vickers D, Nielsen G. Madelung deformity: surgical prophylaxis (physiolysis) during the late growth period by resection of the dyschondrosteosis lesion. *J Hand Surg Br* 1992; **17**: 401–7.

SECTION 5

Decreased joint mobility

General principles of management of decreased joint mobility in children

49

Randall Loder

Introduction

Decreased joint motion occurs in several clinical situations in children. The loss of motion may be associated with pain or there may be painless loss of motion. Reduction in joint motion may involve all movements of the joint or involve only one or more specific movements (Table 49.1).

Table 49.1 ● Various forms of decreased joint mobility seen in children.

Painless or painful	Extent of loss of motion	Movement lost	Examples
Painless	Total loss of motion	All movements	Bony ankylosis
			Congenital synostosis
		Single movement	Congenital quadriceps contracture
	Partial loss	All movements	Chondrolysis
		One or more movements	Contractures of the shoulder following obstetric brachial plexus palsy
Painful	Partial loss	All movements	Arthritis
			Fibrous ankylosis
		One or more movements	Perthes' disease

The pathology giving rise to joint stiffness may be either intra-articular or extra-articular (Figures 49.1–49.4). The commonest cause of extra-articular joint stiffness is contracture of muscles due to various underlying diseases. In general, extra-articular soft issue causes of joint stiffness have a better chance of correction than intra-articular pathology.

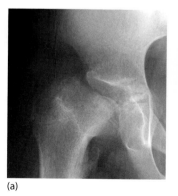 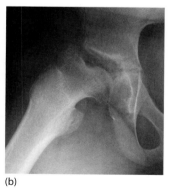

Figure 49.1 ● Intra-articular bony pathology preventing normal range of hip motion. This nine-year-old boy with healed Perthes' disease in the right hip as shown on the anteroposterior **(a)** and frog lateral **(b)** radiographs lacked complete extension, flexion, abduction and internal rotation of the hip.

(a)   (b)

Specific aetiologies causing joint stiffness are congenital deformity (e.g. congenital radio–ulnar synostosis, congenital knee dislocation), post-traumatic or post-infectious arthrofibrosis, intra-articular bony pathology (e.g. osteochondral loose body as in osteochondritis dessicans of the knee, joint incongruity as in healed Perthes' disease), intra-articular soft tissue pathology (e.g. entrapped bucket handle tear of the lateral meniscus), extra-articular bony pathology (e.g. heterotopic bone formation post fracture), extra-articular soft tissue pathology (e.g. soft tissue capsular contracture after an intra-articular elbow fracture, heel cord contracture in a cerebral palsy child). Occasionally both intra-articular and extra-articular pathology may be present, for instance in a child with

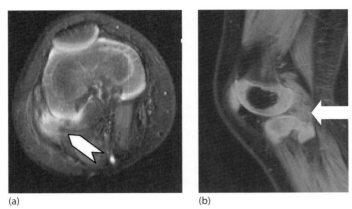

(a)   (b)

Figure 49.2 ● Intra-articular soft tissue pathology preventing normal knee range of motion as shown in this three-year-old child with a Trenaunay-Weber syndrome and a posterolateral intra-articular haemangioma which prevented complete knee extension. In the axial view **(a)** the haemangioma is seen at the level of the meniscus (white arrowhead) with posterior and lateral extension into the soft tissues. On the sagittal view **(b)**, the haemangioma can be seen posteriorly (white arrow).

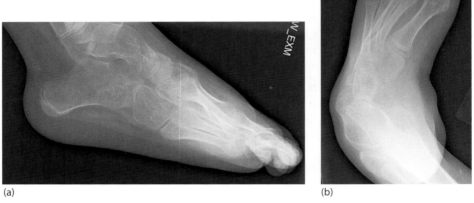

(a)   (b)

Figure 49.3 ● Extra-articular soft tissue pathology preventing normal foot and ankle motion as shown in this 13-year-old boy with spastic quadriplegic cerebral palsy. Note the equinovarus foot deformity which was secondary to a contracture of the Achilles tendon as well as the posterior tibial, flexor hallucis longus and flexor digitorum longus musculotendinous units. The lateral view **(a)** demonstrates the equinus contracture and the anteroposterior view; **(b)** demonstrates varus and supination contractures.

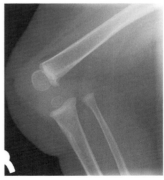

Figure 49.4 ● Both intra-articular and extra-articular pathology preventing normal joint motion. This radiograph is from an eight-month-old girl with a severe pterygium of the knee. Note the soft tissue contracture posteriorly as well as posterior subluxation of the tibia on the femur; both contribute to the knee flexion contracture.

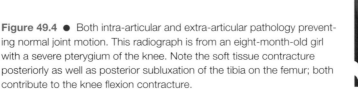

arthrogryposis with both soft tissue contracture and bony incongruity between the femur and tibia resulting in a knee contracture.

In the child with an underlying neuromuscular disorder or syndrome, loss of joint motion can occur for many different reasons, and often reflects the underlying disorder. It is for this reason that the exact type of neuromuscular disorder must be known before starting treatment. In children with cerebral palsy, the soft tissue and bony structures are initially normal, and the deformity and loss of motion is secondary to the underlying spasticity. Since the joints were initially normal it is often possible to improve the range of motion in these children, with therapy (stretching and strengthening exercises), medication (antispasticity agents such as oral diazepam, intrathecal baclofen, intramuscular botulinum toxin) and surgery (tendon lengthening, tenotomies or transfers). In children with arthrogryposis, myelodysplasia and many of the skeletal dysplasias (e.g. diastrophic dwarfism), the joints, capsular structures and muscles are frequently abnormal from birth, and here it is difficult to improve the range of motion of the joint. Instead, intervention should be directed towards maintaining the present motion and, if necessary, repositioning the joint in space by osteotomy so that the arc of motion is in a more functional position.

Problems of management

Loss of function

Although parents and older children may notice diminished motion, the reduced motion may not result in a functional problem. For example, loss of 10° of terminal extension or flexion of the elbow in a child is typically not a functional problem. Similarly, incomplete subtalar joint motion in a child with a subtalar coalition might not represent a functional issue, but rather an issue of activity-related pain. On the other hand, an ankylosed elbow or knee will cause significant functional disability, particularly if the joint is fused in a position that precludes any normal function of the limb.

Deformity

■ At the stiff joint

Often a stiff joint may also be deformed and this further aggravates the loss of function. Even if joint motion cannot be restored, the deformity should be corrected (e.g. equinus deformity in an ankle ankylosed in plantarflexion).

■ Secondary deformity at adjacent mobile joint

It is also important to remember that the joints just proximal and distal to a stiff joint are subjected to abnormal and excessive stresses. As a result of this the adjacent joint may either develop excessive motion (e.g. increased wrist joint motion seen in children with congenital radio-ulnar synostosis) or develop a deformity (e.g. recurvatum deformity that develops at the knee in patients with equinus).

Pain

Pain often indicates underlying joint incongruity, articular cartilage problems or malposition of the joint. In these children, two issues need to be addressed: the loss of joint motion, as well as pain relief. It is often impossible to obtain improvement in both areas as the therapy needed to relieve pain often conflicts with the therapy needed to improve motion. A child with avascular necrosis of the femoral head owing to an unstable slipped capital femoral epiphysis typically demonstrates loss of abduction, internal rotation, and has a fixed flexion, adduction contracture, along with femoral head collapse, articular cartilage breakdown and joint incongruity. In this situation, a hip arthrodesis will correct the abnormal joint position and relieve the pain, but completely limit joint motion. Joint motion cannot be restored aside from total joint arthroplasty which may be contraindicated in a young active child with this disorder. By contrast, a teenager with severe polyarticular chronic juvenile arthritis, minimal ambulatory ability and with a painful destruction of the hip is a good candidate for a total joint arthroplasty because of the limited demands that will be placed on the prosthesis.

Aims of treatment

- Improve function if possible
- Correct deformities that affect function
- Relive pain, if present

Treatment options

Restore movement that is absent and increase the arc of movement at the joint

This would be the ideal option, and it may be feasible in some instances (e.g. release of quadriceps contracture to restore knee flexion or excision of a post-traumatic myositis mass in the brachialis muscle). However, in several instances this may not be possible.

Alter the position of the existing arc of movement without increasing the arc of motion

This may be the only option available in several situations.

Abolish all movement to relieve pain

Pain from a severely damaged joint will persist as long as movement occurs and in such situations arthrodesis of the joint is a logical option.

Avoid any intervention

If the range of motion cannot be improved and the joint is stiff in an acceptable position, no intervention is justified.

While planning treatment the following two questions need to be answered:

1. Can the arc of motion be improved?
2. Can the existing arc of motion be repositioned in space to improve function?

Questions to be answered while planning treatment

It is important to answer these questions for two reasons. First, they guide the orthopaedist to proper treatment. Second, they allow the orthopaedist to convey reasonable expectations to the patient and parents. When considering neuromuscular aetiologies, significant differences exist as to the ability to improve versus reposition the arc of motion. In children with cerebral palsy, the musculotendinous units and periarticular soft tissues were normal at birth, with the loss of motion due to the development of spasticity. In these instances, it is more likely that tendon lengthening will improve the overall joint range of motion. In older children with cerebral palsy, it may be necessary to perform periarticular osteotomies to reposition the joint in space in a better position which will improve the child's physical function (such as a distal femoral extension osteotomy in a teenager with significant knee flexion contracture). However, such osteotomies need to be performed close to skeletal maturity, otherwise recurrence of the deformity frequently occurs secondary to physeal remodelling with continued bony growth. On the other hand, in children with arthrogryposis, the soft tissue contractures and intra-articular joint deformities have been present since before birth, and soft tissue release often repositions the joint arc of motion in space, but does not actually increase the arc of motion, or may even reduce active motion by weakening the muscular motors around the joint. If joint incongruity is due to a bony block, joint motion may be improved if the offending bony anatomy can be repositioned by either removal or osteotomy. Typical examples are a valgus osteotomy in a child with epiphyseal extrusion and hinge abduction in Perthes' disease, or a flexion-rotational osteotomy in a child with a severe slipped capital femoral epiphysis may improve the range of motion of the hip and allow more natural internal rotation, abduction and extension. In some circumstances it is difficult to improve joint motion. One example is a child with a subtalar tarsal coalition; resection of the coalition may result in pain relief, but frequently does not result in improved subtalar joint motion.

Recommended treatment

An outline of treatment of reduced joint motion is shown in Table 49.2.

Table 49.2 ● Outline of treatment of decreased joint mobility in children

INDICATIONS							
Painless loss of motion				**Painful loss of motion**			
Total loss of motion (e.g. bony ankylosis or synostosis) + Position of joint acceptable	Total loss of motion (e.g. bony ankylosis or synostosis) + Position of joint impairing function	Partial loss of motion + Not amenable to treatment that would increase motion + Functional range of motion present	Partial loss of motion + Not amenable to treatment that would increase motion + Range of motion in non-functional range	Partial loss of motion + Amenable to treatment that would increase motion	Underlying pathology amenable to therapy and restoration of motion (e.g. septic arthritis)	Underlying pathology amenable to therapy to arrest progress of disease (e.g. chronic arthritis)	Underlying pathology NOT amenable to therapy to arrest progress of disease (e.g. secondary arthritis)
⇩	⇩	⇩	⇩	⇩	⇩	⇩	⇩
No intervention	Osteotomy to place limb in more functional position	No intervention	Alter arc of motion to more functional range by a metaphyseal osteotomy	Treat underlying cause and restore or improve motion	Appropriate therapy to obtain cure of the disease and retain motion	Appropriate therapy to obtain cure of the disease and restore motion	Abolish painful motion at the joint by formal arthrodesis OR Joint replacement in few situations
TREATMENT							

Congenital radio-ulnar synostosis

Randall Loder

50

Introduction

Congenital radio-ulnar synostosis represents a failure of differentiation in the primitive mesenchymal condensations that occur in the proximal forearm at approximately five weeks of gestation. The humerus, radius and ulna all arise from a shared mesenchymal anlage that later condenses into cartilage and separates into individual bones. Failure of this process to properly occur can result in radio-ulnar synostosis.[1] The process of separation occurs at the time the fetal forearm is in a position of pronation; this explains why in the majority of children with congenital radio-ulnar synostosis the forearm is fixed in pronation. The exact event that causes the failure of separation is unknown. It is an isolated anomaly in one-third of cases and bilateral involvement is seen in 60 percent of affected children.

The development of the forearm occurs early in gestation when many other organ systems are developing; the event that causes the failure of differentiation in the forearm may also affect the development of other organ systems. Therefore, syndromes such as Poland syndrome, Apert syndrome, arthrogryposis, Klinefelter syndrome and many others are associated with congenital radio-ulnar synostosis. Other associated organ system anomalies may also occur.

There are two main types of congenital radio-ulnar synostosis.[2] Type I involves a smooth fusion of the radius and ulna proximally for a variable distance, typically 2–6 cm (Figure 50.1a). Type II is a fusion just distal to the proximal radial epiphysis associated with a congenital dislocation of the radial head (Figure 50.1b). In both types loss of supination is similar; in type II there may also be compromised elbow extension.

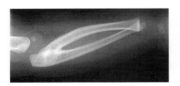 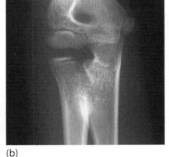 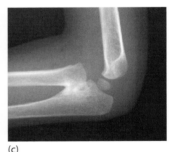

Figure 50.1 ● Radiographs of type I **(a,b)** and type II **(c)** congenital radio-ulnar synostosis.

(a) (b) (c)

Problems of management

Limitation of function of the upper limb

The magnitude of functional limitations imposed by the fixed forearm position depends upon on many factors, including age and occupation, unilateral or bilateral involvement and societal norms (such as eating patterns). All these must be considered when planning therapy.[3,4] Most children demonstrate varying degrees of fixed pronation, which is a good position for writing and keyboard tasks when they become adults. This position, along with increased compensatory rotation at the carpus, wrist and shoulder, often seen in these children, is usually adequate for most activities. In the rare bilateral case with marked fixed pronation, there may be difficulties with using spoons or writing devices, grasping small objects and buckling clothing fasteners. It may also be difficult to get the hand to the mouth or wipe one's face with the palm of the hand (Figure 50.2). Children in Asian cultures, where the rice bowl is held in supination, may experience significant functional limitations.[4]

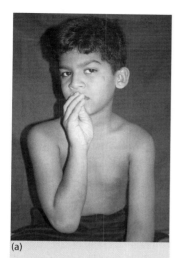

(a)

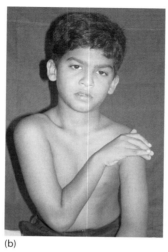

(b)

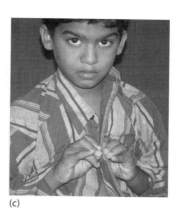

(c)

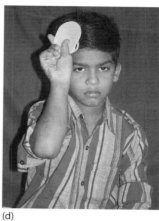

(d)

Figure 50.2 ● Young boy with congenital radio-ulnar synostosis demonstrating activities of daily living. Specific limitations of function can be noted by careful evaluation. He has difficulty in getting his hand to his mouth **(a)** and is unable to touch the opposite shoulder with his palm **(b)**. He manages to button his shirt **(c)** and can comb his hair **(d)** in spite of the fixed pronation deformity.

Risk of complications following surgery

Rotational osteotomies of the forearm for congenital radio-ulnar synostosis are associated with high complication rates; these are nerve palsies, vascular compromise, compartment syndrome and malunion.[1,5,6] Owing to the adaptation of most patients in compensatory rotation through both the carpus and shoulder, and the associated high complication rate of surgery, the risks of surgery rarely outweigh the benefits.[3]

Aims of treatment

- Improving function

Functional limitations are due to two reasons: the first is the limitation of forearm motion and the second is the position of the fused forearm. It is ideal if full motion at the radio-ulnar joints can be restored. If this is not feasible function may be improved by realigning the forearm into a more suitable position.

Treatment options

Resection of the synostosis

Although resection of the synostosis makes considerable sense, the procedure is technically demanding and results are often unsatisfactory. One reason for failure is reformation of synostosis. Interposition of various materials in the resection gap have been tried and of these vascularized fat graft seems to be the most promising.[7] Kanaya[8] reported gratifying short-term results in 12 children on whom he had performed resection of the synostosis and interposed vascularized fat graft and the anconeus muscle. He also performed a shortening angulation osteotomy of the radius to align the radial head towards the capitellum (Figure 50.3). The average motion regained at the radio-ulnar joint was 80°. However, there are no good long-term reports of this method and so most surgeons do not choose this procedure.

Rotational osteotomy

This is the favoured procedure when functional limitations are severe enough to require repositioning of the forearm.

■ The site of osteotomy

The osteotomy can be either through the synostosis[1,5] or in the diaphyses of both bones[9] (Figure 50.4).

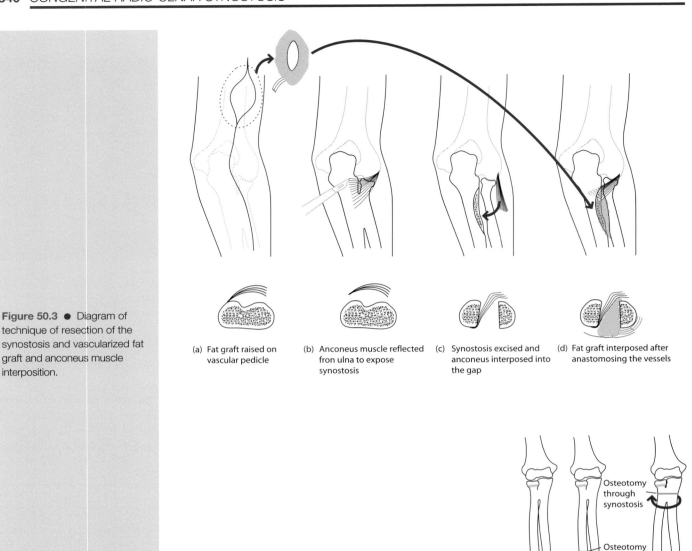

Figure 50.3 ● Diagram of technique of resection of the synostosis and vascularized fat graft and anconeus muscle interposition.

(a) Fat graft raised on vascular pedicle

(b) Anconeus muscle reflected fron ulna to expose synostosis

(c) Synostosis excised and anconeus interposed into the gap

(d) Fat graft interposed after anastomosing the vessels

Figure 50.4 ● Sites of derotation osteotomy for congenital radio-ulnar synostosis.

Osteotomy through synostosis

Osteotomy distal to synostosis

■ The position of fixation

There is no universal agreement on the optimal position of the forearm to be achieved after surgery. In unilateral cases the recommended position of the forearm ranges from 15° of pronation[1] to 35° of supination.[5] It is recommended that in bilateral cases the dominant hand should be left in 20° of pronation, and the non-dominant hand in neutral, unless the patient's career is definitely known,[1] in which case the position of fixation can be tailored to the career.[5] In certain cultures the position of the hand may be different depending upon the needs of the hand in those countries.[3]

The osteotomy should be proximal through the synostosis mass, and also involve slight shortening to reduce the tension on the neurovascular structures during the rotation.[1,5] Fixation should be used, typically an intramedullary Steinmann pin and another cross pin in the younger child; in the older child low profile plate fixation can be considered. In all cases the parents and child must be informed of the significant concern for neurovascular complications and, to some extent, malunion.[2] If the pronation deformity is over 90° one osteotomy through the synostosis mass and a second osteotomy distally has also been recommended.[10]

Factors to be taken into consideration while planning treatment

Current upper limb function and potential function in the future

A very careful assessment of the child's functional limitations for activities of daily living (ADL) must be undertaken with the help of the occupational therapist. While documenting the specific current disability a tentative projection of the functional abilities in different occupations that the child may engage in the future also needs to be explained to the parents. Although the future occupation of the child is difficult to know, it should be borne in mind that in today's society several occupations require keyboard activities. In these occupations a supinated forearm may be more incapacitating than a pronated forearm.

The amount of compensatory carpal supination should also be carefully documented. If there is increased carpal supination, less rotational correction during osteotomy will be needed, which will reduce the risk of complications.[3]

Age of the child

Ideally, any corrective surgery should be undertaken before the child adapts to the current position of the forearm.

Recommended treatment

The outline of treatment of congenital radio–ulnar synostosis is shown in Table 50.1.

Table 50.1 ● Outline of treatment of congenital radio-ulnar synostosis

INDICATIONS		
Unilateral radio-ulnar synostosis OR Bilateral radio-ulnar synostosis + Mild or moderate pronation of the forearm + No demonstrable functional disability for activities of daily living (ADL) ⇩	Bilateral radio-ulnar synostosis + Severe pronation of the forearm + Older child or adolescent + Completely adapted for ADL ⇩	Bilateral radio-ulnar synostosis + Severe pronation of the forearm + Young child (under 5 years of age) + Significant demonstrable functional disability for ADL ⇩
No intervention	No intervention	Derotation osteotomy through fusion mass
TREATMENT		

Rationale of treatment suggested

Why is surgery rarely needed?
Most children and adults demonstrate minimal functional limitations. Similarly, there is increased compensatory motion through the carpus, wrist and shoulder which assists in the function of these patients.

When surgery is considered necessary why is osteotomy preferred to resection of the synostosis?
At present there are no long-term reports of resection of the congenital radio-ulnar synostosis that show consistently good results.[11] In future, if the results of Kanaya can be duplicated, there may be justification to recommend this option.

Why is osteotomy associated with high complication rates?
Since the deformity is congenital, the soft tissues have been contracted since early *in utero*. The neurovascular structures are the most important of the soft tissues, and they are quite sensitive to large amounts of acute rotation that may be performed during the operation. A slight shortening of the osteotomy will help to reduce the tension on the soft tissue structures.

References

1. Simmons BP, Southmayd WW, Riseborough EJ. Congenital radioulnar synostosis. *J Hand Surg [Am]* 1983; **8**: 829–38.
2. Mital MA. Congenital radioulnar synostosis and congenital dislocation of the radial head. *Orthop Clin North Am* 1976; **7**: 375–83.
3. Cleary JE, Omer J, George E. Congenital proximal radio-ulnar synostosis. *J Bone Joint Surg Am* 1985; **67**: 539–45.
4. Ogino T, Hikino K. Congenital radio-ulnar synostosis: compensatory rotation around the wrist and rotation osteotomy. *J Hand Surg [Br]* 1987; **12**: 173–8.
5. Green WT, Mital MA. Congenital radio-ulnar synostosis: surgical treatment. *J Bone Joint Surg Am* 1979; **61**: 738–43.
6. Hankin FM, Smith PA, Kling Jr TF, Louis DS. Ulnar nerve palsy following rotational osteotomy of congenital radioulnar synostosis. *J Pediatr Orthop* 1987; **7**: 103–6.
7. Kanaya F, Ibaraki K. Mobilization of a congenital proximal radio-ulnar synostosis with use of free vascularized fascio-fat graft. *J Bone Joint Surg Am* 1998; **80**: 1186–92.
8. Kanaya F. New approach to radio-ulnar synostosis. In: Gupta A, Kay SPJ, Scheker LR (eds). *The Growing Hand.* London: Mosby, 2000: 237–41.
9. Murase T, Tada K, Yoshida T, Moritomo H. Derotational osteotomy at the shafts of the radius and ulna for congenital radioulnar synostosis. *J Hand Surg [Am]* 2003; **28**: 133–7.
10. Andrisano A, Soncini G, Calderoni PP, Bungaro P. Congenital proximal radio-ulnar synostosis: surgical treatment. *J Pediatr Orthop* 1994; **3**:102–6.
11. Jones ME, Rider MA, Hughes J, Tonkin MA. The use of a proximally based posterior interosseous adipofascial flap to prevent recurrence of synostosis of the elbow joint and forearm. *J Hand Surg [Br]* 2007; **32**: 143–7.

Tarsal coalition

Randall Loder

51

Introduction

Tarsal coalition is an embryologic failure of segmentation of mesenchymal tissue in the hind- and midfoot with secondary failure of formation of the normal hindfoot or midfoot joints.

Tarsal coalitions may be solitary, massive or multiple. Solitary coalitions involve a part of two adjacent bones while massive coalitions involve all of two adjacent tarsals.[1,2] A solitary coalition can range from a minimal fibrous union to complete bony synostosis. Massive coalitions are often associated with other limb anomalies, in particular, fibular hemimelia and proximal focal femoral deficiency. Multiple tarsal coalitions are seen in genetic syndromes such as multiple synostosis syndromes where coalitions of carpal bones, symphalangism and congenital fusion of the elbow may also be present.[1,2]

Solitary tarsal coalitions

The most common solitary coalitions are talocalcaneal (usually involving the middle or anterior facets of the subtalar joint) and calcaneonavicular (Figure 51.1a–d). The exact incidence is unknown as some individuals are asymptomatic and thus the diagnosis is never made. Bilaterality is present in 50–60 percent of affected individuals.

Although solitary coalitions are congenital, they typically do not become symptomatic until the coalition begins to ossify, usually in the early teen years. However, not all coalitions become symptomatic. Children with symptomatic solitary coalitions present with a painful flat foot.[3]

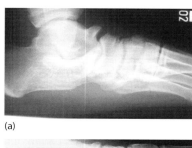
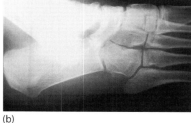
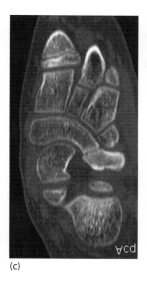
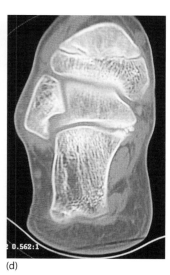

(a)

(b)

(c)

(d)

Figure 51.1 ● Radiographs of a 15-year-old boy with tarsal coalition. In the lateral view **(a)** the 'ant-eater' sign and talar beaking are seen. The oblique view **(b)** shows the complete calcaneonavicular bar. Computed tomography images show the appearance of a calcaneonavicular bar **(c)** and a talocalcaneal bar **(d)**.

Massive tarsal coalitions

Massive tarsal coalitions frequently involve the talus and the calcaneum and are often associated with fibular hemimelia. A proportion of children with this form of tarsal coalition have ball-and-socket ankle joints. Equinovalgus deformity that may be seen in children with fibular hemimelia is on account of the contracted tendoachilles, the tethering of the fibular anlage and the absence of the lateral malleolus. The coalition *per se* does not contribute to the deformity of the foot and ankle.

Multiple tarsal coalitions

Multiple tarsal coalitions are a part of multiple synostosis syndromes. In a small proportion of these patients significant deformities occur at the hind- and midfoot. The deformities which include equinus, equinovarus and forefoot inversion occur at the site of the coalition.[1,2]

Problems of management

Pain

Pain is not a feature of massive or multiple tarsal coalitions. However, it is often a symptom of solitary tarsal coalitions. Pain typically starts when the coalition begins to ossify, reducing subtalar motion and causing pain. This frequently occurs between nine and 14 years in those with calcaneonavicular bars, and slightly later in those with talocalcaneal bars. In due course, pain may also develop on account of degenerative arthritis of the subtalar and midtarsal joints.

Limitation of movement

The severity of limitation of joint movement depends on the site and the extent of tarsal coalition. A talocalcaneal coalition causes marked restriction of subtalar motion while a talonavicular coalition causes some restriction of both subtalar and midtarsal joint motion (Figure 51.2). Children with multiple tarsal coalitions have no movement at all in the subtalar and midtarsal joints.

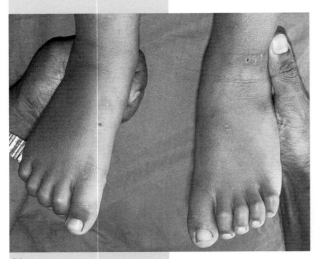

(a)

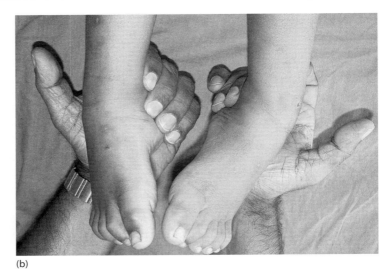

(b)

Figure 51.2 ● Limitation of movement of the subtalar joint is evident in a child with tarsal coalition of the right foot.

Deformity of the foot

Pes planovalgus, and failure to reconstitute a medial longitudinal arch when the child attempts to go into a weight-bearing equinus position, is characteristic of solitary tarsal coalitions (Figure 51.3). This, along with rigidity of foot motion, has been described as a 'peroneal spastic flat foot', but the peroneal muscles are not truly in spasm. Equinovarus deformity or forefoot inversion may occur in some forms of massive and multiple tarsal coalitions.[2]

Degenerative arthritis

Secondary degenerative arthritis may develop in subtalar and midtarsal joints over a period of time in patients with solitary coalitions if they are left untreated. Hence it is important to detect and treat symptomatic coalitions early in an attempt to prevent the development of degenerative arthritis.

Aims of treatment

- Relieve pain, if present
  The primary goal of treatment is to relieve pain in symptomatic children.
- Improve joint motion
  Although theoretically desirable, restoration of joint movement is less important. Again, this is only feasible if the coalition is solitary.
- Correct deformity
  In massive or multiple coalitions, if the foot is not plantigrade, deformities need to be corrected in order to make the foot plantigrade. Similarly, in solitary coalitions, the planovalgus deformity should be corrected.
- Avoid degenerative joint disease
  Although this is a desirable goal, it may not always be realistic.

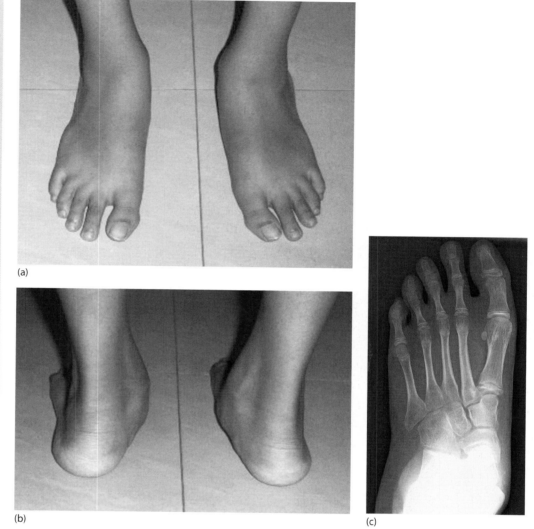

(a)

(b)

(c)

Figure 51.3 ● Planovalgus deformity of the left foot in an adolescent with symptomatic tarsal coalition **(a,b)**. The radiograph shows a relatively uncommon coalition between the medial and intermediate cuneiform bones **(c)**.

Treatment options

Relieving pain

■ Non-operative

Those who present with minimal pain need only simple shoe modifications. These may include heel cups, medial longitudinal arch supports or other orthotics. If more symptomatic, then a trial of immobilization in a short leg walking cast for a few weeks may resolve the symptoms. This is typically followed by a more formal orthosis, such as a UCBL (University of California Biomechanics Laboratory) type.

■ Operative

If the pain is not improved or recurs after a trial of cast immobilization, then surgical resection can be considered. Pain associated with solitary coalitions can be relieved by excising the coalition provided arthritic changes have not developed in the tarsal joints. If degenerative arthritis has already developed, then pain can only be relieved by abolishing all movement in the affected joints by performing an arthrodesis.

■ Resection of the coalition

● The calcaneonavicular coalition: The mainstay procedure is resection of the cartilaginous or osseous bar with interposition of the extensor digitorum brevis muscle belly (Figure 51.4a,b). The muscle is secured in position with the help of a posteromedially directed suture and skin surface button.[4] The raw bone surfaces can also be covered with bone wax to further reduce the risk of coalition reformation. A short leg non–weight-bearing cast is worn for three weeks, after which range of motion exercises and graduated weight bearing is begun.

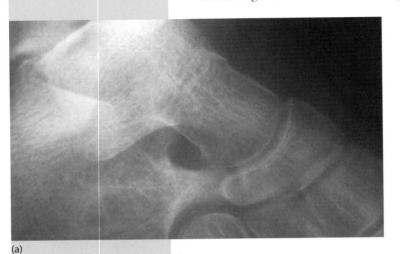
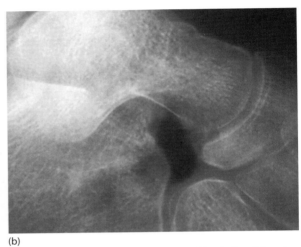

(a) (b)

Figure 51.4 ● Oblique radiographs of a nine-year-old child with a calcaneonavicular coalition before **(a)** and after **(b)** resection and interposition of the extensor digitorum brevis muscle.

● The talocalcaneal coalition: The bar, which involves the anterior and middle facet of the subtalar joint, is identified from a medial approach and excised from a superior direction, leaving the sustentaculum tali untouched. After bar resection, bone wax is first placed onto the raw surfaces, followed by a fat graft. A short leg non–weight-bearing cast is worn for three weeks, after which range of motion exercises and graduated weight bearing is begun.[5–9]

■ Subtalar arthrodesis

This is reserved for a failed resection with minimal talonavicular degenerative arthritis. Another, but uncommon, indication is a large talocalcaneal coalition with no talonavicular degenerative arthritis where the success of resection is likely to be poor due to either the size of the coalition or a varus foot deformity.

■ Triple arthrodesis

This is reserved for failed resections with persistent pain and deformity, or in a symptomatic patient with significant degenerative disease in any of the three joints (subtalar, calcaneocuboid, talonavicular). This is typically seen in the older patient. Standard techniques for any triple arthrodesis are used, followed by gradual weight bearing and ankle motion exercises after cast immobilization has ceased.[6,8,10,11]

Improving joint motion

In children with solitary coalitions, mobility of the subtalar and midtarsal joints may improve once the coalition is resected.

Correction of deformity

Flat foot seen in children with solitary symptomatic coalitions improves and the medial longitudinal arch is restored following resection of the coalition. Correction of deformity in children with massive or multiple coalitions entails performing an osteotomy through the coalition mass.[1,2] The osteotomy is held with Kirschner wires, staples or screws. Union of the osteotomy usually occurs in six to eight weeks. Occasionally, two osteotomies may be needed to correct more complex deformities.[1]

Factors to be taken into consideration while planning treatment

Magnitude of symptoms if the coalition is symptomatic

Children with mild symptoms are initially treated by shoe modifications. Those with more severe symptoms are treated by a short trial of casting and then surgery if there is no relief with casting.

Type of coalition and location of coalition

Initial radiographic examinations consist of standing anteroposterior, lateral radiographs and a non-weight-bearing oblique radiograph. The calcaneonavicular bar is visualized on the oblique radiograph; on the lateral radiograph the 'ant-eater' sign is often seen.[3] This represents the ossified bar as it extends from the calcaneus to the navicular. Talocalcaneal bars are difficult to visualize on the lateral radiograph, and all that is seen is a valgus foot, a C sign and, perhaps, talar beaking. Since talocalcaneal coalitions are rarely seen on these three standard views, the diagnosis is usually not made until a computed tomography (CT) scan is performed. Thus any child with a history and physical examination typical for a tarsal coalition and 'negative' plain radiographs should undergo a fine cut CT examination of the foot to look for a talocalcaneal coalition.[10,12]

Although calcaneonavicular coalitions are often diagnosed with oblique radiographs of the foot, subtalar coalitions may also coexist, and this should be confirmed on the CT scan. For subtalar coalitions, the exact position of the coalition in the subtalar joint should be carefully visualized on the CT scan pre-operatively to guide the surgical planning of the resection.

Since only solitary coalitions are resected it is imperative that the surgeon is sure that one is dealing with a solitary coalition. It is not uncommon to have multiple coalitions,[13] and therefore a CT scan is recommended in all coalitions which on plain radiographs appear to be solitary, to ensure that there are no subtle or small coalitions not previously recognized on plain films.

Coalition size

The success of resection of a talocalcaneal coalition decreases as the size of the coalition increases. Computed tomography scans should be used to quantify the area of the anterior and middle facet, posterior facet and area of coalition, using the techniques of Wilde or Comfort.[6,7,14] From these data the extent of the coalition as a percentage of the total joint surface can be determined. Those patients having less than a third of the total joint surface involved by the coalition have a high likelihood of success with resection (Figure 51.5a–c).

Presence of degenerative changes

When there is significant degenerative joint disease as documented by joint narrowing, subchondral sclerosis and cyst formation, the likelihood of success following resection is less and arthrodesis should be considered as the first procedure. Simple talar neck beaking is not a sign of degenerative changes and is frequently seen in many patients who later have an excellent result from resection.

Is the coalition an isolated deformity or part of a syndrome?

This is an important distinction as many genetic syndromes have other organ system issues which may need to be addressed or investigated. Also, if part of an orthopaedic congenital deformity,[14]

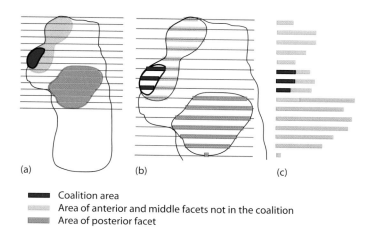

(a) (b) (c)

Figure 51.5 ● Technique of mapping of the extent of the talocalcaneal coalition.

■ Coalition area
▤ Area of anterior and middle facets not in the coalition
▨ Area of posterior facet

the issues of limb length inequality, angular deformity and joint stability need to be evaluated and considered in management.

Recommended treatment

The outline of treatment for tarsal coalition is shown in Table 51.1.

Table 51.1 ● Outline of the recommended management plan for treating tarsal coalition

INDICATIONS						
Asymptomatic Solitary tarsal coalition OR Massive coalition OR Multiple coalitions + Plantigrade foot	Solitary tarsal Coalition + Minimal symptoms	Solitary tarsal coalition + Moderate symptoms of short duration	Calcaneonavicular coalition OR Talocalcaneal coalition involving <50% of articular surface + Symptoms NOT relieved by cast or orthotics OR long duration of symptoms	Failed resection of talocalcaneal coalition OR Talocalcaneal coalition >50% of articular surface OR Degenerative arthritis of only the subtalar joint	Failed resection of calcaneonavicular coalition OR Degenerative arthritis of subtalar and midtarsal joints	Massive or multiple coalitions with a deformity (foot not plantigrade)
⇩	⇩	⇩	⇩	⇩	⇩	⇩
No intervention	Shoe modification	Cast immobilization for 3 weeks followed by orthosis	Resection of coalition and interposition of muscle or fat	Subtalar arthrodesis	Triple arthrodesis	Osteotomy through coalition mass to correct deformity and make foot plantigrade
TREATMENT						

Rationale of treatment choices

Why is non-operative treatment selected in those with minimal symptoms?
Obviously these patients need only minimal intervention to alleviate their symptoms. The risks of surgery are not warranted.

Why bar resection as the first measure?
The long-term goal is to relieve pain. By resecting the bar, the fused portion of the foot may develop some motion, albeit never normal motion. This increase in motion is adequate to relieve the pain; it is also hoped that it will reduce the risk of degenerative joint disease later in life. Proceeding to immediate fusion, although it may relieve pain, will probably result in earlier degenerative joint disease at the ankle, knee and remainder of the joints in the foot.

Why determine the percentage of coalition in the talocalcaneal joint when deciding between resection and arthrodesis?
The results clearly demonstrate that those with a third or less of the subtalar joint involved by the coalition have an approximately 80 percent chance of a good or excellent result with resection of the bar.

Why interpose tissue into the bar resection area?
This is to prevent recurrence of a synostosis between the bony surfaces and to improve the results of resection. This is why both bone wax and soft tissue interposition (e.g. extensor digitorum brevis for calcaneonavicular bar and fat for talocalcaneal bar) are recommended.

Why obtain CT scans on those feet with calcaneonavicular bars prior to resection?
This is to ensure that there is not an associated talocalcaneal bar that should be resected at the same surgery, or if large enough, be more amenable to arthrodesis.

References

1. Rebello G, Joseph B. The foot in multiple synostoses syndromes. *J Foot Ankle Surg* 2003; **9**: 19–24.
2. Rao BS, Joseph B. Varus and equinovarus deformities of the foot associated with tarsal coalition. *Foot* 1994; **4**: 95–9.
3. Vincent KA. Tarsal coalition and painful flatfoot. *J Am Acad Orthop Surg* 1998; **6**: 274–81.
4. Takakura Y, Sugimoto K, Tanaka Y, Tamai S. Symptomatic talocalcaneal coalition. Its clinical significance and treatment. *Clin Orthop Relat Res* 1991; **269**: 249–56.
5. Gonzalez P, Kumar SJ. Calcaneonavicular coalition treated by resection and interposition of the extensor digitorum brevis muscle. *J Bone Joint Surg Am* 1990; **72**: 71–7.
6. Clarke DM. Multiple tarsal coalitions in the same foot. *J Pediatr Orthop* 1997; **17**: 777–80.
7. Wilde PH, Torode IP, Dickens DR, Cole WG. Resection for symptomatic talocalcaneal coalition. *J Bone Joint Surg Br* 1994; **76**: 797–801.
8. Grogan DP, Holt GR, Ogden JA. Talocalcaneal coalition in patients who have fibular hemimelia or proximal femoral focal deficiency. *J Bone Joint Surg Am* 1994; **76**: 1363–70.
9. Mosier KM, Asher M. Tarsal coalitions and peroneal spastic flat foot. *J Bone Joint Surg Am* 1984; **66**: 976–84.
10. Danielsson LG. Talo-calcaneal coalition treated with resection. *J Pediatr Orthop* 1987; **7**: 513–17.
11. Scranton Jr. PE. Treatment of symptomatic talocalcaneal coalition. *J Bone Joint Surg Am* 1987; **69**: 533–8.
12. Oestreich AE, Mize WA, Crawford AH, Morgan Jr. RC. The "anteater nose": a direct sign of calcaneonavicular coalition on the lateral radiograph. *J Pediatr Orthop* 1987; **7**: 709–11.
13. Olney BW, Asher MA. Excision of symptomatic coalition of the middle facet of the talocalcaneal joint. *J Bone Joint Surg Am* 1987; **69**: 539–44.
14. Comfort TK, Johnson LO. Resection for symptomatic talocalcaneal coalition. *J Pediatr Orthop* 1998; **18**: 283–8.

Contractures of muscles

Benjamin Joseph

52

Introduction

Contractures of muscles can be either congenital or acquired. Congenital contractures of muscles are seen in arthrogryposis (multiple congenital contractures) and in association with certain congenital anomalies such as congenital dislocation of the knee, congenital dislocation of the patella, congenital clubfoot and congenital vertical talus. Acquired contractures of muscles may occur in paralytic conditions, following trauma, burns, intramuscular injections and after muscle ischaemia in a compartment syndrome.

Essentially, the contracted muscle may exhibit two types of abnormality: on one hand, the muscle may be of normal architecture and may function normally apart from the fact that it is shorter than normal; on the other hand, the muscle may be partly or completely replaced by fibrous tissue. The first situation may arise as a consequence of the muscle failing to grow normally, as seen in paralytic conditions where a muscle does not grow as the child grows simply due to the lack of stretch stimulus by the antagonist muscle because it is paralysed. The second situation is where muscle fibrosis occurs and a contracture develops because the fibrous tissue retracts and does not stretch as the child grows. This is seen following trauma, burns, intramuscular injections and after muscle ischaemia. The overall function of the muscle depends on the extent of damage to the muscle belly and the extent of muscle fibrosis, which varies in each of these conditions.

Since it is beyond the scope of this chapter to address each and every muscle contracture that may be encountered in paediatric orthopaedic practice, only three selected conditions are discussed in some detail. It is hoped that these examples will give sufficient insight into the recommended approach to decision-making. They are quadriceps contracture, gluteus maximus contracture and ischaemic contracture of the forearm. Muscle contractures that occur in paralytic conditions and contractures seen in association with congenital dislocation of the knee and congenital and habitual patella dislocation are discussed in the relevant chapters.

Consequences of muscle contracture and problems of management

Limitation of movement of the joint

The functional disability due to limitation of joint movement will vary according to the joint involved, the muscle involved and the functional requirements of the patient. For example, consider the implications of 30° loss of elbow extension, 30° loss of knee flexion and 30° loss of knee extension. This degree of loss of elbow extension is likely to cause no significant disability as virtually all activities of daily living can be accomplished quite easily despite this limitation. This degree of loss of knee flexion may not cause any problem in children in many societies while in societies that squat, this could be distressing. Finally, a 30° limitation of knee extension would be a profound disability in everybody as it would be impossible to stand straight with this deformity. It thus becomes very clear that the same magnitude of deformity can have very different implications in different joints and from patient to patient. This needs to be kept in mind while planning treatment.

Joint deformity

Deformities due to contractures of muscles may cause an unsightly appearance but may not result in significant functional disability in certain situations, such as an abduction contracture of the shoulder (Figure 52.1). However, extension contracture of the elbow due to triceps contracture or a quadriceps contracture does cause severe functional limitations although the limb does not look awkward at all (Figure 52.2).

Function of the affected muscle

The function of the affected muscle depends on the underlying condition. In multiple congenital contractures there is inherent muscle weakness. In situations where the muscle has been injured and replaced by fibrous tissue, the degree of weakness is proportional to the area of muscle damaged. Injection fibrosis is usually fairly localized and only a part of the muscle belly is actually fibrotic and hence the muscle is quite strong, whereas following a compartment syndrome a large area of the muscle may be replaced by fibrous tissue and hence the power of the muscle is poor.

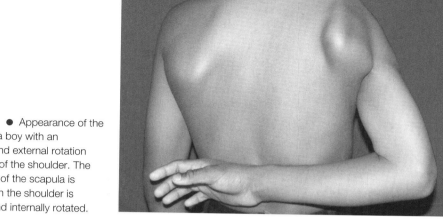

Figure 52.1 ● Appearance of the shoulder in a boy with an abduction and external rotation contracture of the shoulder. The prominence of the scapula is evident when the shoulder is adducted and internally rotated.

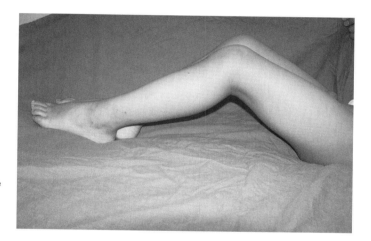

Figure 52.2 ● Appearance of the thigh and leg of a child with quadriceps contracture. The limb looks quite normal.

Aims of treatment

- Improve the range of motion of the joint
  While it is good if the range of movement can be restored to normal, it may be unwise to attempt this if a severe degree of contracture is present as it would lead to muscle weakness.
- Correct deformities
  Release of the contracted muscle will correct the joint deformity in most situations but additional release of contracted soft tissue such as the capsule or ligaments may be needed in some long-standing situations.
- Weaken the muscle as little as possible
  Surgery to relieve the contracture will necessarily entail lengthening the contracted muscle and this should be done in such a manner that the muscle is not unduly weakened by the surgery. In order to achieve this aim, as much of the normal muscle tissue as possible should be left undisturbed, lengthening only the diseased part of the muscle. For example, deltoid contracture following injection fibrosis usually affects only a small group of fibres; these fibres can be located and divided, leaving the major portion of the muscle intact without appreciably weakening the muscle. This may not be feasible in some situations but it must be normal practice whenever possible.

Quadriceps contracture

Quadriceps contracture may develop after post-injection fibrosis, open fractures of the femur and sepsis, either in the knee or the distal femur.

Problems of management

Inability to flex the knee sufficiently to sit comfortably

Often the knee is in complete extension and the child can only sit with the knee extended.

Stiff knee gait resulting in compensatory mechanisms to achieve foot clearance during the swing phase of gait

At least 30° of active knee flexion is needed to enable the toes to clear the ground with ease during the swing phase of gait. The child with a quadriceps contracture will have to vault on the opposite limb or circumduct the affected limb in order to get the toes to clear the ground if knee flexion is far less than 30°.

Weakness of knee extension and extensor lag following surgery

If the muscle is lengthened too much or if too many of the muscle fibres are released, persistent weakness of the muscle can ensue with an extensor lag and inability to keep the knee stable while negotiating stairs.

Problems of wound healing

Some operations that have been described for performing a quadricepsplasty use direct anterior incisions to approach the quadriceps and the femoral shaft.[1] Often these incisions extend onto the front of the proximal tibia to facilitate exposing the knee as well. Once the knee is flexed after surgery, the suture line is under considerable tension. This can result in worrisome wound dehiscence with the attendant risks of deep wound infection.

Adaptive bony changes

If the quadriceps contracture occurs very early in life and if it remains uncorrected for several years, the shape of the femoral condyle may alter and become flattened. It is important to release the contracture in early childhood to prevent the shape of the femur from becoming distorted.

Dislocation of the patella

Contracture of the vastus lateralis can lead to habitual dislocation of the patella. This problem is discussed in detail in Chapter 31, Recurrent and habitual dislocation of the patella.

Aims of treatment

- Improve the range of flexion of the knee sufficiently to facilitate sitting
  The aim of treatment is to obtain at least 90° of knee flexion. This will enable the child to sit comfortably in a chair. However, if the contracture is not very severe to begin with, more flexion may be obtained, especially if the child is from a community that prefers to squat.
- Improve the gait pattern
  If 90° of flexion is achieved the gait pattern reverts to normal provided the quadriceps has not been weakened too much. The compensatory mechanisms of a stiff-knee gait disappear if more than 30° of knee flexion is possible during the swing phase.
- Avoid weakness of the quadriceps following surgery
  If the short diseased muscle fibres alone are released and the normal muscle fibres are left undisturbed, post-operative quadriceps weakness can be minimized. This requires knowledge of the structure of the affected muscle and the site of the contracture. In Figure 52.3a a region of fibrosis of the vastus lateralis is depicted. The effects of releasing the muscle proximally and distally are shown in Figure 52.3b and c, respectively. Far greater numbers of normal muscle fibres are disturbed by a distal release and consequently it is likely that more weakness may ensue after a distal release, as has been confirmed in a clinical study.[2]
  If the contracture is severe, with less than 30° of knee flexion, it is safer to aim to achieve no more than 90° of knee flexion. If a more enthusiastic release is performed, the risk of persistent weakness is greater. On the other hand, if the contracture is less severe and about 60° of flexion is possible prior to surgery, it is probably justified to attempt to obtain greater correction than 90° of knee flexion.
- Ensure satisfactory wound healing
  As an incision that is not under tension is likely to heal more satisfactorily, it is advisable to use an incision that avoids areas which will be under tension when the knee is flexed following surgery.

- Prevent adaptive bony changes
  Early release will prevent adaptive bony changes from occurring. Since established muscle contractures will not respond to any physiotherapy it is futile to persist with any such intervention beyond a year after the contracture is noticed.

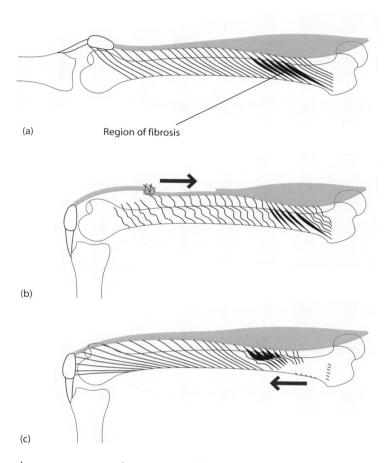

(a)   Region of fibrosis

(b)

(c)

Figure 52.3 ● Diagram showing a region of fibrosis of the quadriceps muscle in the proximal third of the thigh **(a)**. When the muscle is released distally all the fibres of the quadriceps are disturbed and weakened **(b)**. Proximal release of the quadriceps disturbs much fewer normal fibres of the muscle **(c)**.

Treatment options

The only way the contracture can be overcome is by surgery; the choices are only with regard to the nature of the surgery.

Technique of quadricepsplasty

■ Distal release of the quadriceps

Release of the quadriceps in the distal third of the thigh was recommended by Thompson.[1] The operation entails a z-lengthening of the rectus femoris tendon and release of the vasti. When the muscle fibrosis is predominantly in the distal third of the thigh following either an open fracture in the supracondylar region or distal metaphyseal osteomyelitis, a distal release would be more appropriate. In these situations it is important to recognize adherence of the patella if it is present and release intra-articular adhesions. Since incisions placed on the front of the knee are under tension when the knee is flexed, an arthrotomy through a parapatellar incision is best avoided; dealing with the intra-articular adhesions arthroscopically seems a logical alternative.

■ Proximal release of the quadriceps

Techniques of release of the quadriceps from the proximal part of the thigh have been described for treating injection fibrosis.[2–4] One obvious reason for using this technique for injection fibrosis is because the site of the injection is in the proximal part of the thigh. The second important reason for performing a proximal release is because the frequency and the severity of extensor lag noted after the proximal release is less than after a distal release.[2,3] The operation involves releasing the vastus lateralis from the proximal third of the femoral shaft and then progressively releasing fibres of the vastus lateralis and intermedius as required until the knee flexes to 90° (Figure 52.4a–c).

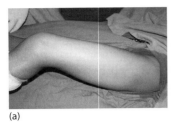
(a)

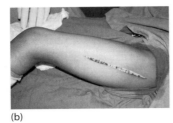
(b)

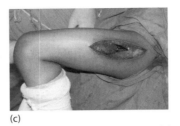
(c)

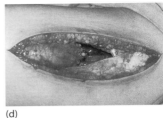
(d)

Figure 52.4 ● Amount of knee flexion possible before surgery in a child with quadriceps contracture due to injection fibrosis **(a)**. The incision **(b)** and the amount of flexion achieved by proximal release of the quadriceps **(c)** and the extent of muscle release **(d)** are shown.

Factors to be taken into consideration while planning treatment

Choice of the incision

The advantages of a lateral incision over an anterior incision are that it overlies the vastus lateralis muscle belly that is most frequently affected and the suture line is not under severe tension when the knee is flexed following the release.

Nature of underlying disease

Injection fibrosis is usually localized to the region surrounding the site of injection. The fibrosis is likely to be more extensive following trauma and infection.

Components of the quadriceps muscle that are contracted

Since injections into the thigh are normally given in the anterolateral or the anterior aspect of the proximal or middle third of the thigh, the fibrosis is most likely to involve the vastus lateralis and the vastus intermedius. The vastus medialis is usually spared. The rectus femoris may be affected if the injection has been given on the anterior aspect of the thigh (Figure 52.5). Quadriceps fibrosis following an open fracture or osteomyelitis is more likely to involve muscle fibres that are in close contact with the bone, and the site of the muscle fibrosis would be most severe at the site of bony involvement.

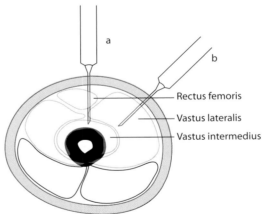

Figure 52.5 ● Diagram showing a cross section of the thigh and the location of the components of the quadriceps muscle. An injection in the anterior aspect of the thigh may cause a contracture of the rectus femoris and the vastus intermedius **(a)**. An injection in the anterolateral aspect of the thigh may cause a contracture of the vastus lateralis while the rectus femoris is spared **(b)**.

Severity of the contracture

Contractures that are mild enough not to cause any disability may be ignored. However, it must be remembered that such a mild contracture seldom attracts the attention of the parents. Any contracture of the quadriceps that does not permit flexion of the knee to nearly 90° needs to be released.

The need to squat or sit cross-legged

In children from societies where squatting is not important, one can accept a degree of contracture of the quadriceps that permits 90° of flexion of the knee. In children from societies where it is necessary to squat, surgery may be considered for even this degree of contracture.

Recommended treatment

The outline of recommended treatment is shown in Table 52.1.

Table 52.1 ● Outline of treatment of acquired quadriceps contracture

INDICATIONS			
Any cause + 90° knee flexion possible + Squatting not needed ⇩ No intervention	Injection fibrosis + Severe contracture (knee flexion <60°) + Irrespective of society and the need to squat ⇩ Proximal quadricepsplasty through lateral incision + Aim for 90° of knee flexion	Injection fibrosis + Mild to moderate contracture (knee flexion 60–90°) + Squatting needed ⇩ Proximal quadricepsplasty through lateral incision + Aim for 110° of knee flexion	Post-traumatic or post-infective quadriceps contracture (fracture or infection in distal femur) ⇩ Distal quadricepsplasty through lateral incision + Release of intra-articular adhesions through arthroscope + Aim for 90° of knee flexion
TREATMENT			

Gluteus maximus contracture

Contracture of the gluteus maximus can develop following intramuscular injections; however, the cause is unclear in several instances.[5] Unlike quadriceps contracture, contracture of the gluteus maximus is usually not so severe as to prevent flexion totally, and the contracture seldom produces major functional disability and thus the approach to treatment is far less aggressive. The child presents with an abnormal awkward sitting posture having to sit with the hips abducted.[5] The extent to which the hips are abducted indicates the severity of the contracture (Figure 52.6a–d). The contracture produces a characteristic pattern of limitation of hip flexion that varies in different positions of the hip and this can be very clearly demonstrated on careful clinical examination (Figure 52.7a–d). Typically, the range of hip flexion reduces as the hip is adducted or internally rotated while the range of hip flexion increases when the hip is abducted and externally rotated.

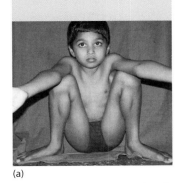 (a) 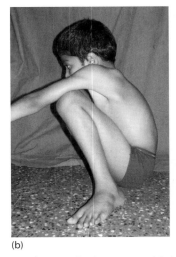 (b) 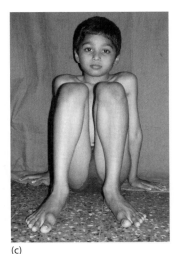 (c) 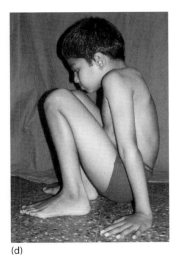 (d)

Figure 52.6 ● This boy with a gluteus maximus contracture was unable to squat with his knees together and had to keep his hips abducted while squatting **(a,b)**. When he squats with his knees together the hip extends and he tends to fall backwards and has to support himself with his hands to avoid falling backwards **(c,d)**.

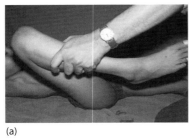
(a)

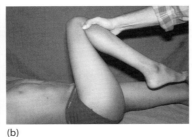
(b)

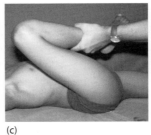
(c)

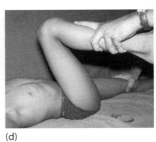
(d)

Figure 52.7 ● Careful examination of the same boy shows that the range of flexion of the hip increases as the hip is abducted **(a)** and decreases as the hip is adducted **(b)**. Similarly, the range of hip flexion increases when the hip is externally rotated **(c)** and decreases as the hip is internally rotated **(d)**. These are characteristic features of contracture of the gluteus maximus muscle.

Problems of management

The problem is usually one of an awkward appearance while sitting. If the contracture is severe it may be difficult for the child to sit in a narrow seat. Milder degrees of contracture do not cause functional limitations.

Aims of treatment

● Enable the child to sit in a narrow seat

Treatment options

The two treatment options are:

● no intervention;
● release of the gluteus maximus.

Recommended treatment

If the contracture is severe enough to prevent the child from sitting comfortably in a narrow seat, the muscle should be released at its insertion. If the contracture is not so severe as to prevent the child from sitting in a narrow seat, treatment can be withheld.

Ischaemic contracture of the forearm

Ischaemic contracture of the muscles of the forearm may follow compartment syndrome that has been inappropriately treated.[6] Unfortunately, this entirely preventable complication occurs frequently enough to warrant a discussion on treatment. Clearly, the severity of contracture is directly related to adequacy and the timing of fascial decompression following the onset of the compartment syndrome.

Since the ischaemia affects all the tissues within the compartment, in addition to damage to muscles, the nerves that traverse the compartment are also affected. Consequently, varying degrees of motor and sensory nerve damage may be seen, and the motor paralysis further compromises function of the muscles that are damaged by ischaemia.

Compartment syndrome of the forearm affects the flexor compartment primarily, although the extensor compartment may be affected in severe cases. Tsuge[7] classified ischaemic contracture of the forearm on the basis of the severity of contracture and the muscles affected (Figure 52.8a–c and Table 52.2). In the mild or localized form only part of the flexor digitorum profundus is involved. In the moderate form the flexor digitorum profundus, the flexor pollicis longus and the superficial flexor muscles are contracted. In severe cases the deep and superficial flexor muscles and some extensor muscles are involved.

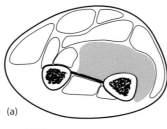
(a)

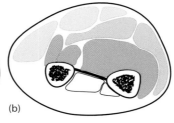
(b)

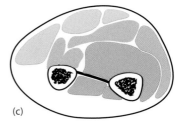
(c)

Figure 52.8 ● Diagram showing the cross section of the forearm and the muscles that are contracted in mild **(a)**, moderate **(b)** and severe ischaemic contracture **(c)**.

MILD
Partial involvement of the flexor digitorum profundus.

MODERATE
Flexor digitorum profundus and flexor pollicus longus severely affected.
Partial involvement of the flexor digitorum superficialis and other superficial flexors.

SEVERE
All flexor muscles affected. Deep extensor muscles also affected.

Table 52.2 ● Classification of ischaemic contracture of the forearm

Severity	Muscles affected	Deformities		Sensory disturbance	Intrinsic muscle paralysis
Mild (localized)	Part of FDP	*Fingers*: Flexion deformity of two or three fingers (usually middle and ring fingers)		No sensory deficit or mild hypoesthesia	Absent or minimal
		Thumb: Nil			
		Wrist: Nil			
Moderate (classic)	FDP FPL + Part of FDS, FCU, FCR	*Fingers*: Flexion deformity of all fingers OR claw deformity (if intrinsic paralysis is present)		Sensory loss in median and ulnar zones	Intrinsic paralysis often present
		Thumb: Flexed and adducted			
		Wrist: Flexion deformity			
Severe	All flexor muscles + Part of extensor muscles	*Fingers*: Claw deformity of all fingers		Sensory loss in median and ulnar zones	Intrinsic paralysis invariably present
		Thumb: Flexed and adducted			
		Wrist: Severe flexion deformity			

Problems of management

Contracture of the flexor muscles of the forearm

Contracture of the flexor muscles produces the characteristic tenodesis sign where the flexion deformity of the fingers is partially or completely corrected when the wrist is flexed while the deformity is accentuated when the wrist is extended (Figure 52.9a,b). The muscles that are most severely affected are the flexor digitorum profundus and the flexor pollicis longus, both of which are situated deep in the flexor compartment.

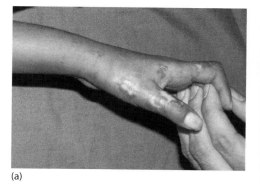
(a)

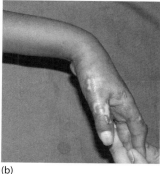
(b)

Figure 52.9 ● The tenodesis sign seen in a child with an ischaemic contracture of the forearm. The flexion deformity of the fingers is accentuated when the wrist is extended **(a)** and decreases when the wrist is flexed **(b)**.

Associated sensory loss on the palm of the hand

The sensations in the zones of the median or ulnar nerves may be compromised as a result of ischaemia of these nerves. The sensory loss may vary from hypoaesthesia to anaesthesia. There may also be some loss of sensation in the forearm and this may increase the risk of plaster sores if sequential casting is being considered as a form of treatment.

Motor weakness

The anterior interosseous nerve is most frequently affected; the median nerve and the ulnar nerve are affected in moderate and severe cases. Consequently, muscles supplied by these nerves may be weak or paralysed. The extent of paralysis, to a large extent, determines the degree of function that may be anticipated following any form of reconstructive surgery.

Scarring of soft tissues

The skin and fascia may also be badly scarred and this may have a bearing on the choice of surgery.

Impaired blood supply

Although some collateral circulation will have been restored in all children who present with forearm contracture following ischaemia of a compartment syndrome, the blood supply to the radius and ulna may not be normal and this may impede bone healing after an osteotomy of these bones.

Aims of treatment

- Improve hand function
  Improvement of the function of the hand is the primary aim of treatment of an ischaemic contracture of the forearm in a child. This should be feasible in the majority of instances despite the seemingly severe nature of deformity.[6]
- Improve the appearance of the wrist and hand
  Improvement of the appearance of the forearm, wrist and hand is the secondary aim in most instances. In the rare situation where function cannot be improved at all, improvement of appearance may be the sole aim.

Treatment options

Any attempt to improve function involves measures both to deal with the paralysis and to relieve the contracture. Options for dealing with paralysis are not included in this chapter as they are discussed elsewhere (see Chapter 60, The paralysed hand and wrist); only options to correct the contracture are discussed here. Most surgeons first deal with the contracture and then, after a time interval, attempt reconstructive surgery to deal with the paralysis.

Excision of the muscle infarct

Seddon[8] has described an operation that entails excision of the part of the muscle belly that is necrotic (which he refers to as the 'muscle infarct'). The unaffected muscle fibres often respond to post-operative stretching and the deformity may improve.

Flexor pronator slide

The release of the origin of the flexor muscles from the medial epicondyle and the proximal ulna, described by Page,[9] relieves moderate degrees of contracture of the flexor muscles. In severe cases extensive release of the muscles from the shafts of the ulna and radius needs to be performed.[7]

Lengthening of flexor tendons in the forearm

Several tendons need to be lengthened in the distal third of the forearm in order to relieve the flexion deformity of the hand. Apart from being a tedious procedure, post-operative adhesions may develop as the bed is already scarred and fibrotic.

Gradual distraction with an external fixator

With the help of an external fixator, gradual distraction of the contracted muscles may be performed. If this is preceded by neurolysis of the median and ulnar nerves the nerves are not at risk of further damage by stretching while they are tethered down by perineural fibrous tissue. The nerves may then have some chance of recovery.

Sequential casting

Sequential casting can be used to correct deformities of the wrist and the fingers if the deformities are mild and after partial correction of severe deformities by surgery. This method of deformity correction is particularly useful before the deformities have become chronic.

Carpectomy

If the contracture is severe, it may occasionally be difficult to correct the deformity of the wrist and hand by release of the contracted muscles alone. In such situations shortening of the skeleton is an option. Shortening of a moderate extent can be achieved by excising a row of carpal bones. This option should be reserved for very severe cases as function of the wrist joint may be poor and pain may develop in the wrist following this procedure. However, if a wrist fusion is being planned as a means of dealing with the paralysis and deformity at the wrist, excising a row of carpal bones will facilitate correction of the deformity and relax the contracted flexor tendons and thus reduce the deformity of the fingers.

Shortening of the radius and ulna

Another option for shortening the skeleton is to shorten the radius and ulna. An appropriate form of stable internal fixation is required after shortening of the bones. The potential risk of delayed union of the osteotomy sites due to the reduced blood flow in the bones must be borne in mind if this option is being considered.

Severity of contracture

The extent of release understandably depends on the severity of the contracture. Mild degrees of contracture that affect two or three fingers can be treated effectively by relatively simple procedures while more severe degrees of contracture require elaborate operations both to overcome the contracture and to deal with the associated muscle paralysis.

Time that has elapsed since the ischaemic insult

After the ischaemia to the muscles has occurred, the area of the muscle belly that is avascular undergoes necrosis and gradually the necrotic area is replaced by fibrous tissue. If the necrotic muscle tissue is excised before the fibrous tissue has formed, the degree of contracture can be minimized. Once the fibrous tissue forms, it retracts as the scar matures. The contracture of the muscle then becomes established within six months of the onset of ischaemia. If there is extensive muscle necrosis the nerves that run through the compartment become caught up in the fibrous cicatrix and this limits the chance of nerve recovery. Efforts to minimize the contracture may be beneficial in the first six months after the compartment syndrome as the contracture is evolving.

The treatment outline recommended for dealing with an ischaemic contracture of the forearm is shown in Table 52.3.

Factors to be taken into consideration while planning treatment

Recommended treatment

Table 52.3 ● Outline of treatment of ischaemic contracture of the forearm

INDICATIONS						
Evolving contracture + Mild type	Evolving contracture + Moderate type	Evolving contracture + Severe type	Established ischaemic contracture Mild type + two fingers involved	Established ischaemic contracture Mild type + three or four fingers involved	Established ischaemic contracture Moderate type	Established ischaemic contracture Severe type
⇩	⇩	⇩	⇩	⇩	⇩	⇩
Sequential casting and splinting	Excision of muscle infarct + Stretching, casting, splinting	Excision of muscle infarct + Neurolysis of median and ulnar nerves + Stretching, casting, splinting	Lengthening of tendons of the flexed fingers in the distal third of the forearm	Muscle slide from humerus and ulna	Muscle slide from humerus, ulna and radius	Excision of fibrotic muscles + Neurolysis of median and ulnar nerves ± Distraction with a fixator OR Proximal row carpectomy and wrist fusion
TREATMENT						

References

1. Thompson TC. Quadricepsplasty to improve knee function. *J Bone Joint Surg Am* 1944; **26**: 366–79.
2. Jackson AM, Hutton PA. Injection-induced contractures of the quadriceps in childhood. A comparison of proximal release and distal quadricepsplasty. *J Bone Joint Surg Br* 1985; **67**: 97–102.
3. Burnei G, Neagoe P, Margineanu BA, Dan D, Burcur PO. Treatment of severe iatrogenic quadriceps retraction in children. *J Pediatr Orthop B* 2004; **13**: 254–8.
4. Sengupta S. Pathogenesis of infantile quadriceps fibrosis and its correction by proximal release. *J Pediatr Orthop* 1985; **5**: 187–91.
5. Shen YS. Abduction contracture of the hip in children. *J Bone Joint Surg Br* 1975; **57**: 463–5.
6. Anderson GA. The child's hand in the developing world. In: Gupta A, Kay SPJ, Scheker LR (eds). *The Growing Hand*. London: Harcourt Publishers Limited, 2000: 1097–114.
7. Tsuge K. Treatment of established Volkmann's contracture. In: Green DP (ed.). *Operative Hand Surgery*. New York: Churchill Livingstone, 1993: 592–603.
8. Seddon HJ. Volkmann's contracture: Treatment by excision of the infarct. *J Bone Joint Surg Br* 1956; **38**: 152–74.
9. Page CM. An operation for the relief of flexion-contracture in the forearm. *J Bone Joint Surg Am* 1923; **5**: 233–4.

SECTION 6

Paralyses

General principles of management of lower motor neuron paralysis

53

Benjamin Joseph

Introduction

Static paralytic problems in children may occur as the result of central nervous system disorders such as spina bifida and poliomyelitis or following disorders of the peripheral nervous system such as obstetric brachial plexus palsy and peripheral nerve injuries.

Progressive paralysis may be encountered in muscular dystrophy and hereditary motor neuropathies.

Although management depends on whether the paralysis is static or progressive and whether it is associated with sensory loss or not, some general principles of management are applicable to all these situations.

Problems of management

Loss of function

The most obvious manifestation of paralysis is the loss of function due to muscle weakness. Muscle paralysis in the lower limb impairs locomotion, while in the upper limb it affects the activities of daily living.

Muscle imbalance

Paralysis of one group of muscles acting on a joint can result in muscle imbalance if the antagonistic muscle group is either unaffected or less severely affected. Muscle imbalance, in turn, can lead to deformities and instabilities at joints.

Deformities

The main cause of joint deformities in paralytic conditions is muscle imbalance, although postural deformities may also occur in paralysed limbs (Figure 53.1). In the growing child, mere correction of paralytic deformity is not enough, the underlying muscle imbalance must also be corrected or else the deformity is likely to recur.

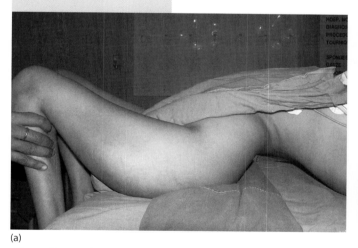
(a)

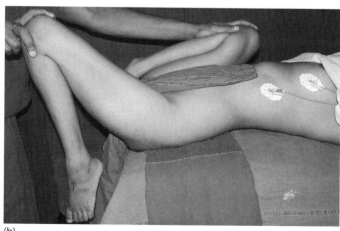
(b)

Figure 53.1 ● Severe flexion deformities of the hips **(a)** and knees **(b)** are seen in an adolescent who had no treatment following an attack of severe poliomyelitis in early childhood. These are predominantly postural deformities.

Instability of joints

Paralysis of all muscles acting on a joint would render the joint flail and unstable in all directions, while paralysis of a group of muscles may result in instability in one direction.

Limb length discrepancy

If paralysis of one limb occurs in a young child, limb length inequality may develop. While some unilateral shortening may not be of much consequence in the upper limb, it may need to be addressed if it occurs in the lower limb.

Aims of treatment

- Restore muscle power if possible
- Correct muscle imbalance
- Prevent deformities and if deformities have already developed correct them
- Restore stability of joints
- Deal with lower limb length inequality

It needs to be emphasized that sometimes it may not be possible to achieve all these aims. It is also important to note that in certain situations it may be wiser to leave some of these problems uncorrected. For example, certain deformities may actually be beneficial (see Chapter 55, The paralysed knee), or a mild degree of shortening may actually facilitate clearance of the paralysed limb during the swing phase of gait. Similarly, some shortening may improve femoral head coverage by the acetabulum when the child stands, if there is a tendency for hip subluxation.

Treatment options

Restoration of muscle power

■ Reinnervation of denervated muscle

Actual restoration of muscle power by reinnervating a paralysed muscle is the best solution. This may be feasible in certain situations (e.g. repair of a severed nerve or neurotization of the musculocutaneous nerve with intercostal nerves to restore function of paralysed elbow flexors). However, in the majority of paralytic situations this may not be possible.

■ Tendon transfer

The next best option is a tendon transfer. A tendon transfer may be considered if the following criteria are fulfilled: the muscle chosen for transfer must have normal power (MRC grade V); transfer of the tendon should not cause any secondary deformity.

If the transfer is likely to cause secondary joint instability, it should be possible to correct the new instability at the time of the tendon transfer.

■ Free muscle transfer

Free transfer of a muscle along with its neurovascular pedicle is yet another way of restoring muscle power. However, there are very limited indications for this procedure.

Correction of muscle imbalance

Muscle imbalance must be corrected even if a deformity can be corrected without rebalancing the muscle power to prevent recurrence of the deformity due to the effect of the muscle imbalance on a proximal joint (Figure 53.2). Muscle imbalance can be restored by either strengthening the weaker muscle group or weakening the stronger muscle group.

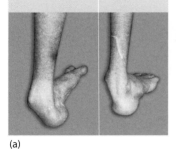
(a)

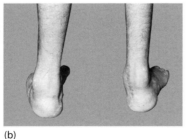
(b)

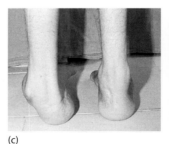
(c)

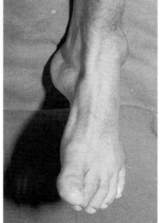
(d)

Figure 53.2 ● An equinovarus deformity of the left foot in an adolescent **(a)** was corrected by triple arthrodesis **(b)**. A varus deformity at the ankle developed over a period of ten years due to muscle imbalance that was not corrected at the time of arthrodesis **(c)**. The tibialis anterior was functioning while the peronei were paralysed **(d)**. The right foot that was flail was also stabilized by a triple arthrodesis; the foot remained plantigrade.

■ Strengthening of the weaker muscle group

Strengthening of the weaker muscle group can be achieved by a tendon transfer. The fact that the power of the transferred muscle will reduce by one grade should be kept in mind when planning the muscle rebalancing procedure.

■ Weakening of the stronger muscle group

When a tendon transfer is performed, weakening of the stronger muscle group occurs since the force of the transferred muscle is removed from the stronger side.

In situations where a tendon transfer is not feasible, weakening of the stronger muscle group can be achieved by tenotomy, tendon lengthening or a muscle slide operation. A tenotomy totally defunctions the muscle but the latter two procedures weaken the muscle by reducing the resting length of the muscle fibres. (Starling's law (1914) states that the force of contraction of a muscle is proportional to the resting length of its fibres.)

Prevention of deformities

If muscle balance is restored soon after the paralysis occurs, deformities may be prevented.

Correction of deformities

Release of contracted tendons should be the first measure to be adopted for correcting paralytic deformity. This may entail a simple tenotomy, intramuscular tendon lengthening, z-lengthening of the tendon or a tendon transfer (Figure 53.3). In situations in which the deforming force of a contracted tendon can be converted to a correcting force by a tendon transfer, it should be considered as the preferred option. Here the tendon should be detached as close to its insertion as possible so as to provide maximum length for appropriate anchorage after it is transferred.

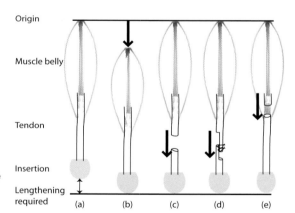

Figure 53.3 ● The diagram shows the various techniques of lengthening a contracted muscle-tendon unit **(a)**: they include muscle slide **(b)**, tenotomy **(c)**, z-lengthening **(d)** and intramuscular lengthening **(e)**.

Z-lengthening of tendons is the most commonly performed procedure for correcting paralytic deformities. The orientation of the 'Z' may be an important consideration when biplanar deformities are corrected (e.g. while correcting an equinovarus deformity the long limb of the Z cut should be in the sagittal plane and the distal limb of the cut is directed medially, but the distal cut should be directed laterally when correcting an equinovalgus deformity – see Chapter 3, Equinovarus). If there is a possibility of the need for a tendon transfer at a later date, intramuscular tendon lengthening is preferred over z-lengthening in order to leave a healthy unscarred tendon for future transfer.

If a tenotomy is the chosen option, it should be performed at the most accessible site.

In more long-standing cases, in addition to releasing contracted tendons, capsulotomy of the joint may be required to correct the deformity. When the deformity is severe, apart from these soft tissue releases, bony surgery may also be required. The aim of bony surgery is to shorten the skeleton sufficiently to relax the contracted soft tissues, thereby correcting the deformity. This often entails a corrective osteotomy performed close to the joint. In general, a closed wedge osteotomy is preferred in order to shorten the bony skeleton. In some situations shortening of the skeleton may be achieved by excision of a segment of the bone or even an entire bone (e.g. talectomy to correct foot deformities, see Chapter 3, Equinovarus).

Stabilization of joints

■ Dynamic stabilization

The best surgical option for correction of joint instability in a single direction is a tendon transfer. A tendon transfer may occasionally be useful in restoring stability when instability in two directions is present (e.g. instability in the sagittal and coronal planes when ankle dorsiflexors and the evertors of the foot are paralysed). A tendon transfer, however, would not be of help in correcting multidirectional instability.

■ Static stabilization

An appropriate orthosis can stabilize a joint externally and may be considered for instability in one or more directions. In general, orthotic stabilization should be considered as an interim option until a more permanent solution can be adopted. It is particularly useful in children who are too young to cooperate with muscle re-education after a tendon transfer. Wherever possible, an effort must be made to find an alternative option by skeletal maturity.

Static stabilization of instability in a single direction may be achieved by a tenodesis (e.g. Westin's tenodesis for calcaneus) or a bone block operation (e.g. posterior bone block at the ankle for foot drop) (see Chapter 56, The paralysed foot and ankle). Arthrodesis is required to surgically stabilize a joint that has multidirectional instability.

It needs to be emphasized that arthrodesis of joints of the foot should be avoided if sensations are lost on the sole as the risk of neuropathic plantar ulceration is much greater if the foot is rendered stiff by arthrodesis even if has been made plantigrade.[1]

Paralytic joint instability may also be improved by:

● realignment of the axis of movement of a joint (e.g. supracondylar femoral extension osteotomy to restore knee stability in quadriceps paralysis, see Chapter 55, The paralysed knee);
● altering the direction of action of functioning muscles (e.g. lateral displacement calcaneal osteotomy to correct varus instability at the ankle joint, see Chapter 56, The paralysed foot and ankle);
● altering the relationship between the articulating surfaces (e.g. proximal femoral varus osteotomy for improving hip stability, see Chapter 25, Paralytic hip dislocation: cerebral palsy; Chapter 26, Paralytic hip dislocation: spina bifida and polio; and Chapter 27, Teratologic hip dislocation in multiple congenital contractures).

These three methods of improving paralytic instability entail osteotomies in the vicinity of the respective joints.

Limb length equalization

Limb length equalization is usually not needed in the upper limb in paralytic situations.

In the lower limb the options for dealing with limb length discrepancy are:

● intentionally avoid equalizing the limb lengths;
● shoe raise;
● shortening of the longer limb;
● lengthening of the short limb.

The principles for choosing the optimal limb equalization option are outlined in the section on management of limb length discrepancy (see Chapter 42, General principles of management of discrepancies of limb length in children; Chapter 43, Length discrepancy of the femur; and Chapter 44, Length discrepancy of the tibia).

Recommended treatment and the rationale for the choice of treatment

In a limb with a lower motor neuron paralysis, an appropriate tendon transfer may enable restoration of muscle power, muscle balance and joint stability and also correct dynamic deformity. No other operation performed on a paralysed limb can restore all these deficits (Table 53.1) and hence, wherever possible, a tendon transfer should be the preferred option. If a tendon transfer is not possible, extra-articular procedures that do not permanently stiffen joints should be considered. An arthrodesis is only selected when these two options are not feasible.

Table 53.1 ● Outline of treatment of a paralysed limb

Operations	Aims of treatment of a paralysed limb that may be fulfilled by each operation			
	Restore muscle power	Restore muscle balance	Restore joint stability	Correct joint deformity
Tendon transfer	Yes	Yes	Yes	Yes (if dynamic and NOT fixed)
Tenodesis	No	No	Yes	Yes
Tendon lengthening	No	Yes	No	Yes
Tenotomy	No	Yes	No	Yes
Arthrodesis	No	No	Yes	Yes
Osteotomy	No	No	Yes	Yes
Bone block	No	No	Yes	No

Reference

1. Maynard MJ, Weiner LS, Burke SW. Neuropathic ulceration in patients with myelodysplasia. *J Pediatr Orthop* 1992; **12**: 786–8.

The paralysed hip

Benjamin Joseph

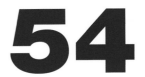

54

Introduction

Paralysis of the muscles around the hip may occur in spina bifida and sacral agenesis, following spinal cord injury, after poliomyelitis and in some forms of muscular dystrophy. Paralysis of all the muscles of both hips would make unaided walking impossible, while paralysis of individual muscles produces distinctive problems related to walking and stability of the hip.

Problems of management

Loss of function

Complete paralysis of the muscles acting on the hip renders the hip flail. Paralysis of the hip flexors makes it difficult to propel the limb forward while walking. Paralysis of hip abductors results in a Trendelenburg gait while paralysis of the hip extensors produces a typical gait pattern where the patient lurches backwards with exaggerated lumbar lordosis.

Muscle imbalance

Quite frequently one muscle group is paralysed while the antagonists are spared, resulting in muscle imbalance.

Deformities

Deformities develop on account of the muscle imbalance or due to the effect of gravity and posture. Deformities that may be encountered in hips that are paralysed include flexion, adduction with internal rotation or abduction with external rotation. Less frequently, an extension deformity of the hip may be seen. An adduction and internal rotation deformity of the hip predisposes to paralytic hip dislocation. An abduction deformity of one hip can cause pelvic obliquity and this can result in the opposite hip dislocating.

Joint instability

Joint instability is quite frequently seen when the abductors and extensors of the hip are paralysed and the flexors and adductors remain functional.

Aims of treatment

- Restore muscle power
  Very few tendon transfers are feasible in the region of the hip and hence restoring muscle power is often not possible. Attempts to improve hip abductor and hip extensor function may, however, be justified.
- Correct deformities
  Deformities of the hip can compromise ambulatory function and also predispose to hip instability and, consequently, such deformities must be corrected. It is important to be aware that some deformities may actually be beneficial. For example, a minor degree of abduction deformity can abolish a Trendelenburg gait even if the gluteus medius and minimus are paralysed.
- Restore joint stability
  Paralytic hip instability should be addressed (see Chapter 25, Paralytic hip dislocation: cerebral palsy; Chapter 26, Paralytic hip dislocation: spina bifida and polio; and Chapter 27, Teratologic hip dislocation in multiple congenital contractures) as dislocation of one or both hips can adversely affect ambulation and sitting balance can be affected if one hip dislocates.

Treatment options

Restoring muscle power

The two muscles that have been used with some measure of success to augment the power of hip abduction are the iliopsoas and the external oblique abdominis (Figure 54.1).

Two techniques of transferring the iliopsoas are the lateral transfer of Mustard[1] and the posterolateral transfer of Sharrard[2] (Figure 54.2). The latter technique was devised with the hope that the transferred tendon would act both as an abductor and an extensor of the hip but this seldom occurs. Evaluation of abductor function after tendon transfers has shown that a proportion of the transfers may, at best, work as a tenodesis without demonstrable active abduction function.[3]

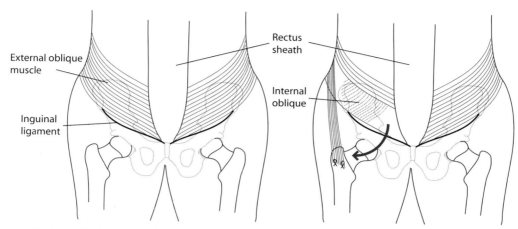

Figure 54.1 ● Diagram illustrating the technique of an external oblique transfer for restoring hip abductor power.

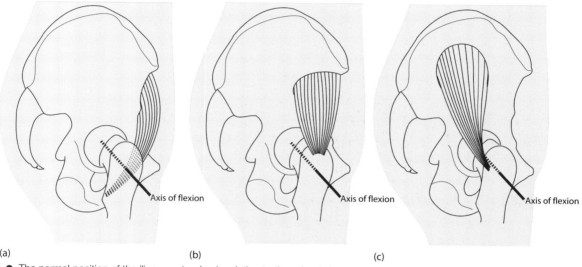

(a)   (b)   (c)

Figure 54.2 ● The normal position of the iliopsoas tendon in relation to the axis of hip flexion is shown **(a)**. It is evident that when a Mustard's transfer is performed the transferred tendon is in line with this axis and hence can act as a pure abductor without either flexing or extending the hip **(b)**. The Sharrard's iliopsoas transfer for hip extensor and abductor paralysis is also shown **(c)**.

The erector spinae transfer for gluteus maximus paralysis improves the lurch[4] but seldom totally restores the power of extension (Figure 54.3).

Correcting deformities

Deformities that are mild or moderate may be treated by releasing contracted soft tissue. However, more severe degrees of deformity require a subtrochanteric osteotomy. The decision on what structures are to be released is taken at the time of surgery. Structures are released in a sequential manner from the deep fascia and the most superficial muscles to the deeper muscles and last of all the capsule of the hip. The effect of the release of each structure is noted by assessing the deformity as the release progresses. Any residual deformity after releasing all these soft tissues should be corrected by an appropriate subtrochanteric osteotomy with internal fixation.

Restoring joint stability

Restoring the stability of the hip entails correction of deformities contributing to instability, correcting muscle imbalance and dealing with the adaptive bony changes that often develop (see Chapter 25, Paralytic hip dislocation: cerebral palsy; Chapter 26, Paralytic hip dislocation: spina bifida and polio; and Chapter 27, Teratologic hip dislocation in multiple congenital contractures).

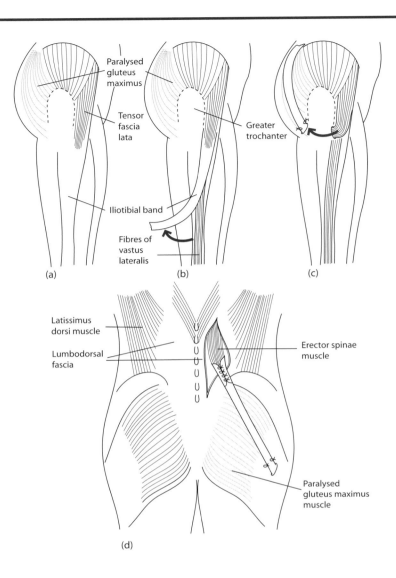

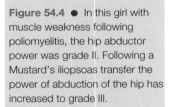

Figure 54.3 ● Diagram illustrating the technique of the erector spinae transfer for restoring power of hip extension.

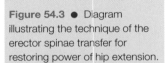

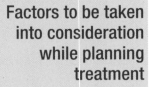

Figure 54.4 ● In this girl with muscle weakness following poliomyelitis, the hip abductor power was grade II. Following a Mustard's iliopsoas transfer the power of abduction of the hip has increased to grade III.

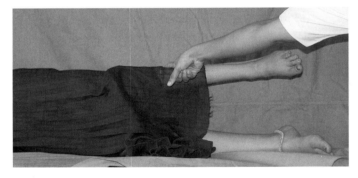

Factors to be taken into consideration while planning treatment

Pre-existing muscle power of the hip and knee

■ Muscle power around the hip

One important factor to consider while planning a tendon transfer for hip abductor paralysis is the pre-existing muscle power. Tendon transfers to improve hip abduction seldom succeed in substantially increasing the power. Often all that can be anticipated is an increase in the power of abduction by one MRC grade. Hence a pre-operative grade II power of the gluteus medius is essential if the aim is to correct the Trendelenburg limp (Figure 54.4).

■ Muscle power around the knee

The indications for performing tendon transfers with the aim of overcoming a Trendelenburg gait are limited to children who have good potential for independent community ambulation with functioning quadriceps. However, a tendon transfer may be considered even if these pre-requisites are not met if the aim is to help restore stability of the hip in a child with a paralytic dislocation of the hip.

Effect of deformities on ambulatory status and hip stability

Minor degrees of deformity at the hip may not require treatment. However, if the deformities are severe enough to compromise the ability to walk, they must be corrected. Any deformity that contributes to instability of the hip must also be corrected. On the other hand, a minor degree of abduction deformity of the hip can provide some stability to the hip and prevent a Trendelenburg gait even if the gluteus medius is completely paralysed and hence it should not be corrected.

Recommended treatment

The recommended treatment of a paralysed hip is shown in Table 54.1.

Table 54.1 ● Management of hip paralysis

INDICATIONS			
Gluteus medius grade II + Functioning quadriceps (grade IV/V) – good prospect for walking ⇩	Gluteus maximus paralysed – severe lurching gait ⇩	Fixed deformities that either preclude walking or compromise hip stability ⇩	Gluteal paralysis with muscle imbalance (strong flexor and adductors) + Hip subluxation ⇩
Mustard's anterolateral iliopsoas transfer	Erector spinae transfer	Contracture release ± Subtrochanteric femoral osteotomy	Mustard's anterolateral iliopsoas transfer
TREATMENT			

Rationale for the choice of treatment

Why is Mustard's transfer preferred to Sharrard's transfer and the external oblique transfer for improving hip abductor power?
There is no strong evidence in the literature to indicate which of these transfers is the most efficient and hence the procedure that is simplest to perform is chosen. Since the iliopsoas muscle and tendon have to be dissected to release the tendon from its insertion in order to restore muscle balance, the additional anterolateral transfer is very easy to do.

References

1. Mustard WT. A follow-up study of iliopsoas transfer for hip instability. *J Bone Joint Surg Br* 1959; **41**: 289–98.
2. Sharrard WJ. Posterior iliopsoas transplantation in the treatment of paralytic dislocation of the hip. *J Bone Joint Surg Br* 1964; **46**: 426–44.
3. Buisson JS, Hamblen DL. Electromyographic assessment of the transplanted ilio-psoas muscle in spina bifida cystica. *Dev Med Child Neurol Suppl* 1972; **27**: 29–33.
4. Cabaud HE, Westin GW, Connelly S. Tendon transfers in the paralytic hip. *J Bone Joint Surg Am* 1979; **61**: 1035–41.

The paralysed knee

Benjamin Joseph

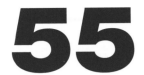

Introduction

Paralysis of the muscles acting on the knee may (1) be confined to the quadriceps alone, (2) involve the hamstrings alone or (3) involve the quadriceps and the hamstrings. Although hamstrings play an important role in the energy transfer during the gait cycle and paralysis of the hamstrings does affect the gait, the disability is far more significant if the quadriceps is paralysed. Unilateral quadriceps paralysis itself is a serious problem and when the extensors of both knees are paralysed the long-term prognosis for independent community ambulation is poor.

Problems of management

Loss of function

Paralysis of the hamstrings results in weakness of active knee flexion. However, since the knee can passively flex due to the effect of gravity, both while walking and sitting down, no treatment is required for hamstring paralysis. Therefore only the treatment of quadriceps paralysis and its associated problems will be considered in this chapter.

Paralysis of the quadriceps results in inability to extend the knee actively.

Muscle imbalance

Isolated paralysis of the quadriceps causes muscle imbalance at the knee.

Deformity

If the hamstrings are functioning in a child with quadriceps paralysis, a flexion deformity of the knee may develop. Genu recurvatum may also be seen in children with quadriceps paralysis. This deformity does not develop because of muscle imbalance but due to posterior thrust of the knee during the latter part of the stance phase. The tendency for recurvatum to develop is much greater when there is an equinus deformity at the ankle joint and when the knee is flail.

Joint instability

Of all the consequences of quadriceps paralysis, knee instability is the most disabling. The quadriceps is an antigravity muscle and its function is vital in stabilizing the knee while walking. During the single limb stance phase of the gait cycle, when the centre of gravity falls behind the axis of the knee, powerful active contraction of the quadriceps is essential to prevent the knee from buckling. A quadriceps that is functioning at grade III power (MRC) may be able to stabilize the knee in single limb stance while walking on a smooth level surface. However, while walking on uneven ground, walking up or down an incline or negotiating stairs, the knee is likely to give way such that these children will have to adopt a hand-to-thigh gait (Figure 55.1).

Figure 55.1 ● A child with paralysis of the quadriceps secondary to poliomyelitis walks with a hand-to-thigh gait **(a)**. An area of hyperpigmentation and hyperkeratosis is evident on the front of the thigh due to the repetitive friction while walking in this fashion **(b)**.

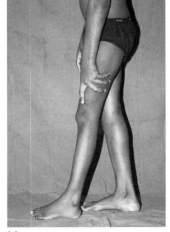
(a)

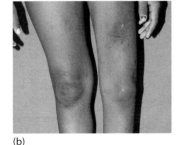
(b)

Aims of treatment

- Restore muscle power
  If possible, the power of active knee extension must be restored. This is possible by means of a hamstring transfer, but would weaken knee flexion quite considerably.
- Prevent and correct deformity
  Flexion deformity of the knee, however mild, should be corrected if the quadriceps is paralysed. Minor degrees of genu recurvatum should be left uncorrected if the quadriceps is paralysed but severe genu recurvatum must be corrected.
- Restore stability
  By far, the most important aim is to ensure the stability of the knee during the stance phase of gait.

Treatment options

Restoring muscle power

Power of knee extension can be restored by performing a hamstring tendon transfer; however, not all patients with quadriceps paralysis are candidates for this transfer. Schwartzmann and Crego[1] defined the criteria that must be fulfilled before performing the transfer. These prerequisites are normal power (grade V) of the hamstrings, gastrocsoleus and the gluteus maximus and the absence of either a flexion deformity or recurvatum at the knee. If these criteria are satisfied, the biceps femoris and the semitendinosus tendons may be transferred to the patella (Figure 55.2).

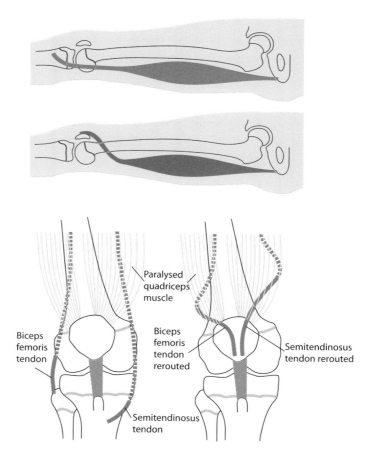

Figure 55.2 ● Technique of performing a hamstring transfer.

Labels in figure: Paralysed quadriceps muscle; Biceps femoris tendon; Biceps femoris tendon rerouted; Semitendinosus tendon rerouted; Semitendinosus tendon

Correcting deformities

As mentioned earlier, even minor degrees of flexion deformity of the knee must be corrected in any patient in whom the quadriceps is paralysed. This is because in the presence of a flexion deformity, the weight-bearing line passes posterior to the axis of motion of the knee and it is impossible for the paralysed knee to remain stable (Figure 55.3a,b). The techniques of correction of flexion deformities at the knee are discussed in Chapter 13, Flexion deformity of the knee. On the other hand, genu recurvatum of up to 15° may actually be beneficial when the quadriceps is paralysed. The weight-bearing line will pass anterior to the axis of knee motion if there is genu recurvatum and this will stabilize the knee and prevent it from buckling (Figure 55.3c). However, excessive degrees of genu recurvatum should be corrected.

Restoring joint stability

The stability of the knee can be restored dynamically by performing a hamstring transfer, while static restoration of joint stability can be achieved by either the use of an orthosis or surgery. A supracondylar extension osteotomy which creates a 10° recurvatum can restore stability (Figure 55.3c). However, if this procedure is performed in a skeletally immature child, remodelling of the osteotomy site is likely to occur with recurrence of instability of the knee. Hence this surgery is reserved for the skeletally mature patient.

A patient with paralysed quadriceps can stabilize the knee if there is a fixed equinus deformity. With initial toe contact the weight-bearing line passes anterior to the axis of the knee and the knee remains stable (Figure 55.3d). In this situation correcting the equinus deformity completely will make the knee unstable. Hence, if severe equinus deformity in a child with quadriceps paralysis is being corrected, it is desirable to leave 10–15° residual equinus uncorrected.

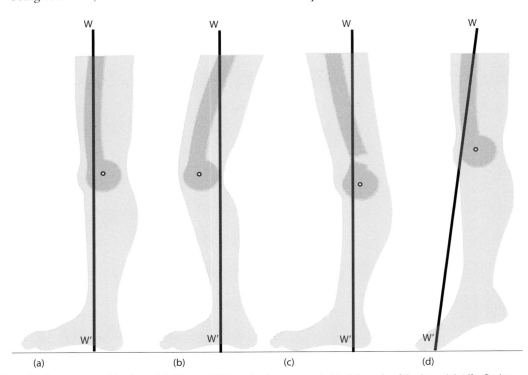

(a)   (b)   (c)   (d)

Figure 55.3 ● Diagram illustrating the axis of movement of the knee **(a)**. The weight-bearing line passes behind the axis of the knee joint if a flexion deformity of the knee is present **(b)**. The knee cannot remain stable if the quadriceps muscle is paralysed. The weight-bearing line passes anterior to the axis of the knee joint when a genu recurvatum deformity is present **(c)**. This enables the knee to remain stable even if the quadriceps is paralysed. Similarly, a supracondylar extension osteotomy sufficient to produce a 10 or 15° recurvatum deformity can stabilize a paralysed knee. An equinus deformity can also stabilize a knee with a paralysed quadriceps by ensuring the weight-bearing line passes in front of the axis of the knee joint **(d)**.

A floor-reaction orthosis (FRO) (Figure 55.4a) or a knee-ankle-foot orthosis (KAFO) with a knee lock (Figure 55.4b) can be used to stabilize the knee. The FRO has the advantages of leaving the knee unlocked during the swing phase of gait and permitting knee flexion while sitting down without having to manipulate a knee lock.[2]

Factors to be taken into consideration while planning treatment

Factors to be considered while planning treatment include the age of the patient, the presence of associated deformities of the hip, knee and ankle of the same limb and the muscle power at the hip, knee and ankle of both the limbs.

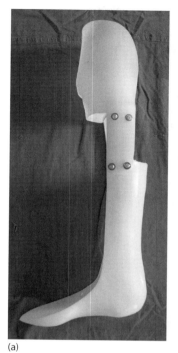 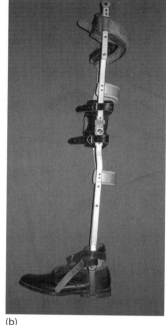 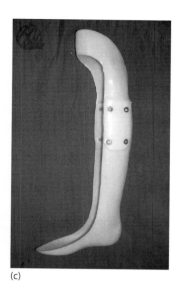

(a)   (b)   (c)

Figure 55.4 ● **(a)** A floor-reaction orthosis which is used to stabilize the paralysed knee. The orthosis is moulded with the ankle in about 10° of plantarflexion. **(b)** A knee-ankle-foot orthosis used for quadriceps paralysis. The knee is locked in extension when the patient is upright. **(c)** A Lehneis modification of a floor-reaction orthosis used to stabilize the paralysed knee and prevent the knee from hyperextending.

The age of the patient

As mentioned earlier, a supracondylar extension osteotomy to restore knee stability is not recommended in skeletally immature children on account of the tendency for remodelling. Conversely, every attempt must be made to facilitate the abandoning of an orthosis once skeletal maturity has been reached.

Deformities of the hip, knee and ankle

Hamstring transfer is not justified in the presence of a flexion deformity of the hip and, if present, the hip flexion deformity should be corrected before performing the hamstring transfer. Similarly, flexion or recurvatum deformities of the knee must also be corrected prior to performing a hamstring transfer.

If an equinus deformity is present at the ankle, and if the knee is remaining stable on account of this deformity, no intervention is needed for the paralysed knee. However, if for some reason complete correction of the equinus is considered essential, then the quadriceps weakness has to be dealt with as outlined here.

A floor-reaction orthosis is ineffective in the presence of even a minor degree of flexion deformity at the knee. Hence it is essential that the flexion deformity is corrected prior to fitting an FRO. Similarly an FRO should be avoided if a severe degree of genu recurvatum is present because the orthosis stabilizes the knee by exerting an extension force at the knee, which can aggravate the deformity. However, genu recurvatum associated with quadriceps paralysis can be effectively controlled by using the Lehneis modification of the FRO (Figure 55.4c).

Pre-existing muscle power of the knee

Hamstring transfer is not recommended in patients in whom the quadriceps power is less than grade II. This is because this non-phasic transfer does not function well if the power of the quadriceps is grade 0 or I to begin with. Hence, patients with very weak power of the quadriceps should be treated by an osteotomy or bracing.

Muscle power of the hip

A hamstring transfer should only be considered if the hip extensor power is grade V. This is because the hamstrings are secondary hip extensors and once they are transferred hip extension can only be brought about by the gluteus maximus.

Muscle power of the opposite limb

Most patients cannot manage to walk with FROs on both limbs and hence if both the knees are paralysed and require bracing, a traditional KAFO needs to be used on one limb. Since the overall stability provided by a locked KAFO is greater than that of an FRO, the former is used on the weaker limb (Figure 55.5).

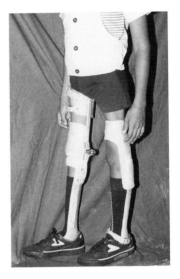

Figure 55.5 ● A boy with paralysis of both knees wearing a floor-reaction orthosis on one limb and a knee-ankle-foot orthosis on the weaker limb.

Recommended treatment

The recommended treatment for quadriceps paralysis is shown in Table 55.1.

Table 55.1 ● Management of quadriceps paralysis

INDICATIONS				
Any age: Quadriceps power grade II/III + Grade V power of the gluteus maximus, gastrocsoleus and hamstrings + No deformity at the knee, hip or ankle	Skeletally mature: Quadriceps power grades 0–III + Power of the gluteus maximus, gastrocsoleus or hamstrings less than grade V ± Flexion deformity of the knee	Skeletally immature: Quadriceps power grades 0–III + Power of the gluteus maximus, gastrocsoleus or hamstrings less than grade V + Flexion deformity of the knee	Skeletally immature: Quadriceps power grades 0–III + Power of the gluteus maximus, gastrocsoleus or hamstrings less than grade V + No flexion deformity at the knee + Opposite limb does not require bracing of the knee	Skeletally immature: Quadriceps power grades 0–III + Power of the gluteus maximus, gastrocsoleus or hamstrings less than grade V + No flexion deformity at the knee + Opposite limb also paralysed and requires bracing of the knee
⇩	⇩	⇩	⇩	⇩
Transfer of semitendinosus and biceps femoris to the patella	Supracondylar extension osteotomy of the femur to create 10° of recurvatum	Correct flexion deformity and provide orthosis	Floor-reaction orthosis (Lehneis modification if there is a recurvatum deformity >15°)	Knee-ankle-foot orthosis for the weaker limb AND Floor-reaction orthosis for the stronger limb
TREATMENT				

References

1. Schwartzmann JR, Crego CH. Hamstring tendon transplantation for quadriceps paralysis in residual poliomyelitis: a follow-up study of 134 cases. *J Bone Joint Surg Am* 1948; **30**: 541–52.

2. Joseph B, Rajasekaran S. Poliomyelitis. In: Bulstrode C, Buckwalter J, Carr A *et al.* (eds). *The Oxford Textbook of Orthopedics and Trauma*. Oxford: Oxford University Press, 2002: 1511–32.

The paralysed foot and ankle

Benjamin Joseph

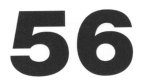

Introduction

The foot and ankle are very commonly affected in various paralytic conditions and paralysis of different muscles acting on the foot results in characteristic gait aberrations. Apart from the awkward appearance, foot deformities may result in secondary deformities of the knee (e.g. an equinus deformity may cause a genu recurvatum to develop) or increase the risk of neuropathic plantar ulceration if sensation is also lost.

Problems of management

Loss of function

During normal gait, the heel initially makes contact with the ground. The rest of the foot is then lowered to the ground so that in mid-stance the entire weight-bearing part of the sole is in firm contact with the ground (the foot is plantigrade). In the terminal part of the stance phase the heel is lifted off the ground and then active, powerful contraction of the triceps surae facilitates forward propulsion of the limb into the swing phase (the push-off). In the swing phase of gait, active dorsiflexion of the ankle is essential to help the toes clear the ground. Two common problems encountered in paralytic conditions are paralysis of the ankle dorsiflexors resulting in foot drop and paralysis of the triceps surae resulting in a weak push-off.

Muscle imbalance

Muscle imbalance around the axes of the ankle and subtalar joints can produce either static or dynamic deformities.

Deformities

Static (or fixed) deformities of the ankle, subtalar and midtarsal joints prevent the normal weight-bearing part of the sole from resting on the ground (the foot is no longer plantigrade).

Instability of joints

Instability of the subtalar joint makes it difficult to walk on uneven terrain, while instability of the ankle prevents a normal gait pattern. If the dorsiflexors of the ankle are functioning while the triceps surae is paralysed, in terminal stance uncontrolled ankle dorsiflexion occurs. This characteristic, unsightly gait abnormality is referred to as a calcaneal hitch. Abnormally high shearing forces, which are generated under the heel when this occurs, contribute to neuropathic ulceration if sensations on the sole are lost.

Limb length discrepancy

Although the major component of the shortening occurs in the femur and the tibia, the foot also contributes to lower limb length inequality.

Aims of treatment

- Make the foot plantigrade
- Restore active dorsiflexion during the swing phase of gait. If this is not possible, prevent the foot from 'dropping' into plantar flexion during swing
- Ensure that the ankle and subtalar joints are stable throughout the stance phase of gait
- Facilitate a powerful push-off at the terminal part of the stance phase. If this is not possible, at least prevent a calcaneal hitch in terminal stance

The specific aims of treatment in each patient depend on the pattern and the severity of paralysis that is present and hence the aims are likely to vary, as illustrated in these examples.

■ Aims of treatment of a flail foot

The flail foot is usually plantigrade as there is no muscle imbalance; no tendon transfer is feasible and so active dorsiflexion cannot be restored; the ankle and subtalar joints are unstable; the power of push-off cannot be restored and there is no tendency for a calcaneal hitch as the dorsiflexors of the ankle are paralysed. Here, the aims of treatment are to prevent foot drop during the swing phase and to ensure that the subtalar joint is stable in stance.

■ Aims of treatment of a foot with a common peroneal nerve palsy

The paralysis of the dorsiflexors and evertors result in a foot drop, equinovarus deformity and instability of the subtalar joint. There is no weakness of push-off. Here, the aims are to restore a plantigrade foot, restore active dorsiflexion, prevent foot drop and to stabilize the subtalar joint during stance.

■ Aims of treatment of a foot with a deep peroneal nerve palsy

The isolated paralysis of the ankle and toe dorsiflexors causes a foot drop. The foot is plantigrade during stance and there is no instability of the subtalar joint or weakness of push-off. Here, the sole aim is to restore active ankle dorsiflexion.

Pre-operative assessment for planning treatment

In order to determine what treatment options are available in a particular patient, it is imperative that a careful clinical assessment of the foot is done. Based on the clinical assessment, these questions need to be answered before planning treatment:

- What are the muscles that are paralysed?
- What is the power of each muscle that is functioning?
- Is there muscle imbalance at the ankle, subtalar or midtarsal joints that has either already produced a deformity or has the potential to produce a deformity in future?
- Are there any muscles of grade V power that can be spared for a tendon transfer without producing a fresh imbalance or instability?

To facilitate responses to these questions, the muscle power of each muscle can be charted on the template shown in Figure 56.1. The graphic representation of the muscle balance around the axes of the ankle and subtalar joints will be clearly evident when each tendon is shaded according to the power of the respective muscle as shown.

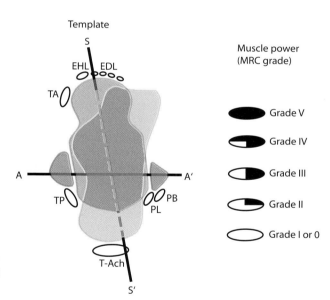

Figure 56.1 ● Template for charting the power of muscles acting on the ankle and the subtalar joint.

This assessment clarifies whether a tendon transfer is a feasible option. If a tendon transfer is considered feasible, then the following questions also need to be answered.

- Is there a fixed, static deformity that needs to be corrected prior to a tendon transfer?
- If a tendon transfer were performed, would the child be capable of comprehending and cooperating with the post-operative muscle re-education programme?

Treatment options

Making the foot plantigrade

In order to restore a plantigrade tread, dynamic and static (fixed) deformities need to be corrected. Dynamic deformities may be corrected by weakening the deforming force (by tenotomy or tendon lengthening) or by redirecting the deforming force into a corrective force (by a tendon transfer).

Static deformities, if present, should be corrected as outlined in Chapters 2–7.

Enabling active dorsiflexion during swing

If the paralysed dorsiflexor cannot be reinnervated, a tendon transfer is needed to restore active dorsiflexion. The tendon of the tibialis posterior or one of the peroneal tendons may be transferred to the dorsum of the foot.

Ensuring stability of the ankle and subtalar joints during stance

Performing a tendon transfer can often restore stability of the subtalar joint. If this is not possible an orthosis may be required until the child is old enough for an arthrodesis.

Facilitating a strong push-off or at least preventing a calcaneal hitch

Tendon transfers are seldom effective in restoring powerful push-off if the triceps surae is paralysed. This is because no muscle in the calf has power comparable to that of the normal triceps surae.[1] Despite this, tendon transfers are justified in order to reduce the muscle imbalance. An appropriate tendon transfer should prevent the calcaneus deformity from progressing[2] and provide some power of push-off. If no muscle is available for the transfer, tenodesis of the Achilles tendon may at least prevent the calcaneus deformity from progressing and also prevent the calcaneal hitch while walking.[3]

Since the problems vary with each individual pattern of paralysis, the options for treatment also vary with each pattern.

To illustrate how to choose the treatment in a child with paralysis of the foot an example is presented here. Figure 56.2a shows the equinovarus deformity of the foot of a boy with spina bifida. The equinovarus deformity is passively correctable (Figure 56.2b). The scar of a neuropathic plantar ulcer under the base of the fifth metatarsal can be seen in Figure 56.2c.

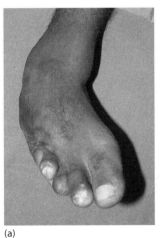
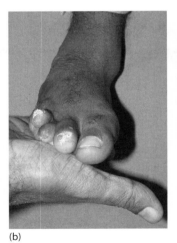
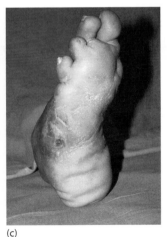

Figure 56.2 ● **(a)** Equinovarus deformity in a boy with spina bifida. **(b)** The deformity is passively correctable. **(c)** A scar of a healed neuropathic ulcer is seen under the base of the fifth metatarsal.

(a)   (b)   (c)

The power of muscles around the foot and ankle is depicted in Figure 56.3a. All muscles other than the tibialis anterior and the tibialis posterior are paralysed.

Figure 56.3b shows the way muscle balance can be restored by transfer of the tibialis posterior tendon.

Transfer of the tibialis posterior to the peronei behind the ankle restores muscle balance across the axes of both the ankle and the subtalar joints. This transfer also corrects the varus deformity as part of the unopposed inversion force has now been converted to an eversion force. The subtalar joint, which was unstable, has now been stabilized. By obtaining a plantigrade foot the risk of recurrence of the neuropathic plantar ulcer has been minimized. All this has been achieved without performing an arthrodesis (which is contraindicated when plantar sensation is absent).

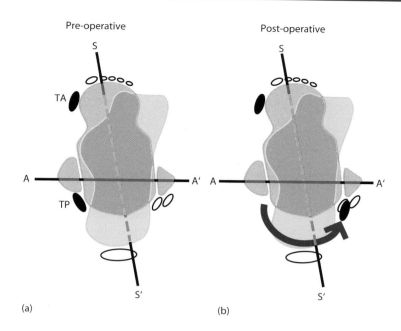

Figure 56.3 ● **(a)** The power of muscles around the foot and ankle is shown on the template. **(b)** The proposed tendon transfer, the site of attachment of the transferred tendon and the anticipated muscle balance across the axes of the ankle and subtalar joints are shown.

Recommended treatment

The recommended treatment for dealing with a paralysed foot is outlined in Tables 56.1–56.4.

The more common patterns of paralysis encountered in various paralytic conditions are listed below in Table 56.1. The problems of management, the tendon transfer that may be performed

Table 56.1 ● Tendon transfers for restoring muscle balance in paralysed feet

Paralysis	Problems	Muscle balance before and after tendon transfer	Tendon transfer	Effect of transfer
Tibialis Anterior + Extensor hallucis + Extensor digitorum	*Muscle weakness:* Foot drop *Muscle imbalance:* Plantarflexion > dorsiflexion *Potential deformity:* Equinus	**Figure 56.4a** **Figure 56.4b**	Tibialis posterior transfer OR Peroneus longus transfer	Can correct foot drop and restore active dorsiflexion + Improves muscle balance + Can prevent equinus deformity

Tibialis anterior + Extensor hallucis + Extensor digitorum + Peroneus longus + Peroneus brevis	*Muscle weakness:* Foot drop No power of eversion *Muscle imbalance:* Plantarflexion > dorsiflexion and Inversion > eversion *Deformity:* Equinovarus	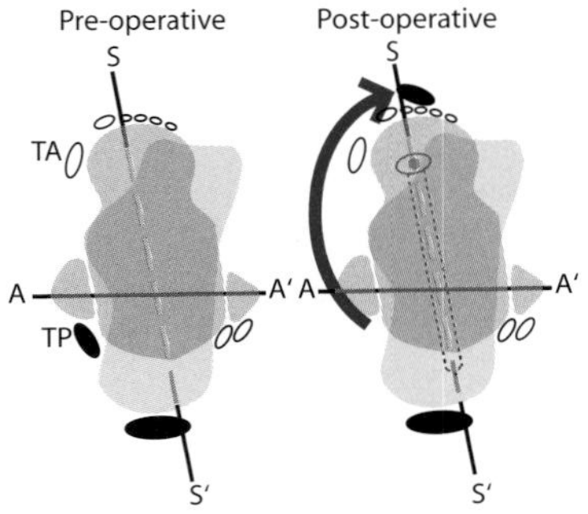 **Figure 56.4c** [a]Additional procedure needed (Subtalar arthrodesis)	Tibialis posterior transfer	Can correct foot drop and restore active dorsiflexion + Improves muscle balance across ankle but makes the subtalar joint flail[a] + Can correct equinovarus deformity
Tibialis anterior + Extensor hallucis + Extensor digitorum + Tibialis posterior	*Muscle weakness:* Foot drop No inversion *Muscle imbalance:* Plantarflexion > dorsiflexion and Eversion > inversion *Deformity:* Equinovalgus	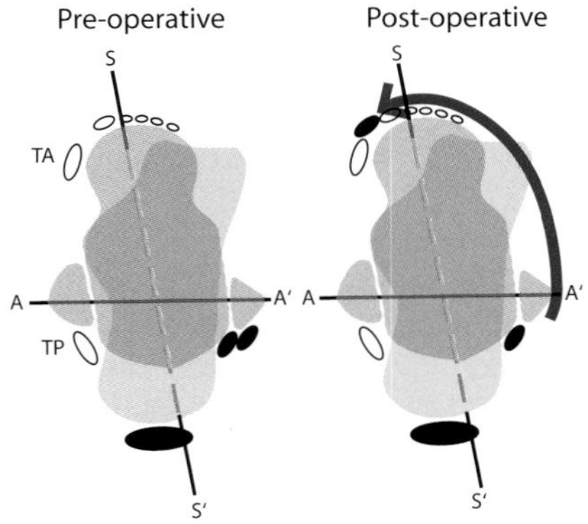 **Figure 56.4d**	Peroneus longus transfer OR Peroneus brevis transfer	Can correct foot drop and restore active dorsiflexion + Improves muscle balance across ankle and subtalar joint + Can correct equinovalgus deformity
Triceps surae + Tibialis posterior	*Muscle weakness:* Plantarflexor power lost Invertor weakness *Muscle imbalance:* Dorsiflexion > plantarflexion and Eversion > inversion *Deformity:* Calcaneovalgus	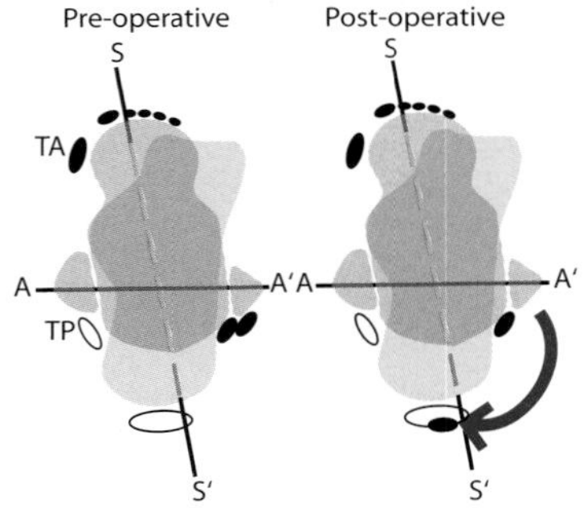 **Figure 56.4e**	Peroneus longus translocation through groove in tuberosity of calcaneum	Can prevent calcaneal hitch and restore weak push-off + Improves muscle balance + Can prevent progression of calcaneus deformity
Tibialis posterior	*Muscle weakness:* Inversion weak *Muscle imbalance:* Eversion > inversion *Deformity:* Planovalgus	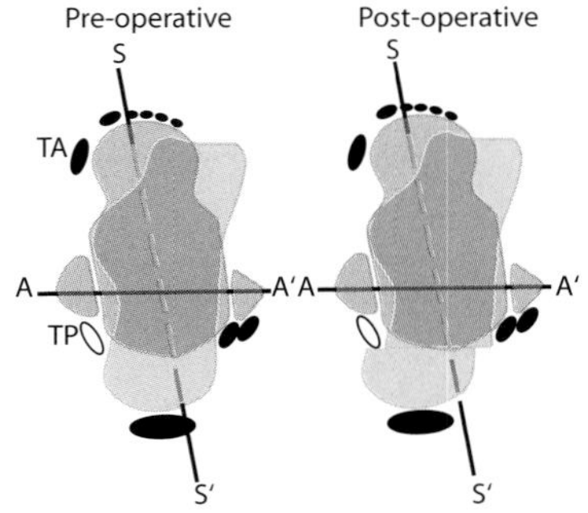 **Figure 56.4f** [b]Not a true tendon transfer but has the effect of a tendon transfer	Medial displacement osteotomy of the calcaneum[b] produces the effect of medial shift of the Achilles tendon	Improves muscle balance + Improves the hindfoot valgus deformity

Figures referenced: Pre-operative / Post-operative diagrams labelled S, S', A, A', TA, TP.

and the anticipated effects of the transfer in each situation are enumerated in the table and illustrated in Figures 56.4a–f.

While it is clear that a well-planned tendon transfer is a valuable option in dealing with several paralytic problems around the foot and the ankle, it may not be feasible. In such situations other options need to be considered. Tables 56.2–56.4 summarize the recommended management plan for dealing with each of the problems associated with paralysis of the foot and ankle.

Management of paralytic deformities of the foot and the management of shortening are dealt with in Chapters 2–7, Chapter 43 and Chapter 44.

Table 56.2 ● Treatment outline for restoration of muscle power around the foot and ankle

INDICATIONS			
If direct repair of the nerve is feasible (as in a peripheral nerve injury)	Re-innervation of muscle not feasible + Muscle of grade V power available for tendon transfer + NO fixed deformity of ankle or subtalar joint present + Transfer of the tendon will not produce fresh instability	Muscle of grade V power available for tendon transfer + Fixed deformity of ankle or subtalar joint present	Muscle of grade V power available for tendon transfer + Transfer of the tendon will produce fresh instability
⇩	⇩	⇩	⇩
			Fusion of joint made unstable by the transfer + Tendon transfer
Direct repair of the nerve	Tendon transfer	Correction of fixed deformity + Tendon transfer	
TREATMENT			

Table 56.3 ● Treatment outline for restoration of muscle balance around the foot and ankle

INDICATIONS		
Tendon transfer feasible and likely to restore muscle balance	Tendon transfer not feasible + Muscle imbalance mild (1 or 2 MRC grade difference between antagonistic muscle groups)	Tendon transfer not feasible + Muscle imbalance severe (3 or more MRC grade difference between antagonistic muscle groups)
⇩	⇩	⇩
		Tenotomy of tendon of stronger muscle
Tendon transfer	Lengthening of tendon of stronger muscle	
TREATMENT		

Table 56.4 ● Treatment outline for restoring stability of joints of the foot and ankle in the presence of paralysis

INDICATIONS					
Foot drop OR Calcaneus (Unidirectional instability of the ankle) ± Unidirectional instability of the subtalar joint (varus OR valgus instability) + Tendon of muscle of grade V power available for transfer	Foot drop (Unidirectional instability of the ankle) + Bi-directional instability of the subtalar joint (varus AND valgus instability) + Tendon of muscle of grade V power available for transfer + Child over 5 years of age	Foot drop (Unidirectional instability of the ankle) + No instability at subtalar joint + No suitable tendon available for transfer	Calcaneus (Unidirectional instability of the ankle) + No suitable tendon available for transfer + Skeletally immature child	Multi-directional instability of foot and ankle + Skeletally mature child + No tendons available for restoring stability + Sensation on the sole intact	Multidirectional instability of foot and ankle + In skeletally immature child OR Bidirectional instability of the subtalar joint + In a child under 5 years of age (too young for subtalar arthrodesis) OR Sensations lost on the sole of the foot
⇩	⇩	⇩	⇩	⇩	⇩
Tendon transfer	Tendon transfer to restore ankle stability + Arthrodesis of subtalar joint	Ankle–foot orthosis OR Posterior bone block operation	Tenodesis of Achilles tendon	Triple arthrodesis (Elmslie type of fusion for calcaneovalgus OR Lambrinudi type for flail foot)	Ankle-foot orthosis
TREATMENT					

References

1. Silver RL, de la Garza J, Rang M. The myth of muscle balance. A study of relative strengths and excursions of normal muscles about the foot and ankle. *J Bone Joint Surg Br* 1985; **67**: 432–7.
2. Banta JV, Sutherland DH, Wyatt M. Anterior tibial transfer to the os calcis with Achilles tenodesis for calcaneal deformity in myelomeningocele. *J Pediatr Orthop* 1981; **1**: 125–30.
3. Westin GW, Dingeman RD, Gausewitz SH. The results of tenodesis of the tendo Achilles to the fibula for paralytic calcaneus. *J Bone Joint Surg Am* 1988; **70**: 320–28.

The paralysed elbow

Benjamin Joseph

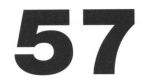

Introduction	Paralysis of the elbow is commonly seen in children with obstetric brachial plexus palsy and in children with multiple congenital contractures (MCC). In obstetric palsy, the elbow flexors, the elbow extensors or both the flexors and extensors may be paralysed. In MCC, generally either the flexors or the extensors are paralysed.

Introduction

Paralysis of the elbow is commonly seen in children with obstetric brachial plexus palsy and in children with multiple congenital contractures (MCC). In obstetric palsy, the elbow flexors, the elbow extensors or both the flexors and extensors may be paralysed. In MCC, generally either the flexors or the extensors are paralysed.

Problems of management

Loss of function

Paralysis of the biceps brachii and the brachialis results in inability to get the hand to the mouth. Paralysis of the triceps does not permit overhead activities as the elbow cannot be held extended. Triceps paralysis may preclude the use of crutches in children with associated paralysis of the lower limbs.

Muscle imbalance and deformities

In MCC, flexion deformity of the elbow may be seen when the triceps is paralysed, while an extension deformity may occur when the biceps is paralysed.

Paralysis of flexors of the elbow

Aims of treatment

- To restore active elbow flexion and to correct the extension deformity, if present

Treatment options

Restoring active elbow flexion

■ Steindler flexorplasty

In children in whom the wrist and hand flexors are of normal power, a simple option for restoring active elbow flexion is to transfer the common flexor origin from the medial epicondyle proximally onto the humeral shaft (Figure 57.1a,b). Although active flexion is restored by this operation, the power seldom exceeds grade III. There may be a tendency for the wrist to flex excessively when the child attempts to flex the elbow following the transfer. Children who can simultaneously contract the radial wrist extensor while attempting elbow flexion can prevent excessive wrist flexion following this operation. In MCC, wrist extensors are often paralysed and,

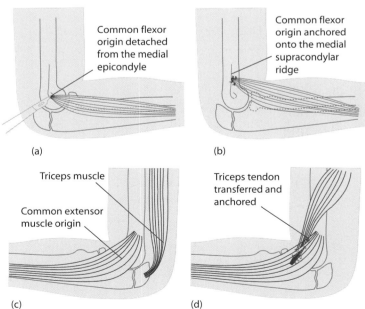

(a)

Common flexor origin detached from the medial epicondyle

(b)

Common flexor origin anchored onto the medial supracondylar ridge

(c)

Triceps muscle

Common extensor muscle origin

(d)

Triceps tendon transferred and anchored

Figure 57.1 ● **(a,b)** Technique of performing a Steindler flexorplasty. **(c,d)** Technique of performing a triceps transfer. The triceps tendon is sutured to the common extensor muscles.

frequently, there is a flexion deformity of the wrist. In these children the wrist deformity can become accentuated following a Steindler flexorplasty.

■ Triceps transfer

Transfer of the entire triceps to the radial tuberosity was recommended by Bunnell.[1] However, transferring the triceps to the common extensors is easier to perform and is also as effective[2] in restoring reasonable flexion strength (Figure 57.1c,d). Since a fresh imbalance is created by a triceps transfer, a flexion deformity of the elbow may develop in some children. If transfer of the triceps is done only on one elbow in a child with arthrogryposis and then post-operatively a flexion deformity develops, bimanual activity may be hampered as one elbow will be flexed and the other would remain extended. On the other hand, if flexion deformities of both elbows develop after triceps transfers are performed on both elbows it may become impossible to get either hand to the perineum for independent personal hygiene.

■ Transfer of the long head of the triceps

Mennen *et al.*[2] have suggested that the long head of the triceps alone can be transferred to restore the power of elbow flexion. This part of the triceps has a separate neurovascular pedicle and it can be separated from the other two heads fairly easily. A fascia lata graft is used to facilitate attachment of the muscle in the forearm. Long-term results of this operation on a large number of patients are as yet not available. The theoretical advantage of this operation is that elbow extensor power is retained as two heads of the triceps are not disturbed.

■ Pectoralis major transfer

Unipolar and bipolar transfers of the pectoralis major have been described. The unipolar transfer has the disadvantage that the direction of pull is not optimal. While attempting to flex the elbow after the unipolar transfer, strong adduction of the limb tends to occur. Bipolar transfer of the pectoralis major mobilized on its neurovascular pedicle can overcome this problem. However, a strong adductor is sacrificed and this may be disabling if the child has to use crutches or a wheelchair. In addition, unsightly scars and asymmetry of the chest wall and the breast may be a problem in girls.

■ Bipolar latissimus dorsi transfer

The entire latissimus dorsi is mobilized on its neurovascular pedicle. This transfer is not ideal for children with MCC as the muscle is often fibrotic. The latissimus dorsi is an important muscle that is necessary for walking with crutches and should not be transferred if the child needs crutches to walk.

■ Free functioning muscle transfer

Free microvascular transfer of the rectus femoris or gracilis muscle may be done[3] when other simpler options are not feasible.

Restoring passive elbow flexion

The triceps is lengthened by performing a V–Y plasty of the triceps aponeurosis with a posterior capsulotomy of the elbow as necessary, after protecting the ulnar nerve.

Power of elbow flexors

If the power of the biceps is less than grade II, a Steindler flexorplasty is unlikely to improve the elbow flexor power sufficiently for efficient elbow function and hence a more powerful muscle needs to be transferred.

Power of wrist and finger flexors

The power of the wrist and finger flexors should be grade V if a Steindler flexorplasty is to work efficiently.

Power of muscles of the shoulder girdle

If the muscles of the shoulder girdle are paralysed, transfer of the pectoralis major or the latissimus dorsi is not appropriate.

Power of the muscles of the lower limb

If extensive paralysis of the lower limb is present and the child needs either a wheelchair or crutches for walking, the triceps should not be transferred as its function is important for effective wheelchair transfer and for walking with crutches.

Presence of fixed extension deformity of the elbow

If an extension deformity due to a contracture of the triceps is present, it must be corrected before performing any tendon transfer to restore elbow flexion. However, if a triceps transfer is planned, detaching the triceps from its insertion will correct the deformity at the time of the tendon transfer.

Is the weakness symmetrical?

If bilateral symmetrical paralysis of elbow flexion is present, the functional disability and adaptive mechanisms already used by the child for activities of daily living must be carefully evaluated. Bilateral elbow flexor paralysis is frequently seen in MCC. One view is to attempt to restore active elbow flexion in the dominant limb while leaving the non-dominant limb in extension. This enables the child to get one hand to the mouth and face, and the other hand to the perineum for personal hygiene;[4] however, the wisdom of this approach has been questioned.[5] In MCC there is often poor grasp; in the absence of strong unilateral grasp, it is very important to retain bimanual activity. One elbow fixed in extension and the other in flexion may prevent bimanual function.

Recommended treatment

The treatment recommendations for dealing with flexor paralysis of the elbow are shown in Table 57.1.

Table 57.1 ● Treatment options for dealing with flexor paralysis of the elbow

INDICATIONS				
Elbow flexor power grade II + Wrist and finger flexors grade V + No flexion deformity at wrist + Unilateral or bilateral elbow flexor weakness	Elbow flexor power grade I or 0 + Triceps power grade V + Child would not need crutches or wheelchair for mobility + Unilateral elbow flexor weakness	Elbow flexor power <grade III in both upper limbs + Poor wrist and finger flexors + Child would not need crutches or wheelchair for mobility	Elbow flexor power <grade III in both upper limbs + Crutches or wheelchair needed for mobility + Extension deformity of elbow	Elbow flexor power <grade III + Associated weakness of the shoulder girdle muscles, triceps and wrist and finger flexors
⇩ Steindler flexorplasty	⇩ Triceps transfer	⇩ Transfer of long head of triceps OR Triceps transfer	⇩ Tricepsplasty to correct extension deformity	⇩ Free functional muscle transfer
TREATMENT				

Paralysis of extensors of the elbow

Although active extension of the elbow can be restored by performing an appropriate tendon transfer, surgery for restoring the power of extension is far less frequently performed than surgery for restoring active elbow flexion.

Treatment options

The options available for restoring active elbow extension are posterior transfer of the muscle belly of the brachioradialis, transfer of the posterior part of the deltoid and a latissimus dorsi transfer. Of these, the brachioradialis transfer is the simplest. None of these transfers are likely be feasible in MCC.

Brachioradialis transfer

The brachioradialis transfer has advantages in that it is a relatively simple procedure and that it does not weaken movement of either the elbow or the wrist in any plane. The proximal part of the belly of muscle is transposed posterior to the axis of the elbow joint (Figure 57.2a). The power of extension is unlikely to be greater than grade III after this transfer.

Posterior deltoid transfer

The posterior part of the deltoid is separated from the rest of the muscle, detached from its insertion and attached to a tongue of the triceps aponeurosis that has been raised from the olecranon and reversed (Figure 57.2b). This transferred part of the deltoid can now extend the elbow through its attachment to the triceps. The advantage of this transfer is that the transferred

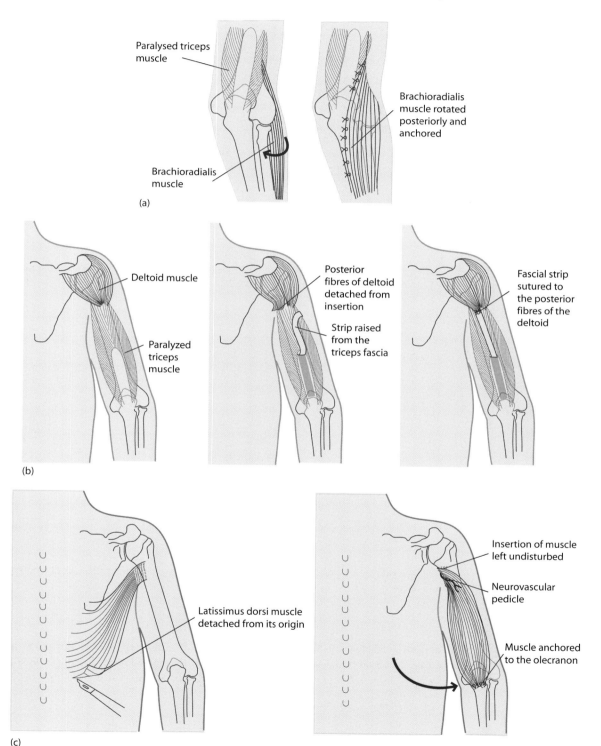

Figure 57.2 ● Techniques for restoring power of elbow extension: brachioradialis transfer **(a)**; transfer of the posterior deltoid **(b)**; latissimus dorsi transfer **(c)**.

part of the deltoid will be acting when the shoulder is abducted and this will stabilize the elbow during overhead activity.

Latissimus dorsi transfer

The Hovnanian technique of the latissimus dorsi transfer is likely to provide strong extensor power. The origin of the muscle is transferred to the radius while the original insertion of the muscle is not disturbed (Figure 57.2c).

References

1. Mennen U. Surgical aspects of neuromuscular disorders of the upper extremity. In: Gupta A, Kay SPJ, Scheker LR (eds). *The Growing Hand*. London: Mosby, 2000: 443–6.
2. Mennen U, van Heest A, Ezaki MB, Tonkin M, Gericke G. Arthrogryposis multiplex congenita. *J Hand Surg [Br]* 2005; **30**: 468–74.
3. Chung DC, Carver N, Wei FC. Results of functioning free muscle transplantation for elbow flexion. *J Hand Surg [Am]* 1996; **21**: 1071–7.
4. Axt MW, Niethard FU, Doderlein L, Weber M. Principles of treatment of the upper extremity in arthrogryposis multiplex congenita type I. *J Pediatr Orthop B* 1997; **6**: 179–85.
5. Ezaki M. Treatment of the upper limb in the child with arthrogryposis. *Hand Clin* 2000; **16**: 703–11.

The paralysed shoulder in the child

Benjamin Joseph

58

Introduction

Paralysis of muscles of the shoulder in children is most frequently seen following obstetric brachial plexus injuries. Non-progressive shoulder paralysis may also be seen following poliomyelitis. Reconstructive surgery for the shoulder is often needed in these two situations, but the clinical problems are different in the two conditions due to the distinctly differing patterns of recovery. In infants with brachial plexus injuries some recovery may be anticipated after axonotmesis and even neurotmesis as the gaps between the severed nerves are small and hence nerve regeneration across these gaps is often possible. However, as recovery occurs, cross-innervation frequently develops due to misdirection of the regenerating axons. Cross-innervation causes co-contraction of synergistic and antagonistic muscle groups.[1] This adds to the problems of paresis, muscle imbalance, deformities and joint instabilities that occur in all paralytic conditions.

Problems of management

Loss of function

Shoulder paralysis can be quite incapacitating. Deltoid paralysis may make it impossible to get the hand to the head. If elbow flexor weakness is present in addition to shoulder paralysis it may not even be possible to get the hand to the mouth for feeding. Internal rotator weakness may make it impossible to get the hand to the back.

Deformities

Fixed deformities of the shoulder are infrequently seen in poliomyelitis but are very common in obstetric brachial plexus palsy.

The deformities secondary to muscle imbalance that are seen in obstetric palsy vary from patient to patient depending on the pattern of paralysis. Each of the deformities is masked by compensatory positioning of the scapula. Attempting to stretch the contracted muscles causes the scapula to stand out prominently. The scapular elevation signs of Putti and Zancolli (Figure 58.1) are examples of this phenomenon. Zancolli[2] noted deformities in 82 percent of children with obstetric palsy and classified the patterns of deformities and the muscle contractures in each type (Table 58.1).

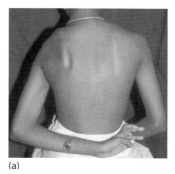
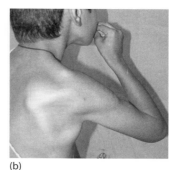

(a)   (b)

Figure 58.1 ● The scapular elevation sign signifies that there is a contracture of a muscle acting on the shoulder. The angle of the scapula elevates when the shoulder is moved in a direction opposite to the direction of action of the contracted muscle. In this adolescent girl there is contracture of the external rotators of the shoulder **(a)**, while in this boy there is an adduction contracture **(b)**.

Joint instability

Posterior dislocation of the shoulder is often encountered in children with internal rotation contracture while a proportion of children with external rotation contracture develop anterior instability. It is important to identify instability as its presence will influence the treatment.

Table 58.1 ● Patterns of contractures in obstetric palsy

Deformity	Muscle contracture	Scapular elevation sign
Internal rotation Adduction 63%	Subscapularis Teres major Latissimus dorsi Pectoralis major	*Positive in*: Abduction and external rotation
External rotation Abduction 14%	Infraspinatus Teres minor	*Positive in*: Adduction and internal rotation
Internal rotation External rotation 3%	Subscapularis Teres major Latissimus dorsi Pectoralis major Infraspinatus Teres minor	*Positive in*: Adduction and internal rotation and Abduction and external rotation
Abduction 2%	Supraspinatus	*Positive in*: Adduction

The frequency with which each deformity is encountered is shown in percentages in column 1.

Co-contraction of antagonistic muscles

Four patterns of co-contraction have been identified in obstetric paralysis,[1] three of which affect the shoulder.

1. Co-contraction between shoulder abductors and shoulder adductors results in limitation of shoulder abduction. Co-contraction of shoulder abductors with the adductors (pectoralis major, teres major and the latissimus dorsi) can be demonstrated very easily by palpating the anterior and posterior axillary folds while the child attempts to abduct the shoulder. If the muscles stand out taut in the axillary folds co-contraction is present (Figure 58.2a,b).
2. Co-contraction between the elbow flexors and extensors.
3. In co-contraction between the shoulder abductors and elbow flexors, when the child attempts to take his or her hand to the mouth, the shoulder abducts involuntarily (Figure 58.2c,d). The

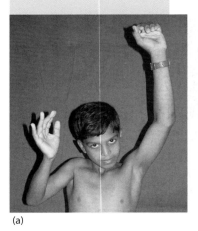 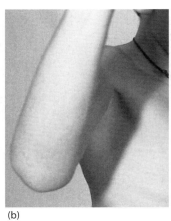 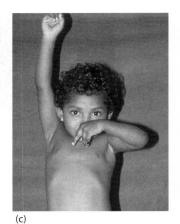 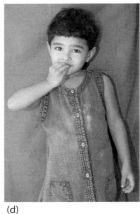

(a) (b) (c) (d)

Figure 58.2 ● Active abduction of the right shoulder in this boy is limited **(a)** although the passive abduction was near normal and the deltoid muscle was functioning well. A closer look **(b)** shows that the pectoralis major is standing out prominently in the anterior axillary fold indicating that there is co-contraction of the abductors and adductors of the shoulder. **(c,d)** As this child attempts to abduct both shoulders, the left elbow flexes involuntarily **(c)**. Similarly, as this child flexes the elbow to get her right hand to her mouth the shoulder involuntarily abducts **(d)**. This trumpet sign is due to co-contraction of the shoulder abductors and the elbow flexors.

posture of the limb is similar to that adopted while holding a trumpet and hence is referred to as the 'trumpet sign'.[1]

4. In co-contraction between the shoulder abductors, elbow flexors and finger flexors, when the child attempts to abduct the shoulder, the elbow and fingers flex involuntarily.

Aims of treatment

- Improve shoulder function
  An attempt must be made to improve shoulder function by increasing the power and the range of movement of the shoulder. Tendon transfers, release of contractures and overcoming co-contraction is necessary to achieve this. In about 20 percent of children with obstetric paralysis, and some children with polio, the shoulder is flail. In these children arthrodesis of the shoulder is a reasonable option.
- Correct deformities and muscle imbalance
  Deformities need to be corrected in order to reduce the tendency for scapular elevation, thus improving the appearance of the shoulder and back. Restoration of muscle balance will minimize the risk of recurrence of deformity.
- Restore joint stability
  Joint stability needs to be restored before the articular surfaces of the humeral head and the glenoid undergo irreversible changes. Once the articular surfaces are deformed the joint will become incongruous.

Treatment options

Improving shoulder function

■ Restoring muscle power

Attempts at reinnervating paralysed muscles of the shoulder by repair of the brachial plexus are not justified after the age of one year in children with obstetric palsy. Hence, tendon transfers are needed to improve power in older children.

■ Restoring the power of abduction

Two transfers currently used for augmenting the power of abduction of the shoulder are the trapezius transfer and the transfer of the clavicular head of the pectoralis major (Figure 58.3).

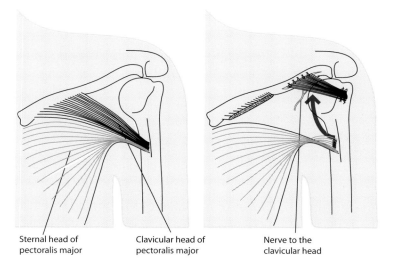

Figure 58.3 ● Technique of bipolar transfer of the clavicular head of the pectoralis major.

Sternal head of pectoralis major   Clavicular head of pectoralis major   Nerve to the clavicular head

■ Restoring the power of external rotation

Often there is weakness of external rotation of the shoulder and commonly transfer of the teres major and the latissimus dorsi is performed to restore the power of external rotation (Figure 58.4).

■ Relieving co-contraction

Correction of co-contraction by releasing or transferring antagonist muscles increases the range of movement.

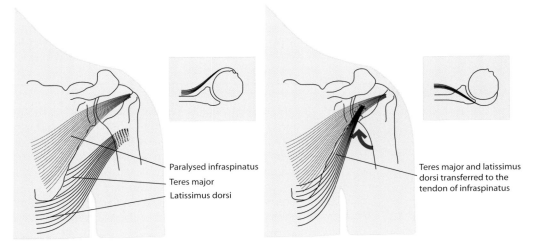

Paralysed infraspinatus
Teres major
Latissimus dorsi

Teres major and latissimus dorsi transferred to the tendon of infraspinatus

Figure 58.4 ● Technique of transfer of the teres major and the latissimus dorsi to the infraspinatus in order to improve the power of external rotation of the shoulder.

■ Shoulder arthrodesis

In children in whom the shoulder is flail, arthrodesis of the shoulder can improve shoulder function quite dramatically. After arthrodesis, the scapulothoracic muscles can move the arm in all directions by elevating, depressing, protracting, retracting and rotating the scapula on the rib cage. In the past, most surgeons preferred to defer arthrodesis until the child had reached skeletal maturity. The reasons for this trend included the potential difficulty in achieving sound fusion, the risk of damaging the proximal humeral growth plate and the impression that the position of fusion can change with growth. However, it has been shown that arthrodesis can be achieved in children as young as seven years of age without damage to the growth plate.[3] Although there is no agreement on what the optimal position of fusion ought to be, the position of arthrodesis should be such that it enables the hand to reach the head. In order to achieve this, the humerus must be held in at least 30° of abduction, 30° of flexion and 30° of internal rotation in relation to the vertebral border of the scapula. In the younger child a greater degree of abduction may be chosen since some loss of abduction may occur with growth.

Correcting deformity and restoring muscle balance

Weakening internal rotation and augmenting external rotation of the shoulder not only improves the power of external rotation but also reduces the risk of posterior dislocation.

Release of contractures responsible for producing scapular elevation improves the appearance even if function does not improve.

Restoring joint stability

Release of an internal rotation contracture can improve stability in a shoulder that is subluxating posteriorly while release of an external rotation contracture improves anterior subluxation.

Power of muscles of the shoulder, elbow, hand and thorax

The extent of paralysis of muscles of the shoulder, elbow and hand and the power of the scapulothoracic muscles are all of vital importance.

If the shoulder is flail, the only available option to improve shoulder function is an arthrodesis. On the other hand, if only some muscles are paralysed there may be scope for tendon transfers.

If the muscles of the forearm and hand are so severely paralysed that reconstruction is not feasible, there is no justification to undertake surgery to improve shoulder function.

The scapulothoracic muscles need to be of normal power if an arthrodesis of the shoulder is to function well.

Stability of the shoulder

The stability of the shoulder must be assessed and any instability should be corrected if the humeral head is not deformed.

Factors to be taken into consideration while planning treatment

Shape of the humeral head

If the shape of the humeral head is altered the congruity of the humeral head and the glenoid must be assessed before considering reduction of the deformed head into the glenoid.

Age of the child

If arthrodesis is being considered, the child must be at least seven years old. In younger children the humeral head and glenoid are too small to obtain sound fusion.

Recommended treatment

The outline of treatment of shoulder paralysis is shown in Table 58.2.

Table 58.2 Outline of treatment of the paralysed shoulder in children

INDICATIONS								
Isolated deltoid paralysis + Hand and elbow function satisfactory	Shoulder power not normal but adequate + Hand and elbow function satisfactory + Contracture producing scapular elevation	Shoulder abduction power satisfactory + External rotator power weak + Internal rotation contracture + Hand and elbow function satisfactory	Co-contraction of shoulder abductor and adductors + Weak abductor and external rotators + Hand and elbow function satisfactory	Internal rotator contracture causing posterior subluxation/ dislocation of humeral head + Humeral head not distorted + Hand and elbow function satisfactory	Internal rotator contracture causing posterior subluxation/ dislocation of humeral head + Humeral head distorted + Hand and elbow function satisfactory	Flail shoulder + Good scapulothoracic muscle power + Hand and elbow function satisfactory + Child over 7 years of age	Flail shoulder + Paralysed scapulothoracic muscles + Hand and elbow function satisfactory	Any form of shoulder paralysis + Hand function too poor to salvage by reconstruction
⇩	⇩	⇩	⇩	⇩	⇩	⇩	⇩	⇩
Trapezius transfer to restore shoulder abduction	Release of contracted muscle responsible for scapular elevation	Contracture release and transfer of teres major and latissimus dorsi to infraspinatus	Transfer of clavicular head of pectoralis major to the rotator cuff + Teres major and latissimus dorsi to infraspinatus	Internal rotator contracture release	Derotation osteotomy of proximal humerus	Shoulder arthrodesis	No intervention to improve shoulder function	No intervention to improve shoulder function
TREATMENT								

Rationale of treatment suggested

Why should hand function be satisfactory before considering shoulder reconstruction?
The primary function of the shoulder is to facilitate positioning of the hand to perform its activity at the chosen point in space. Hence, if the hand itself is non-functional there is no justification in undertaking reconstructive surgery on the shoulder.

Why is a trapezius transfer advocated only if there is isolated paralysis of the deltoid and not in situations where, in addition to deltoid paralysis, other muscles are also paralysed?

Shoulder arthrodesis is a salvage option for dealing with a paralysed shoulder should other options fail. It is desirable to leave all muscles that move the scapula untouched in case an arthrodesis becomes necessary in children with more extensive paralysis.

References

1. Chuang DC, Ma HS, Wei FC. A new strategy of muscle transposition for treatment of shoulder deformity caused by obstetric brachial plexus palsy. *Plast Reconstr Surg* 1998; **101**: 686–94.
2. Zancolli EA. Classification and management of the shoulder in birth palsy. *Orthop Clin North Am* 1981; **12**: 433–57.
3. Makin M. Early arthrodesis for a flail shoulder in young children. *J Bone Joint Surg Am* 1977; **59**: 317–21.

The paralysed shoulder and elbow in the infant

59

Benjamin Joseph

Introduction

Paralysis of the shoulder and elbow following obstetric brachial plexus injury occurs with upper arm and whole-arm types of lesions. Fortunately, the majority of obstetric brachial plexus injuries are neurapraxia and, consequently, these palsies are transient with complete recovery of function.[1] The more severe degrees of injury include axonotmesis and neurotmesis (Figure 59.1a–c).

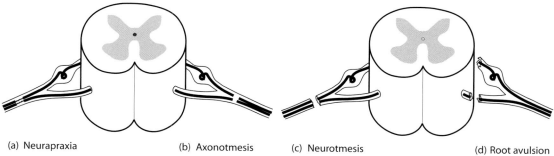

(a) Neurapraxia   (b) Axonotmesis   (c) Neurotmesis   (d) Root avulsion

Figure 59.1 ● Diagrammatic representation of the different patterns of injuries of the brachial plexus that may be seen in obstetric brachial plexus palsy. They include neurapraxia **(a)**, axonotmesis **(b)**, neurotmesis **(c)** or root avulsion **(d)**.

In early infancy it is difficult to differentiate between these different types of injuries and, unfortunately, electrodiagnostic tests are not entirely reliable. Hence prognosis is predicted on the basis of the extent and timing of recovery of function. It has been shown that if antigravity power of the biceps is restored by two months of age, full recovery will occur within two years. If antigravity strength of the biceps recovers between three and six months of age, some degree of limitation of joint movement and development of joint contractures appear to be inevitable.[1] The most severe form of injury is an avulsion of the roots from the cord proximal to the posterior root ganglion (Figure 59.1d). A pre-ganglionic avulsion of the roots of the plexus may be suspected if the infant has an associated Horner syndrome or phrenic nerve avulsion with paralysis of the hemidiaphragm.

Prognosis for recovery depends on whether the injury to the brachial plexus is pre-ganglionic or post-ganglionic (extraforaminal). Similarly, the feasibility of repair of the severed root is also restricted to post-ganglionic injury as any form of repair within the spinal canal would not be possible (Figure 59.2).

Figure 59.2 ● The injury to the plexus may be extraforaminal (post-ganglionic injury) or within the spinal canal (pre-ganglionic injury).

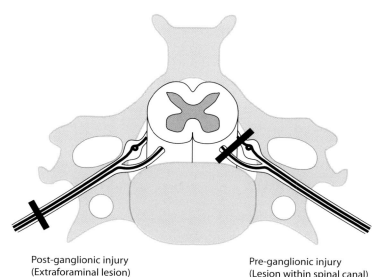

Post-ganglionic injury (Extraforaminal lesion)   Pre-ganglionic injury (Lesion within spinal canal)

Problems of management

Timing of intervention

Since the clinician has to wait till some recovery occurs before predicting the prognosis, it is imperative that one is aware of how long one can safely wait before intervening. Any attempt at repair of the brachial plexus should be undertaken before there is irreparable damage to the motor end plates of the paralysed muscles. It is estimated that motor end plates completely degenerate around 18-24 months after nerve injury. It is also well established that nerve regeneration following surgical restoration of neural continuity proceeds only at the rate of 1 mm per day. Hence if useful function following repair of the injured brachial plexus is to be expected, surgery must be done sufficiently early to enable the regenerating neurons to reach the target muscles before degeneration of the motor end plates occurs. Thus, if the aim is to re-innervate muscles of the elbow, the repair of the plexus needs to be performed by six to nine months of age.

Aims of treatment

- Restore nerve supply to the paralysed muscles
  The aim of treatment is to attempt to reinnervate the paralysed muscles before permanent damage to the motor end plates occurs.
- Preserve normal joint motion and prevent joint contractures and shoulder subluxation or dislocation
  Since there is a very high risk of these children developing contractures of the shoulder, every effort must be made to prevent them.

Treatment options

Observe for recovery

All infants with obstetric brachial plexus injuries should be kept under close observation for the first three months after birth to document the extent and timing of recovery of motor power.

Neurolysis of the brachial plexus

Although neurolysis was popular in the past, most surgeons have abandoned performing this as the definitive procedure since the results were not very satisfactory.[2]

Nerve grafting after neuroma resection

With the help of an operating microscope the neuroma is resected and sural nerve grafts are used to bridge the gap between the ends of the nerve.[1]

Nerve transfers (neurotization) to reinnervate the paralysed muscles

In cases of pre-ganglionic avulsions nerve transfers in conjunction with nerve grafting is performed. The nerves that may be used for such transfers include the intercostal nerves (T2–T4), a branch of the spinal accessory nerve after it innervates the trapezius muscle, phrenic nerve, contralateral C7 root and the hypoglossal nerve.[3]

Passive exercises to prevent contractures

Passive range-of-motion exercises need to be performed every day on a very regular basis to prevent contractures from developing in all children with obstetric brachial plexus injuries. In particular, passive external rotation exercises must be performed religiously to prevent an internal rotation contracture which is the prime reason for posterior subluxation and dislocation of the shoulder. These exercises must be performed while the scapula is stabilized. Children in whom surgical repair of the plexus has been carried out should also do these exercises to prevent contractures from developing by the time the muscles become reinnervated.

Factors to be taken into consideration while planning treatment

Site of injury to the plexus (pre-ganglionic or post-ganglionic)

Pre-ganglionic avulsions of the plexus cannot be repaired by nerve grafting and thus children with these severe injuries need to be treated by nerve transfers. Once it is clear that the injury is pre-ganglionic, there is no justification in waiting for signs of recovery until six or nine months. Children with pre-ganglionic injuries should be offered surgical intervention by three months of age.

Age of the child

Infants under the age of three months are not subjected to surgery on the brachial plexus. Children over the age of nine months are not candidates for repair of the plexus as it is probably too late.

Extent of spontaneous recovery and the potential for further recovery

If grade III (MRC) power of elbow flexion is restored spontaneously by two months of age, no surgical intervention is justified as full recovery is anticipated. If grade III muscle power is restored by six months of age, again, exploration of the brachial plexus is not necessary, but care needs to be taken to minimize the extent of joint contractures. If antigravity power (grade III) of the elbow flexors is not restored by six to nine months of age in infants with post-ganglionic lesions, exploration of the brachial plexus is indicated. Since no spontaneous recovery can be expected in infants with pre-ganglionic injuries, exploration of the plexus and nerve transfers should be considered by three months of age.

Recommended treatment

The recommended outline of treatment for obstetric brachial plexus injury in the infant is shown in Table 59.1.

Table 59.1 ● Outline of treatment of the paralysed shoulder and elbow in the infant

INDICATIONS				
Pre-ganglionic or post-ganglionic injury Infant under 3 months of age	Pre-ganglionic injury Infant 3 months of age	Post-ganglionic injury + Spontaneous recovery of grade III flexion of elbow by 2 months of age	Post-ganglionic injury + Spontaneous recovery of grade III flexion of elbow by 3–6 months of age	Post-ganglionic injury + No spontaneous recovery of grade III flexion of elbow by 6 months of age
				⇩
		⇩	⇩	Resection of neuromas and sural nerve grafting by 9 months of age + Post-operative physiotherapy to prevent contractures
⇩	⇩	No surgery on plexus + Physiotherapy to prevent contractures by the time full recovery of muscle power occurs	No surgery on plexus + Physiotherapy to prevent contractures + Deal with residual weakness in the older child	
Physiotherapy to prevent contractures prior to surgery	Nerve transfers to reinnervate the paralysed muscles + Post-operative physiotherapy to prevent contractures			
TREATMENT				

References

1. Waters PM. Update on management of pediatric brachial plexus palsy. *J Pediatr Orthop B* 2005; **14**: 233–44.
2. Clarke HM, Al-Qattan MM, Curtis CG, Zuker RM. Obstetrical brachial plexus palsy: results following neurolysis of conducting neuromas-in-continuity. *Plast Reconstr Surg* 1996; **97**: 974–84.
3. El-Gammal TA, Fathi NA. Outcomes of surgical treatment of brachial plexus injuries using nerve grafting and nerve transfers. *J Reconstr Microsurg* 2002; **18**: 7–15.

The paralysed hand and wrist

Benjamin Joseph

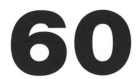

Introduction

Non-progressive paralysis of the hand can be seen in children after peripheral nerve injuries due to lacerations or nerve injuries that may complicate fractures of the humerus, elbow, forearm or wrist. Although in many instances the nerve injury associated with a fracture is transitory and complete recovery occurs, occasionally, permanent paralysis may ensue. Paralysis of the hand may also occur following lower arm or the more severe whole arm type of obstetric brachial plexus palsy or after poliomyelitis or Hansen's disease. Paralysis of the muscles of the hand also occurs as part of a compartment syndrome of the forearm, and this may persist if prompt decompression of the fascial compartment is not performed.

Associated sensory loss is seen in peripheral nerve injuries, brachial plexus palsies, Hansen's disease and following compartment syndrome. Problems of motor paralysis and sensory loss are further compounded by muscle contracture if ischaemic contracture has occurred following a compartment syndrome.

Problems of management

Loss of function

The two most important functions of the hand are to grasp objects firmly in the palm of the hand and to hold small objects between the pulps of the thumb, index and middle fingers as in writing with a pencil (Figure 60.1). The latter posture of the thumb and fingers is referred to as the tripod pinch.

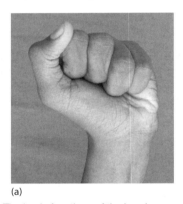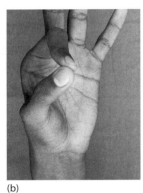

(a) (b)

Figure 60.1 ● The basic functions of the hand are grasp and pinch. When an object is grasped firmly the wrist is extended and the fingers are flexed at the metacarpophalangeal and interphalangeal joints **(a)**. The typical 'tripod pinch' posture is adopted while holding a fine object between the thumb and the index finger. The pulps of the thumb and the index finger meet **(b)**.

In order to grasp large objects firmly, there must be sufficient power in the wrist extensors and the finger flexors. For effective pinch, thumb opposition should be strong and the flexors of the metacarpophalangeal (MCP) and interphalangeal (IP) joints of the index and middle finger should be functional. At the same time, the MCP and IP joint of the thumb should remain stable as the flexed fingers push against the terminal phalanx of the thumb.

In order to get an object into the palm of the hand or between the tips of the thumb and fingers so as to hold it, the fingers and thumb have to extend sufficiently to encircle the object before the actual grasping or pinching action can be initiated. Similarly, after placing an object in a desired position, to let go of the object the thumb and fingers need to extend. This movement is referred to as release.

Grasp or pinch is affected when either the intrinsic or extrinsic muscles of the hand are paralysed and release is affected when the extrinsic finger and thumb extensors are paralysed.

Muscle imbalance and deformity

Paralysis of the intrinsic muscles of the fingers when the long finger flexors and extensors (the extrinsic muscles) are functioning results in muscle imbalance at all three joints of the fingers.

The extensor digitorum acts unopposed on the MCP joint as the lumbrical muscle and the interossei (that flex the MCP joint) are paralysed and the long finger flexors act unopposed at the IP joints as the interossei and lumbricals (that extend the IP joints) are paralysed. Consequently, the MCP joint hyperextends and the IP joints flex producing the characteristic claw deformity.

When the intrinsic muscles of the thumb are paralysed the characteristic deformity is the 'ape thumb' deformity and the main feature is inability to oppose the thumb. The child is unable to perform the tripod pinch; the pulp of the thumb comes into contact with the lateral side of the terminal phalanx of the index finger while attempting to oppose the thumb to the index finger.

Joint instability

Occasionally the MCP or IP joint of the thumb is unstable and may collapse into flexion or hyperextension; this makes it impossible to oppose the thumb effectively against the index and middle fingers.

Aims of treatment

- Restore strong grasp
  Since a strong wrist extensor is essential for grasping objects firmly, it is important to restore the power of wrist extension if there is radial nerve palsy. It is also necessary to ensure active flexion of the MCP and IP joints of the fingers. If the fingers are clawed due to intrinsic muscle paralysis, flexion of the MCP joints of the fingers must be restored.
- Restore a tripod pinch
  If the opponens pollicis is paralysed the opposition of the thumb must be restored. Since opposition is a complex movement involving abduction, internal rotation and flexion of the thumb, it is important that all three of these movements are restored.
- Restore release
  The power of finger and thumb extension should be restored if these muscles are paralysed.
- Ensure that the joints of the thumb are stable
  If any of the joints of the thumb is unstable, efficient pinch will not be possible and hence stability needs to be restored.

Treatment options

Restoring wrist extension

■ Tendon transfer

The pronator teres may be transferred to the extensor carpi radialis brevis to restore active extension of the wrist.

■ Orthosis

If the pronator teres is not strong enough to be transferred, a splint that prevents the wrist drop may be considered.

■ Tenodesis

Tenodesis of the tendons of the paralysed wrist extensors to the radius can prevent the wrist drop.

■ Arthrodesis

In the skeletally mature adolescent the wrist may be fused in extension. Fusion of the wrist can help in two ways. First, the stable wrist in extension will facilitate a strong grasp provided the finger flexors are strong. Second, if the flexors of the wrist are functioning, following wrist arthrodesis these tendons will be available for transfers to improve hand function now that they have no function at the wrist. However, one disadvantage of a wrist arthrodesis is the loss of the tenodesis effect that assists finger extension.

Restoring metacarpophalangeal joint flexion

As mentioned earlier, paralysis of the lumbrical and interossei muscles results in deformities at the MCP and IP joints; however, it is not necessary to attempt to correct deformities at each of the three joints independently. If the MCP joint can be made to remain in a few degrees of flexion the extensor digitorum can extend the IP joints through the dorsal digital expansion. Thus, mere restoration of flexion of the MCP joint will succeed in correcting clawing of the finger. Flexion of the MCP joint may be restored by a tendon transfer (dynamic correction) or by a procedure that produces a mild flexion deformity at the MCP joint (static correction) when a dynamic correction is not feasible.

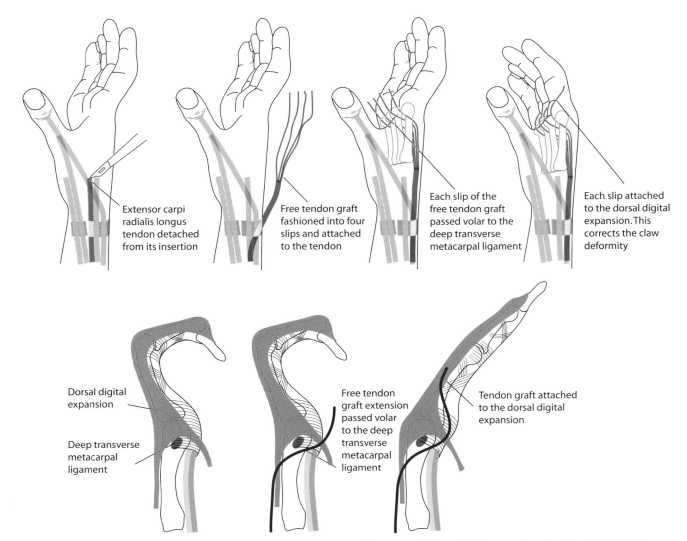

Figure 60.2 ● Diagram showing the technique of performing the extensor-to-flexor four-tailed transfer for correcting claw hand. Note that the transferred tendon strips are passed volar to the axis of the metacarpophalangeal (MCP) joints. Only then will the transferred tendon produce active flexion of the MCP joint.

■ Tendon transfer

Several tendon transfers have been described for restoring active flexion of the MCP joint.[1,2] Among these, the transfer of a wrist extensor to the proximal phalanges of the fingers, described by Brand,[3] is widely used. This extensor-to-flexor four-tailed transfer (EF4T) entails the use of a free tendon graft passed volar to the axis of the MCP joint to ensure flexion of the joint (Figure 60.2). The success of the operation depends both on the appropriate tension of the transfer and the post-operative rehabilitation as re-educating the transferred muscle is vitally important.

■ Lasso procedure

Zancolli[4] described an operation in which the flexor sublimis tendon is passed through the fibrous flexor sheath distal to the axis of the MCP joint and stitched back on itself with sufficient tension to produce a mild flexion deformity of the MCP joint. No free tendon graft is needed and, consequently, the operation is simpler than the EF4T (Figure 60.3a). Muscle re-education is also more simple after this procedure.

■ Pulley advancement

Palande[5] described an elegant procedure that did not involve any tendon transfer but still enabled active flexion of the MCP joint. The proximal pulley of the fibrous flexor sheath is excised so that the mouth of the flexor sheath is moved from a point proximal to the axis of the MCP joint to a point distal to the axis of the joint. By so doing, the flexor tendon bowstrings which increases its

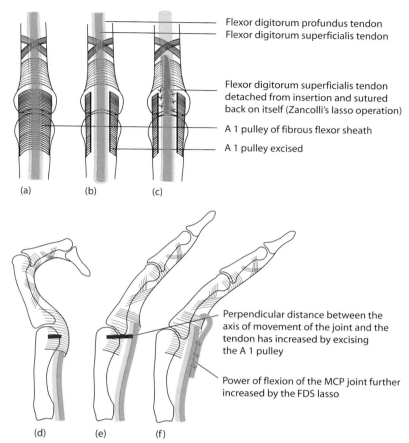

Figure 60.3 ● Diagram showing the technique of correcting a claw deformity **(a)** by performing pulley advancement **(b)** and the Zancolli lasso procedure **(c)**. Note that in the lasso procedure, the flexor digitorum sublimus tendon that normally flexes the proximal interphalangeal joint is converted to a flexor of the metacarpophalangeal (MCP) joint. By advancing the mouth of the fibrous flexor sheath the flexor digitorum tendons bowstring and this increases their flexor moment arms at the MCP joint.

flexor moment at the MCP joint. This is sufficient to enable the flexor tendons to actively flex the MCP joint (Figure 60.3b).

■ Capsulorraphy

Another operation advocated by Palande[5] is a capsulorraphy of the MCP joint that may be done in conjunction with pulley advancement. By excising a portion of the volar capsule of the MCP joint and closing the gap a mild flexion deformity of the MCP joint is created (Figure 60.4).

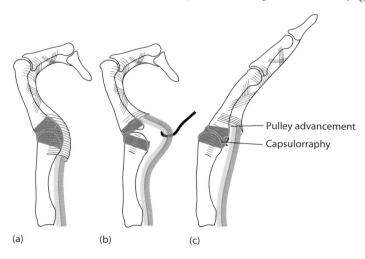

Figure 60.4 ● Capsulorraphy of the MCP joint produces a flexion deformity of the MCP joint.

■ Splintage

A knuckleduster splint that holds the MCP joints flexed may be an acceptable option as a temporary measure, encouraging the child to use the hand more while waiting for a more permanent solution.

Restoring thumb opposition

■ Tendon transfer (opponensplasty)

Several tendon transfers have been described for restoring active opposition of the thumb. Transfer of the sublimis tendon of the ring finger is one option that is widely used.[6] Another tendon that is often used for an opponensplasty is the extensor indicis proprius. Two critical aspects of performing an opponensplasty are the direction of routeing of the tendon and the point of attachment of the transferred tendon on the thumb. If care is taken in getting both these two technical points correct, then the transferred tendon should be able to abduct and internally rotate the thumb (Figure 60.5).

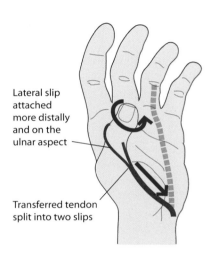

Lateral slip attached more distally and on the ulnar aspect

Transferred tendon split into two slips

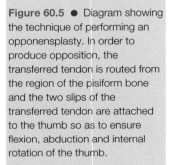

Figure 60.5 ● Diagram showing the technique of performing an opponensplasty. In order to produce opposition, the transferred tendon is routed from the region of the pisiform bone and the two slips of the transferred tendon are attached to the thumb so as to ensure flexion, abduction and internal rotation of the thumb.

■ Arthrodesis

If there is no tendon available to transfer for restoring dynamic opposition of the thumb, the thumb may be arthrodesed in a position of opposition. Although it will suffice if the carpometacarpal joint of the thumb is fused, it may be difficult to get this joint to fuse in a child. Another option is to fuse the first and second metacarpals together with a bale graft after ensuring that the thumb is held opposed. The index and middle fingers can then oppose against a stable thumb post. The disadvantage of this procedure, however, is that the thumb will always remain in an opposed position and this may be a hindrance in some situations, such as putting the hand into a pocket.

■ Splintage

A splint that holds the thumb in opposition may be used as a temporary measure to decide whether hand function can be improved by ensuring opposition. It may be used for longer periods in children who need an arthrodesis but are too young for this option.

Restoring release

Power of active extension of the thumb can be provided by transferring the palmaris longus tendon to the thumb and the flexor carpi ulnaris to the extensor digitorum tendons. If the palmaris longus is absent the flexor carpi ulnaris may be transferred to the finger extensors and the thumb extensor.

Restoring stability of the thumb

If muscle balance is restored across the MCP and IP joints of the thumb, these joints should be stable. However, in situations where there is extensive paralysis arthrodesis of the carpometacarpal joint, the MCP or the IP joint may be needed.

Age of the child

Children under the age of seven years are unlikely to be able to comprehend the instructions for muscle re-education that is essential for rehabilitation following a tendon transfer. Hence, tendon transfers should be reserved for children who are old enough to cooperate with the post-operative rehabilitation regimen.

Arthrodesis of joints of the hand in children is better avoided as growth arrest due to physeal damage can easily occur. For this reason, if an arthrodesis is considered essential, it should be performed after skeletal maturity. Tenodesis operations that may work well in the adult may not be predictable as the tension on the tenodesis may alter with growth of the skeleton.

Pattern of paralysis and availability of muscles for transfer

The choice of the tendon transfer is governed by the extent of paralysis and the muscles that are still functioning. When a single nerve is paralysed there is a choice of tendons available for transfers. However, when both intrinsic and extrinsic muscles of the hand are paralysed or when there are multiple nerve palsies, a sufficient number of functioning muscles may not be available for transfer in order to restore function.

Feasibility of post-operative muscle re-education

If efficient rehabilitation services to supervise the child's post-operative rehabilitation are not available or if the child cannot either comprehend or cooperate with the re-education programme, it is wiser to select a procedure that has little or no need for muscle re-education.

Associated sensory loss

Attempts at making a paralysed hand functional may be influenced by the extent of sensory loss that might be present. If even protective sensation is not present over most of the palmar surface of the hand it may not be worthwhile embarking on reconstructive surgery unless the child is old enough to understand the consequences of sensory loss and is capable of caring for the insensate hand.

The recommended approach to the management of the paralysed hand in a child is shown in Tables 60.1–60.3.

Table 60.1 ● Outline of treatment of claw hand in children

INDICATIONS			
Young child + Severe sensory loss in palm of the hand + Child not old enough to care for the anaesthetic hand	Any age + No muscle available for dynamic transfer + Weak long finger flexors	Child unable to comprehend or cooperate with post-operative rehabilitation programme	Older child in whom capsulorraphy and pulley advancement unsuccessful + Extensors of wrist and fingers and the extrinsic finger flexors are functioning well ⇩
⇩	⇩	⇩	Zancolli's lasso OR EF4T (if surgeon is experienced in hand surgery)
Delay intervention	Capsulorraphy	Capsulorraphy + Pulley advancement	
TREATMENT			

Table 60.2 ● Outline of treatment of opponens paralysis in children

INDICATIONS				
Young child + Severe sensory loss in palm of the hand + Child not old enough to care for the anaesthetic hand	Child unable to comprehend or cooperate with post-operative rehabilitation programme	Skeletally immature child + No muscle available for transfer	Child capable of cooperating with post-operative rehabilitation programme + Functioning flexor digitorum sublimus AND profundus	Skeletally mature + No muscle available for transfer
⇩	⇩	⇩	⇩	⇩
Delay intervention	Delay surgery + Opponens splint	Delay surgery + Opponens splint	Opponensplasty with FDS4 (flexor digitorum sublimis tendon to the ring finger)	Arthrodesis of the thumb with an intermetacarpal graft between the first and second metacarpals
TREATMENT				

Table 60.3 ● Outline of treatment of wrist and finger drop in children

INDICATIONS			
Pronator teres, flexor carpi ulnaris and palmaris longus functioning normally	Pronator teres not functioning + Skeletally immature child	Pronator teres not functioning + Skeletally mature + Other muscles around the wrist functioning well	Pronator teres not functioning + Skeletally mature + Paralysis of several muscles of the hand requiring other tendon transfers
⇩	⇩	⇩	⇩
Pronator teres transfer to extensor carpi radialis brevis + Flexor carpi ulnaris transfer to extensor digitorum + Palmaris longus transfer to the thumb abductor and extensor	Cock-up splint	Tenodesis of wrist extensors to radius	Wrist arthrodesis
TREATMENT			

References

1. Anderson GA. The child's hand in the developing world. In: Gupta A, Kay SPJ, Scheker LR (eds). *The Growing Hand*. London: Mosby, 2000: 1097–114.
2. Nanchahal J, Wolff TW. Reconstructive surgery in peripheral nerve palsy. In: Gupta A, Kay SPJ, Scheker LR (eds). *The Growing Hand*. London: Mosby, 2000: 825–30.
3. Brand PW. Tendon grafting. Illustrated by a new operation for intrinsic paralysis of the fingers. *J Bone Joint Surg Br* 1961; **43**: 444–53.
4. Zancolli EA. Claw hand caused by paralysis of the intrinsic muscles. *J Bone Joint Surg Am* 1957; **39**: 1076–80.
5. Palande DD. Correction of paralytic claw finger in leprosy by capsulorraphy and pulley advancement. *J Bone Joint Surg Am* 1976; **58**: 59–66.
6. Palande DD. Opponensplasty in intrinsic muscle paralysis of the thumb in leprosy. *J Bone Joint Surg Am* 1975; **57**: 489–93.

General principles of management of upper motor neuron paralysis

61

Benjamin Joseph

Introduction

Spastic paralysis in children is most commonly seen in cerebral palsy. However, it can occur following meningitis, encephalitis, traumatic brain injury and asphyxiation (e.g. near drowning). Apart from these forms of static encephalopathies, rare forms of progressive encephalopathies can occur in children. The principles of management of static encephalopathies are discussed in this chapter.

Problems of management

Spasticity

Spasticity is one of the most important manifestations of motor system involvement following brain damage due to injury or disease. It may be defined as a velocity-dependent hyperactivity of stretch reflexes.[1] If untreated, the spastic muscle may undergo myostatic contracture. This is because stretch is the stimulus that enables muscle growth to keep pace with the growth of the skeleton[2] and the opposing muscles are not strong enough to stretch the spastic muscle.

Oral medication currently available is largely ineffective in adequately reducing spasticity without an unacceptable degree of side effects.

Muscle imbalance

Paresis of one group of muscles or spasticity in the opposing group (even in the absence of paresis) can result in muscle imbalance which, in turn, can produce deformity at the intervening joint.

Incoordination

Varying degrees of incoordination may be seen in children with cerebral palsy. It is far more pronounced if there is associated dystonia, athetosis, tremors or ataxia.

Involuntary movements

Involuntary movements such as athetoid or dystonic movements compound the problem of spasticity and make surgical intervention far more unpredictable.

Loss of selective control

While normal individuals can contract a single muscle at a time, children with cerebral palsy may be unable to do so and may have to rely on the mass action of a group of muscles in order to produce the desired movement. A good example of this phenomenon is seen in the tibialis anterior. Normal children can be instructed to actively dorsiflex the ankle at will while seated with the legs hanging over the edge of a couch. Children with cerebral palsy are often unable to do this and would have to flex the thigh against resistance in order to activate the tibialis anterior (Figure 61.1).

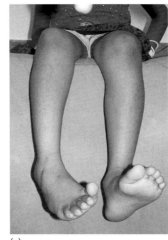
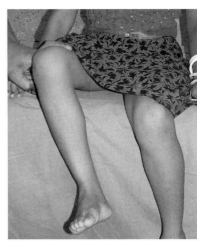

Figure 61.1 ● **(a)** A child with right hemiplegic cerebral palsy attempts to dorsiflex her ankles. The normal left ankle dorsiflexes while the right side does not. This is on account of her lack of selective control over the tibialis anterior muscle of the right side. **(b)** As the child flexes her hip against resistance the right ankle dorsiflexes.

(a)   (b)

Co-contraction of antagonistic muscles

In normal individuals when a group of muscles contract, there is reciprocal inhibition of the antagonistic muscles to facilitate movement at the joint. In cerebral palsy simultaneous contraction of both opposing muscle groups can occur. An example of this is seen at the knee where the rectus femoris and the hamstrings contract simultaneously, resulting in a stiff-knee gait.[3]

Deformities

Spasticity and muscle imbalance result in deformities at joints, which further compromise function of the limbs. Although the deformities are initially due to muscle contractures, over a period of time, adaptive bony changes will supervene.

Joint dislocation

The hip, in particular, is vulnerable to this complication as the result of a combination of spasticity, muscle imbalance and deformities (see Chapter 25, Paralytic hip dislocation: cerebral palsy). Less frequently, paralytic dislocation of the shoulder or the radial head may also occur.

The combination of all of these problems results in difficulty in ambulation when the lower limb is involved, while upper limb involvement results in difficulty in performing the activities of daily living.

Among the various problems that may be seen with upper motor neuron lesions, spasticity, muscle imbalance, deformities and the effect of co-contraction and dislocation of the hip may be altered by orthopaedic intervention. Involuntary movements may be improved by medication or neurosurgical intervention. However, there is no treatment for incoordination and the lack of selective control.

Long-term aims of management

The long-term aims of management will be to either achieve maximum function for independent living, improve function to minimize the degree of dependence or facilitate the care of the totally dependent child.

After evaluating the child, the goals of treatment must be clearly defined. It is necessary to determine whether, in due course, the child can be made to function independently in society. If this is not likely, the aim will be to improve function sufficiently to at least reduce the extent to which the child is dependent on the care giver. In some instances no functional improvement may be anticipated. Even in these patients treatment may be justified if it is likely to make it easier for the care giver to look after the totally dependent child.

To achieve these long-term goals, orthopaedic surgery may be indicated as follows.

- Improve function
  The function of the upper limbs is to fulfil the activities of daily living, while that of the lower limbs is to walk. Surgery should ideally improve these functions. However, it needs to be emphasized that in cerebral palsy improvement of function cannot be achieved in many instances.
- Improve appearance
  Even if function cannot be improved, there is a definite role for correcting deformities even if the only obvious benefit is improvement in appearance. It is unfair to assume that children with disabilities are not concerned about appearance. Body image is important and correction of deformities may go a long way in improving the self-esteem of the child.
- Facilitate personal hygiene
  Correction of severe adduction deformities of the hip will facilitate perineal hygiene. Release of severe flexion deformities of the fingers or a severely adducted thumb will relieve maceration of the palmar skin and reduce skin infections. Such surgery is clearly indicated even if no functional gain is envisaged.
- Prevent or treat complications
  The prime example of a preventable complication in cerebral palsy is hip dislocation. Surgery as a measure to prevent dislocation of the hip is not only justified but is of paramount importance since a proportion of dislocated hips become painful and, in turn, pain increases spasticity quite profoundly. Surgery is also indicated to remedy the situation once a dislocation has occurred.

Short-term aims of management

- Reduce spasticity
- Restore muscle balance
- Reduce involuntary movements
- Overcome the effects of co-contraction of antagonistic muscles
- Correct deformities
- Prevent or reduce joint dislocations

Treatment options

Reducing spasticity

■ **Physiotherapeutic measures**

One of the main ways of reducing spasticity is slow repetitive passive stretching of the spastic muscles and appropriate posturing. The repetitive stretching of the spastic muscle also provides the stimulus to enable the muscle to grow as the skeleton grows. Hence, physiotherapy needs to be continued on a regular basis until skeletal maturity.

■ **Tone inhibition casting**

A short period of immobilization in a cast can reduce spasticity temporarily. This is particularly useful in controlling spasticity of the gastrocsoleus muscle.

■ **Orthotics**

Splintage has a similar effect to casting and may be useful in situations where a tone inhibition cast has been found to be effective. In general, bracing is restricted to the ankle and foot in the lower limb and the wrist and hand in the upper limb.

■ **Myoneural blocks**

One way of reducing spasticity is to weaken the overactive muscle by partial temporary denervation. This can be achieved by injecting drugs either in the vicinity of the nerve supplying the spastic muscle or into the muscle belly in the region of its motor point. (The motor point of a muscle is the point at which electrical stimulation would produce the maximal response.) The perineural injection is usually done with the help of an electrical stimulator that can deliver a low voltage current through a needle that is passed towards the nerve based on surface landmarks. Demonstrable visible contraction of the muscle in response to an electrical stimulus indicates that the tip of the needle is in contact with the nerve and then the agent can be injected there. The second method does not require an electrical stimulator since the injection is given into the muscle belly. The site of injection ideally should be at the motor point which is the site at which stimulation would produce the strongest contraction for a given strength of current. The motor points of muscles of the upper and lower limbs have been mapped out by physiologists in the past, and the site of injection may be selected from these maps.

Phenol, 40 percent alcohol[4] and botulinum toxin[5] have been used for this purpose. Of these, phenol is seldom used now on account of the tissue damage that can occur following the injection. Botulinum toxin and alcohol, when injected into the motor point of the muscle, have a similar effect of reducing spasticity that lasts for six to nine months.

This approach is particularly effective in young children and appears to delay the need for surgery. Botulinum toxin is very expensive and, for this reason, alcohol may be preferred in less affluent societies. However, alcohol injection is painful and requires a short anaesthetic at the time of injection.

■ **Intrathecal baclofen**

Intrathecal administration of baclofen from an implanted pump is effective in controlling spasticity.[6] This overcomes the problem of side effects that are seen with oral administration as much smaller doses of the drug are needed to control spasticity when given intrathecally. Cost and technical issues related to the pump are major limiting factors.

■ **Selective dorsal rhizotomy**

Selective division of posterior rootlets that carry afferent impulses from spastic muscles has been shown to reduce spasticity.[7] This method entails a lumbar laminectomy which may increase susceptibility to developing spinal deformities and spondylolisthesis.[8]

■ Neurectomy

Truncal neurectomy of nerves supplying spastic muscles which used to be practised in the past has now been abandoned. However, division of some branches of nerves to a spastic muscle may be considered as a means of reducing spasticity.

■ Surgery on spastic muscle-tendon unit

Surgery on the muscle-tendon unit is the most widely used approach to dealing with spasticity. The offending muscle is weakened by either lengthening the tendon or by releasing the muscle fibres from its proximal origin and permitting them to slide distally. The effect of both these operations is to reduce the resting length of the muscle fibres, thereby weakening the muscle.

Restoring muscle balance

■ By strengthening the weaker muscle group

Theoretically, physiotherapy should help increase the strength of weak muscles; in reality, it seldom works in these children. The next option is to transfer the tendon of one of the spastic muscles to the weaker side. While the outcome of a tendon transfer is usually predictable in lower motor neuron paralysis, the results are often quite unpredictable in upper motor neuron paralysis. The transferred muscle may not function at all due to lack of selective control, which makes muscle re-education very difficult. The transfer may occasionally result in overcorrection as the transferred spastic muscle may overact and produce an imbalance in the opposite direction (Figure 61.2).

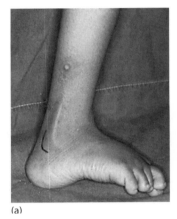
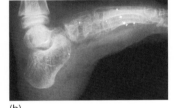

Figure 61.2 ● A tibialis posterior transfer to the dorsum of the foot was performed one year earlier to correct an equinovarus deformity in a boy with cerebral palsy. A calcaneovalgus deformity has developed **(a,b)**. The transferred tendon had to be divided in order to correct the new deformity.

(a)   (b)

■ By weakening the spastic, stronger muscle group

This is currently the mainstay of surgery aimed at restoring muscle balance in spastic situations. A decision needs to be made if a spastic muscle should be totally defunctioned by performing a tenotomy or whether it should be merely weakened by tendon lengthening or a muscle slide. This will depend on the degree of muscle imbalance that is present. There is always a risk of weakening the muscle group too much and then the muscle imbalance may be reversed. For example, excessive lengthening of the Achilles tendon to correct a spastic equinus results in excessive dorsiflexion of the ankle and a crouch gait.

Reducing involuntary movements

Medication or neurosurgery may help to reduce involuntary movements. It is seldom possible to get rid of the involuntary movements totally.

Overcoming the effects of co-contraction of antagonistic muscles

If co-contraction of antagonistic spastic muscles can be demonstrated it may help if one of the muscles is transferred so that both muscles work in unison.[3]

Correcting deformities

In several instances, mild deformities will correct once the contracted tendons are released. In more long-standing cases, osteotomies or shortening of the bone may be needed to correct the deformities.

Preventing or reducing joint dislocations

The approach to preventing and reducing spastic hip dislocation is discussed in Chapter 25.

Recommended treatment

An outline of the treatment of spastic equinus is presented in Table 61.1 to illustrate the following principles.

Table 61.1 ● Outline for management of spastic equinus

INDICATIONS					
Spastic equinus without any contracture	Poor response to physiotherapy	Good response to tone inhibition casting	Poor response to tone inhibition casting	Poor response to myoneural block	Recurrence of equinus with a contracture
					⇩
				⇩	Lengthening of the Achilles tendon
			⇩	Aponeurotic lengthening of gastrocsoleus	
		⇩	Myoneural block		
	⇩	Ankle–foot orthosis			
⇩	Tone inhibition cast				
Physiotherapy					
TREATMENT					

Rationale for treatment choice

In view of the risk of overcorrection and unpredictable response to surgery it is advisable to initially choose the least invasive method.

It is preferable to choose a treatment that has a low risk of overcorrection and few reported complications.

It is safer to undercorrect rather than overcorrect muscle imbalance.

References

1. Young RR, Wiegner AW. Spasticity. *Clin Orthop Relat Res* 1987; **219**: 50–62.
2. Ziv I, Blackburn N, Rang M, Koreska J. Muscle growth in normal and spastic mice. *Dev Med Child Neurol* 1984; **26**: 94–9.
3. Perry J. Distal rectus transfer. *Dev Med Child Nurol* 1987; **29**: 153–8.
4. Carpenter EB, Seitz DG. Intramuscular alcohol as an aid in the management of spastic cerebral palsy. *Dev Med Child Neurol* 1980; **22**: 497–501.
5. Cosgrove AP, Graham HK. Botulinum toxin A in the management of spasticity with cerebral palsy. *Br J Surg* 1992; **74**:135–6.
6. Albright AL, Cervi A, Singletary J. Intrathecal baclofen for spasticity in cerebral palsy. *J Am Med Assoc* 1991; **265**: 1418–22.
7. Peacock WJ, Staudt LA. Functional outcomes following selective posterior rhizotomy in children with cerebral palsy. *J Neurosurg* 1991; **74**: 380–85.
8. Johnson MB, Goldstein L, Thomas SS *et al.* Spinal deformity after selective dorsal rhizotomy in ambulatory patients with cerebral palsy. *J Pediatr Orthop* 2004; **24**: 529–36.

The spastic foot and ankle

Benjamin Joseph

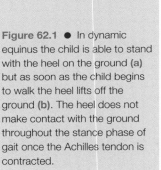

62

Deformities of the foot and ankle that occur very frequently in cerebral palsy include equinus, equinovarus, varus and valgus. Calcaneus deformity is encountered less frequently and this may be seen as a complication of the treatment of equinus.

Equinus is by far the most common deformity encountered in the lower limb in cerebral palsy. The deformity may either be dynamic due to spasticity of the gastrocsoleus or a fixed equinus due to a contracture of the muscle.

Loss of the normal heel–toe sequence of the gait cycle

The child with an equinus will be unable to dorsiflex the ankle during the swing phase of gait and the toe will make initial contact with the ground instead of the heel. If the deformity is dynamic the heel will come down and make contact with the ground by mid-stance. If the gastrocsoleus is contracted the heel will not touch the ground throughout the gait cycle (Figure 62.1).

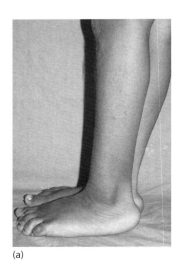
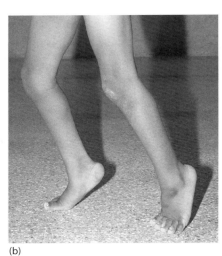

(a)   (b)

Figure 62.1 ● In dynamic equinus the child is able to stand with the heel on the ground **(a)** but as soon as the child begins to walk the heel lifts off the ground **(b)**. The heel does not make contact with the ground throughout the stance phase of gait once the Achilles tendon is contracted.

Development of secondary deformities at the knee and foot

Secondary deformities at the knee and foot can develop in children with severe spasticity or a contracture of the gastrocsoleus. These secondary deformities are recurvatum deformity at the knee, valgus deformity of the hindfoot (valgus ex-equino) and a break in the midfoot. If a genu recurvatum deformity develops the child will be able to get the heel to the ground although, in reality, the foot remains plantarflexed at the ankle (Figure 62.2a). In children with valgus deformity of the hindfoot secondary to equinus, it can be demonstrated that passive dorsiflexion of the ankle is restricted if the range of motion is tested with the foot held in inversion (Figure 62.2b). If the foot is not inverted while testing, an erroneous impression of ankle dorsiflexion may be obtained.

It is important that the underlying equinus deformity is corrected before adaptive bony changes occur at the sites of these secondary deformities.

Weakness of the gastrocsoleus after surgery to correct equinus

If the gastrocsoleus is lengthened too much the muscle is weakened excessively and this can have disastrous consequences. Excessive lengthening of the gastrocsoleus can lead to a calcaneus deformity and severe crouch gait and, occasionally, the child may be unable to walk. Therefore, lengthening of the muscle should be performed very carefully, ensuring that the extent of lengthening should be just sufficient to get the ankle dorsiflexed to 10° beyond the neutral position.

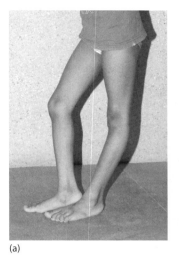
(a)

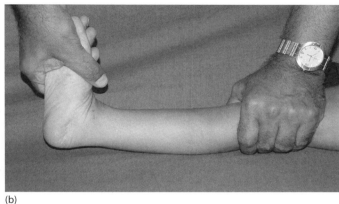
(b)

Figure 62.2 ● **(a)** Genu recurvatum that has developed in a child with spastic equinus. **(b)** The contracture of the Achilles tendon may not be evident if dorsiflexion is attempted without holding the foot in inversion. The ankle cannot be dorsiflexed when the foot is held inverted; consequently, it is important to test for tightness of the Achilles tendon while the foot is held inverted.

Aims of treatment

- Correct equinus to facilitate a heel–toe sequence of gait
- Correct the secondary deformities that may have developed due to the underlying equinus
- Prevent excessive weakening of the gastrocsoleus

Treatment options

Physiotherapeutic options

■ Stretching exercises

Repeated, gentle, slow stretching of the gastrocsoleus helps to reduce the spasticity and also helps in preventing a contracture from developing or recurring after surgical release.

■ Tone inhibition casting

A below-knee walking cast that is well moulded and extends to the tips of the toes is applied and retained for three weeks. Quite appreciable reduction in spasticity of the gastrocsoleus is often noted when the cast is removed. However, the effect is short-lived.[1] Nevertheless, this period of reduction in spasticity may be very useful in facilitating more effective physiotherapy and will also help to decide the potential benefits of bracing.

Orthotic options

In children with a dynamic equinus who respond favourably to tone inhibition casting an ankle–foot orthosis may be considered. A choice must be made whether to use a rigid or an articulated ankle–foot orthosis. An orthosis may be used as the primary form of treatment of the spastic equinus or may be used after a myoneural block or after surgery in order to maintain the improvement obtained by the block or surgery.

■ Rigid ankle–foot orthosis

A rigid ankle–foot orthosis moulded in 10° of dorsiflexion of the ankle is prescribed if there is a tendency for a genu recurvatum.[2] A rigid orthosis may be preferred if there is an associated dynamic varus or valgus deformity as it splints the subtalar joint more efficiently than an articulated orthosis.

■ Articulated ankle–foot orthosis

An articulated ankle–foot orthosis is preferred in most instances as the orthosis will permit dorsiflexion but prevent plantarflexion. The gait pattern is closer to normal with an articulated ankle–foot orthosis than with a rigid orthosis.

Myoneural blocks

Myoneural block of the gastrocnemius with either botulinum toxin or alcohol reduces the spasticity of the muscle. The effect is temporary with the beneficial effect lasting for around six to nine months. The blocks are ineffective once there is an established contracture of the muscle.

Surgical options

Once there is an established equinus contracture, a distinction needs to be made between isolated contracture of the gastrocnemius and contracture of both the soleus and the gastrocnemius. If both the muscles are contracted, lengthening of the tendo Achilles is performed but if the gastrocnemius alone is contracted, aponeurotic lengthening of the gastrocnemius is performed. As emphasized earlier, it is extremely important to ensure that the gastrocsoleus is not over-lengthened as it will result in a calcaneus deformity and a crouch posture which is very difficult to treat. The risk of over-lengthening may be more when the tendo Achilles is lengthened than when aponeurotic lengthening is done. For this reason, some surgeons, in all cases, prefer not to lengthen the tendo Achilles at all and only lengthen the gastrocnemius.

■ Gastrocnemius lengthening

Lengthening of the gastrocnemius can be done close to the musculotendinous junction by any one of the techniques illustrated in Figure 62.3. In the past, release of the two heads of the gastrocnemius from their femoral attachment was popular but currently this is not recommended.

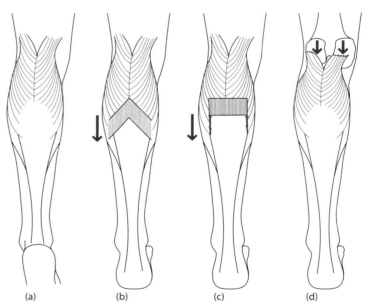

(a)   (b)   (c)   (d)

Figure 62.3 ● Various techniques of lengthening of the contracted gastrocnemius muscle **(a)** include aponeurotic release at its musculotendinous junction **(b,c)** and release of the origin of the heads of the muscle from the femoral condyles **(d)**.

■ Tendo Achilles lengthening

The options for lengthening the tendo Achilles include open Z-plasty and percutaneous lengthening either by White's technique or by Hoke's technique (Figure 62.4).

The percutaneous techniques are preferred as the risk of overcorrection may be less than with open lengthening.

Contribution of spasticity and contracture

It is important to distinguish between spasticity and contracture of the gastrocsoleus before embarking on treatment. It may not be easy to make this distinction if there is severe spasticity. In such situations either a myoneural block with local anaesthetic or examination of the child under general anaesthesia may be attempted. The myoneural block or administration of general anaesthetic will abolish the spasticity and any residual equinus can then be attributed to contracture of the muscle.

Factors to be taken into consideration while planning treatment

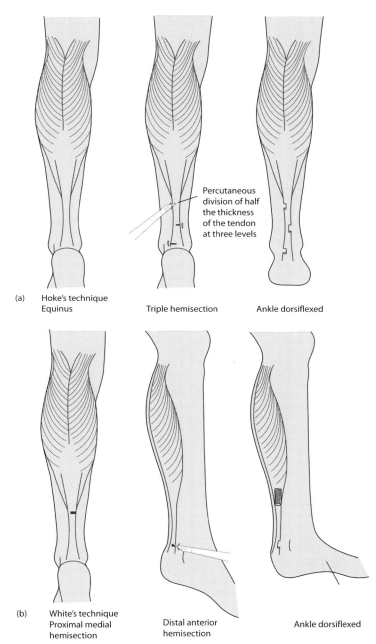

(a) Hoke's technique
Equinus

Triple hemisection

Percutaneous division of half the thickness of the tendon at three levels

Ankle dorsiflexed

(b) White's technique
Proximal medial hemisection

Distal anterior hemisection

Ankle dorsiflexed

Figure 62.4 ● Techniques of lengthening the Achilles tendon in cerebral palsy.

If an equinus contracture is present, the true extent of the contracture may be masked if the knee is flexed or if the hindfoot is free to evert. Hence, while testing for contracture of the gastrocsoleus, the knee must be held extended and the foot held in inversion.

Response to stretching and bracing

Milder degrees of spasticity will respond to non-operative methods of treatment while surgical intervention is necessary for spasticity not responsive to physiotherapy, bracing and myoneural blocks.

Presence of secondary deformities

The choice of the type of orthosis will be influenced by the presence of a genu recurvatum; a rigid orthosis moulded in mild dorsiflexion is used if there is a tendency for recurvatum while an articulated orthosis is preferred if there is no recurvatum.

Presence of associated deformities

In the presence of an associated varus or valgus deformity of the hindfoot a rigid orthosis may be preferred to an articulated orthosis.

The parts of the muscle that are contracted

In the rare situation where there is a contracture of the soleus, lengthening of the Achilles tendon will be necessary while in the majority of instances, where a gastrocnemius contracture is responsible for the equinus, release of the gastrocnemius alone should be done.

The recommended treatment for spastic equinus is shown in Table 62.1.

Recommended treatment

Table 62.1 ● Recommended treatment of spastic equinus

INDICATIONS							
Dynamic equinus	Dynamic equinus + Poor response to stretching	Dynamic equinus + Good response to tone inhibition cast	Dynamic equinus + Dynamic varus or valgus deformity + Good response to tone inhibition cast	Dynamic equinus + Genu recurvatum deformity + Good response to tone inhibition cast	Dynamic equinus + Inadequate response to tone inhibition cast and bracing	Contracture of the gastrocnemius	Contracture of the soleus and gastrocnemius
⇩	⇩	⇩	⇩	⇩	⇩	⇩	⇩
Stretching exercises	Tone inhibition cast	Articulated ankle–foot orthosis	Rigid ankle–foot orthosis with trim lines anterior to the malleoli	Rigid ankle–foot orthosis molded in 10° of dorsiflexion	Myoneural block of gastrocnemius	Gastrocnemius lengthening	Achilles tendon lengthening
TREATMENT							

Varus

Varus deformity of the foot may develop on account of spasticity or contracture of the tibialis anterior or the tibialis posterior and is often seen in association with equinus in children with hemiplegic cerebral palsy.

Problems of management

Loss of plantigrade posture

If the deformity is dynamic, the foot will be plantigrade while resting on the ground and the varus deformity will be noted only in the swing phase of gait (Figure 62.5). A dynamic varus may not interfere with walking ability but once these tendons become contracted, the foot will no longer remain plantigrade. The lateral border of the foot makes contact with the ground and a painful callosity may develop over the base of the fifth metatarsal bone. If the contracted tendons are not released, adaptive changes in the tarsal bones develop and then correction of the deformity will only be possible if bony surgery is performed in addition to the tendon release.

Aims of treatment

- Correct the varus deformity of the hindfoot and restore a plantigrade foot

Treatment options

Ankle–foot orthosis with trim lines anterior to the malleoli

A light-weight thermoplastic ankle–foot orthosis with trim lines running anterior to the malleoli can adequately control dynamic varus deformity, particularly in the young child. While this is

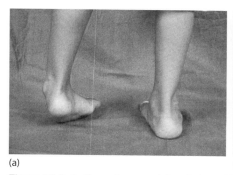 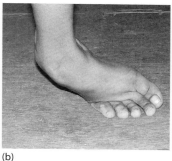 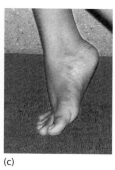

(a) (b) (c)

Figure 62.5 ● Dynamic varus deformity in a child with cerebral palsy that is evident in the swing phase of gait **(a)**. Varus deformity secondary to contracture of the invertors will be present even in the stance phase of gait **(b,c)**.

effective, it is best avoided as a long-term measure since rigid bracing of the ankle joint increases energy consumption.

An orthosis is recommended for a few months post-operatively following a tendon transfer in order to prevent the transferred tendon from stretching too much until its full strength is restored.

Myoneural block

Myoneural block of the tibialis posterior can reduce the spasticity of the muscle and thus remedy the tendency for hindfoot varus. However, it is technically difficult to inject the muscle as it is deep in the posterior compartment of the calf.

Intramuscular lengthening of the tibialis posterior

Intramuscular lengthening of the tibialis posterior tendon weakens the muscle and thus reduces the varus deformity. The tendon is divided within the substance of the muscle belly a few centimetres above the ankle.[3] This ensures that excessive lengthening of the tendon does not occur. Another important advantage of this technique of tendon lengthening is that the tendon distal to the lowest muscle fibres is left undisturbed. If a tendon transfer is needed at a later date it would be easy to perform as there will be no fibrosis or adherence of the tendon.

Split tibialis anterior transfer

If the tibialis anterior is considered to be the muscle primarily responsible for the varus deformity, the lateral half of the tendon is transferred either to the cuboid bone or to the tendon of the peroneus brevis.[4,5] This operation reduces the deforming inversion force and converts some force of the muscle into a correcting force (Figure 62.6a).

Split tibialis posterior transfer

If the tibialis posterior is considered to be the muscle at fault and if the tendency for varus persists even after intramuscular lengthening of the tibialis posterior, the lateral half of the tendon is transferred[6] to the peroneal tendon from across the back of the ankle joint (Figure 62.6b).

Transfer of the tibialis posterior

The entire tendon of the tibialis posterior can be transferred to the dorsum of the foot to correct an equinovarus deformity. However, the tendon transfer may not function at all since phase conversion is less likely to occur in cerebral palsy. There is also a risk of overcorrection.

Tenotomy of the tibialis posterior

A tenotomy may weaken the invertors too much and this can result in a valgus deformity. Tenotomy of the tibialis posterior, however, may be considered as an option in the adolescent with a recurrent, rigid varus deformity.

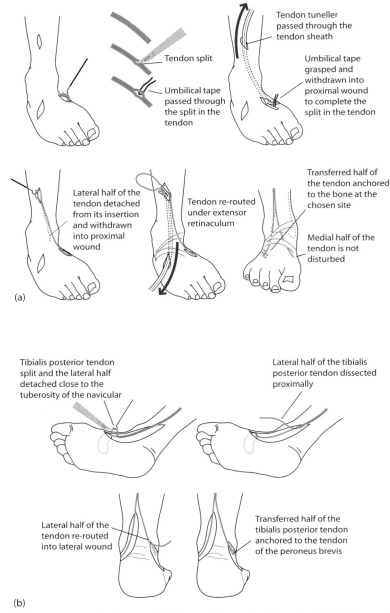

Figure 62.6 ● Technique of performing a split tibialis anterior transfer **(a)** and a split tibialis posterior transfer **(b)**.

Factors to be taken into consideration while planning treatment

Which invertor muscle is primarily at fault?

Careful assessment is needed to determine which muscle is at fault. Dynamic electromyography with fine wire electrodes could theoretically identify inappropriate activity of the tibialis posterior during the swing phase of gait. However, this facility is not available in many centres and children may find the use of needle electrodes distressing. If the tibialis posterior is at fault, the foot tends to go into plantar flexion and inversion during the swing phase and the deformity is mainly in the hindfoot. If a spastic tibialis anterior is at fault, the hindfoot and the forefoot tend to invert without appreciable plantar flexion in the swing phase.

Contribution of spasticity and contracture

Milder degrees of spasticity may be managed without surgery while surgery is necessary for severe spasticity and established contracture.

Age of the child and duration of the deformity

In the younger child adaptive bony changes will not have occurred and so surgery can be limited to the soft tissues. In older children with adaptive bony changes, soft tissue release will have to be combined with surgery on the tarsal bones in order to restore a plantigrade tread.

Recommended treatment

The treatment of spastic varus of the hindfoot is outlined in Table 62.2.

Table 62.2 ● Management of spastic varus deformity of the foot

INDICATIONS					
Mild dynamic varus + Young child	Dynamic varus + Good response to stretching exercises	Dynamic varus + Not responding to stretching and splinting	Static varus + Older child + Inversion and plantarflexion during swing phase	Static varus + Older child + NO inversion and plantarflexion during swing phase	Long-standing static varus + Adolescent + Adaptive bony changes present ⇩ Tibialis posterior release + Midtarsal osteotomy + Split tibialis anterior transfer + Protect transfer with AFO with trim lines anterior to the malleoli for 6 months
⇩ Stretching exercises	⇩ Rigid thermoplastic ankle–foot orthosis (AFO) with trim lines anterior to the malleoli	⇩ Intramuscular lengthening of tibialis posterior + Followed by: AFO with trim lines anterior to the malleoli	⇩ Split tibialis posterior transfer + Protect transfer with AFO with trim lines anterior to the malleoli for 6 months	⇩ Split tibialis anterior transfer + Protect transfer with AFO with trim lines anterior to the malleoli for 6 months	
TREATMENT					

Valgus

Valgus deformity can develop secondary to a contracture of the gastrocsoleus; this is referred to as valgus ex-equino. Spasticity of the peronei also contributes to this deformity.

Problems of management

Altered mechanics of the foot

The valgus pronated foot looks unsightly and is poorly adapted to support the weight of the body. The mechanical advantage of the calcaneal lever arm is considerably reduced and, consequently, the power of push-off is diminished.

Loss of the medial longitudinal arch

The medial longitudinal arch of the foot collapses and, in severe cases, the head of the talus is palpable in the instep. Pain may develop in this region when weight is borne on the talar head.

Concomitant deformity of the midtarsal joint

When the valgus deformity of the hindfoot develops, pronation and abduction of the forefoot occur at the midtarsal joint (Figure 62.7).

Valgus instability of the subtalar joint

In long-standing cases, even after dealing with the spastic and contracted tendons, the deformity may persist due to stretching of the capsule of the subtalar joint or to adaptive bony changes. In older children with severe involvement, ankle valgus can also develop and then treatment becomes even more difficult.

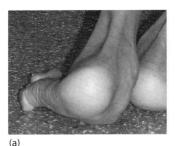 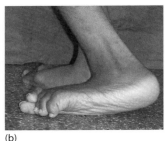

Figure 62.7 ● Spastic valgus deformity in a child with cerebral palsy. In addition to the valgus deformity of the hindfoot **(a)**, the foot is pronated and abducted at the midtarsal joint **(b)**.

(a) (b)

Associated external tibial torsion

External tibial torsion can aggravate the valgus deformity of the foot and this may also need to be addressed.

<table>
<tr><td>

Aims of treatment

</td><td>

- Correct the valgus deformity of the hindfoot along with the pronation and the forefoot abduction
- Restore the stability of the subtalar joint
- Prevent ankle valgus and adaptive bony changes in the tarsal bones

</td></tr>
</table>

Treatment options

Ankle–foot orthosis

A supple valgus deformity of the foot can be controlled in an ankle–foot orthosis with trim lines anterior to the malleoli.

Lengthening of the gastrocsoleus

If the gastrocsoleus is contracted it should be lengthened.

Lengthening of the peronei

If the peronei are spastic, intramuscular lengthening of the peroneal muscles can be performed.

Lengthening of the calcaneum

In a patient with a rigid valgus deformity, lengthening of the spastic muscle and lengthening of the calcaneum can improve the appearance of the foot. The lateral column is lengthened by inserting bone graft in the form of a wedge into the lateral aspect of an osteotomy made between the anterior and middle facets of the subtalar joint[7] (Figure 62.8a).

Extra-articular subtalar fusion

In the older child and in long-standing cases mere reduction of the spasticity may not correct the deformity even if muscle imbalance has been corrected. In such cases fusion of the subtalar joint is an option to consider (Figure 62.8b). In the skeletally immature child, an extra-articular technique of fusion is followed.[8]

Derotation osteotomy of the tibia at the supramalleolar region

If the child has associated external tibial torsion, tibial derotation osteotomy should be considered in addition to specific treatment for the valgus deformity, as outlined in Table 62.3.

Factors to be taken into consideration while planning treatment

Age of the child

In the young child bracing is likely to suffice while in the older child and the adolescent adaptive changes in the bones and the subtalar joint may make it necessary to undertake bony surgery in order to improve the alignment of the foot.

Presence of contracture of the gastrocsoleus

If the gastrocsoleus is contracted, it needs to be released, in addition to dealing with the spastic peronei.

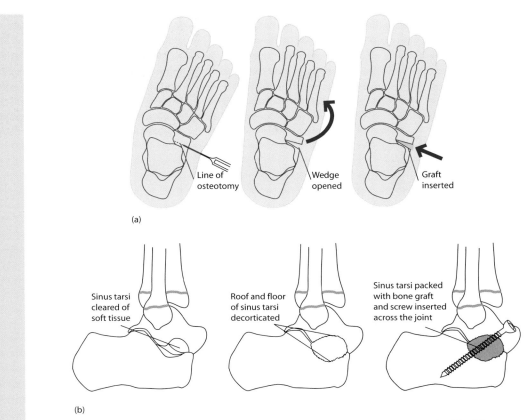

(a)

(b)

Figure 62.8 ● Technique of lengthening of the calcaneum **(a)** and fusion of the subtalar joint **(b)**.

Table 62.3 ● Management of spastic valgus deformity of the foot

INDICATIONS					
Mild dynamic valgus + Young child	Dynamic valgus + Good response to stretching exercises	Static valgus + Not responding to stretching and splinting + Demonstrable tightness of the gastrocsoleus	Static valgus + Not responding to stretching and splinting + NO tightness of the gastrocsoleus	Static valgus persisting even after lengthening of the gastrocsoleus OR the peronei + Passively correctable deformity	Long-standing static valgus + Adolescent + Adaptive bony changes present + Deformity not passively correctable
					⇩
			⇩	⇩	Triple arthrodesis + Peroneal lengthening
			Intramuscular lengthening of the peronei + Followed by: AFO with trim lines anterior to the malleoli	Extra-articular subtalar arthrodesis	
⇩	⇩	⇩			
Stretching exercises	Rigid thermoplastic AFO with trim lines anterior to the malleoli	Aponeurotic lengthening of gastrocnemius			
TREATMENT					

Persistence of the valgus after release of the tendons of the spastic or contracted muscles

If a valgus deformity persists after releasing the underlying contracture of either the peronei or the gastrocsoleus, it may indicate that structural changes have occurred in the subtalar joint or the talus and calcaneum.

Recommended treatment

The plan of treatment for spastic valgus deformity of the hindfoot is outlined in Table 62.3.

Calcaneus

A small number of older children and adolescents develop severe fixed calcaneus deformity that is usually associated with some valgus deformity both at the ankle and subtalar joints. This deformity pattern may be seen in children who have undergone excessive lengthening of the Achilles tendon.

Problems of management

Severe crouch

The main consequence of the calcaneus deformity is the severe aggravation of any pre-existing crouch to a degree that may make walking exceedingly difficult.

Inability to passively plantarflex the ankle

Initially the ankle can be passively plantarflexed; over time, the tibialis anterior becomes contracted and then the ankle cannot be passively plantarflexed.

Over-lengthened Achilles tendon

The Achilles tendon is invariably stretched. This is usually an iatrogenic problem, although it may occasionally develop in children with long-standing severe crouch in whom lengthening of the gastrocsoleus has not been done.

Aims of treatment

- Correct the calcaneus deformity
  The aim of treatment is to correct the calcaneus deformity and ensure that the tibia is perpendicular to the sole of the foot to enable the child to stand erect without any tendency to crouch.
- Prevent excessive dorsiflexion of the ankle
  Mere correction of a rigid calcaneus deformity may not improve the posture on account of muscle imbalance. In order to improve the muscle balance the ankle dorsiflexors need to be weakened.
- Restore normal length of the Achilles tendon
  The overstretched or over-lengthened Achilles tendon renders the gastrocsoleus weak and ineffective. Restoration of the length of the Achilles tendon can increase the tension of the muscle fibres and thus augment the power of plantarflexion.

Treatment options

Rear-entry floor reaction orthosis

Gage and Novacheck described a rear-entry floor reaction orthosis that prevents the ankle from dorsiflexing while permitting plantarflexion.[9] This may be attempted in children in whom the ankle can be passively plantarflexed.

Lengthening of the ankle dorsiflexors and plication of the Achilles tendon

When passive plantarflexion of the ankle is not possible owing to contracture of the ankle dorsiflexors, the tendon of the dorsiflexors can be lengthened. The Achilles tendon can be plicated simultaneously.

Tibiotalocalcaneal arthrodesis

Once the rigid deformities of the ankle and subtalar joints become severe, soft tissue procedures aimed at improving muscle balance will not succeed. At this stage tibiotalocalcaneal arthrodesis has been shown to improve the posture and gait.[10]

Factors to be taken into consideration while planning treatment

Age of the child

Arthrodesis should ideally be reserved for children who are approaching skeletal maturity in order to minimize the risk of damage to the growth plate of the distal tibia.

Presence of contracture of the dorsiflexors of the ankle

Once the dorsiflexors of the ankle are contracted, a rear-entry orthosis will not be effective.

Presence of ankle valgus

If the deformity has been present long enough for secondary changes in the ankle to also develop, soft tissue procedures will not correct the deformity.

Recommended treatment

The outline of treatment of calcaneus deformity is shown in Table 62.4.

Table 62.4 ● Treatment of spastic calcaneus deformity

INDICATIONS		
Passively correctable deformity + Young child	Deformity not passively correctable (demonstrable contracture of the dorsiflexors of the ankle) + No ankle valgus + Skeletally immature	Deformity not passively correctable (demonstrable contracture of the dorsiflexors of the ankle) + Ankle valgus present + Skeletally mature ⇩
⇩	⇩	Tibiotalocalcaneal arthrodesis
Gage's rear-entry floor reaction orthosis	Lengthening of the tendons of the ankle dorsiflexors + Plication of the Achilles tendon + Gage's rear-entry floor reaction orthosis	
TREATMENT		

References

1. Watt J, Sims D, Harckham F *et al.* A prospective study of inhibitive casting as an adjunct to physiotherapy for cerebral-palsied children. *Dev Med Child Neurol* 1986; **28**: 480–88.
2. Rosenthal RK, Deutsch SD, Miller W, Schumann W, Hall JE. A fixed-ankle, below-the-knee orthosis for management of genu recurvatum in spastic cerebral palsy. *J Bone Joint Surg Am* 1975; 57: 545–7.
3. Majestro TC, Ruda R, Frost HM. Intramuscular lengthening of the posterior tibialis muscle. *Clin Orthop Relat Res* 1971; **79**: 59–60.
4. Hoffer MM. Reiswig JA, Garett AM, Perry J. The split anterior tibial tendon transfer in the treatment of spastic varus hindfoot of childhood. *Orthop Clin North Am* 1974; **5**: 31–8.
5. Barnes MJ, Herring JA. Combined split anterior tibial tendon transfer and intramuscular lengthening of the posterior tibial tendon. Results in patients who have a varus deformity of the foot due to spastic cerebral palsy. *J Bone Joint Surg Am* 1991; **73**: 734–8.
6. Kling TF Jr, Kaufer H, Hensinger RN. Split posterior tibial-tendon transfers in children with cerebral spastic paralysis and equinovarus deformity. *J Bone Joint Surg Am* 1985; **67**: 186–94.
7. Noritake K, Yoshihashi Y, Miyata T. Calcaneal lengthening for planovalgus foot deformity in children with spastic cerebral palsy *J Pediatr Orthop B* 2005; **14**: 274–9.
8. Alman BA, Craig CL, Zimbler S. Subtalar arthrodesis for stabilization of the valgus hindfoot in patients with cerebral palsy. *J Pediatr Orthop* 1993; **13**: 634–41.
9. Gage JR, Novacheck TF. An update on the treatment of gait problems in cerebral palsy. *J Pediatr Orthop* 2001; **10**: 265–74.
10. Muir D, Angliss RD, Nattrass GR, Graham HK. Tibiotalocalcaneal arthrodesis for severe calcaneovalgus deformity in cerebral palsy. *J Pediatr Orthop* 2005; **25**: 651–6.

The spastic knee

Benjamin Joseph

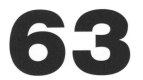

Introduction

Common problems at the knee in children with cerebral palsy include flexion deformity, recurvatum and a stiff-knee gait.

Flexion deformity of the knee

Flexion of the knee while standing and a crouch gait may develop owing to problems at the knee itself or they can develop secondarily because of problems at the hip or the ankle. Spasticity or contracture of the hamstrings are the most common causes of crouch, but crouch may also be secondary to flexion of the hip, quadriceps inefficiency or a calcaneus deformity of the ankle. Apart from being unsightly, crouch gait results in very high energy expenditure when walking.[1]

Problems of management

Hamstring spasticity or contracture

Hamstring spasticity commonly manifests when the child is around seven years of age and unless regular stretching is practised the hamstrings are prone to develop a contracture quite rapidly.

Quadriceps weakness

Spasticity of the hamstrings creates a tendency to stand with the knee flexed (Figure 63.1). Unless the quadriceps muscle power is adequate to counteract this tendency, a crouch gait will ensue. Whenever the hamstrings are contracted the quadriceps muscle is weak. Once the hamstring contracture is released, the quadriceps power can increase with appropriate strengthening exercises, provided the patellar tendon has not been overstretched.

Lengthening of the patellar tendon and patella alta

In children with long-standing flexion deformity the ligamentum patellae becomes stretched and patella alta develops (Figure 63.2). In these children the crouch will persist even after releasing the hamstrings. The quadriceps muscle will be incapable of extending the knee fully as the quadriceps mechanism is ineffective due to the elongated patellar tendon.

Flexion deformity

If the crouch gait persists a fixed flexion deformity of the knee can develop and over a period of time the deformity, if uncorrected, can become severe.

Aims of treatment

- Reduce hamstring spasticity and contracture
  The overactive spastic hamstrings need to be weakened sufficiently to restore muscle balance between the flexors and extensors of the knee.
- Restore the power of knee extension
  The power of the quadriceps must be augmented sufficiently to ensure that the muscle is capable of stabilizing the knee in extension during the stance phase of gait.
- Correct the flexion deformity
  Even minor degrees of flexion deformity need to be corrected in order to enable the child to stand straight.

Treatment options

Physiotherapy (hamstring stretching and quadriceps strengthening)

If the crouch gait is due to spasticity of the hamstrings without demonstrable contracture, quadriceps strengthening exercises and hamstring stretching should be done regularly.

Myoneural block of hamstring muscles

Physiotherapy may be supplemented with a myoneural block of the hamstrings if there is no contracture. These measures can help to delay surgical intervention.

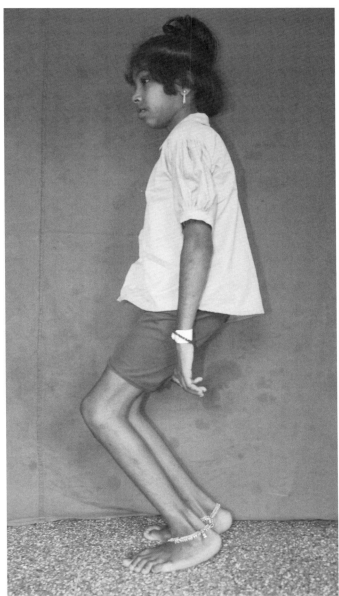

Figure 63.1 ● Hamstring spasticity results in a crouch posture and flexion deformity of the knee.

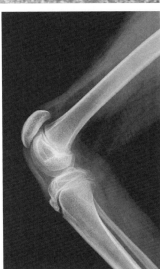

Figure 63.2 ● Lateral radiograph of the knee of a child with cerebral palsy and long-standing crouch. The patella alta is clearly seen.

Floor-reaction orthosis

A floor–reaction orthosis produces a backward thrust onto the front of the proximal tibia when the child bears weight. This orthosis is useful when crouch persists after adequate release of the hamstrings (Figure 63.3).

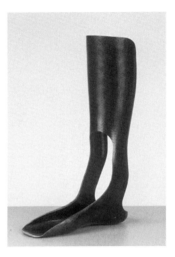

Figure 63.3 ● A floor-reaction orthosis used to treat crouch. Courtesy of Professor Kerr Graham, Melbourne, Australia.

Hamstring release

Once the hamstrings are contracted they need to be released. The most widely recommended method of hamstring release is the fractional lengthening technique.[2] The technique entails aponeurotic lengthening of the semimembranosus and biceps femoris and Z-plasty of the semitendinosus.

Hamstring transfer

Two methods of hamstring transfer have been employed. The rationale of both these transfers is to convert the transferred tendons from flexors of the knee to extensors of the hip. As the transferred muscle extends the hip the femur is pulled backwards and this in turn extends the knee (Figure 63.4).

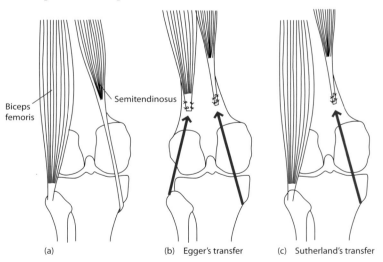

Biceps femoris

Semitendinosus

(a) (b) Egger's transfer (c) Sutherland's transfer

Figure 63.4 ● Egger's transfer of the hamstrings **(b)** and Sutherland's transfer of the semitendinosus to the back of the femur **(c)**.

■ Egger's transfer

Egger recommended transfer of the medial and lateral hamstrings into the back of the distal femur. This operation is currently not favoured because of an unacceptable frequency of genu recurvatum developing after surgery.[3]

■ Sutherland's transfer

Sutherland's transfer is based on the same principle as Egger's transfer but only the semitendinosus is transferred to the back of the femur. Sutherlands's transfer is preferred as it has a lower risk of producing a recurvatum since only one tendon is transferred to the femur rather than two as in the operation described by Egger.

Correcting the flexion deformity

In long-standing cases with a fixed flexion deformity, release of the hamstrings alone will not suffice to correct the deformity. In such instances a femoral supracondylar extension osteotomy may be needed. If the flexion deformity is severe, some shortening of the femur may reduce the risk of sciatic nerve stretch.

Correcting patella alta

The two options for correcting patella alta are plication of the patellar tendon and distal transfer of the tibial tuberosity (Figure 63.5).

■ Plication of the patellar tendon

Plication of the patellar tendon is the preferred option in the skeletally immature child.

■ Distal transfer of the tibial tuberosity

In the skeletally mature child the tibial tuberosity can be shifted distally. The transplanted tuberosity must be fixed securely to avoid the spastic muscle from pulling the fragment free.

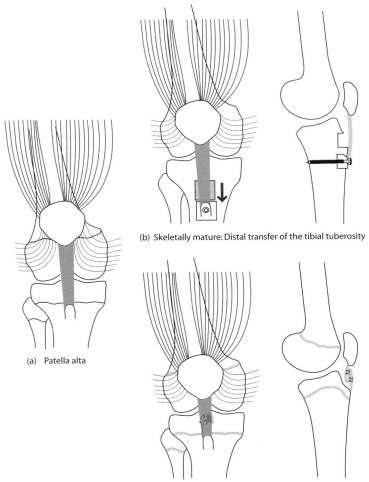

(a) Patella alta

(b) Skeletally mature: Distal transfer of the tibial tuberosity

(c) Skeletally immature: Plication of the patellar tendon

Figure 63.5 ● The techniques of correcting patella alta **(a)** are distal transfer of tibial tuberosity along with the insertion of the tendon **(b)** and plication of the patellar tendon **(c)**.

Correcting flexion deformity of the hip

Since a child with spastic flexion deformity of the hip will tend to stand with the hips and knees flexed it is important to correct both the hip and knee deformity in order to ensure that the knee remains straight.

Correcting the calcaneus deformity of the ankle

A calcaneus deformity can compound a crouch posture, and even after addressing the knee deformity the child will continue to crouch unless the ankle dorsiflexion is addressed. (The options for dealing with calcaneus are shown in Table 62.4 of Chapter 62, The spastic foot and ankle.)

Age of the child

The degree of deformity and the extent of adaptive changes like patella alta increase with age and hence the approach will have to be more aggressive in the older child and the adolescent.

Presence of contracture of the hamstrings

If the hamstrings are spastic and no contracture of the muscle is present, non-operative methods of treatment may be adopted. However, once there is demonstrable contracture of the hamstrings, surgical intervention is need.

Power of the quadriceps

If the quadriceps muscle is weak, the power of knee extension will need to be augmented by a tendon transfer.

Presence of fixed flexion deformity of the knee and the severity of the deformity

In more long-standing cases fixed flexion deformity will need to be addressed. If the flexion deformity is severe, shortening of the femur should be performed to minimize the risk of sciatic nerve damage.

Presence of patella alta

If patella alta is present, it must be corrected to enable the quadriceps to effectively extend the knee.

The recommended treatment outline for dealing with spastic crouch gait is shown in Table 63.1.

Factors to be taken into consideration while planning treatment

Recommended treatment for spastic flexion deformity of the knee

Genu recurvatum

Genu recurvatum may develop in children with spasticity or contracture of the gastrocsoleus, or after surgery for crouch gait.

If the gastrocsoleus is spastic and the ankle can be dorsiflexed passively beyond neutral, the genu recurvatum can be controlled effectively by using an ankle-foot orthosis that has been suitably modified. A flexor moment at the knee can be created by holding the ankle in 10° of dorsiflexion in an orthosis that has been moulded in this position. The other way to create a flexor moment at the knee is to fix a heel on an ankle-foot orthosis that has been moulded with the ankle in neutral position (Figure 63.6). If there is a contracture of the gastrocsoleus, lengthening of the gastrocnemius or the tendo Achilles should be undertaken to prevent the genu recurvatum from progressing.

Stiff-knee gait

Stiff-knee gait is characterized by decreased sagittal plane movement of the knee during the swing phase. To clear the ground the child either circumducts the limb or vaults on the opposite leg. The cause of this particular gait abnormality is co-spasticity of the rectus femoris and the hamstrings.[4] On the basis of the information gleaned from gait analysis, Perry[4] recommended transferring the distal end of the rectus femoris muscle posterior to the axis of knee motion. The rectus femoris is detached close to its insertion into the patella and is transferred either medially to the semitendinosus or laterally to the iliotibial band (Figure 63.7). This procedure has been shown to increase knee flexion during swing.[5]

Table 63.1 ● The outline of treatment of spastic flexion deformity of the knee and crouch gait

INDICATION

Young child + Crouch gait + No fixed deformity + Spastic hamstrings + Strong quadriceps	Young child + Crouch gait persisting despite stetching + No fixed deformity + Spastic hamstrings + Strong quadriceps	Older child + Crouch gait + No fixed deformity + Hamstring spasticity or contracture + Weak quadriceps	Adolescent + Crouch gait + Flexion deformity (moderate/mild) + Hamstring contracture + Weak quadriceps	Adolescent + Crouch gait + Flexion deformity (severe) + Hamstring contracture + Weak quadriceps	Adolescent + Crouch gait + Flexion deformity (severe) + Hamstring contracture + Patella alta	Adolescent + Crouch gait + No fixed flexion deformity of the knee + Calcaneus deformity of the ankle	Persistent crouch gait after release or transfer of hamstrings + No fixed flexion deformity of the knee + Weak quadriceps
⇩	⇩	⇩	⇩	⇩	⇩	⇩	⇩
Hamstring stretching + Quadriceps strengthening	Myoneural block to hamstrings + Quadriceps strengthening	Sutherland's transfer + Quadriceps strengthening	Femoral supracondylar osteotomy + Sutherland's transfer and quadriceps strengthening	Femoral shortening + Sutherland's transfer and quadriceps strengthening	Femoral shortening + Sutherland's transfer and quadriceps strengthening + Patellar tendon plication	Treat as outlined in Chapter 62 (Table 62.4)	Floor-reaction orthosis

TREATMENT

Whenever the Sutherland transfer is performed, fractional lengthening of the aponeurosis of the semimembranosus and biceps femoris is also done.

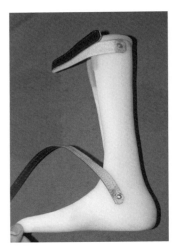

Figure 63.6 ● An AFO that is moulded in 10° of dorsiflexion can control genu recurratum.

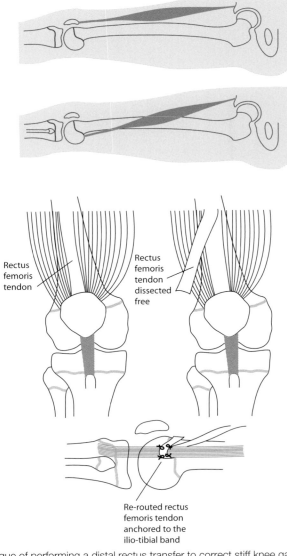

Rectus femoris tendon

Rectus femoris tendon dissected free

Re-routed rectus femoris tendon anchored to the ilio-tibial band

Figure 63.7 ● Technique of performing a distal rectus transfer to correct stiff knee gait.

References

1. Raja K, Joseph B, Benjamin S, Minocha V, Rana B. Physiological cost index in cerebral palsy. Its use as an outcome measure of the efficiency of ambulation. *J Pediatr Orthop* 2007; **27**: 130–6.

2. Green WT, McDermott LJ. Operative treatment of cerebral palsy of the spastic type. *JAMA* 1942; **118**: 434–40.

3. Evans EB, Julian JD. Modifications of the hamstring transfer. *Dev Med Child Neurol* 1966; **8**: 539–51.

4. Perry J. Distal rectus transfer. *Dev Med Child Neurol* 1987; **29**: 153–8.

5. Gage JR, Perry J, Hicks RR, Koop S, Werntz JR. Rectus femoris transfer to improve knee function in children with cerebral palsy. *Dev Med Child Neurol* 1987; **29**: 159–66.

The spastic hip

Benjamin Joseph

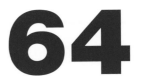

Common problems of the hip in cerebral palsy include adduction deformity, flexion deformity, internal rotation gait and hip subluxation and dislocation. Although these problems may occur in combination, each problem will be discussed separately for the sake of simplicity. Hip dislocation in cerebral palsy is discussed elsewhere in the book (Chapter 25, Paralytic hip dislocation: cerebral palsy).

Adduction deformity

A spastic adduction deformity of the hip may be dynamic due to spasticity of the muscles that adduct the hip (the adductor muscles and the gracilis muscle) or there may be a true contracture of these muscles. It is important to differentiate between spasticity and contracture and treatment should be planned accordingly. Although this differentiation can often be made by careful clinical examination, sometimes it may be difficult to do so if the spasticity is severe. In such situations the child may be examined under anaesthesia, when spasticity will be overcome and any limitation of passive hip abduction can be attributed to a contracture of the adductors. When testing for adduction contracture the hips and knees should be held in extension.

Problems of management

Scissor gait

Spasticity of adductors of the hip results in a characteristic scissoring gait pattern with the limbs crossing the line of progression. This gait pattern is both unsightly and energy inefficient.

Tendency for hip subluxation and dislocation

Adductor spasticity and contracture predispose to hip subluxation and dislocation (see Chapter 25, Paralytic hip dislocation: cerebral palsy).

Interference with perineal hygiene

When contracture of the adductors becomes severe, separation of the thighs sufficiently for proper perineal hygiene becomes impossible. This degree of contracture is usually encountered in severely disabled children with total body involvement who are non-walkers.

Recurrence of deformity

Despite adequate initial treatment there is a tendency for the adduction deformity to recur in about 10 percent of patients.[1] This tendency can persist until skeletal maturity and hence it is important that measures are taken to minimize the risk of recurrence and to detect early recurrence as soon as it manifests.

Overcorrection of deformity

Overzealous weakening of the adductors can have very serious consequences if the abductor muscles are strong. The hips may go into wide abduction making it difficult to walk or to sit in a wheelchair.[2]

Aims of treatment

- Correct the scissor gait in ambulant children
  Overcoming scissoring of the hips will improve the appearance and the efficiency of gait by reducing energy consumption.
- Facilitate perineal hygiene
  Restoring passive abduction of the hips will achieve this aim. This alone may be of great help to the care giver of a totally dependent child.
- Prevent or correct hip subluxation
  Reducing adductor spasticity before the hip has begun to subluxate may prevent this complication. Once subluxation has occurred, prompt measures to reduce spasticity of the adductors may help to prevent the subluxated hip from dislocating.[3] If the range of passive abduction of the hip is less than 30°, the hip is at risk for subluxation. Children in whom this degree of restriction of abduction is noted should have a radiograph of the pelvis to see if early

subluxation is present (Figure 64.1). It is recommended that all children with cerebral palsy are screened for impending hip instability on a regular basis since early detection of instability can minimize the extent of surgery for these children.[4]

- Avoid overcorrection

  It is important to choose interventions that have little risk of overcorrection as the consequences of overcorrection can be disastrous.

- Minimize the risk of recurrence

  Adequate physiotherapy and maintenance of appropriate posture can reduce the risk of recurrence of adduction contracture following surgery and hence the need for such measures cannot be overemphasized.

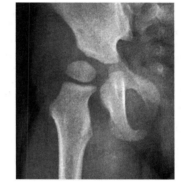

Figure 64.1 ● Radiograph of the pelvis of a child with cerebral palsy showing early subluxation of the hip. The Shenton's line is broken, the medial joint space is increased and there is uncovering of the femoral head.

Treatment options for dealing with adduction deformity and scissoring

Stretching exercises and modification of sitting and lying posture

This is the mainstay of treatment for the vast majority of young children with adductor spasticity. A daily regimen of passive slow stretching of the adductors is instituted. Care is taken to ensure that the hips of non-ambulant children are kept abducted with the help of padded blocks or cushions while the child sits and lies.

Myoneural blocks

Local anaesthetics, 40 percent alcohol, phenol or botulinum toxin may be used. Local anaesthetic action is very short-lived and hence it is not useful as a definitive measure of reducing adductor spasticity. However, local anaesthetics may be used to enable the clinician to evaluate the effect of a more long-lasting agent. The effects of alcohol and botulinum toxin last for six to nine months.

Adductor tenotomy

This operation entails release of the adductor longus and the gracilis muscles from their respective origins from the pubic bone. If the adduction contracture is severe, some fibres of the adductor brevis may also have to be released.

Adductor tenotomy and obturator neurectomy

In the past, obturator neurectomy was routinely performed in conjunction with release of the adductors. However, since this may weaken the adductors excessively, an obturator neurectomy is currently reserved for recurrences and if the hip abductors are very weak.

Adductor transfer

The adductor muscles are erased from their origin on the pubic bone and transferred more posteriorly onto the ischium. The rationale of the operation is to abolish the adductor action and enhance the hip extensor power. The procedure is more extensive and more complicated than the simple adductor release and the results have not been superior to the adductor release.[5,6]

Factors to be taken into consideration while treating adduction deformity

Spasticity or contracture

The first and foremost issue is to differentiate between spasticity and contracture of the adductor muscles.

If a contracture is present, surgery is indicated, whereas the initial treatment of spastic adductors is essentially non-operative.

Response to non-operative measures

If there is poor response to non-operative measures, spastic adductors will have to be weakened by surgery.

Stability of the hip

If there is radiological evidence of hip subluxation (with an increased medial joint space, a break in Shenton's line and excessive uncovering of the femoral head) surgery is required irrespective of whether or not there is contracture of the adductors (Figure 64.1).

Power of the abductor muscles

If surgery is being contemplated, a careful assessment of hip abductor power should be done. If the abductor power is grade III or greater (MRC) then an obturator neurectomy should be avoided.

Ambulatory status of the child

The posture of the non-ambulant child can contribute to recurrence of an adduction deformity and attention must be paid to ensuring an optimal posture following surgery. The consequences of overcorrection of an adduction deformity are most serious in the ambulant child and hence greater care needs to be exercised while deciding upon treatment in these children.

Recommended treatment and its rationale

The recommended treatment plan for dealing with adduction deformity is shown in Table 64.1.

If the adduction deformity is dynamic with no true contracture of the muscles, physiotherapy to stretch the adductors should be rigorously practised. In children demonstrating a lot of spasticity, myoneural block of the adductors will supplement the physiotherapy. When seated, a wedge should be placed between the thighs to keep the hips abducted. If the response to these measures is poor, it is necessary to surgically weaken the adductors.

Among the surgical options listed, adductor tenotomy alone should suffice in most instances. Obturator neurectomy is best avoided due to the risk of weakening the adductors too much and producing an abduction deformity. As the results of transferring the adductors to the ischium are no better than that of adductor release, the additional surgery is not warranted.

It needs to be emphasized that, irrespective of the treatment adopted, physiotherapy needs to be continued regularly in order to avoid an early recurrence of adduction deformity.

Flexion deformity

Flexion deformity of the hip results in a lordotic posture and secondary knee flexion while walking. It also increases the risk of hip instability. Flexion deformity develops on account of either spasticity or contracture of the iliopsoas or the rectus femoris. It is important to ensure that the flexion at the hip that may be seen while the child is standing is not a compensatory mechanism for a flexed knee. If the child can kneel without excessive lumbar lordosis the hips flexors are not at fault.

Problems of management

Abnormal posture and gait

Children who develop a flexion deformity of the hip either walk with hip flexion and compensatory knee flexion or with the knee straight and compensatory lumbar lordosis. Both these postures are undesirable.

Tendency for hip instability

Hip flexion deformity predisposes to hip subluxation and dislocation.

Excessive weakening of the hip flexor

It is important to be aware that excessive weakening of the hip flexors can hamper forward propulsion of the limb during the initial part of the swing phase of gait. This needs to be avoided when undertaking surgery to treat spastic hip flexion.

Table 64.1 ● Outline of treatment of spastic adduction deformity

INDICATION						
Dynamic deformity (no contracture)	Dynamic deformity (no contracture) + Poor response to stretching exercises	Dynamic deformity (no contracture) + Poor response to stretching exercises AND myoneural block OR Hip subluxation	Adduction contracture in non-ambulant child (sitter) + Interference with personal hygiene OR Impending hip subluxation (passive hip abduction <30°) OR Hip subluxation	Adduction contracture in non-ambulant child (bed ridden) + Interference with personal hygiene OR Impending hip subluxation (passive hip abduction <30°) OR Hip subluxation	Ambulant child + Scissor gait OR Impending hip subluxation (passive hip abduction <30°) OR Hip subluxation + grade III or more hip abductor muscle power	Ambulant child + Scissor gait OR Impending hip subluxation (passive hip abduction <30°) OR Hip subluxation + Hip abductor muscle power <grade III
⇩	⇩	⇩	⇩	⇩	⇩	⇩
Stretching exercises	Myoneural block	Adductor tenotomy	Adductor tenotomy + Seating modification with hips abducted	Adductor tenotomy + Pillow between thighs to keep hips abducted	Adductor tenotomy	Adductor tenotomy + Anterior obturator neurectomy
TREATMENT						

Aims of treatment

- In the ambulant child the aim is to overcome the flexion deformity of the hip without excessively weakening the hip flexor power
- In the non-ambulant child the aim is to correct the flexion deformity and thereby reduce the risk of hip instability

Treatment options for dealing with spastic hip flexion deformity

Stretching exercises

Stretching of the hip flexors may be effective in reducing spasticity and preventing a contracture in young children.

Myoneural blocks

Although injecting the iliopsoas is technically difficult, methods have been described to facilitate injection of the muscle as a measure of reducing its spasticity.[7]

Iliopsoas tenotomy

Division of the iliopsoas tendon close to its insertion into the lesser trochanter is fraught with the risk of weakening the power of hip flexion too much, although it effectively relieves a contracture of this muscle.

This is of importance in the ambulant child but of less relevance in the non-ambulant child. On the contrary, if there is associated hip dislocation in the non-ambulant child, it may be desirable to divide the tendon at its insertion and transfer it to the greater trochanter. This may improve the muscle balance and thus facilitate a more stable reduction of the unstable hip (see Chapter 25, Paralytic hip dislocation: cerebral palsy).

Intramuscular release of psoas at the pelvic brim

Release of the psoas tendon at the brim of the pelvis avoids disturbing the iliacus and will ensure that sufficient hip flexor power is retained.[8]

Rectus femoris release

If the Duncan-Ely test confirms contracture of the rectus femoris it should be released. In the ambulant child, if the spastic rectus femoris is also causing a stiff-knee gait the muscle can be released distally and transferred (see Chapter 63, The spastic knee). In the non-ambulant child the rectus femoris may be released from its proximal attachment to the anterior inferior iliac spine along with the release of the iliopsoas.

Factors to be taken into consideration while treating spastic hip flexion deformity

Ambulatory status of the child

In an ambulant child the flexion deformity needs to be corrected without compromising the hip flexor power too much, while this is not a consideration in the non-ambulant child. In the non-ambulant child the flexion deformity is often seen in association with an adduction deformity; in this case the iliopsoas can be released from the lesser trochanter through the medial incision made for the adductor release.

Presence of associated deformities at the knee

If in addition to the hip flexion deformity there is a hamstring contracture in an ambulant child, the deformities at the hip and knee need to be corrected simultaneously or else the child will continue to stand with the hip and knee flexed. As mentioned earlier, if the rectus femoris is contributing to the hip flexion deformity, the site of release of the rectus will depend on whether the rectus is producing a stiff-knee gait.

Stability of the hip

If release of the hip flexion contracture is part of the procedure to reduce a spastic hip dislocation, the options for dealing with the iliopsoas tendon include tenotomy and transfer.

Recommended treatment for spastic hip flexion deformity

The outline of treatment of spastic hip flexion deformity is shown in Table 64.2.

Table 64.2 ● The outline of treatment of spastic hip flexion deformity

INDICATIONS					
Ambulant child + Iliopsoas contracture (no rectus contracture)	Ambulant child + Iliopsoas contracture + Rectus femoris contracture + Stiff-knee gait	Ambulant child + Iliopsoas contracture + Rectus femoris contracture + Hamstring contracture	Non-ambulant child + Iliopsoas contracture + Rectus femoris contracture	Non-ambulant child + Iliopsoas contracture + Adductor contracture	Non-ambulant child + Iliopsoas contracture + Hip dislocation
⇩	⇩	⇩	⇩	⇩	⇩
Intramuscular release of the psoas tendon at the pelvic brim	Intramuscular release of the psoas tendon at the pelvic brim + Distal rectus transfer	Intramuscular release of the psoas tendon at the pelvic brim + Distal rectus transfer + Hamstring release	Intramuscular release of the psoas tendon at the pelvic brim + Proximal rectus release (single incision)	Iliopsoas release from lesser trochanter + Adductor release (single incision)	Iliopsoas release from lesser trochanter + Adductor release + Iliopsoas transfer to greater trochanter
TREATMENT					

Internal rotation gait

Internal rotation gait is quite common in children with cerebral palsy. Mild degrees of internal rotation gait may be of little consequence but more severe degrees of internal rotation gait can be both awkward and energy inefficient. Among the causes for an internal rotation gait are excessive femoral anteversion, spasticity of the medial hamstrings and spasticity of the internal rotators of the hip.

Aim of treatment

- The aim of treatment is to restore a normal foot-progression angle without producing weakness of the abductors of the hip

Treatment options for internal rotation gait

Femoral derotation osteotomy

If the internal rotation is due to femoral anteversion, derotation osteotomy of the femur with internal fixation is recommended after the child is at least eight years old. The site most commonly chosen for performing the derotation osteotomy is the proximal femur. This site permits the use of strong internal fixation devices that will allow early ambulation. However, the derotation can also be performed at the supracondylar level.

Medial hamstring release

Since spasticity or contracture of the medial hamstrings can contribute to an internal rotation gait, it is important that contracted hamstrings are released to see whether the internal rotation gait improves before considering a derotation osteotomy.

Anterior and medial transfer of gluteus medius

Steel demonstrated a clinical sign to identify spasticity of the anterior fibres of the gluteus medius and minimus.[9] He recommended anterior and medial transfer of the insertion of the gluteus medius (Figure 64.2). While the internal rotation gait improved in most of these patients, a quarter of them developed a Trendelenburg gait. Since a Trendelenburg gait is unacceptable, this operation cannot be recommended.

Selective internal rotator release

An operation to selectively weaken the internal rotator power without interfering with the abductor power has been described.[10] The advantage of this procedure is that the abductor power is not affected as only the internal rotator fibres of the gluteus medius are transferred posteriorly at their origin, while the pure abductor fibres remain untouched (Figure 64.3).

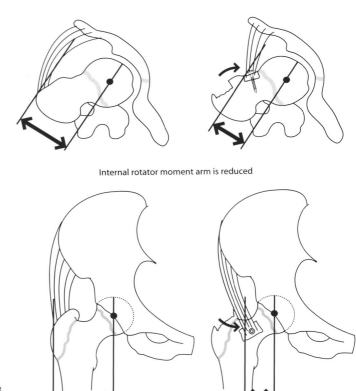

Internal rotator moment arm is reduced

Abductor moment arm is also reduced

Figure 64.2 ● Technique of medial transfer of the insertion of gluteus medius and minimus. The abductor moment arm is reduced quite markedly.

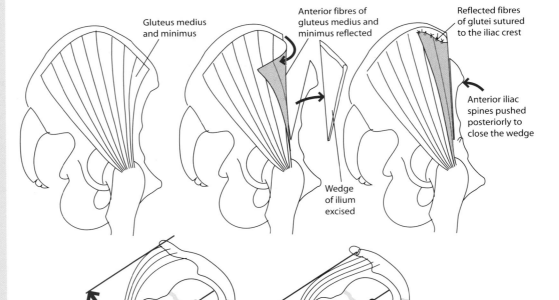

Gluteus medius and minimus

Anterior fibres of gluteus medius and minimus reflected

Reflected fibres of glutei sutured to the iliac crest

Wedge of ilium excised

Anterior iliac spines pushed posteriorly to close the wedge

Internal rotator moment arm is reduced but abductor moment is not altered

Figure 64.3 ● Technique of performing release of the origin of the internal rotator fibres of the gluteus medius and minimus. The internal rotator moment is reduced but the abductor fibers are not disturbed.

Recommended treatment

The treatment of internal rotation gait is outlined in Table 64.3.

Table 64.3 ● Outline of treatment of internal rotation gait in cerebral palsy

INDICATIONS		
Internal rotation gait + Medial hamstring contracture	Internal rotation gait + Steel's test positive + No hamstring tightness OR No improvement of gait after hamstring release ⇩	Internal rotation gait + Steel's test negative + No hamstring tightness ⇩
⇩	Selective internal rotator release	Femoral derotation osteotomy at the intertrochanteric or the subtrochanteric level with rigid internal fixation
Hamstring release		
TREATMENT		

References

1. Samilson RL, Carson JJ, James P, Raney FL Jr. Results and complications of adductor tenotomy and obturator neurectomy in cerebral palsy. *Clin Orthop Relat Res* 1967; **54**: 61–73.
2. Pollock GA. Treatment of adductor paralysis by hamstring transposition. *J Bone Joint Surg Br* 1958; **40**: 534–7.
3. Presedo A, Oh CW, Dabney KW, Miller F. Soft tissue releases to treat spastic hip subluxation in children with cerebral palsy. *J Bone Joint Surg Am* 2005; **87**: 832–41.
4. Dobson F, Boyd RN, Parrott J, Nattrass GR, Graham HK. Hip surveillance in children with cerebral palsy. *J Bone Joint Surg Br* 2002; **84**: 720–26.
5. Terjesen T, Lie GD, Hyldmo AA, Knaus A. Adductor tenotomy in spastic cerebral palsy. A long-term follow-up study of 78 patients. Acta Orthop 2005; **76**: 128–37.
6. Reamers J, Poulson S. Adductor transfer versus tenotomy for stability of the hip in spastic cerebral palsy. *J Pediatr Orthop* 1984; **4**: 52–4.
7. Willenborg MJ, Shilt JS, Smith BP *et al.* Technique of ultrasound-guided eletromygraphy-directed boulinum a toxin injection in cerebral palsy. *J Pediatr Orthop* 2002; **22**: 165–8.
8. Bleck EE. Surgical management of spastic hip flexion gait patterns with special reference to iliopsoas recession. *J Bone Joint Surg Am* 1970; **52**: 829–30.
9. Steel HH. Gluteus medius and minimus insertion advancement for correction of internal rotation gait in spastic cerebral palsy. *J Bone Joint Surg Am* 1980; **62**: 919–27.
10. Joseph B. Treatment of internal rotation gait due to gluteus medius and minimus overactivity in cerebral palsy: Anatomical rationale of a new surgical procedure and preliminary results in twelve hips. *Clin Anat* 1998; **11**: 22–8.

The spastic forearm and hand

Benjamin Joseph

Introduction

The upper limb is affected predominantly in children with cerebral palsy who have a hemiplegic pattern of topographical involvement and in children with quadriplegic or total body involvement. Subtle involvement of the upper limb may occur in a diplegic pattern of cerebral palsy but intervention in this case is not necessary.

Although it would be desirable to improve the function of the hand in all children with upper limb involvement, this may not be possible in several instances and it is important to identify the children in whom functional improvement may not occur following intervention. Despite the poor chance of functional improvement, surgical intervention may still be justified in order to achieve a less impressive aim. The anticipated benefit of surgery must be clearly explained to the parents of the child before embarking on surgery.

Although the thumb is often affected in conjunction with the forearm and hand, the approach to management of the thumb will be dealt with in Chapter 66, The spastic thumb.

Problems of management

Spasticity and contracture of the pronators of the forearm and flexors of the wrist and fingers

The muscles in the forearm that demonstrate most spasticity are the pronators of the forearm and the flexors of the wrist and fingers. In some children all these muscles may be spastic, in others the forearm pronators are spastic while the flexors are less spastic and in some children the flexors are overactive while the pronators are not. Depending on which muscles are spastic, the corresponding deformities of the forearm will be seen (Figure 65.1).

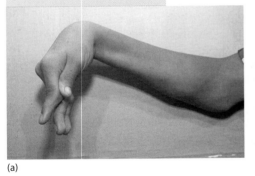 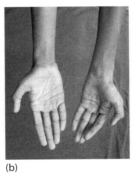 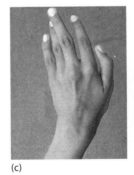 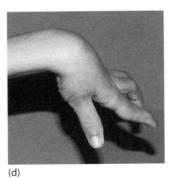

(a) (b) (c) (d)

Figure 65.1 ● Common deformities of the forearm and wrist seen in cerebral palsy include pronation with limited active supination **(a,b)**, ulnar deviation **(c)** and flexion of the wrist **(d)**.

Weakness of supination and wrist extension

The antagonistic muscles are weak and even if no pronation or flexion contracture is present the child may have demonstrable weakness of active forearm supination and wrist extension.

Weak grasp

As a consequence of the muscle imbalance, most children with upper limb involvement demonstrate weakness of grasp which can vary from total inability to grasp an object to mild reduction of grip strength.

Poor release

Some children have weakness of finger extension and in these children the release is compromised. This inability of release may only be demonstrable when the wrist is passively held in extension. It is extremely important to test for the ability to release in this position if any surgery aimed at augmenting wrist extensor power is being contemplated (Figure 65.2).

Unacceptable appearance

Apart from the compromised function of the hand, a flexed wrist and hand is quite unsightly.

Problems with hygiene and clothing

In children with severe involvement and no useful hand function at all, there may be severe contractures of the fingers to such a degree that the palm cannot be cleaned.

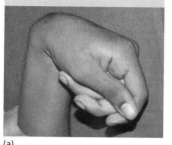
(a)
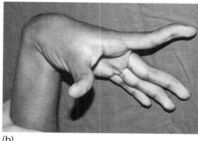
(b)
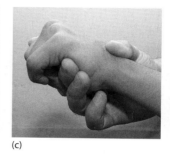
(c)
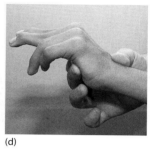
(d)

Figure 65.2 ● If a tendon transfer aimed at improving the power of wrist extension is being planned for a child with poor hand function **(a,b)** the improvement in the grasp **(c)** and the ability to release should be tested with the wrist held passively in extension **(d)**.

Aims of treatment

- To improve function of the hand by improving the power of grasp and at the same time ensuring ease of release

  It may never be feasible to achieve fine prehensile hand function in children with cerebral palsy. A more basic function of the hand is to grasp and release objects, and an attempt must be made to achieve this degree of function wherever possible. The need to improve hand function is even more pressing in non-ambulant children, in whom functioning of both hands are vital in order to make them more independent in the activities of daily living and for propelling their wheelchair. While it is of paramount importance to improve the grip strength so that the child can grasp objects, it is equally important to ensure that the ability to release the object is not impaired.

- Improve appearance of the limb by correcting the visible deformity

  If the function cannot be improved, it may be justified to perform surgery to simply straighten out a severely deformed wrist in order to improve the appearance of the limb in a child who is self-conscious about the deformity.

- Improve the hygiene of the hand

  Surgery may be needed to facilitate washing and cleaning of the palm and for greater ease of clothing in severely affected children in whom no functional improvement is envisaged at all.

Treatment options

Non-surgical options

■ Stretching exercises and bimanual activity

To begin with, in the younger child, spasticity of the flexors and the pronators can be treated by stretching exercises. If this is practised on a regular basis the onset of contractures can be delayed and the severity of contractures minimized. In addition to these exercises, the child is stimulated to use the affected hand by encouraging bimanual activity. This will help to prevent the child from ignoring the weak hand totally. This is very important because if the child ignores the limb, any surgery at a later date may be ineffective in improving function.

■ Splintage

If there are no contractures, dynamic deformities can be controlled by the use of light-weight splints. The child is then encouraged to use the hand with the splint (Figure 65.3). Splintage is useful

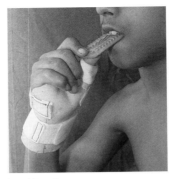

Figure 65.3 ● A splint may improve hand function.

as a temporary measure and definitive surgery may be needed in most children who show improved hand function with splintage. Splintage is useful as a pre-operative measure of anticipated outcome following surgery. As the child uses the hand while wearing the splint it will give both the surgeon and the parents an idea of the extent of improvement that may ensue following surgery. Finally, splintage is often needed in the post-operative period until function improves.

■ Myoneural blocks

Temporary reduction of spasticity can be achieved by injecting the muscles with botulinum toxin.[1] The application of splints and stretching of the spastic muscles during physiotherapy is facilitated by the block.

Surgical options

■ Flexor carpi ulnaris transfer to the extensor carpi radialis brevis

This tendon transfer, described by Green,[2] attempts to remove the principal deforming force (that produces flexion and ulnar deviation of the wrist) and convert it to a corrective force that facilitates active supination and wrist extension (Figure 65.4). The tendon is detached from its insertion into the pisiform and re-routed around the medial border of the ulna onto the dorsum of the wrist and attached to the tendon of the extensor carpi radialis brevis with moderate tension as the wrist is held in dorsiflexion.

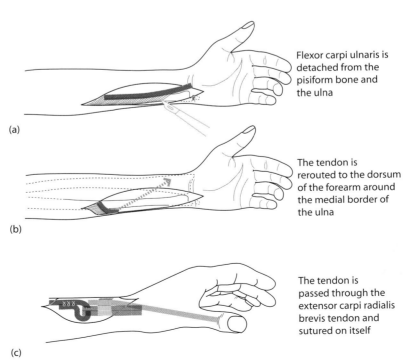

(a) Flexor carpi ulnaris is detached from the pisiform bone and the ulna

(b) The tendon is rerouted to the dorsum of the forearm around the medial border of the ulna

(c) The tendon is passed through the extensor carpi radialis brevis tendon and sutured on itself

Figure 65.4 ● Diagram showing the technique of flexor carpi ulnaris transfer to the wrist extensor.

■ Flexor carpi ulnaris transfer to the extensor digitorum

Children who have weakness of release and are unable to release their fingers when the wrist is held dorsiflexed could benefit from a transfer of the flexor carpi ulnaris tendon to the extensor digitorum tendons. This transfer will remove the deforming force and improve active supination and finger extension. Hoffer *et al.*[3] suggested that the decision to perform this transfer could be made with the help of dynamic electromyography. If the flexor carpi ulnaris fires when the child is attempting release of the fingers this transfer would be appropriate.

■ Pronator transfer or release

If wrist deformity is not present and hand function is satisfactory, the pronator overactivity may be reduced by lengthening the pronator teres tendon. If it is felt that the power of supination needs to be augmented, the pronator teres may be re-routed around the radius so as to make the muscle supinate the forearm.[4] A supination deformity of the forearm should be avoided and hence it is important that power of supination is assessed prior to the transfer and the transfer should be performed only if supination is demonstrably weak.

■ Flexor aponeurotic release

In a child who has good potential for functional improvement with predominant flexor spasticity and no pronator spasticity, aponeurotic release of the flexor muscles is recommended (Figure 65.5).[5]

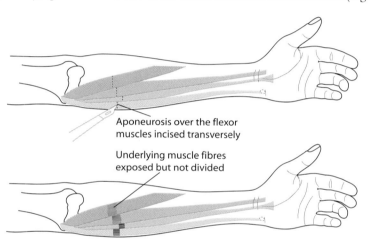

Aponeurosis over the flexor muscles incised transversely

Underlying muscle fibres exposed but not divided

Figure 65.5 ● Diagram showing the technique of performing an aponeurotic release of the flexors of the wrist and fingers.

■ Flexor pronator slide

If there is contracture of the flexors and pronators or if there is severe spasticity of these muscles releasing, the common flexor origin from the medial epicondyle and sliding the muscles distally[6] is the procedure of choice (Figure 65.6).

■ Superficialis to profundus transfer

If no functional outcome is anticipated in a child with very severe flexion contracture without any pronator contracture, the tendons of all the superficial flexors are sectioned at one level, while all the tendons of the flexor profundus are sectioned at another level. The proximal stumps of the superficial tendons are then tagged to the distal stumps of the profundus tendons.[7] At the same time the wrist flexors are tenotomized (Figure 65.7). This operation is recommended in the non-functional hand in adult stroke patients but can be equally useful in the adolescent with cerebral palsy.

Likelihood of improving function

Before undertaking surgery on the upper limb with the aim to improve hand function, detailed assessment of the child's hand and level of comprehension is essential.

■ Assess the ability to grasp and release independently

If the child has some independent grasp and release function, although not of normal strength or dexterity, there is a fair chance that surgery may improve function. On the other hand, the prognosis for functional improvement should be guarded if the child does not show any attempt at all to grasp and release.

Factors to be taken into consideration while planning treatment

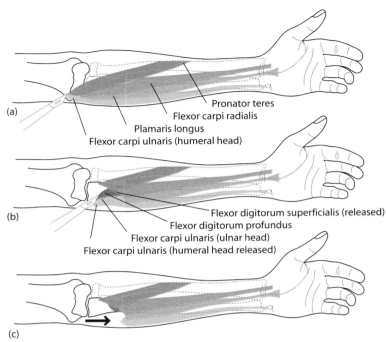

(a)

Pronator teres
Flexor carpi radialis
Plamaris longus
Flexor carpi ulnaris (humeral head)

(b)

Flexor digitorum superficialis (released)
Flexor digitorum profundus
Flexor carpi ulnaris (ulnar head)
Flexor carpi ulnaris (humeral head released)

(c)

Figure 65.6 ● Technique of performing a flexor pronator slide.

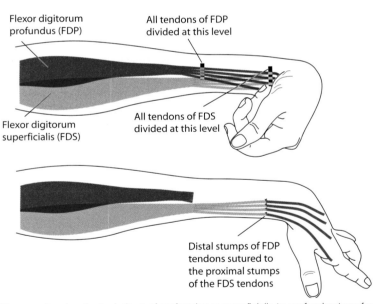

Flexor digitorum profundus (FDP)

All tendons of FDP divided at this level

Flexor digitorum superficialis (FDS)

All tendons of FDS divided at this level

Distal stumps of FDP tendons sutured to the proximal stumps of the FDS tendons

Figure 65.7 ● Diagram showing the technique of performing a superficialis to profundus transfer.

■ Assess the integrity of fine sensations in the fingers

Although it is often assumed that there is no sensory impairment in cerebral palsy, it is important to be aware that finer sensations such as stereognosis, two-point discrimination and the ability to appreciate textures may be affected. These sensations, which are of vital importance in ensuring optimal hand function, must be carefully tested. It has been suggested that the likelihood of improving hand function by surgery is greater in children who do not have significant impairment of these fine sensations.[8]

■ Record the age of the child

Surgery directed to improving hand function often entails a tendon transfer, and following surgery muscle re-education is essential in optimizing function. A child of average intelligence should be around the age of seven years to be able to cooperate with the rehabilitation.

■ Assess the intelligence of the child

Unless the child's IQ is above 70 they may not be able to comprehend instructions for post-operative muscle re-education.

In summary, some improvement of hand function following surgery may be anticipated in children over the age of seven years, with an IQ of at least 70, with independent grasp and release and in whom the finer sensations are intact (Figure 65.8). If these criteria are not fulfilled, the chances of obtaining functional improvement after surgery are poor although the appearance of the limb may improve.

The choice of the operative procedure often depends on whether there is a chance of functional improvement. If function is envisaged, care must be taken to avoid weakening the muscles too much. Hence the muscle slide operation or the superficialis to profundus transfer which considerably weaken the flexors are reserved for children with little chance of functional improvement.

Ability to release with the wrist extended

If the child is unable to extend the fingers while the wrist is passively held in extension, transfer of the flexor carpi ulnaris to the wrist extensor is contraindicated.

Pattern of deformities

The choice of surgical procedure will also depend on which muscles are spastic and the pattern of deformities that are present.

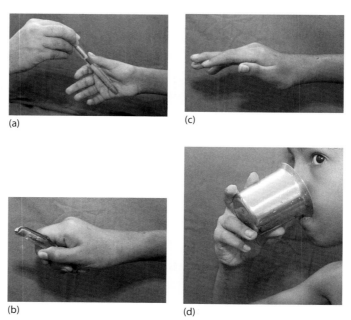

(a)

(c)

(b)

(d)

Figure 65.8 ● Improved hand function with satisfactory grasp and release of the hand seen in a child who has undergone a transfer of the flexor carpi ulnaris to the wrist extensor.

Recommended treatment

The outline of recommended treatment is shown in Table 65.1.

Table 65.1 ● Outline of treatment of the spastic forearm and hand

INDICATIONS								
Spasticity of flexors and pronators in child under 7 years	Spasticity of flexors and pronators in child under 7 years + Poor response to stretching	Spasticity of flexors and pronators + Child either awaiting surgery or post-operative	Flexor spasticity OR contracture + No pronator contracture or spasticity + Functional improvement anticipated	Pronator spasticity OR contracture + No flexor contracture or spasticity + Functional improvement anticipated + Supination weak	Flexor and pronator spasticity or contracture + Able to release fingers with wrist extended + Functional improvement anticipated	Flexor and pronator spasticity or contracture + Poor release with wrist extended + Functional improvement anticipated	Flexor and pronator spasticity or contracture + Minimal or no functional improvement anticipated	Flexor contracture + No pronator contracture + No functional improvement anticipated
⇨	⇨	⇨	⇨	⇨	⇨	⇨	⇨	⇨
Stretching exercises + Encourage use of affected hand	Myoneural block (Botox) + Encourage use of affected hand	Splintage + Encourage use of affected hand	Flexor aponeurotic release	Pronator transfer	Flexor carpi ulnaris transfer to the extensor carpi radialis brevis	Flexor carpi ulnaris transfer to the extensor digitorum	Flexor pronator slide	Superficialis to profundus transfer
TREATMENT								

References

1. Cosgrove AP, Graham HK. Botulinum toxin A in the management of spasticity with cerebral palsy. *Br J Surg* 1992; **74**: 135–6.

2. Green WT. Tendon transplantation of the flexor carpi ulnaris for pronation flexion deformity of the wrist. *Surg Gynecol Obstet* 1942; **75**: 337–42.

3. Hoffer M, Perry J, Melkonian GJ. Dynamic electromyography and decision making for surgery of the upper extremity of patients with cerebral palsy. *J Hand Surg [Am]* 1979; **4**: 424–31.

4. Sakellarides HT, Mital MA, Lenzi ND. Treatment of pronation contractures of the forearm in cerebral palsy by changing the insertion of the pronator radii teres. *J Bone Joint Surg Am* 1981: **63**: 645–52.

5. Tonkin M, Gschwind C. Surgery for cerebral palsy: Part 2. Flexion deformity of the wrist and fingers. *J Hand Surg [Br]* 1992; **17**: 260–67.

6. Inglis AE, Cooper W. Release of the flexor-pronator origin for flexion deformities of the hand and wrist in spastic paralysis. *J Bone Joint Surg* 1966; **48**: 847–57.

7. Keenan MA, Korchek JI, Botte MJ, Smith CW, Gartland DE. Results of transfer of the flexor digitorum superficialis tendons to the flexor digitorum profundus tendons in adults with acquired spasticity of the hand. *J Bone Joint Surg* 1987; **69**: 1127–32.

8. Goldner JL, Ferlic DC. Sensory status of the hand as related to reconstructive surgery of the upper extremity in cerebral palsy. *Clin Orthop Relat Res* 1966; **46**: 87–92.

The spastic thumb

Benjamin Joseph

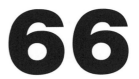

Introduction

The characteristic deformity that occurs when muscles acting on the thumb are spastic is the thumb-in-palm deformity. This deformity may be due to spasticity of the intrinsic muscles of the thumb, spasticity and weakness of the extrinsic muscles of the thumb or a combination of both. Depending on which muscles are at fault the deformity at the carpometacarpal (CMC) joint, the metacarpophalangeal (MCP) joint and the interphalangeal (IP) joint will vary. Based on the pattern of deformities seen, different types of thumb-in-palm deformity have been described.[1] If only the adductor pollicis is spastic, the first metacarpal is adducted at the CMC joint but the MCP and IP joints are extended. Spasticity of the flexor pollicis brevis will cause the MCP joint to flex. If, in addition to this, the flexor pollicis longus is spastic, the IP joint will also be flexed (Figure 66.1).

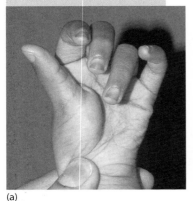

(a)

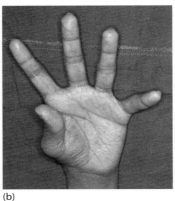

(b)

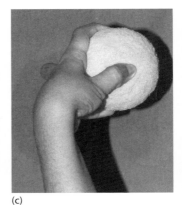

(c)

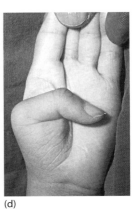

(d)

Figure 66.1 ● **(a)** Type I thumb-in-palm deformity. The first metacarpal is adducted due to spasticity of the adductor pollicis muscle. **(b)** Type II thumb-in-palm deformity. The first metacarpal is adducted and the metacarpophalangeal (MCP) joint is flexed. Here the adductor pollicis and the flexor pollicis brevis are spastic. **(c)** Type III thumb-in-palm deformity. In addition to spasticity of the adductor pollicis and the flexor pollicis brevis, there is instability of the MCP joint. **(d)** Type IV thumb-in-palm deformity. The adductor pollicis, the flexor pollicis brevis and the flexor pollicis longus are spastic. Here the first metacarpal is adducted and there is flexion of both the MCP and IP joints of the thumb.

Problems of management

Adduction of the thumb

As a consequence of spasticity of the adductor pollicis the thumb remains adducted. In order to grasp a large object in the palm the thumb needs to abduct while the hand is positioned over the object and then the thumb has to adopt a position of opposition in order to grasp the object. Opposition is a composite movement occurring predominantly at the CMC joint of the thumb entailing abduction, internal rotation and flexion of the first metacarpal. It is clear that both for opening the hand to receive the object in the palm and for grasping it efficiently, abduction of the thumb is essential and if hand function is to improve abduction of the spastic thumb must be facilitated.

Flexion of the thumb

If, in addition to spasticity of the adductor pollicis, the flexor pollicis brevis is also spastic, the thumb will lie across the palm. This makes it even more difficult to grasp an object as the thumb has already occupied the palm even before the object can be held.

Instability of the joints of the thumb

In order to fulfil any prehensile function effectively, the index and middle fingers need to oppose against a stable thumb post. In some children the MCP joint of the thumb may hyperextend on account of muscle imbalance and this renders the joint unstable.

Aims of treatment

- Facilitate thumb radial abduction
  In order to enable active radial abduction of the thumb, spasticity and contracture of the adductor muscle must be overcome and if the abductor muscles of the thumb are weak they need to be augmented.
- Prevent the thumb from lying in the palm while attempting to grasp an object
  If contractures of the adductor and flexors of the thumb and spasticity of these muscles are overcome the thumb will not lie in the palm.
- Ensure a stable thumb post
  The MCP and IP joint of the thumb should be made stable either by rebalancing the muscles acting across these joints or, if this fails, the unstable joint may need to be arthrodesed.

Treatment options

Adductor pollicis release from its origin

The most common operation performed for an adducted thumb is the release of the adductor pollicis from its origin.[2] An incision is made in the thenar crease and the adductor pollicis muscle can be identified simply by retracting medially the flexor tendon to the index finger. The muscle is erased from its origin on the shaft of the third metacarpal bone and the flexor retinaculum (Figure 66.2).

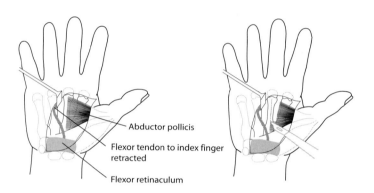

Abductor pollicis

Flexor tendon to index finger retracted

Flexor retinaculum

Figure 66.2 ● Technique of release of the adductor pollicis from its origin.

Adductor pollicis tenotomy

The adductor pollicis along with the flexor pollicis brevis may be detached from their insertion. This is not preferred as it may weaken the muscle too much.

Flexor pollicis brevis release from its origin

If the MCP joint is flexed, the flexor pollicis brevis muscle needs to be released. This can be done by erasing the fibres of the muscle at its origin when the release of the adductor pollicis is performed.

Flexor pollicis longus lengthening

If the IP joint is flexed, indicating spasticity of the flexor pollicis longus, its tendon is lengthened in the distal third of the forearm.

Tendon transfer to augment radial abductor power

If the power of thumb abduction is weak, in addition to releasing the spastic adductor, a tendon transfer may be done. Various tendon transfers have been described for strengthening the power of abduction of the thumb, including transfer of the flexor pollicis longus[3] and the extensor pollicis longus.[4] Yet another simple way of augmenting the power of abduction is to translocate the tendon of the extensor pollicis longus laterally by releasing its sheath and letting it shift away from Lister's tubercle (Figure 66.3). This will decrease the normal adductor moment of the tendon. This operation is recommended rather than a formal tendon transfer as it is very simple to perform and does not involve detachment and reattachment of a tendon. Furthermore, no muscle re-education is necessary after this procedure. If further augmentation of abduction is needed at a later date because of persistent radial abduction weakness, a formal transfer can be done as this operation does not 'burn any bridges'.

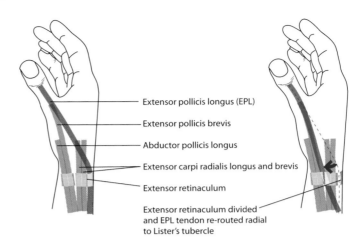

Extensor pollicis longus (EPL)

Extensor pollicis brevis

Abductor pollicis longus

Extensor carpi radialis longus and brevis

Extensor retinaculum

Extensor retinaculum divided
and EPL tendon re-routed radial
to Lister's tubercle

Figure 66.3 ● Technique of translocation of the extensor pollicis longus from around Lister's tubercle.

Stabilization of the thumb

If the MCP joint remains unstable after muscle rebalancing, a tenodesis of the joint may be done in skeletally immature children. In the skeletally mature child an arthrodesis may be required.[5]

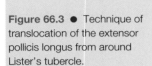

Factors to be taken into consideration while planning treatment

The type of thumb-in-palm

The structures that are spastic or contracted determine the type of thumb–in–palm deformity and, accordingly, the structures will have to be released.

Power of radial abduction of the thumb

If the power of radial abduction is demonstrably weak after release of the spastic muscles acting on the thumb, a tendon transfer will be needed to enable the thumb to abduct actively.

Table 66.1 ● Outline of treatment of spastic thumb-in-palm deformity

INDICATIONS							
Any type (types I–IV) of thumb-in-palm + Child under 5 years of age	Any type (types I–IV) of thumb-in-palm + Child between 5 and 7 years	Type I OR Type III thumb-in-palm + Child over 7 years	Type I OR Type III thumb-in-palm + Child over 7 years + Weakness of active thumb abduction persists after adductor pollicis release	Type II thumb-in-palm + Child over 7 years	Type IV thumb-in-palm + Child over 7 years	Type III thumb-in-palm + Persistent instability of the MCP joint following procedures as shown in column 3 or 4	Any type of thumb-in-palm + Persistent weakness of thumb abduction even after procedures as shown in column 4, 5 or 6
							⇩
					⇩	⇩	Formal tendon transfer to strengthen abduction thumb
			⇩	⇩	Release of adductor pollicis AND flexor pollicis brevis origins + FPL lengthening + EPL translocation	MCP tenodesis in skeletally immature child OR Arthrodesis in the skeletally mature child	
⇩	⇩	⇩	Augmentation of thumb abduction by EPL translocation	Release of adductor pollicis AND flexor pollicis brevis origins + EPL translocation			
Stretching exercises	Splintage	Release of adductor pollicis origin					
TREATMENT							

Age of the child

The choice of the technique of stabilization of the MCP joint is governed by the age of the child. If a tendon transfer that requires muscle re-education is contemplated, the child should be at least seven years of age in order to cooperate with post–operative rehabilitation.

Recommended treatment

The outline of treatment of the spastic thumb is shown in Table 66.1.

References

1. House JH, Gwathney FH, Fidler MO. A dynamic approach to the thumb-in-palm deformity in cerebral palsy. *J Bone Joint Surg* 1981; **63**: 216–25.
2. Matev I. Surgery for the spastic thumb-in-palm deformity. *J Hand Surg [Br]* 1991; **16**: 127–32.
3. Smith RJ. Flexor pollicis longus abductor-plasty for spastic thumb-in-palm deformity. *J Hand Surg [Am]* 1982; **7**: 327–34.
4. Manske PR. Redirection of extensor pollicis longus in the treatment of spastic thumb-in-palm deformity. *J Hand Surg [Am]* 1985; **10**: 553–60.
5. Goldner JL, Koman LA, Gelberman R, Levin S, Goldner RD. Arthrodesis of the metacarpophalangeal joint of the thumb in children and adults. An adjunctive treatment of thumb-in-palm deformity in cerebral palsy. *Clin Orthop Relat Res* 1990; **253**: 75–89.

SECTION 7

Epiphyseal and Physeal Problems

Blount's disease

Randall Loder

67

Introduction

Blount's disease, or tibia vara, is a progressive varus deformity occurring at the medial part of the proximal tibial physis. There are two main types: infantile Blount's which begins during the early childhood years, and late-onset or adolescent Blount's which begins in late childhood and the early teen years.[1] The aetiology is not completely known, but most researchers feel that Blount's disease represents an overload phenomenon on the proximal medial tibial physis owing to supra-physiologic compressive forces from the severe obesity that is so common in these children.[2,3]

The natural history of infantile Blount's disease is quite different from late-onset adolescent Blount's disease (Table 67.1). It is important to be aware of the differences in the natural history and evolution of the disease in young children and adolescents as the approach to management of these two types will differ on account of these differences.

Table 67.1 ● Differences between infantile Blount's disease and adolescent Blount's disease

Feature	Infantile Blount's disease	Adolescent Blount's disease
Physeal changes	Progressive and often severe	Mild
Physeal bar formation	Frequent	Does not occur
Metaphyseal changes	Progressive changes	No changes seen
Joint deformity	Common	Rare
Internal tibial torsion	Common	Rare
Recurrence	Often seen	Seldom seen

Infantile Blount's disease

Infantile Blount's involves definite radiographic changes in both the proximal tibial physis and metaphysis that are progressive. These changes have been classified into six stages by Langenskiöld (Figure 67.1); this staging has relevance for both treatment planning and predicting prognosis.

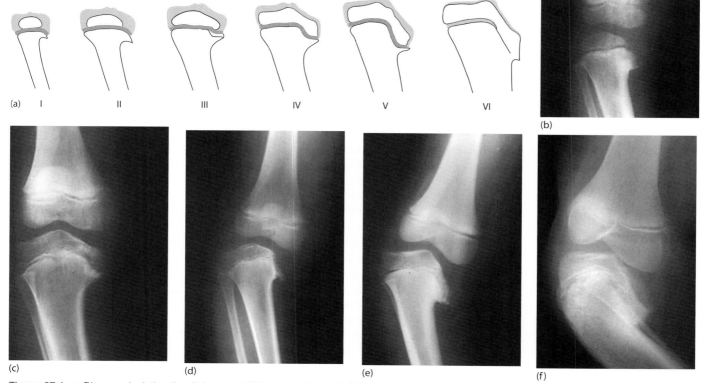

Figure 67.1 ● Diagram depicting the six Langenskiöld stages of infantile Blount's disease (a). Depression of the articular surface of the medial tibial plateau is evident in stages IV, V and VI and premature physeal arrest is seen in stage VI. Radiographs of examples of stage II (b), stage III (c), stage IV (d), stage V (e) and stage VI (f) disease.

Problems of management

Tibial deformity

Apart from the varus deformity of the proximal tibia, there is usually some degree of associated internal tibial torsion; both these deformities need to be addressed.

Joint deformity

Depression of the medial tibial plateau (epiphysis) occurs in the later stages of the disease and this can lead to joint instability, recurrence of deformity and early degenerative joint disease.

Physeal bar formation

The normal physeal architecture gets lost in the medial part of the physis (Figure 67.2). In due course, complete physeal arrest and a bony bar may develop. Dealing with the physeal bar is extremely problematic as the results of physeal bar resection in children with infantile Blount's disease may be very disappointing.

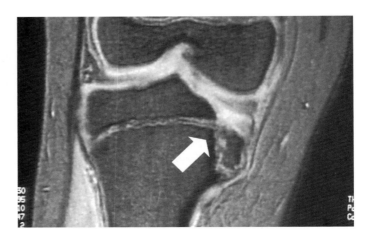

Figure 67.2 ● A magnetic resonance scan of a seven-year five-month-old child with severe infantile tibia vara. Note the complete loss of physeal architecture (white arrow) in the medial tibial physis at the level of the metaphyseal depression.

Limb length inequality

In unilateral infantile Blount's there can be significant physeal growth retardation in the involved side. Owing to the underlying joint instability and deformity, limb lengthening is not a good option. The patient must be closely followed so that the opportune window for an epiphyseodesis of the opposite extremity is not missed.

Recurrence of deformity

Children with infantile Blount's have a significant risk of recurrence and progression of the disease, including physeal bar formation, even when the initial surgical correction is excellent.[4,5] The chances of recurrence are greater as the stage of the disease increases. This emphasizes the need for early diagnosis and intervention.

Neurovascular complications

Proximal tibial osteotomies are associated with a high frequency of compartment syndrome and peroneal nerve palsy. Extreme diligence is required to watch for these complications, and all children undergoing a proximal tibial osteotomy for Blount's disease should have an anterior compartment fasciotomy at the time of the index procedure.[6]

Aims of treatment

- Restore normal alignment of the tibia
  Restoring the normal alignment of the tibia and restoring the normal mechanical axis of the limb is the foremost important goal. However, in some large, older children this is impossible due to the massively large thigh girth which prevents them from standing in a normal mechanical axis alignment.[7]
- Correct joint deformity
  If the tibial articular surface is depressed it needs to be corrected. In severe cases, elevation of the medial tibial epiphyseal depression should be considered along with proximal tibial osteotomy.[8]

- Equalize limb length
  It is important to minimize the limb length inequality as differing knee levels might be yet another predisposing factor for the early development of degenerative joint disease.
- Maintain correction and prevent recurrence
  In infantile disease, recurrence is commonly encountered.[4,5] Unfortunately, there are no known post-operative programmes (e.g. post-operative orthotics) that are successful in preventing recurrence. The best chance of preventing recurrence is to correct the deformity in the very early stages of the disease.
- Prevent neurovascular complications
  Appropriate care needs to be taken to minimize the risk of neurovascular complications.

Treatment options

Non-operative

In young children with infantile Blount's and Langenskiöld stage I or II, full time use of a knee-ankle-foot orthosis can be considered.[9] The success rate, however, is variable. If the child has not achieved complete correction by the age of four years or has progressed to Langenskiöld stage III disease, then immediate tibial osteotomy is indicated.[4,5]

Proximal tibial osteotomy

Proximal tibial osteotomy is the most widely used surgery. In children with infantile involvement, it must be below the level of the tibial tuberosity. In the young child with stage III disease the internal tibial torsion and the tibia vara can be corrected by an oblique osteotomy[10] as shown in Figure 67.3. In older children transverse proximal tibial osteotomy to correct both the varus and internal tibial torsion deformities, anterior compartment fasciotomy and fixation is recommended. In young children simple cross pins can be used while in the older child a plate and screws may be used (Figure 67.4b). However, in older children external fixators are desirable due to their ability to 'fine tune' the correction post-operatively if necessary (Figure 67.4c).

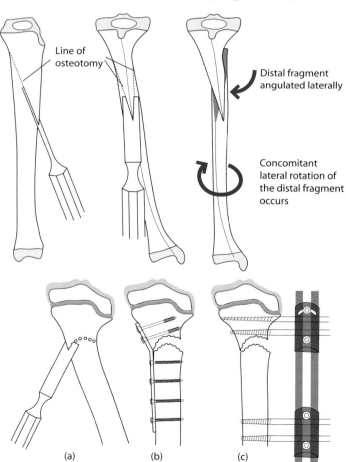

Figure 67.3 ● Diagram showing the technique of performing an oblique osteotomy that can correct both the varus deformity and the internal tibial torsion.

Figure 67.4 ● Proximal tibial osteotomy **(a)** can be stabilized with a plate and screws **(b)** or with an external fixator **(c)**.

(a)   (b)   (c)

Proximal medial tibial epiphyseal elevation

In children in whom there is significant depression of the medial tibial epiphysis, elevation of the epiphysis by an intra-epiphyseal osteotomy, sparing the physis, can be performed (Figure 67.5a). If performed at the initial surgery, a proximal tibial osteotomy to achieve proper alignment must also be performed.[8] When the child is approaching skeletal maturity or if there is evidence of premature physeal arrest, a transphyseal osteotomy with elevation of the tibial plateau can be performed (Figure 67.5b).

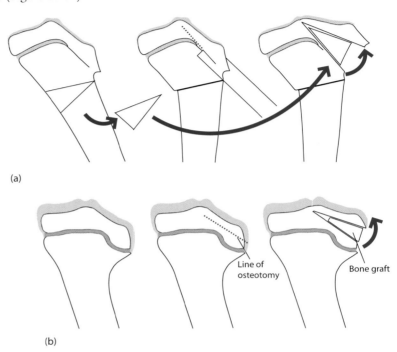

(a)

Line of osteotomy

Bone graft

(b)

Figure 67.5 ● (a) Transepiphyseal osteotomy elevating the tibial plateau. **(b)** Intra-epiphyseal osteotomy elevating the depressed medial tibial plateau.

Physeal bar resection

In children with infantile Blount's who are young and have developed a proximal medial tibial physeal bar, resection can be considered, along with repeat osteotomy.[11] The results are often disappointing.

Epiphyseodesis and later limb lengthening by angular correction with external fixators

In children with 'malignant' infantile Blount's disease who have recurrence following several proximal tibial osteotomies or other surgery, this option can be considered. The implications of the gradual correction of deformity with the external fixator must be fully explained to the parents as it requires excellent patient compliance.

Factors to be taken into consideration while planning treatment

Stage of the disease

The Langenskiöld stage needs to be considered while planning treatment. The earliest stages may be amenable to non-operative treatment, while the more advanced stages need aggressive surgical intervention.

Unilateral or bilateral involvement

If bilateral, the risk of limb length inequality is less for those with infantile Blount's disease. When considering surgery, bilateral osteotomies place significant mobility issues on the child and family, especially in the older, massively obese child.

Amount of growth remaining

In bilateral cases, if there is minimal remaining growth in the proximal tibial physis, then transphyseal procedures can be considered. Similarly, if there is a negligible amount of growth remaining and the deformity is unilateral, then a transphyseal procedure with contralateral epiphyseodesis can be considered.

Presence of a physeal bar

In later Langenskiöld stages, it may be prudent to evaluate for the presence of a physeal bar with a magnetic resonance imaging scan.

General medical health

In the massively obese child, concern about obesity-associated problems must be kept in mind; these include type II diabetes and sleep apnoea.

Recommended treatment

The recommended treatment for infantile Blount's disease is shown in Table 67.2.

Table 67.2 ● Outline of treatment of infantile Blount's disease

INDICATIONS					
Langenskiöld stage I or II + Under 4 years of age ⇩ Full-time use of knee-ankle-foot orthosis	Langenskiöld stage III + 4 or 5 years of age ⇩ Rab's oblique osteotomy + Fasciotomy	Langenskiöld stage III + >5 years of age ⇩ Proximal tibial osteotomy with derotation (over correct by 10°) + Fasciotomy	Langenskiöld stage IV/V + Not near skeletal maturity ⇩ Proximal tibial osteotomy with derotation (over correct by 10°) + Intra-epiphyseal osteotomy to elevate the medial tibial plateau + Fasciotomy	Langenskiöld stage IV/V + Near skeletal maturity OR Physeal arrest evident ⇩ Proximal tibial osteotomy with derotation + Transepiphyseal osteotomy to elevate the medial tibial plateau + Fasciotomy	Multiple recurrences ⇩ Epiphyseodesis of the proximal tibia and fibula + Proximal tibial osteotomy with derotation + Fasciotomy + Limb lengthening ± OR Contralateral epiphyseodesis at the appropriate time
TREATMENT					

Adolescent Blount's disease

Late-onset Blount's usually involves mild changes in the tibial physis, no metaphyseal changes and gradually progressive genu varus (Figure 67.6).

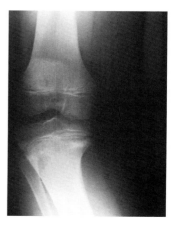

Figure 67.6 ● Radiograph of an adolescent with late-onset Blount's disease. Physeal and metaphyseal changes are minimal.

Problems of management

Aim of treatment

Treatment options

Tibial deformity and mechanical axis deviation

The varus deformity and the malalignment of the limb need to be corrected in order to prevent early degenerative arthritis of the knee.

- Correct the tibial deformity and restore the mechanical axis
  As in the case of infantile Blount's, restoring the mechanical axis may be difficult in the very obese individual. However, if the alignment is restored the deformity generally does not recur.

Proximal tibial valgus osteotomy

Correction of the deformity can be achieved by performing an osteotomy at the infrapatellar level, and anterior compartment fasciotomy is performed simultaneously. External fixator immobilization is desirable to allow fine tuning of the correction;[12] AO plate fixation may also be used[13] (Figure 67.7). Simple cross-pin fixation should not be used.[14]

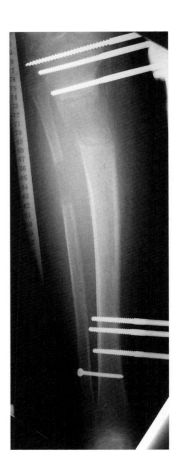

Figure 67.7 ● Correction of adolescent tibia vara with an external fixator.

Proximal tibial osteotomy and gradual correction with external fixator

Particularly in unilateral cases, precise correction of the deformity can be achieved by gradual correction with an external fixator.

Proximal lateral tibial epiphyseodesis

In a child with adolescent Blount's and who has adequate remaining growth, proximal lateral tibial physeal arrest with either staples or hemiepiphyseodesis may result in sufficient correction due to continued medial tibial physeal growth. Although the results are variable, it is a much smaller procedure than osteotomy and should be performed if possible.[7]

Growth remaining

If more than two years of remaining growth is present and the deformity is mild, lateral tibial physeal arrest should be performed. This author recommends formal epiphyseodesis, assuming that the family will report for regular follow-up to ensure that overcorrection does not occur.[9]

In children with more severe deformity who have minimal growth remaining, the osteotomy can be above the tibial tuberosity and ablating the physis; otherwise the osteotomy can be just below the tibial tuberosity.

Severity of deformity

If the severity of the deformity is mild and sufficient remaining growth is present, lateral tibial epiphyseodesis would be the preferred option. On the other hand, if the deformity is severe, full correction of the deformity would not occur by epiphyseodesis and in such a situation a formal corrective osteotomy would be required to achieve complete correction.

Unilateral or bilateral involvement

In unilateral adolescent Blount's disease, gradual correction of the deformity by hemicallotasis would ensure that the limb length is maintained.

The outline of treatment of adolescent Blount's disease is shown in Table 67.3.

Table 67.3 ● Outline of treatment of adolescent Blount's disease

INDICATIONS			
Unilateral/bilateral + Mild deformity + >2 years growth remaining	Unilateral + Mild deformity + <2 years growth remaining OR Severe deformity (that is unlikely to correct by staple epiphyseodesis)	Bilateral + <2 years growth remaining	Bilateral + >2 years growth remaining
⇩	⇩	⇩	⇩
Lateral staple epiphyseodesis of proximal tibia + Follow up to ensure that over correction is not occurring	Hemicallotasis with external fixator	Closed wedge proximal tibial osteotomy performed proximal to the tibial tuberosity	Closed wedge proximal tibial osteotomy performed distal to the tibial tuberosity
TREATMENT			

Why perform the osteotomy below the tibial tuberosity in the older adolescent child?
The ideal immobilization is use of an external fixator. The pins or wires needed for the fixator require adequate bone for fixation; a transphyseal osteotomy does not allow adequate room for placement of the pins or wires necessary for an external fixator.

Why not use simple cross-pin fixation with long leg cast in the older child undergoing osteotomy?
Owing to the large size of these children, it is difficult to ensure the desired alignment intra-operatively, and the complication rate of malunion and pin track infection is unacceptable.

Why perform an anterior compartment fasciotomy after proximal tibial osteotomy?
The risk of neurovascular complications is high in children undergoing proximal tibial osteotomy. A prophylactic anterior compartment fasciotomy reduces the chances of compartment syndrome.

Why strive for overcorrection after proximal tibial osteotomy in infantile Blount's and anatomic alignment in adolescent Blount's disease?

The ligamentous laxity associated with the long-term varus deformity in the infantile condition, along with the high risk of recurrence, requires slight overcorrection of the deformity. Ligament laxity and recurrence are seldom seen in adolescent Blount's disease.

References

1. Greene WB. Infantile tibia vara. *J Bone Joint Surg Am* 1993; **75**: 130–43.
2. Henderson RC, Greene WB. Etiology of late-onset tibia vara: is varus alignment a prerequisite? *J Pediatr Orthop* 1994; **14**: 143–6.
3. Davids JR, Huskamp M, Bagley AM. A dynamic biomechanical analysis of the etiology of adolescent tibia vara. *J Pediatr Orthop* 1996; **16**: 461–8.
4. Loder RT, Johnston II CE. Infantile tibia vara. *J Pediatr Orthop* 1987; **7**: 639–46.
5. Schoenecker PL, Meade WC, Pierron RL, Sheridan JJ, Capelli AM. Blount's disease: a retrospective review and recommendations for treatment. *J Pediatr Orthop* 1985; **5**: 181–6.
6. Slawski DP, Schoenecker PL, Rich MM. Peroneal nerve injury as a complication of pediatric tibial osteotomies: a review of 255 osteotomies. *J Pediatr Orthop* 1994; **14**: 166–72.
7. Henderson RC, Kemp Jr. GJ, Greene WB. Adolescent tibia vara: alternatives for operative treatment. *J Bone Joint Surg Am* 1992; **74**: 342–50.
8. Gregosiewicz A, Wosko I, Kandzierski G, Drabik Z. Double-elevating osteotomy of tibiae in the treatment of severe cases of Blount's disease. *J Pediatr Orthop* 1989; **9**: 178–81.
9. Zionts LE, Shean CJ. Brace treatment of early infantile tibia vara. *J Pediatr Orthop* 1998; **18**: 102–9.
10. Rab GT. Oblique osteotomy fro Blount's disease (tibia vara). *J Pediatr Orthop* 1988; **8**: 715–20.
11. Beck CL, Burke SW, Roberts JM, Johnston II CE. Physeal bridge resection in infantile Blount disease. *J Pediatr Orthop* 1987; **7**: 161–3.
12. Price CT, Scott DS, Greenberg DA. Dynamic axial external fixation in the surgical treatment of tibia vara. *J Pediatr Orthop* 1995; **15**: 236–43.
13. Martin SD, Moran MC, Martin TL, Burke SW. Proximal tibial osteotomy with compression plate fixation for tibia vara. *J Pediatr Orthop* 1994; **14**: 619–22.
14. Loder RT, Schaffer JJ, Bardenstein MB. Late-onset tibia vara. *J Pediatr Orthop* 1991; **11**: 162–7.

Perthes' disease

Benjamin Joseph

68

Introduction

Perthes' disease is a self-limiting form of osteochondrosis of the capital femoral epiphysis of unknown aetiology that develops in children commonly between the ages of five and 12 years.[1] Children under five and adolescents are affected much less frequently.[1,2] The blood supply to part or all of the epiphysis becomes interrupted, leading to necrosis of the involved part. The blood supply is restored spontaneously and the necrotic epiphysis heals over a period of two to four years, providing the onset of the disease is not in adolescence. The process of healing in children can be clearly identified on plain radiographs and the evolution of the disease can be quite reliably divided into discrete stages on the basis of plain radiographic appearances.[3] These stages are those of avascularity (stage I), fragmentation (stage II), regeneration (stage III) and complete healing (stage IV). The first three stages of the disease can be further subdivided into early (substage a) and late (substage b) parts of each respective stage (Figures 68.1a–g).

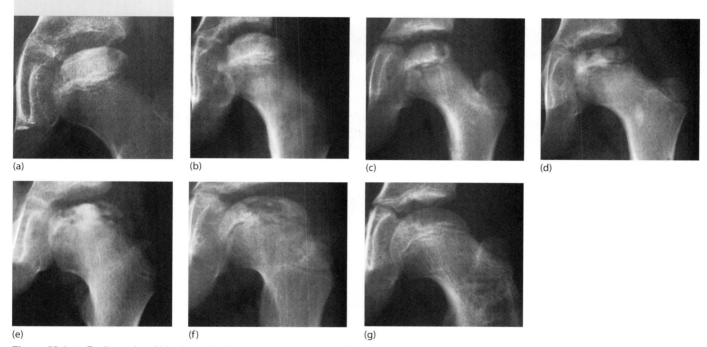

(a)   (b)   (c)   (d)

(e)   (f)   (g)

Figure 68.1 ● Radiographs of hips in each of the stages of evolution of Perthes' disease. In stage Ia the epiphysis is sclerotic but the height of the epiphysis is equal to that of the uninvolved hip **(a)**. In stage Ib the epiphysis is sclerotic and there is some loss of epiphyseal height but the epiphysis is in one piece **(b)**. In stage IIa early fragmentation of the epiphysis is evident with one or two vertical fissures in the epiphysis **(c)**. In stage IIb the epiphysis is in several fragments **(d)**. In stage IIIa early new bone formation is evident at the periphery of the epiphysis. At this stage the new bone is immature woven bone and is not of normal density on the radiograph **(e)**. Mature bone covers at least a third of the circumference of the epiphysis in stage IIIb **(f)**. The disease is considered to have healed when there is no avascular bone visible on the radiograph **(g)**.

In adolescents there does not appear to be any spontaneous ability for the blood supply to be re-established and consequently the disease does not pass through the stages of evolution seen in younger children.[2]

Problems of management

Deformation of the femoral head

In a proportion of children the femoral head becomes deformed during the process of revascularization of the epiphysis (Figure 68.2a). Among the factors that seem to contribute to the propensity for femoral head deformation, extrusion of the femoral head outside the margins of the acetabulum appears to be the most important.[3,4] There is evidence to suggest that irreversible deformation occurs either in the latter part of the stage of fragmentation or very early in the stage of regeneration.[3]

Enlargement of the femoral head

The femoral head becomes enlarged as the disease progresses (Figure 68.2b) and the extent of this enlargement is proportional to the degree of its deformation.[3]

Capital physeal growth impairment

The avascularity of the epiphysis impairs normal growth at the capital femoral physis and, as a result of this, in some older children the femoral neck is foreshortened. The trochanter continues to grow normally and as a consequence the greater trochanter outgrows the femoral head and neck (Figure 68.2c). This results in altered mechanics of the hip and a Trendelenburg gait.

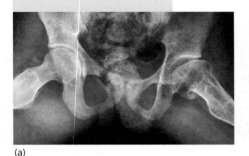
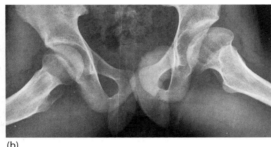
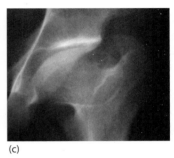

(a) (b) (c)

Figure 68.2 ● **(a)** Radiograph of the hip of a young adult with healed Perthes' disease that was not treated. The femoral head is deformed and the acetabular and femoral articular surfaces are no longer congruent. **(b)** Radiograph of the pelvis of a child with healed Perthes' disease showing enlargement of the femoral head. **(c)** Radiograph of the hip of a young adult with healed Perthes' disease in whom retardation of capital physeal growth has resulted in foreshortening of the femoral neck and 'overgrowth' of the greater trochanter. The tip of the trochanter is at a higher level than the centre of the femoral head and consequently this young man had a Trendelenburg gait.

Secondary degenerative arthritis of the hip

All three morphological changes in the proximal femur listed above can contribute independently or collectively to the development of secondary degenerative arthritis.[5,6] However, the most important factor that predisposes to the development of degenerative arthritis is deformation of the shape of the femoral head.[7]

Aims of treatment

- Prevent deformation of the femoral head
  This is the most important aim of treatment of Perthes' disease. In order to plan treatment aimed at preventing this complication it is necessary to understand the pathogenesis of femoral head deformation. Weight-bearing and muscular contraction produce stresses that are transmitted across the acetabular margin onto the extruded part of the avascular femoral capital epiphysis. The avascular epiphysis is particularly vulnerable to deformation when subjected to these stresses. Studies have shown that if extrusion of the femoral head exceeds 20 percent by the time the disease has progressed to the latter part of the stage of fragmentation there is a high risk of femoral head deformation[3,4] (Figure 68.3). Hence every effort must be made to prevent extrusion of the femoral head, and if extrusion does occur it should be corrected before the latter part of the stage of fragmentation if deformation of the femoral head is to be prevented.[8]
- Minimize enlargement of the femoral head
  Since the degree of enlargement of the femoral head is related to the severity of deformation of the femoral head, intervention that succeeds in preventing femoral head deformation is likely to succeed also in minimizing the extent of enlargement of the femoral head.[9,10]
- Prevent or correct greater trochanteric overgrowth
  Although the interference with normal femoral capital physeal growth appears to be related to the severity of the disease, there is no way of identifying which children will develop this

complication. Hence, treatment is directed at dealing with trochanteric overgrowth – the effect of retardation of femoral capital physeal growth. It is possible to prevent overgrowth of the trochanter by arresting its growth. It is also possible to restore the normal relationship between the centre of the femoral head and the trochanter once overgrowth of the trochanter has occurred. The aim of treatment is to ensure that the tip of the trochanter is at or below the level of the centre of the femoral head in order to prevent a Trendelenburg gait.

- Prevent secondary degenerative arthritis of the hip
  By ensuring that the femoral head remains spherical and by minimizing the extent to which it enlarges, the chances of developing late degenerative arthritis can be reduced.

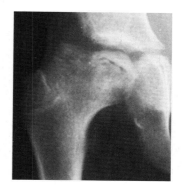

Figure 68.3 ● Radiograph of the pelvis of a child with Perthes' disease showing more than 20 percent extrusion of the femoral head. Deformation of the portion of the femoral head directly under the lateral margin of the acetabulum is clearly seen.

Treatment options

Weight relief

In the past, treatment was primarily directed at avoiding weight-bearing for a prolonged period with the hope that this would prevent the femoral head from becoming deformed. However, there is little evidence to suggest that this method of treatment is effective in preventing femoral head deformation.

Containment by bracing or casting

'Containment' aims at repositioning the extruded anterolateral part of the femoral epiphysis into the confines of the acetabulum. This can be achieved either by abducting and flexing the hip or by abducting and internally rotating the hip. Various forms of braces have been designed to hold the hip in the desired position during the active stages of the disease (Figure 68.4). Containment needs to be ensured until the healing progresses beyond the stage where the epiphysis is vulnerable to deformation, i.e. until the late part of the stage of regeneration (stage IIIb). It follows that the brace needs to be worn for up to two years if it is to be effective.

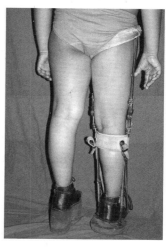

Figure 68.4 ● Various forms of braces that keep the affected hip abducted or abducted and internally rotated have been used to achieve containment in Perthes' disease. A splint that attempts to also reduce the weight-bearing stresses on the hip is the paten-ended caliper seen here; the sole raise on the opposite side ensures some abduction of the affected hip.

A broomstick cast (Figure 68.5) which also holds the hips abducted and flexed or internally rotated may be used as a temporary form of containment until more definitive treatment can be instituted.

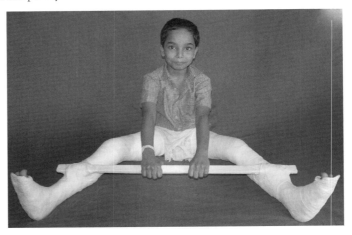

Figure 68.5 ● A child with Perthes' disease who has been put in a broomstick cast as a temporary method of containment.

Surgical containment

Containment can be achieved either by performing a femoral osteotomy or by surgery on the pelvic bone. Femoral osteotomies are designed so as to ensure that the proximal fragment is either abducted and internally rotated (when a femoral derotation osteotomy is performed) or abducted and flexed (when a varus extension osteotomy is performed). Surgery on the pelvis attempts to either augment the acetabulum or re-orient it in order to improve the coverage of the anterolateral part of the femoral epiphysis.

■ Femoral osteotomies

■ Varus derotation osteotomy

A varus derotation osteotomy is one of the most widely used methods of achieving containment (Figure 68.6a). It entails an intertrochanteric or subtrochanteric osteotomy wherein the distal fragment is adducted and externally rotated to the same degree of abduction and internal rotation of the hip required to achieve containment. Some surgeons decide the extent of abduction and internal rotation needed by performing a pre-operative arthrogram to determine which position of the hip provides the best containment. However, 20° of varus angulation and about 20–30° of derotation appear to be sufficient for obtaining adequate containment in most instances[9] and thus arthrographic verification may not be essential. The osteotomy is held with a plate and screws. In children up to

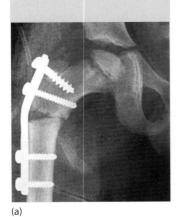

(a)

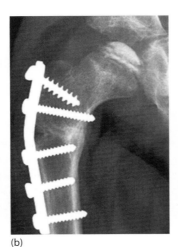

(b)

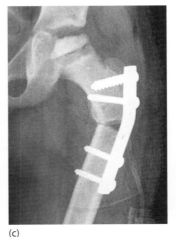

(c)

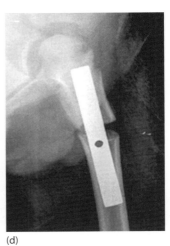

(d)

Figure 68.6 ● **(a)** Radiograph of the hip of a child who has undergone a varus derotation osteotomy. **(b)** Radiograph of the hip of a ten-year-old boy six weeks after an open wedge varus derotation osteotomy showing callus filling the gap and union of the osteotomy progressing very well. Anteroposterior **(c)** and lateral **(d)** radiographs of the hip of a child who has undergone a varus extension osteotomy. The distal fragment has been adducted and extended by 20° and the epiphysis is well contained.

the age of 12 years an open wedge osteotomy may be performed without running the risk of delayed union of the osteotomy[9] (Figure 68.6b). Since the amount of permanent shortening can be minimized if an open wedge osteotomy is performed, it is preferred to a closed wedge osteotomy.

It is important to ensure that all hip movements are restored to normal before the varus derotation surgery is performed and this is usually possible if the child is kept in traction for a few days. If after a period of traction internal rotation alone remains restricted, a varus extension osteotomy may be performed. If other movements also remain restricted, surgery is not justified. In such cases, a broomstick cast is applied under anaesthesia with the hips in wide abduction. Six weeks later the cast is removed and the hip is mobilized. Often the movements are fully restored by this time and surgery can then be safely undertaken.

■ Varus extension osteotomy

If passive internal rotation of the hip remains restricted after a period of traction or after the broomstick cast is removed a varus extension osteotomy is performed (Figure 68.6c,d).

■ **Pelvic surgery**

■ Shelf operation

This procedure which entails creating a bony shelf to cover the extruded part of the epiphysis has been recommended in the older child.[11]

■ Redirectional osteotomy

Reorienting the acetabulum by a Salter's osteotomy so that it increases coverage of the anterolateral aspect of the femoral epiphysis is another way of improving containment.[12]

■ Displacement osteotomy

A Chiari osteotomy is yet another way of improving coverage of the femoral head.

Greater trochanteric arrest

Growth of the greater trochanter can be slowed down by performing an epiphyseodesis when a varus osteotomy is performed. This has been routinely recommended in the older child[9,13] as a measure to prevent greater trochanteric overgrowth. The epiphyseodesis can be performed by drilling the growth plate of the greater trochanter or by a transfixing the trochanteric growth plate with a screw (Figure 68.7).

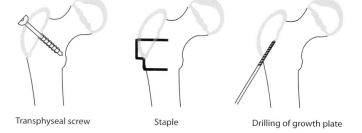

Transphyseal screw　　　Staple　　　Drilling of growth plate

Figure 68.7 ● Diagram showing the techniques of performing a trochanteric epiphyseodesis.

Factors to be taken into consideration while planning treatment

Age of the child

The older the child, the poorer is the prognosis[1,7] for several reasons. First, the tendency for the femoral head to extrude is clearly greater in the older child[3] and consequently there is a greater risk of the femoral head deforming in older children. Second, the disease is more severe in older children with more extensive epiphyseal involvement and hip stiffness.[14] Third, if the femoral head does become deformed some remodelling can occur between healing of the disease and skeletal maturity, but the potential for remodelling becomes poorer with the increasing age of the child. It follows that more aggressive treatment may be warranted in the older child.

Extent of epiphyseal involvement

The prognosis is poorer when the entire epiphysis is avascular than when only part of the epiphysis is avascular.[1] The tendency for the femoral head to extrude is also greater when a greater part of the epiphysis is avascular.[3] The outcome is generally favourable even without treatment when less than half the epiphysis is avascular.

Stage of evolution of the disease

Since the treatment of Perthes' disease is aimed at preventing deformation of the femoral head it is essential that any intervention that is planned is instituted before this complication develops. Irreversible deformation of the femoral head occurs either by the late fragmentation stage (stage IIb) or in the early stage of regeneration (stage IIIa) and containment should be achieved before the disease progresses to this stage.[8]

Range of movement of the hip

Hip stiffness is a poor prognostic sign and containment is not likely to be effective if the hip is stiff, hence containment is not justified in the presence of hip stiffness. In some children restriction of internal rotation alone may persist despite a period of traction and in these children containment cannot be achieved by abduction–internal rotation. In such children abduction with flexion of the hip is the position that would ensure containment of the anterolateral part of the femoral capital epiphysis.

Presence of epiphyseal extrusion

As mentioned earlier, the most important factor that influences the outcome in Perthes' disease is extrusion of the epiphysis. Extrusion tends to increase gradually as the disease progresses from onset to the early part of the fragmentation stage (stage IIb). Thereafter an abrupt increase in extrusion occurs in untreated children.[3] Extrusion occurs almost invariably in children who are over the age of seven years at the onset of the disease[15] and it exceeds 20 percent in the majority of these older children.[3]

The recommended treatment plan for children with Perthes' disease who are under the age of 12 years at the onset of symptoms is shown in Table 68.1.

Recommended treatment to prevent femoral head deformation

Table 68.1 ● Treatment for Perthes' disease in children under 12 years of age

INDICATIONS					
Under 5 years of age at onset + Any degree of epiphyseal involvement + No extrusion + In stage I, II or III of the disease	Under 5 years of age at onset + Half or more of epiphysis involved + Extrusion present In stage I or II + of the disease	Under 12 years of age at onset + Less than half the epiphysis involved + No extrusion[a] + In stage I, II or III of the disease	5–7 years of age at onset + Half or more of epiphysis involved + Extrusion present + In stage I or stage II of the disease	7–12 years of age at onset + Half or more of epiphysis involved + Extrusion present OR absent + In stage I or II of the disease	Under 12 years of age at onset + Half or more of epiphysis involved + Extrusion present + In stage III of the disease + Hip pain
⇩	⇩	⇩	⇩	⇩	⇩
No active intervention Periodic review until healing	Contain with a brace in abduction and flexion or abduction and internal rotation	No active intervention Periodic review until healing	Varus derotation femoral osteotomy (if all hip movements are restored) OR Varus extension femoral osteotomy (if internal rotation alone is limited)	Varus derotation femoral osteotomy (if all hip movements are restored) OR Varus extension femoral osteotomy (if internal rotation alone is limited) + Trochanteric arrest	Treat pain with rest and traction until pain is relieved + Treat residual problems by salvage procedures (see Table 68.2)
TREATMENT					

[a] Extrusion does not usually occur in children in whom less than half the epiphysis is involved.

Rationale of treatment

Why is a femoral osteotomy preferred to a pelvic osteotomy for achieving containment?
Apart from being a simpler operation, the femoral osteotomy appears to hasten healing of the disease.[10] In older children, if the femoral osteotomy is performed at the stage of avascular necrosis (stage I) the stage of fragmentation may be completely bypassed in about a third of children. In virtually every child in whom the stage of fragmentation is bypassed the femoral head remains spherical.[10] There is no evidence in the literature to suggest that an innominate osteotomy would have these effects on the natural history of the disease.

Why is an open wedge osteotomy recommended?
Since any angulation osteotomy results in some degree of shortening of the bone, a technique that produces the least amount of shortening is preferred.

Why is surgical containment not recommended in the stage of regeneration (stage III)?
Containment in the stage of regeneration is not likely to prevent deformation of the femoral head as deformation occurs by the commencement of this stage of evolution of the disease. Results of containment at this stage of the disease are too poor to justify it.[8]

Why is containment recommended in children over the age of seven years even if there is no extrusion?
Extrusion of the epiphysis will occur sooner or later in these older children[3,15] and since the results of surgery early in the course of the disease (in stages Ia, Ib or IIa) are distinctly superior to the results of surgery later in the disease,[8] containment is recommended even before there is any demonstrable extrusion in children over the age of seven years at the onset of symptoms.

Salvage surgery for sequelae of Perthes' disease

Some children with Perthes' disease are not candidates for treatment directed at preventing femoral head deformation simply because they are seen too late in the course of the disease. However, treatment may be justified in some of these patients.

Aims of treatment

In children with sequelae of Perthes' disease the aims of treatment are very different to those of treating early Perthes' disease. Here the aims are to:

- Relieve pain
- Correct Trendelenburg gait
- Minimize the risk of development of degenerative arthritis

Salvage options

Valgus osteotomy

A small proportion of children develop a phenomenon referred to as hinge abduction,[16] where abduction of the hip does not occur around its normal anteroposterior axis of rotation passing through the centre of the femoral head. Instead, the femoral head hinges on the acetabular margin, the medial joint space increases and the hip opens out medially (Figure 68.8). Frequently this abnormal movement is associated with pain. It has been shown that the pain can be relieved by performing a valgus osteotomy of the proximal femur.[16]

Joint distraction

Arthrodiatasis or joint distraction with the help of an articulated external fixator has been tried as a method of treatment for children with severe Perthes' disease.[17] A fixator that permits uniaxial motion (flexion and extension) is applied with proximal screws in the ilium and distal screws in the femur with the axis of the joint of the fixator aligned to correspond to the axis of movement of the hip joint. The joint is distracted and the fixator is retained for a few months and then removed. Although the procedure may possibly facilitate healing and prevent collapse of the epiphysis, it is unclear as to how long the fixator needs to be retained.

Arthrodesis

This is an option in adolescents if the hip is very painful and grossly distorted[2] (Figure 68.9). Excellent function can be anticipated in these patients although motion is abolished.[18]

Cheilectomy

This operation attempts to improve the shape of the femoral head once the femoral head is irreversibly deformed. It involves removing the bump on the lateral aspect of the head. This theoretically

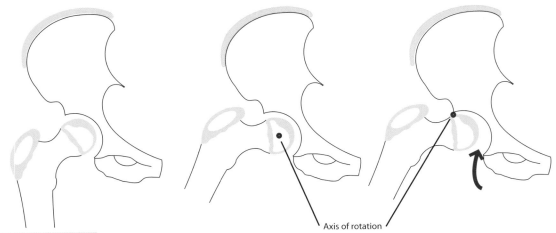

Figure 68.8 ● Diagram showing normal abduction and hinge abduction of the hip. As hinge abduction occurs the medial joint space increases (curved arrow) and the articular surfaces of the acetabulum and the femoral head are not concentric.

Figure 68.9 ● **(a)** Radiograph of the hip of an adolescent with Perthes' disease with gross destruction of the articular surface of the femur. **(b)** An intra-articular arthrodesis has been performed and sound union has occurred.

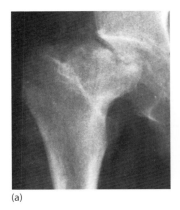
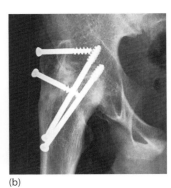

(a)   (b)

improves the shape of the head and removes one obvious cause of hinge abduction. However, there is a risk of joint stiffness after this operation and the long-term results are not good.[19]

Greater trochanteric advancement

If the greater trochanter has overgrown to such an extent that a Trendelenburg gait is present, distal and lateral transfer of the greater trochanter is recommended (Figure 68.10). The transfer augments the abductor lever arm by virtue of lateralization of the insertion of the gluteus medius. In addition, the distal transfer increases the resting length of the fibres of the gluteus medius. As a result of this the Trendelenburg gait is corrected and the stresses on the hip are also reduced. The operation is preferably done in patients in whom the femoral head contour is spherical.

Lengthening of the femoral neck

This is a complex operation entailing distal transfer of the greater trochanter and simultaneous lengthening of the femoral neck. Although this operation attempts to correct both the shortened

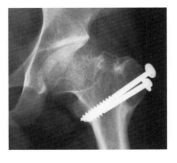

Figure 68.10 ● Distal and lateral transfer of the greater trochanter has been performed on this hip. The Trendelenburg gait was corrected following the operation.

neck and the overriding of the trochanter, the results do not appear to be appreciably better than isolated greater trochanteric advancement, which is a much simpler operation.[20]

Improving acetabular coverage of the femoral head

Improving acetabular coverage over an enlarged femoral head may reduce the risk of degenerative arthritis by reducing the stress on the femoral head. Acetabular coverage may be improved by a periacetabular osteotomy that permits the acetabular roof to be rotated over the femoral head or by fashioning a shelf over the uncovered part of the femoral head.

Presence of pain

Pain is usually due to mechanical impingement of the femoral head against the acetabular rim in patients with hinge abduction or due to arthritic changes in a grossly deformed hip.

The shape of the femoral head

If the femoral head is spherical it is justified to improve the acetabular coverage and improve the mechanics of the hip by distal transfer of the elevated greater trochanter. This may minimize the risk of development of degenerative arthritis. On the other hand, if the femoral head is grossly deformed, these measures may be of little use.

The size of the femoral head

If the femoral head is enlarged, acetabular coverage may be considered provided the shape of the head is not grossly distorted.

The congruity of the hip

If the femoral head and the acetabulum are congruent, acetabular coverage can be improved by a redirectional innominate osteotomy. However, if the hip is not congruent acetabular coverage may be improved by a shelf operation or by a Chiari osteotomy.

An outline of recommended treatment is shown in Table 68.2.

Factors to be considered while planning treatment of sequelae of Perthes' disease

Recommended treatment for sequelae of Perthes' disease

Table 68.2 ● Treatment for the sequelae of Perthes' disease

INDICATIONS				
Healing not complete OR Healed disease + Pain present on abduction + Spherical head + Hip congruent in adduction + Demonstrable hinge abduction ⇩ Valgus intertrochanteric osteotomy	Healed disease + No pain + Large spherical femoral head with uncovering + Hip congruent ⇩ Innominate osteotomy OR Shelf operation OR Acetabular augmentation to improve femoral head coverage	Healed disease + No pain + Large flattened femoral head with uncovering + Hip not congruent ⇩ Shelf operation OR OR Chiari osteotomy to improve femoral head coverage	Healed disease + No pain + Spherical head + Hip congruent + Coxa breva (short neck) + Trochanteric overgrowth with Trendelenburg gait ⇩ Trochanteric advancement	Healed disease + Pain + Irregular femoral head + Hip not congruent + Arthritic changes ⇩ Arthrodesis
TREATMENT				

References

1. Catterall A. *Legg-Calve-Perthes' Disease*. Edinburgh: Churchill Livingstone, 1982: 60–1.
2. Joseph B, Mulpuri K, Verghese G. Perthes' disease in the adolescent. *J Bone Joint Surg Br* 2001; **83**: 715–20.
3. Joseph B, Varghese G, Mulpuri K, Rao NLK, Nair NS. The natural evolution of Perthes' disease: a study of 610 children under 12 years of age at disease onset. *J Pediatr Orthop* 2003; **23**: 590–600.
4. Green NE, Beuchamp RD, Griffin PP. Epiphyseal extrusion as a prognostic index in Legg-Calve-Perthes disease. *J Bone Joint Surg Am* 1981; **63**: 9000–5.
5. Bowen JR, Foster BK, Hartzell CR. Legg-Calve-Perthes disease. *Clin Orthop Relat Res* 1984; **185**: 97–108.
6. Bajaj HN, Joseph B, Chacko V. Radiological changes in late untreated Perthes' disease. *Ind J Radiol Imaging* 1988; **42**: 385–8.
7. Stulberg SD, Cooperman DR, Wallensten R. The natural history of Legg-Calve-Perthes' disease. *J Bone Joint Surg Am* 1981; **63**: 1095–1108.
8. Joseph B, Nair NS, Rao NLK, Mulpuri K, Varghese G. Optimal timing for containment surgery for Perthes' disease. *J Pediatr Orthop* 2003; **23**: 601–6.
9. Joseph B, Srinivas G, Thomas R. Management of Perthes' disease of late onset in southern India: the evaluation of a surgical method. *J Bone Joint Surg Br* 1996; **78**: 625–30.
10. Joseph B, Rao N, Mulpuri K, Varghese G, Nair S. How does a femoral varus osteotomy alter the natural evolution of Perthes' disease? *J Pediatr Orthop B* 2005; **14**: 10–15.
11. Daly K, Bruce C, Catterall A. Lateral shelf acetabuloplasty in Perthes' disease: a review at the end of growth. *J Bone Joint Surg Br* 1999; **81**: 380–4.
12. Salter RB. The present status of surgical treatment for Legg-Perthes' disease. *J Bone Joint Surg Am* 1984; **66**: 961–6.
13. Matan AJ, Stevens PM, Smith JT, Santora SD. Combination trochanteric arrest and intertrochanteric osteotomy for Perthes' disease. *J Pediatr Orthop* 1996; **16**: 10–14.
14. Chacko V, Joseph B, Seetharam B. Perthes' disease in south India. *Clin Orthop Relat Res* 1986; **209**: 95–9.
15. Muirhead-Allwood W, Catterall A. The treatment of Perthes' disease: the results of a trial of management. *J Bone Joint Surg Br* 1982; **64**: 282–5.
16. Quain S, Catterall A. Hinge abduction of the hip. Diagnosis and treatment. *J Bone Joint Surg Br* 1986; **68**: 61–4.
17. Segev E, Ezra E, Weintroub S, Yaniv M. Treatment of severe late onset Perthes disease by soft tissue release and articulated hip distraction: early results. *J Pediatr Orthop B* 2004; **13**: 158–65.
18. Iobst CA, Stanitski CL. Hip arthrodesis revisited. *J Pediatr Orthop* 2001; **21**: 130–4.
19. Rowe SM, Jung ST, Cheon SY *et al.* Outcome of cheilectomy in Legg-Calve-Perthes disease – minimum 25-year follow-up of five patients. *J Pediatr Orthop* 2006; **26**: 204–10.
20. Schneidmueller D, Carstens C, Thomsen M. Surgical treatment of overgrowth of the greater trochanter in children and adolescents. *J Pediatr Orthop* 2006; **26**: 486–90.

Slipped capital femoral epiphysis

Randall Loder

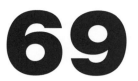

69

Introduction

Slipped capital femoral epiphysis (SCFE) is an anterior, superior and external rotational displacement of the proximal femoral metaphysis relative to the fixed epiphysis which occurs through the physis during the prepubescent and adolescent growth spurt. The average age of presentation in boys is 13 years and in girls 12 years. It is deemed to be a common cause of degenerative hip disease in adult life. It is slightly more common in boys than girls and tends to occur in children who are obese (>95th percentile weight for age, or BMI >25 kg/m^2). The natural history is one of gradual increase in the SCFE as time passes and, as the severity of the SCFE increases, so does the incidence of degenerative hip disease later in life.[1] Thus early diagnosis and appropriate intervention when the slip is less severe is desirable.

Slipped capital femoral epiphysis may occur without any obvious underlying disease (idiopathic SCFE) or may be associated with underlying endocrine abnormality or renal failure.

Slipped capital femoral epiphysis can be classified as stable (able to walk with or without crutches) and unstable (unable to walk, with or without crutches).[2] The vast majority of SCFEs are stable (around 95 percent); unstable SCFEs are plagued by a markedly increased incidence of avascular necrosis (AVN) which is devastating to the hips in these young people.

Problems of management

Progression of slip

If untreated, the slip can progress[3] and a small proportion of unstable SCFEs can progress despite seemingly adequate treatment.

Risk of AVN

Unstable SCFE inherently has a high risk of AVN (Figure 69.1) and attempts at forceful reduction can increase this risk. When AVN develops, there are many approaches to the problem, none of which offer spectacular results.

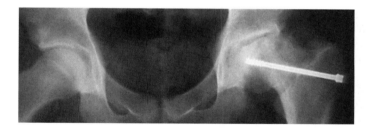

Figure 69.1 ● Avascular necrosis in a 17-year-old boy who had sustained an unstable slipped capital femoral epiphysis at age 13 years.

Risk of chondrolysis

Another serious complication of SCFE is chondrolysis (Figure 69.2) which is a poorly understood phenomenon.[4] It can occur in untreated SCFEs, is more frequent in more severe SCFEs, and is increased if there is permanent penetration of the joint with internal fixation devices. The quoted incidence is 5–7 percent. The natural history of chondrolysis follows that of two major paths: some children will undergo a late reconstitution of the joint space to a certain degree while others will undergo nearly complete ankylosis, often in a bad position.

Late degenerative arthritis of the hip

Slipped capital femoral epiphysis is felt to be a common cause of degenerative hip disease in adult life. As the severity of the SCFE increases so does the incidence of degenerative hip disease later in life; thus diagnosis at a lesser degree of SCFE is desirable.

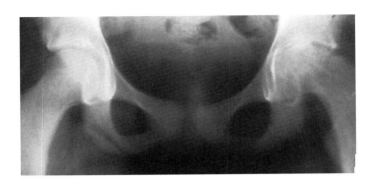

Figure 69.2 ● Chondrolysis in a 13-year-old girl with a left slipped capital femoral epiphysis that had been previously treated by screw fixation in which there was joint penetration.

Aims of treatment

- Halt progression of the SCFE
  This can be achieved by either ensuring stable fixation of the epiphysis or by facilitating early fusion of the physis.
- Minimize the risk of AVN
  Although this may not be within the control of the surgeon, some measures may help to reduce the risk of AVN. Choosing surgical procedures that have a low risk of producing AVN and avoiding forceful manipulation to achieve reduction of the slip are two such measures.
- Minimize the risk of chondrolysis
  Care should be taken to avoid penetration of the joint by the implant.
- Minimize the risk of degenerative arthritis
  Restoring the anatomy of the proximal femur to as near normal as possible theoretically reduces the risk of degenerative arthritis if performed without complications.

Treatment options

In situ fixation

In situ fixation involves placement of a single cannulated screw in the centre of the epiphysis in both anteroposterior (AP) and lateral views, and gives excellent results in stopping SCFE progression with minimal risk of chondrolysis.[5] Technically it is performed on a fracture table with movement of the C-arm from AP to lateral views, rather than moving the limb. Skin lines are made using the technique of Canale. At the intersection of the lines, a small incision is made. A guide pin is inserted into the centre of the epiphysis on both AP and lateral views. A cannulated screw is inserted over this guide pin, coming no closer than 0.5–1 cm to the subchondral bone (Figure 69.3).

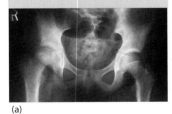
(a)

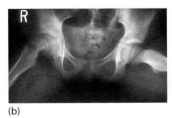
(b)

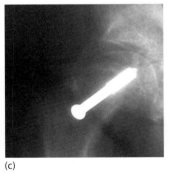
(c)

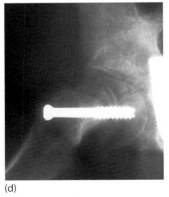
(d)

Figure 69.3 ● The anteroposterior (AP) **(a)** and frog lateral radiographs **(b)** of a child with a right slipped capital femoral epiphysis (SCFE). Both AP and lateral radiographs of both hips must be obtained whenever evaluating a child with a stable SCFE, so as not to miss an SCFE on the opposite side that might be asymptomatic. Post-operative radiographs demonstrate the presence of a single cannulated screw in the centre of the epiphysis on both AP **(c)** and lateral **(d)** projections, crossing the physis and 1 cm from the subchondral bone.

Reduction and fixation

The more severe degrees of unstable SCFEs may be reduced by gentle repositioning and internally fixed with cannulated screws.

Bone graft epiphyseodesis

Bone graft epiphyseodesis techniques can be either open or minimally invasive. The concept is to place a bone graft across the physis which acts as both an internal fixation device and also incites a rapid physeal closure (Figure 69.4), thus preventing the SCFE from progressing.[6]

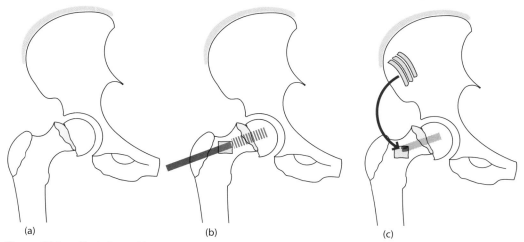

Figure 69.4 ● Technique of bone graft epiphyseodesis for slipped capital femoral epiphysis **(a)**. A thick drill is passed across the physeal plate **(b)**. Iliac bone graft is then placed across the physis in the hole created by the drill **(c)**.

Spica cast application

Spica cast immobilization will typically stop SCFE progression while in the cast, but often progression again ensues once the cast has been removed. It also treats the opposite hip, and may result in a lower incidence of bilaterality compared to *in situ* fixation. It is associated with an extremely high incidence of chondrolysis and has thus been abandoned by most surgeons.

Osteotomy

When children present with stable, severe SCFEs >50 or 60°, some authors recommend proceeding with osteotomy as the initial treatment. Osteotomy will reposition the epiphysis relative to the more distal femur. Osteotomy locations are at the physis (cuneiform) (Figure 69.5), basilar neck and intertrochanteric or subtrochanteric.[7] Although osteotomy at the physeal level makes the most orthopaedic and mechanical sense, the incidence of AVN increases as the osteotomy approaches the physis. The potential problem with more distal osteotomies (e.g. intertrochanteric) is that they are compensatory and may pose problems for later total hip arthroplasty owing to a deformed femur. When planning osteotomy, the size of the bone and the availability of appropriate internal fixation implants are paramount. Not having the appropriate size and type of implants gives poor results as these children are typically large and require rigid fixation devices. Templating is strongly encouraged before osteotomy.

The factors that need to be considered while planning treatment are stability of the SCFE (stable or unstable) the aetiology of the slip, severity of the slip, the age of the child, and the state of the proximal femoral physis. These factors are predictive of (1) risk of degenerative joint disease later in adult life, (2) risk of the epiphysis of the opposite hip also slipping, (3) risk of complications (AVN and chondrolysis) and (4) potential for remodelling and/or the need for later reconstructive osteotomy.

Stability of the slip

The first and foremost factor to be considered is the stability of the SCFE. Stability of the SCFE is very important in imparting prognosis with regard to the risk of AVN and subsequent hip deterioration. Children with unstable SCFE should be treated urgently, admitted upon diagnosis, placed on complete bed rest, and internal fixation within the following day. Treating unstable SCFE as an emergency should hopefully decrease the risk of AVN.[8] However, the patient and parents must

Factors to be taken into consideration while planning treatment

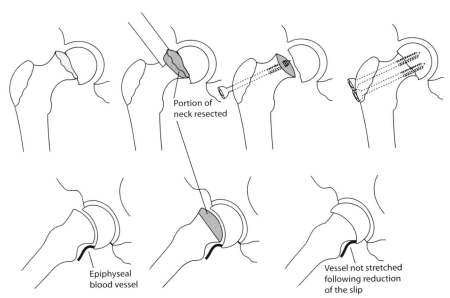

Figure 69.5 ● Diagram showing an osteotomy of the neck of the femur performed to reduce a slipped capital femoral epiphysis.

be counselled regarding the potentially negative outcome in unstable slips despite early treatment. Similarly, fixation of a stable SCFE is not an elective procedure, as there are many cases of children who have tripped or fallen with a stable SCFE becoming unstable and resulting in AVN.

Aetiology of the slip

The aetiology of the slip has a bearing on the chances of bilateral involvement. The incidence of bilaterality in children with idiopathic SCFE ranges from 15 to 60 percent, and is higher if a child presents at a younger age with the index SCFE. The incidence of bilaterality in children with underlying metabolic disorders is much higher, and may approach 100 percent. If the risk of bilaterality is high, then the physician must weigh the risk/benefit ratio of prophylactic treatment for the opposite hip when presented with a child with a newly diagnosed unilateral SCFE.[9]

Severity of the slip

Severity of the SCFE in the stable SCFE directly correlates with the adult risk of degenerative hip disease.[1] Slipped capital femoral epiphysis can be quantified by the epiphyseal–shaft angle as measured on the frog lateral radiograph[10] (Figure 69.6). Those with a SCFE angle <30° are considered mild, 30–50° moderate and >50° severe. The natural history of children with SCFE is gradual deterioration into degenerative hip disease in adult life; this deterioration is more rapid in the more severe SCFEs.

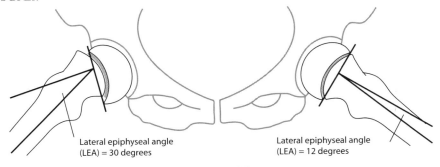

Slip angle : 30 − 12 = 18 degrees

Figure 69.6 ● Method of determining slipped capital femoral epiphysis (SCFE) severity using the lateral epiphyseal-shaft angle as described by Southwick.[10] On both hips, seen in the frog lateral view, three lines are drawn: a line connecting the anterior and posterior tips of the epiphysis; a perpendicular to the epiphyseal line and a line along the long axis of the femoral shaft. The difference between the normal and SCFE side lateral epiphyseal angle (LEA) is the slip angle (LEA slip − LEA normal), which is a measure of the severity of the slip.

Age of the child

If the child is young (<10 years of age) prophylactic fixation of the opposite hip should be strongly considered on account of a higher risk of bilateral involvement.[11]

In younger children with SCFE, remodelling after fixation *in situ* may occur. However, this is controversial, with diverse opinions regarding the potential for remodelling.

State of the capital femoral physis

If a child presents with a severe deformity and the proximal femoral physis is nearly closed, then there is no potential for remodelling. This then raises the question of treatment: fixation *in situ* or a redirectional osteotomy. Redirectional osteotomy in a child with a severe SCFE improves the arc of motion, position of the limb in space, and increases the percentage of articular cartilage of the femoral head in contact with the acetabulum. It seems logical that this would therefore decrease the risk of degenerative joint disease and prolong the longevity of the hip. This, however, remains to be seen as long-term follow-up of children with osteotomy using modern techniques of surgery and fixation is not yet available.

Recommended treatment

The outline of recommended management of SCFE in various situations is given in Table 69.1 and summarized below.

Table 69.1 ● Outline of treatment of slipped capital femoral epiphysis

INDICATIONS			
Stable + Idiopathic SCFE + Slip of any degree of severity + In an adolescent	Stable + Idiopathic SCFE + Severe slip + In an adolescent + Parents opt for correction of the malalignment	Stable + Idiopathic SCFE + Slip of any degree of severity + Child <10 years of age OR SCFE with underlying metabolic or endocrine dysfunction	Unstable slip
⇩	⇩	⇩	⇩
In situ fixation with a single cannulated centrally placed screw	*In situ* fixation with a single cannulated centrally placed screw + Intertrochanteric osteotomy after physeal closure	*In situ* fixation with a single cannulated centrally placed screw + Prophylactic fixation of the uninvolved hip	Immediate bed rest + Traction + Gentle reduction of slip + Emergent fixation within 24 hours with two cannulated screws + Joint decompression + Delayed weight-bearing
TREATMENT			

Stable SCFE

If the physis is open, *in situ* fixation is recommended for all SCFEs in an urgent fashion. A single, centrally placed cannulated screw is used for fixation. After physeal closure, and in a more leisurely fashion, the risk/benefits of osteotomy can be discussed with the family and carried out if desired by all involved. If the family opts for osteotomy, an intertrochanteric osteotomy of Müller with rigid AO blade plate fixation is performed (Figure 69.7).

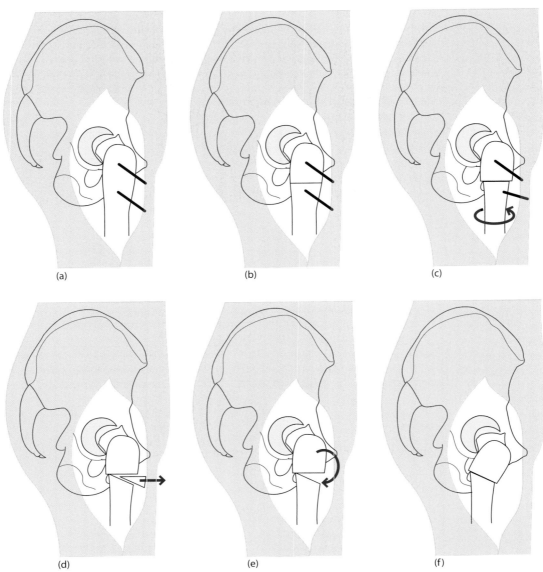

(a) (b) (c)

(d) (e) (f)

Figure 69.7 ● Technique of performing flexion-internal rotation intertrochanteric osteotomy as described by Mueller for the treatment of slipped capital femoral epiphysis.

Unstable SCFE

The author recommends gentle repositioning with one or two cannulated screws for fixation, mini-arthrotomy for joint decompression and guarded activity until adequate callus is seen prior to weight-bearing (Figure 69.8).

Rationale of treatment suggested

Stable SCFE

Why in situ fixation? Why a single screw?
The results with *in situ* fixation using a single, centrally placed cannulated screw are excellent, with minimal morbidity, excellent stabilization of the SCFE with minimal progression and an extremely low risk of AVN and chondrolysis.

Why is routine osteotomy not advocated?
The long-term improvement in the natural history of children with severe SCFEs treated by modern techniques of osteotomy is still unknown, and thus osteotomy is not yet routinely recommended for all severe SCFEs.

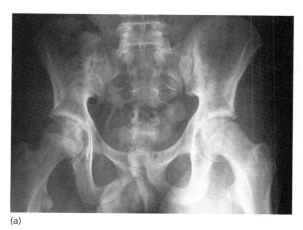
(a)

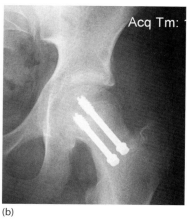
(b)

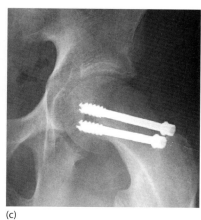
(c)

Figure 69.8 ● The radiograph of a 14-year-old boy with an unstable left slipped capital femoral epiphysis **(a)**. He was treated with emergent gentle repositioning, internal fixation with two cannulated screws and mini-arthrotomy for joint decompression. Post-operative anteroposterior **(b)** and lateral radiographs **(c)**.

If an osteotomy is performed, why at the intertrochanteric level?
An osteotomy at the intertrochanteric level carries an extremely low risk of AVN.

Why is bone graft epiphyseodesis not preferred?
Bone graft epiphyseodesis is associated with a higher incidence of SCFE progression compared to *in situ* fixation, and when performed open, results in increased morbidity. For that reason most physicians today will perform *in situ* fixation and not bone graft epiphyseodesis.

Why is routine prophylactic fixation of the opposite hip not recommended?
The role of prophylactic fixation is controversial and must be considered on an individual basis. Factors that must be weighed are the aetiology of the SCFE, age of the child, ability/compliant nature of the patient and family to follow through on symptoms in the opposite hip, and the ability of the family to follow through on routine return visits.

Unstable SCFE

Why is it imperative that emergent surgery be done?

Why is reduction recommended?

Why are two screws used?

Why is joint decompression by a mini-arthrotomy advocated?
To minimize the potential risk of AVN, newer data seem to suggest that developing gentle repositioning, fixation and joint decompression may offer the best outcome,[8] hence this is the present recommended treatment. However, the numbers in any series are quite small, and there is still considerable controversy as to the exact timing of fixation, number of fixation devices (e.g. one or more cannulated screws), exact role of arthrotomy or joint decompression, role of reduction, and if reduction is performed, the type (e.g. open or gentle closed repositioning), and magnitude of reduction (e.g. strive for complete reduction or simply enough to permit screw fixation).

References

1. Carney BT, Weinstein SW, Noble J. Long-term follow-up of slipped capital femoral epiphysis. *J Bone Joint Surg Am* 1991; **73**: 667–74.
2. Loder RT, Richards BS, Shapiro PS, Reznick LR, Aronson DD. Acute slipped capital femoral epiphysis: the importance of physeal stability. *J Bone Joint Surg Am* 1993; **75**: 1134–40.
3. Carney BT, Weinstein SL. Natural history of untreated chronic slipped capital femoral epiphysis. *Clin Orthop Relat Res* 1996; **322**: 43–7.
4. Lubicky JP. Chondrolysis and avascular necrosis: complications of slipped capital femoral epiphysis. *J Pediatr Orthop B* 1996; **5**: 162–77.
5. Aronson DD, Carlson WE. Slipped capital femoral epiphysis: a prospective study of fixation with a single screw. *J Bone Joint Surg Am* 1992; **74**: 810–19.

6. Weiner DS, Weiner S, Melby A, Hoyt Jr WH. A 30-year experience with bone graft epiphysiodesis in the treatment of slipped capital femoral epiphysis. *J Pediatr Orthop* 1984; **4**: 145–52.

7. Crawford AH. Role of osteotomy in the treatment of slipped capital femoral epiphysis. *J Pediatr Orthop B* 1996; **5**: 102–9.

8. Gordon JE, Abrahams MS, Dobbs MB, Luhmann SJ, Schoenecker PL. Early reduction, arthrotomy, and cannulated screw fixation in unstable slipped capital femoral epiphysis treatment. *J Pediatr Orthop* 2002; **22**: 352–8.

9. Kocher MS, Bishop JA, Hresko MT *et al.* Prophylactic pinning of the contralateral hip after unilateral slipped capital femoral epiphysis. *J Bone Joint Surg Am* 2004; **86**: 2658–65.

10. Southwick WO. Osteotomy through the lesser trochanter for slipped capital femoral epiphysis. *J Bone Joint Surg Am* 1967; **49**: 807–35.

11. Segal LS, Davidson RS, Robertson WWJ, Drummond DS. Growth disturbance after pinning of juvenile slipped capital femoral epiphysis. *J Pediatr Orthop* 1991; **11**: 631–7.

Physeal bars represent an area of physeal growth arrest with subsequent bony bar formation across a portion of the physis. The bars result in a tether to normal longitudinal bone growth and can result in angular deformity, limb length discrepancy, or both.[1] They usually occur as the result of trauma (Figure 70.1). They may also occur due to sepsis (osteomyelitis, purpura fulminans and meningococcaemia), neoplasia, environmental exposure (e.g. thermal and electrical burns, frostbite), congenital deformities (e.g. infantile tibia vara) and sequelae to medical treatment (e.g. physeal arrest in developmental hip dysplasia, cruciate ligament reconstruction, internal fixation in physeal fractures, irradiation for malignancy, inadvertent intravenous extravasation).

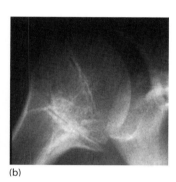

Figure 70.1 ● A proximal humeral epiphyseal injury at the age of six years and three months **(a)** that resulted in a peripheral lateral physeal arrest. The appearance at age 11 years 10 months **(b)**.

(a)   (b)

Physeal bars can be peripheral, central or linear (Figure 70.2); the location and the size of the bar determines the effect on normal growth of the physis.

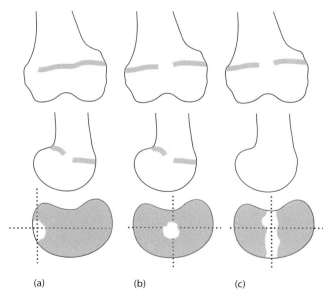

Figure 70.2 ● Various locations of physeal bars: peripheral **(a)**, central **(b)** and linear **(c)**.The appearance of sagittal sections (centre row) and coronal sections (top row) through the bars.

(a)   (b)   (c)

Cessation of linear growth

Once a physeal bar develops, that region of the physis cannot contribute to linear growth of the bone. However, whether this will affect the overall growth at the physis with resultant growth arrest will depend on the size and location of the bar and on the amount of growth remaining in the physis. The amount of growth is unique to each of the long bone physes and the amount of growth contributed to each physis must be known.[2–7]

Angular deformity

When there is significant remaining growth a physeal bar will result in an angular deformity if peripherally located. Central bars usually result in a tenting of the articular surface, with varying amounts of angular deformity, if the bar is eccentrically located.

Limb length discrepancy

A large centrally placed bar in a child who has significant growth remaining will result in considerable shortening of the limb. If the limb length discrepancy is minimal at diagnosis, then a successful physeal bar resection will not require limb equalization procedures (e.g. contralateral epiphyseodesis, unilateral limb lengthening) assuming that resumption of normal longitudinal growth occurs after bar resection. However, that does not always occur, and there is often incomplete resumption of growth as well as late deceleration or premature cessation of growth.

Determining the size and location of the bar

The size of the bar can be determined by many different means, depending upon the technology available. This author prefers magnetic resonance imaging (MRI) evaluation with calculation of the physeal bar area using specific software available on many MRI scanners.[8,9] If this is not available, then a helical computed tomography scan with appropriate reconstructions into both coronal and sagittal reconstructions or traditional anteroposterior and lateral tomograms can be used, and the bar size and location plotted on a physeal bar map.[10]

Aims of treatment

- Equalization of limb length
  If the physeal bar has resulted in limb length inequality this should be corrected. The ideal limb length discrepancy at skeletal maturity is within 2 cm; in the upper extremity this can be slightly more.
- Correction of angular deformity
  Angular deformities that result from a laterally placed physeal bar also need to be addressed. In the lower extremity significant pathologic angular deformity at skeletal maturity (especially around the knee) is likely to result in early degenerative joint disease.
- Ablation or resumption of growth
  If there is significant growth remaining in a child with a physeal bar, resumption of growth is a major aim of treatment. In the child with minimal growth remaining, complete growth ablation instead may be the goal of treatment.

Treatment options

Observation

This is selected if the remaining growth is minimal and if the bar is not likely to contribute to significant angular deformity or limb length discrepancy.

Epiphyseodesis

If the physeal bar involves over 25–50 percent of the physeal area, there is no associated angular deformity, and there is between 2 and 4 cm of lower extremity limb length discrepancy projected at skeletal maturity, then an epiphyseodesis of the corresponding contralateral physis is recommended.[4,11,12] On occasion, epiphyseodesis of the remaining open physis on the affected side is also necessary. Rarely, the child's projected height at skeletal maturity is short enough that the parents may not wish to lose the 2–4 cm of height that will result from an epiphyseodesis and may then elect for limb lengthening.

Physeal bar resection with spacer interposition

The Langenskiöld procedure[13–15] is indicated when the physeal bar is <50 percent of the cross-sectional area and when there is >2 cm of growth remaining in the involved physis. The underlying concept is to remove the bony tether between the metaphysis and physis, in the hope that normal longitudinal bone growth will resume from the remaining physis assumed to be normal and healthy. After resection, the void must be filled with a spacer (a bone growth retardant) to prevent reformation of the bony bar. The spacers used are fat and methylmethacrylate cement.

The choice of spacer depends upon the surgeon's preference and mechanical stability (i.e. a small bar resection is easily filled with fat, a large resection with significant loss of metaphyseal bone which will lead to structural weakness is better filled with methylmethacrylate cement).[16,17] One theoretical advantage of autogenous fat is that the 'spacer' can grow and hypertrophy with the resumption of longitudinal bone growth. After resection, bony markers must be placed in both the epiphysis and metaphysis so that growth can be measured in order to monitor the success or failure of the resection. Peripheral bars are simpler to resect due to easier surgical approach and exposure (Figure 70.3 and 70.4). Central bars require large amounts of metaphyseal bone resection with innovative visualization techniques (small dental mirrors or arthroscopes)[18,19] (Figure 70.5). Even when technically well performed, the results of physeal bar resection are often disappointing.[20]

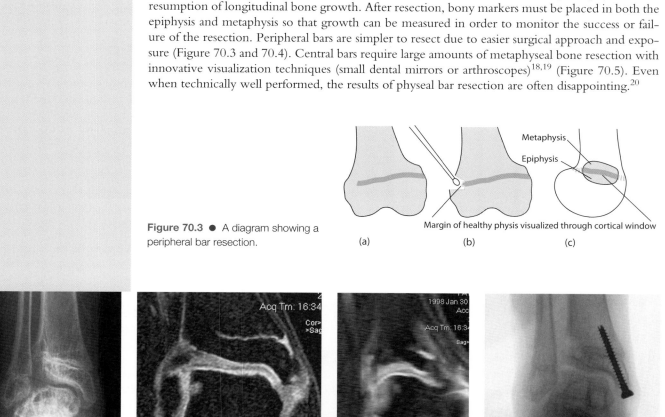

Figure 70.3 ● A diagram showing a peripheral bar resection.

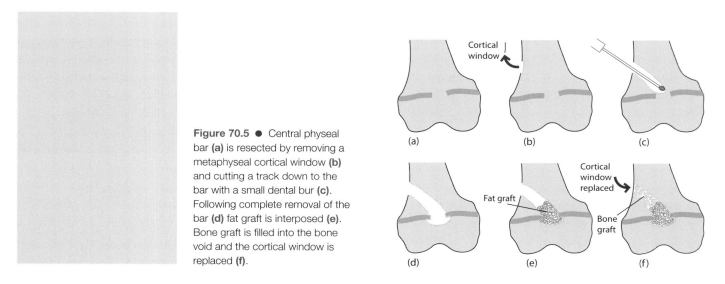

Figure 70.4 ● This lateral distal tibial physeal bar occurred in a girl with fulminant sepsis, purpura fulminans, multiorgan failure and who was on extracorporeal membrane oxygenation life support for a prolonged time. The anteroposterior radiograph at the age of eight years and nine months **(a)**, the magnetic resonance scans **(b,c)**. Appearance after bar resection, autogenous buttock fat graft interposition and medial tibial screw hemiepiphyseodesis **(d)**.

Figure 70.5 ● Central physeal bar **(a)** is resected by removing a metaphyseal cortical window **(b)** and cutting a track down to the bar with a small dental bur **(c)**. Following complete removal of the bar **(d)** fat graft is interposed **(e)**. Bone graft is filled into the bone void and the cortical window is replaced **(f)**.

Corrective osteotomy with or without physeal bar resection or epiphyseodesis

In patients with significant angular deformity (>5–10°) a corrective osteotomy is also necessary; an opening wedge osteotomy (if safe considering skin and neurovascular issues) will assist in improving a mild limb length discrepancy.[21] In those with a moderate limb length discrepancy at skeletal maturity, a contralateral epiphyseodesis is also necessary (Figures 70.6 and 70.7).

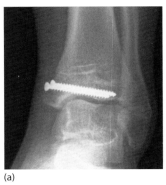
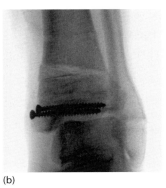

(a)   (b)

Figure 70.6 ● Corrective osteotomy without physeal bar resection in a skeletally mature 16-year-old boy who had sustained a Salter-Harris III fracture of the distal tibia at age 13 treated with open reduction and internal fixation. The fracture healed uneventfully, but a medial physeal growth arrest with bony bar and subsequent varus deformity occurred. The limb length discrepancy was only 1 cm, the ankle was in varus with complete closure of the distal tibial physis **(a)**. Appearance of the ankle after opening wedge osteotomy with bone graft interposition and ipsilateral distal fibular epiphyseodesis **(b)**. The epiphyseal screws were embedded in bone and could not be removed.

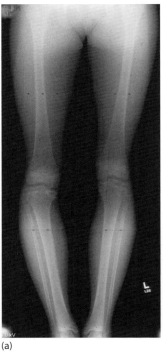
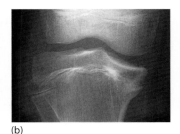
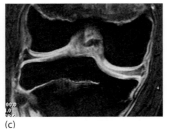

(a)   (b)   (c)

Figure 70.7 ● This 13-year-old cheerleader presented with a gradually progressive genu varus deformity on the right, with no significant history of trauma other than repetitive jumping from her cheerleading. The right lower extremity was 1 cm shorter than the left. **(a)** A standing long leg radiograph demonstrating the varus deformity. **(b)** An anteroposterior knee radiograph demonstrating the medial tibial physeal bar. **(c)** Magnetic resonance scan confirming the physeal bar. Owing to less than 2 cm of remaining longitudinal growth in the remaining portion of the proximal tibial physis, physeal bar resection was not performed. Instead, epiphyseodesis of the remainder of the proximal tibial physis with a concomitant proximal tibial osteotomy and contralateral proximal tibial epiphyseodesis was performed. The normal mechanical axis alignment was restored and at skeletal maturity the leg length discrepancy was negligible.

Limb lengthening with or without physeal bar resection or epiphyseodesis

In patients with a major limb length discrepancy projected at skeletal maturity, physeal bar resection will again be inadequate, and an ipsilateral limb lengthening with or without a contralateral epiphyseodesis is selected.

Aetiology of the physeal bar

This is important since physeal bars due to sepsis may be associated with several bars in the same extremity. Also, the results of bar resection tend to be better for those that are the result of a traumatic event rather than those from sepsis, tumour or irradiation. It is important to know if there are other physeal arrests in the same extremity, as the results of physeal bar resection at multiple locations are quite poor.

How much remaining growth is there in the involved physis?

This is very important to know. A simple way is to determine if there is less than two years of remaining growth;[2–7] if so, then many surgeons favour terminating the remaining growth and dealing with the limb length difference with an epiphyseodesis of the opposite extremity or a lengthening osteotomy of the involved limb if a concomitant angular deformity is present. The likelihood of growth resumption after bar resection must also be taken into account.

Which physis is involved?

It is important to know which physis is involved (e.g. distal humerus, distal femur, etc.) and the amount of growth contributed from each physis to the overall length of the bone must be kept in mind. Those physes with minimal contribution to longitudinal growth of the involved bone (e.g. distal humerus) typically result in angular deformities with minimal limb length discrepancy. Those physes with significant contribution to longitudinal growth (e.g. distal femur) will not only often have an angular deformity but a significant limb length inequality at skeletal maturity if the physeal arrest develops when there is significant remaining growth.

Size of the physeal bar

This is very important to know so that a decision regarding bar resection can be made. The exact amount of bar that can be successfully resected with resumption of normal longitudinal growth is debatable, but it is a fair statement that the smaller the bar, the greater the chance of successful growth restoration after resection. Bars involving >50 percent of the physeal area should not even be considered for resection, and arrests involving >25 percent of the physeal area are unlikely to resume normal longitudinal growth after resection.

Location of the physeal bar

The surgical approach varies depending upon the location of the bar. Peripheral bars are usually easily accessible; central or linear bars are more problematic and require more invasive resection methods, which may influence the selected treatment (i.e. epiphyseodesis with limb lengthening being recommended rather than bar resection).

Associated angular deformity

If there is a significant angular deformity associated with the bar, it is probable that bar resection will not completely correct it. A corrective osteotomy, either at the same time or at a later date, is likely to be needed. As a usual rule, deformities in the plane of motion of the joint correct better than those not in the plane of motion. It is for this reason (among others) that many surgeons will recommend physeal bar resection and then perform angular corrective osteotomy at a later date. This allows for the success of the bar resection to become apparent as well as healing/filling in of the metaphyseal bone removed during the bar resection; good bone stock in that area is necessary in order to perform the osteotomy as well as to obtain fixation.

Associated limb length discrepancy

If there is or will be a significant limb length discrepancy (>2 cm), resection alone will be inadequate in restoring limb length equality. Ipsilateral limb lengthening and/or contralateral epiphyseodesis is likely to be necessary.

Recommended treatment

Physeal bar resection alone is indicated when the physeal bar size is <50 percent of the cross-sectional area and there is significant remaining growth (2 cm or more in this author's opinion).

If there is an angular deformity of >5–10° an osteotomy will also be necessary. This can either be performed at the time of the bar resection or as a secondary procedure. The timing of the osteotomy is often determined by mechanical factors – will there be enough bone left after the resection to permit the necessary fixation to hold the osteotomy in the appropriate position until osteotomy union or not?

If the projected limb length discrepancy at skeletal maturity is between 2 and 4 cm, then a contralateral epiphyseodesis is performed at the appropriate time (determined using standard epiphyseodesis guidelines – although the amount of growth that will occur after physeal bar resection can be variable and can make this determination even more of a 'guesstimate' than in standard epiphyseodesis timing situations).

If the projected limb length discrepancy at skeletal maturity is >4 or 5 cm, then a limb lengthening will often be necessary.

If there are multiple unilateral physeal bars at an early age, then limb reconstruction using guidelines for congenital limb deformities is recommended (e.g. analogous to proximal femoral focal deficiency).

The outline of treatment is summarized in Table 70.1.

Table 70.1 ● Outline of treatment of a physeal bar

INDICATIONS					
Area of bar <25% + <2 cm remaining growth + No angular deformity	Area of bar <25% + 2–4 cm remaining growth OR projected limb length discrepancy + No angular deformity	Area of bar <25% + 2–4 cm remaining growth OR projected limb length discrepancy + Angular deformity present	Area of bar <25% + >4 cm remaining growth OR projected limb length discrepancy + Angular deformity present	Area of bar 25–50%	Area of bar 50%
⇩	⇩	⇩	⇩	⇩	⇩
Complete epiphyseodesis of remainder of physis	Physeal bar resection with spacer interposition + Contralateral epiphyseodesis	Physeal bar resection with spacer interposition + Contralateral epiphyseodesis + Corrective osteotomy (either simultaneously or later)	Physeal bar resection with spacer interposition + Contralateral epiphyseodesis + Limb lengthening + Corrective osteotomy (either simultaneously or later)	Complete epiphyseodesis of involved epiphysis + Manage limb length inequality (as outlined in Chapters 42–48)	Follow guideline for 25–50% (but outcomes are guarded) more complex reconstructions are likely to be necessary that include complete epiphyseodesis, contralateral epiphyseodesis limb lengthening and angular deformity correction
TREATMENT					

Rationale of treatment suggested

Why perform an epiphyseodesis if there is <2 cm remaining growth?
Minimal limb length inequalities are easily treated with the very simple percutaneous epiphyseodesis with very predictable results, compared to the more technically difficult and less predictable outcomes with physeal bar resections.

Why is it necessary to know the size of the physeal bar and the location of the bar?
Bars with <25 percent physeal surface area have a reasonable success rate from resection; those larger than that have a very poor success rate from resection and are better treated with other methods (e.g. completion of epiphyseodesis and limb lengthening). The anatomic location of the

bar (e.g. peripheral, central, linear) is necessary in order to plan the surgical approach to any bar resection.

Why is it necessary to perform an angular corrective osteotomy after bar resection?
An angular deformity of >5–10° is unlikely to respond and remodel even with a successful physeal bar resection that restores normal longitudinal bone growth.

References

1. Khoshhal KI, Kiefer GN. Physeal bridge resection. *J Am Acad Orthop Surg* 2005; **13**: 47–58.
2. Paley D, Bhave A, Herzenberg JE, Bowen JR. Multiplier method for predicting limb length discrepancy. *J Bone Joint Surg Am* 2000; **82**: 1432–46.
3. Aguilar JA, Paley D, Paley J *et al.* Clinical validation of the multiplier method for predicting limb length at maturity, part I. *J Pediatr Orthop* 2005; **25**: 186–91.
4. Aguilar JA, Paley D, Paley J *et al.* Clinical validation of the multiplier method for predicting limb length discrepancy and outcome of epiphyseodesis, part II. *J Pediatr Orthop* 2005; **25**: 192–6.
5. Anderson M, Green WT, Messner MB. Growth and predictions of growth in the lower extremities. *J Bone Joint Surg Am* 1963; **45**: 1–14.
6. Anderson M, Messner MB, Green WT. Distribution of lengths of the normal femur and tibia in children from one to eighteen years of age. *J Bone Joint Surg Am* 1964; **46**: 1197–202.
7. Moseley CF. A straight line graph for leg length discrepancies. *Clin Orthop Relat Res* 1978; **136**: 33–40.
8. Ecklund K. Magnetic resonance imaging of pediatric musculoskeletal trauma. *Top Magn Reson Imaging* 2002; **13**: 203–18.
9. Lohman M, Kivisaari A, Vehmas T *et al.* MRI in the assessment of growth arrest. *Pediatr Radiol* 2002; **32**: 41–5.
10. Carlson WO, Wenger DR. A mapping method to prepare for surgical excision of a partial physeal arrest. *J Pediatr Orthop* 1984; **4**: 232–8.
11. Horton GA, Olney BW. Epiphyseodesis of the lower extremity: results of the percutaneous technique. *J Pediatr Orthop* 1996; **16**: 180–2.
12. Gabriel KR, Crawford AH, Roy DR, True MS, Sauntry S. Percutaneous epiphyseodesis. *J Pediatr Orthop* 1994; **14**: 358–62.
13. Langenskiöld A. An operation for partial closure of an epiphyseal plate in children, and its experimental basis. *J Bone Joint Surg Br* 1975; **57**: 325–30.
14. Broughton NS, Dickens DRV, Cole WG, Menelaus MB. Epiphyseolysis for partial growth plate arrest. Results after four years or at maturity. *J Bone Joint Surg Br* 1989; **71**: 13–16.
15. Williamson RV, Staheli LT. Partial physeal growth arrest: treatment by bridge resection and fat interposition. *J Pediatr Orthop* 1990; **10**: 769–76.
16. Bueche MJ, Phillips WA, Gordon J, Best R, Goldstein SA. Effect of interposition material on mechanical behavior in partial physeal resection: a canine model. *J Pediatr Orthop* 1990; **10**: 459–62.
17. Langenskiöld A, Österman K, Valle M. Growth of fat grafts after operation for partial bone growth arrest: demonstration by computed tomography scanning. *J Pediatr Orthop* 1987; **7**: 389–94.
18. Marsh JS, Polzhofer GK. Arthroscopically assisted central physeal bar resection. *J Pediatr Orthop* 2006; **26**: 255–9.
19. Jackson AM. Excision of the central physeal bar: a modification of Langenskiöld's procedure. *J Bone Joint Surg Br* 1993; **75**: 664–5.
20. Hasler CC, Foster BK. Secondary tethers after physeal bar resection. A common source of failure? *Clin Orthop Relat Res* 2002; **405**: 242–9.
21. Scheffer MM, Peterson HA. Opening-wedge osteotomy for angular deformities of long bones in children. *J Bone Joint Surg Am* 1994; **76**: 325–34.

SECTION 8

Infections

Acute septic arthritis

Benjamin Joseph

71

Introduction

Septic arthritis is more common than osteomyelitis in infancy and childhood. Although any joint can be involved, the hip and knee are the most frequently affected and they account for almost two-thirds of all cases of septic arthritis. Involvement of multiple joints occurs in about 5 percent of children with septic arthritis[1] and some of the less commonly involved joints may be affected when there is multiple joint involvement. Children under the age of five years appear to be far more susceptible to developing septic arthritis and account for 75 percent of all cases of acute septic arthritis.

It is useful to be aware of these general facts regarding the pattern of involvement as this knowledge may be invaluable in diagnosis of the condition.

Among the organisms that cause septic arthritis, the most common is *Staphylococcus aureus*. Other bacteria including group A and group B streptococci, *Streptococcus pneumoniae* and *Haemophilus influenzae* are implicated less frequently.[2,3] Neonates are more susceptible to group B streptococcal infection.[3] There has been a recent upsurge of septic arthritis caused by methicillin-resistant strains of *Staphylococcus aureus* (MRSA). These infections were once thought to be predominantly hospital-acquired, but of late, several cases of community-acquired MRSA have been identified.[3]

Problems of management

Apart from the effects of the infection on the child's general health, the joint *per se* is prone to considerable damage.

Destruction of articular and epiphyseal cartilage

Potent proteolytic enzymes are released by the bacteria and by activated polymorphs, synovial cells and chondrocytes during the inflammatory reaction in response to the infection in the joint. These enzymes cause degradation of the hyaline cartilage with depletion of the collagen and the glucosaminoglycans.

Experimental evidence suggests that cartilage degradation begins within eight hours of bacterial colonization.

Damage to the growth plate in the vicinity of the joint

A combination of vascular damage and proteolytic degradation contribute to damage to the growth plate.

Dislocation of the joint

Capsular distension occurs due to the effusion that develops soon after the onset of the infection. Further stretch of the capsular ligaments occurs due to the intense hyperaemia that occurs with the infection. Muscle spasm that develops in response to the pain in the joint causes the capsule to stretch even more as the limb is held in a posture dictated by the muscles that are in spasm. A combination of these factors makes the capsular stabilizing mechanism of the joint ineffective and subluxation or dislocation of the joint ensues.

Damage to the blood supply of the bone within the joint

In children with septic arthritis of the hip, the blood supply to the femoral head may be disrupted by tamponade due to the increased intra-articular pressure that develops as pus accumulates in the joint.

The potential long-term consequences of these complications include joint instability, joint stiffness, deformity, limb length inequality and secondary degenerative arthritis.

Problems of establishing a diagnosis

Since cartilage destruction commences very soon after onset of infection it becomes exceedingly important to establish a diagnosis as soon as possible and to institute treatment within a day or two of the onset of symptoms.

It needs to be emphasized that no imaging modality can confirm the diagnosis of a septic infection in the joint. At best, imaging may enable the clinician to confirm the presence of an effusion in the joint and that there is inflammation in the joint.

Similarly, laboratory investigations such as blood counts, erythrocyte sedimentation rate (ESR) and C-reactive protein (CRP) may help in suggesting that there is an infective process going on but cannot definitely confirm the diagnosis of septic arthritis.

The only way the joint infection can be conclusively diagnosed is by demonstrating bacteria in the fluid removed from the joint. However, an organism may only be cultured in approximately 60 percent of cases of true septic arthritis. Thus it is evident that no single test can be relied upon for confirming the diagnosis of septic arthritis.

On the basis of a careful clinical examination, a tentative diagnosis of septic arthritis needs to be made. If joint aspiration does not yield fluid with bacteria demonstrable either in a Gram-stained smear or on culture, a presumptive diagnosis may be made with the help of the results of other laboratory tests in conjunction with clinical findings.

Kocher *et al.*[4] identified clinical and laboratory predictors of septic arthritis: history of fever, inability to bear weight on the limb, ESR >40 mm/hour and a white blood cell (WBC) count >12 000/mL. They noted that the predicted probability of septic arthritis was 0.2 if none of these predictors was present and that the probability of a diagnosis of septic arthritis was 40, 93.1 and 99.6 percent if two, three or four of these predictors, respectively, were present. In another study, temperature >37°C, ESR > 20 mm/hour, CRP > 1 mg/dL, WBC > 11 000/mL and an increased joint space >2 mm were identified as independent multivariate predictors of septic arthritis.[5]

Realizing the limitations of investigations in confirming the diagnosis of septic arthritis, it is imperative that treatment is commenced on the basis of a high index of suspicion. Definitive treatment should not be withheld for want of confirmatory laboratory tests.

Aims of treatment

- Control and eradicate infection
  It is vital that infection is controlled as soon as possible in order to prevent complications.
- Prevent cartilage damage
  In order to prevent destruction of articular, epiphyseal and physeal cartilage the inflammation needs to be controlled and the bacterial load rapidly minimized so that the proteolytic enzymes in the joint reduce dramatically.
- Prevent damage to the growth plate
  If the bacterial load and the inflammation are reduced the risk of growth plate damage can be minimized.
- Prevent dislocation of the joint
  The capsular distension needs to be reduced by adequately draining the joint. In addition, muscle spasm and inflammation should be reduced.
- Prevent avascular necrosis
  Reduction of the intra-articular pressure by prompt decompression of the joint can reduce the risk of vascular compromise.

Treatment options

Controlling and eradicating infection with antibiotics

■ The choice of antibiotics

The antibiotic selected should be effective against the organism responsible for the infection. Since Gram-positive organisms are most frequently responsible for the infection, an antibiotic that is effective against these organisms should be started empirically.

■ The route of administration

To begin with, the intravenous route of administration of antibiotic is preferred. Once a satisfactory clinical response is obtained, the antibiotic may be given orally. The other route of administration used by some surgeons is the intra-articular route. The disadvantage of this route of administration is that repeated arthrocentesis is needed and this itself is potentially fraught with the risk of introduction of fresh infection into the joint. In addition to this potential risk, the antibiotic may be an irritant to the synovium and may actually increase the inflammatory response.

■ **The duration of therapy**

In the past it was recommended that treatment with antibiotics should be continued for six weeks. However, recent studies suggest that the duration of medication may be reduced to four weeks or less without adverse outcome in the long term.[6,7]

Decompression of the joint

Decompression of the joint relieves pain and reduces the stretch of the capsule. Once pain subsides, the muscle spasm also reduces. Reduction of the muscle spasm and capsular distension will reduce the tendency for joint subluxation and dislocation. In the hip, the risk of vascular tamponade can also be minimized by decompressing the joint. Decompression of the joint may be done either by aspirating the joint or by a formal arthrotomy.

■ **Aspiration**

Aspiration may need to be repeated as the effusion in the joint may re-collect within a day.

■ **Arthrotomy**

An arthrotomy is the most definitive way of decompressing the joint. The additional advantage of a formal arthrotomy is that it enables the surgeon to inspect the articular surfaces to determine whether the cartilage is damaged. The capsule is not closed following the arthrotomy and this ensures that an effusion does not collect again.

Joint lavage

Lavage of the joint helps to remove cellular debris and reduce the bacterial load.

The lavage can be done in one of three ways: repeated aspiration and wash-out, lavage at the time of a formal arthrotomy or lavage through an arthroscope. Arthroscopic lavage is particularly useful in the older child with septic arthritis of the knee. In smaller children and for infection of smaller joints arthroscopic lavage may not be feasible.

Immobilization of the joint

Rest to the joint either by immobilization in a plaster cast or by traction helps to reduce pain. Once the infection is under control and the inflammation has reduced, active mobilization of the joint should be resumed in order to avoid joint stiffness.

Duration of symptoms

As cartilage degradation commences soon after the onset of infection it is mandatory that appropriate treatment is instituted as soon as possible. It follows that if the symptoms have been present for more than two days and the clinical signs strongly suggest infection in the joint, it may be safer to drain the joint soon after starting antibiotics. On the other hand, if the symptoms have been present for less than a day, the clinical response to intravenous antibiotics may be carefully monitored and drainage of the joint may be deferred for a day. If resolution of symptoms is not clearly evident within a day of commencing antibiotics the joint must be drained.

Age of the child

The consequences of cartilage destruction in the neonate are far more catastrophic than in an older child and hence the permissible window for observation for response to antibiotics is shorter. Furthermore, neonates are often already on antibiotics in an intensive care unit when the infection in the joint develops. Thus, a more proactive approach is needed in neonates and early decompression of the joint should be considered.

Source of infection

If the infection develops in hospital it is possible that more virulent organisms or organisms that are resistant to certain antibiotics are responsible for the infection. In such a situation early drainage of the joint should be considered.

Joint affected

A superficial joint such as the knee can be easily monitored for response to treatment and drainage may be withheld whereas a deep-seated joint like the hip is more difficult to evaluate and thus drainage of the hip should be considered earlier rather than later. Yet another reason for considering early drainage of the hip is because complications of septic arthritis are far more common in the hip than in other joints.

Associated disease

The presence of other systemic disease that impairs immunity and host resistance increases the chances of an unfavourable outcome. In such situations it is probably more appropriate to consider early drainage of the joint.

Number of predictors of possible septic arthritis

If three of the predictors of septic arthritis as suggested by Kocher *et al.* are present, arthrotomy should be considered, especially if the hip joint is affected.[8]

Recommended treatment

The outline of treatment of acute septic arthritis is shown in Table 71.1.

Table 71.1 ● Outline of treatment of acute septic arthritis of the hip

INDICATIONS			
Neonate with pseudoparalysis + Tenderness and swelling over a joint	Child with 1-day history of acute joint pain + 3 or 4 of Kocher's criteria present + Superficial joint affected + Community-acquired infection	Child with 1-day history of acute joint pain + 3 or 4 of Kocher's criteria present + Hip joint affected (community-acquired infection) OR Any joint if hospital-acquired infection ⇩ Intravenous antibiotics	Child with >1-day history of acute joint pain + 3 or 4 of Kocher's criteria present + Any joint affected + Community- OR hospital-acquired infection ⇩ Intravenous antibiotics
⇩	⇩ Intravenous antibiotics	+	+
Intravenous antibiotics + Arthrotomy and lavage + Immobilization in a cast	+ Careful monitoring of clinical response for resolution of symptoms	Arthrotomy + Lavage + Cast/traction	Arthrotomy + Lavage + Cast/traction
TREATMENT			

Rationale of recommended treatment

The author has recommended a seemingly aggressive approach to treatment involving arthrotomy and drainage in all but a very select group of children with community-acquired infection of no longer than a day's duration affecting a superficial joint. The reason for such an approach is because the risks of delayed drainage far outweigh the benefits of waiting and watching for a response to antibiotics.

References

1. Shaw BA, Kasser JR. Acute septic arthritis in infancy and childhood. *Clin Orthop Relat Res* 1990; **257**: 212–25.
2. Morrey BF, Bianco AJ, Rhodes KH. Septic arthritis in children. *Orthop Clin North Am* 1975; **6**: 923–34.
3. Arnold, SA, Elias D, Buckingham SC *et al.* Changing patterns of acute hematogenous osteomyelitis and septic arthritis. Emergence of community-associated Methicillin-resistant Staphylococcus aureus. *J Pediatr Orthop* 2006; **26**: 703–8.

4. Kocher MS, Zurakowski D, Kasser JR. Differentiating between septic arthritis and transient synovitis of the hip in children: an evidence-based clinical prediction algorithm. *J Bone Joint Surg Am* 1999; **81**: 1662–70.

5. Jung ST, Rowe SM, Moon ES *et al.* Significance of laboratory and radiological findings for differentiating septic arthritis and transient synovitis of the hip. *J Pediatr Orthop* 2003; **23**: 368–72.

6. Vinod MB, Mattussek J, Curtis N, Graham HK, Carapetis JR. Duration of antibiotics in children with osteomyelitis and septic arthritis. *J Pediatr Child Health* 2002; **38**: 363–7.

7. Kim HK, Alman B, Cole WG. A shortened course of parenteral antibiotic therapy in the management of acute septic arthritis of the hip. *J Pediatr Orthop* 2000; **20**: 44–7.

8. Frick SL. Evaluation of the child who has hip pain. *Orthop Clin North Am* 2006; **37**: 133–40.

Acute osteomyelitis

Benjamin Joseph

72

Acute osteomyelitis commonly occurs in the first decade of life and boys appear to be more commonly affected.[1] In infants, acute osteomyelitis and septic arthritis can coexist.

Staphylococcus aureus still remains the most common organism responsible for acute osteomyelitis; streptococci, *Kingella kingae*, Gram-negative organisms and salmonella are far less frequently responsible. Streptococcal osteomyelitis may follow infected skin lesions of measles and chickenpox and children with sickle cell disease are prone to develop salmonella osteomyelitis.

Spread of infection

The infection usually begins in the metaphyseal region of bone. If infection is not controlled pus will collect there and then may track into the medullary cavity or under the periosteum. Pus may also track into an adjacent joint if the metaphysis is intra-articular (Figure 72.1).

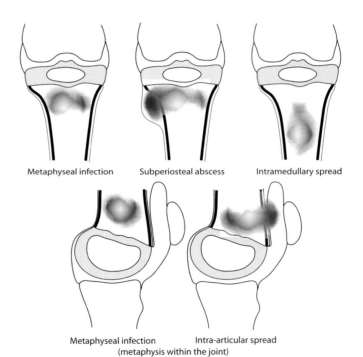

Metaphyseal infection   Subperiosteal abscess   Intramedullary spread

Metaphyseal infection   Intra-articular spread
(metaphysis within the joint)

Figure 72.1 ● Diagram demonstrating how the pus from the metaphysis can track subperiosteally, into the medullary cavity and into the adjacent joint if the metaphysis is situated within the joint capsule.

Progression to chronic infection of bone

If frank suppuration occurs and the pus is not drained promptly, the entire medullary cavity will become filled with pus and the periosteum may also get stripped off from the cortex circumferentially by the subperiosteal collection. Once this occurs the diaphysis is devoid of both endosteal and periosteal blood supply and becomes a sequestrum; the infection then becomes chronic.

Pathological fracture

The bone in the metaphyseal region becomes weakened and can fracture if not protected (Figure 72.2). This risk of fracture increases once the cortex has been drilled or windowed as part of treatment.[2]

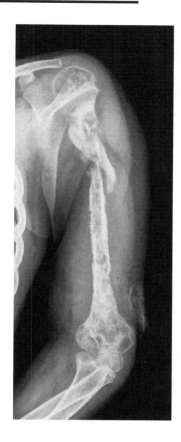

Figure 72.2 ● Pathological fracture in a child with osteomyelitis.

Growth arrest

Since the infection is located in the vicinity of the growth plate, damage to the growth plate can occur. The damage may be localized to a part of the physis, and the location and the area of damage will determine whether growth arrest will occur. When the damage is severe enough to produce growth arrest, limb length discrepancy or angular deformities can develop. The frequency of growth plate damage following osteomyelitis has been estimated to be around 3 percent in children[2] and the frequency appears to be higher in neonates.[3]

Aims of treatment

- Control and eradicate infection
  With appropriate prompt treatment the infection can be controlled and eradicated in the majority of instances; in only about 5 percent of cases does recurrence of infection occur. The recurrence is often within one year following primary treatment.[4] However, eradication of the infection can become exceedingly difficult once the acute infection passes to the chronic stage.
- Prevent spread of infection
  If the infection remains localized to the metaphysis, the likelihood of control of the infection and prevention of complications are good. Once the infection breaks out of the cortex the treatment will necessarily have to be more aggressive in order to prevent complications.
- Prevent progression to chronic osteomyelitis
  The likelihood of preventing chronic osteomyelitis is directly related to how soon after the onset of symptoms treatment is begun.
- Prevent complications
  Pathological fracture can be prevented by protecting the weakened bone in a cast. Diaphyseal sequestration can be avoided if subperiosteal collection of pus is drained before the entire periosteum is stripped off the cortex (Figure 72.3). This will only be possible if the subperiosteal abscess is recognized early and drained.

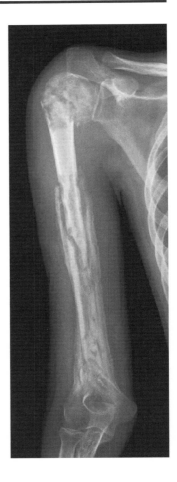

Figure 72.3 ● Extensive diaphyseal sequestration seen in a child who had inadequate treatment of acute osteomyelitis.

Establishing the diagnosis

Trueta[5] divided the clinical stages of acute osteomyelitis into three. In stage I there is severe bone pain and profound local tenderness without any soft tissue inflammation. In stage II the systemic and local signs are more pronounced; this corresponds to the development of a subperiosteal abscess. In stage III there is pus in the soft tissues and in this stage it is difficult to distinguish osteomyelitis from cellulitis.

The provisional diagnosis of acute osteomyelitis should be made on clinical grounds alone, and every effort must be made to establish a definite diagnosis in stage I of the disease itself. Acute localized tenderness in the region of the metaphysis of a long bone in the presence of fever should be sufficient grounds to make a tentative diagnosis of acute osteomyelitis.

Plain radiographs are of little use in the diagnosis of acute osteomyelitis. In stage I there are no plain radiographic changes either in the soft tissue planes or in the bone. In stages II and III there is loss of definition of soft tissue planes indicative of oedema. However there are still no changes in the bone; bone changes appear 10–14 days after the onset of infection in children or a little sooner in neonates. The radiograph is useful to distinguish acute osteomyelitis from Ewing's sarcoma.

Ultrasound scanning is useful for diagnosis of a subperiosteal abscess and should be done in all cases.[6] Magnetic resonance imaging (MRI) can detect early bone oedema; the characteristic features are reduced signal intensity in the marrow on the T1-weighted image and increased signal intensity on the T2-weighted image.[7] MRI can also delineate a subperiosteal abscess. It is particularly useful for diagnosing osteomyelitis of pelvic bones but is seldom needed to diagnose osteomyelitis of bones of the limbs.

Elevated leukocyte count, erythrocyte sedimentation rate and C-reactive protein help in the diagnosis but none of these tests can confirm the diagnosis of osteomyelitis. Blood cultures may be positive in around 40 percent of patients.

The most valuable test in confirming the diagnosis of acute osteomyelitis is aspiration, which can be done within hours of admission to hospital.

A 16- or 18-gauge spinal needle is advanced up to the cortex of the bone at the site of maximal tenderness. Aspiration is attempted from the subperiosteal space. If pus is encountered it is sent immediately for Gram stain and culture. If no pus is aspirated from the subperiosteal plane, the needle is advanced into the metaphysis and intra-osseous aspiration is attempted. Fluid from within the bone is sent for Gram stain and culture. A positive yield on aspiration can be anticipated in around 60 percent of instances.[8]

Treatment options

Antibiotics

It is essential to administer appropriate antibiotics that are effective against the causative organism early in the course of the disease to control the infection. Once aspiration is performed, intravenous antibiotics are started; the choice of the antibiotic is based on the most probable organism.

Drainage of subperiosteal abscess

Surgical drainage is indicated if a subperiosteal abscess is demonstrated on the ultrasound or MR scan, or if pus is aspirated from the subperiosteal plane.[2,8] Early drainage of the abscess is essential to prevent circumferential stripping of the periosteum and total loss of periosteal blood supply of the diaphysis.

Decompression of bone

Decompression of the bone has been recommended in all cases of acute osteomyelitis by some surgeons[9] while others have questioned the need to decompress the bone.[10,11] Cole *et al.*[11] suggest that surgery should be restricted to children with symptoms lasting more than five days and that the surgery be limited to drainage of the abscess.

If decompression of the bone is considered necessary it is done through a small skin incision. The periosteum is incised and a couple of drill holes are made in the cortex. Often, a few beads of pus exude through the drill holes; if the suppuration is extensive, a great deal of pus may ooze out of the drill holes. If a large quantity of pus is drained, a small window can be made in the cortex to facilitate irrigation of the bone.

Splintage or casting

If the bone appears soft and moth-eaten, or if the cortex has been drilled or windowed, the limb is protected in a cast in order to prevent a fracture.

Factors to be taken into consideration while planning treatment

Age of the child

Acute osteomyelitis tends to be more severe and complications more frequent in neonates than when it occurs in older children. Hence, surgical intervention may be justified more frequently when dealing with neonates with osteomyelitis.

Duration of symptoms

If the duration of symptoms is less than 24–48 hours there is a fair chance that the infection may be controlled with antibiotic therapy. On the other hand, if the duration of symptoms is greater than 72 hours it is likely that a subperiosteal abscess may have already collected.

Associated illness

The symptoms may be masked or atypical in a child who is on treatment for septicaemia and then develops osteomyelitis. Furthermore, since the osteomyelitis has developed while the child is already on antibiotics it may not be safe to rely on antibiotics alone for resolution of the bone infection. In such situations it may be necessary to consider early surgical decompression of the bone.

Presence of a subperiosteal abscess

It is universally acknowledged that the presence of a subperiosteal abscess is an indication for drainage.

Recommended treatment

The outline of treatment is shown in Table 72.1.

Table 72.1 ● Treatment of acute osteomyelitis

INDICATIONS				
<24 hours of symptoms + Fever and localized tenderness over involved bone + No subperiosteal abscess demonstrable on ultrasound scan (stage I of Trueta)	1–3 days of symptoms + Fever and localized tenderness over Involved bone + Small subperiosteal abscess demonstrable on ultrasound scan (stage II of Trueta)	3–5 days of symptoms + Tenderness of the involved bone + Inflamed soft tissue overlying the bone + Large subperiosteal abscess ± Pus in the soft tissue planes (stage III of Trueta)	>5 days of symptoms + Tenderness of the involved bone + Inflamed soft tissue overlying the bone + Large subperiosteal abscess + Pus in the soft tissue planes	Acute osteomyelitis developing in a neonate or child already on treatment for septicaemia
⇩	⇩	⇩	⇩	⇩
i.v. antibiotics + Bed rest + Observe for clinical response for 36 hours + Repeat ultrasound to ensure that no subperiosteal abscess is collecting	i.v. antibiotics + Bed rest + Drainage of subperiosteal abscess	i.v. antibiotics + Bed rest + Drainage of subperiosteal abscess + Decompression of bone by drilling + Splintage of the limb	i.v. antibiotics + Bed rest + Drainage of subperiosteal abscess + Decompression of bone by making a window in the cortex + Lavage + Splintage of the limb	Continue antibiotics + Decompression of bone + Splintage
TREATMENT				

Rationale of treatment suggested

Why is surgery being advocated only if a subperiosteal abscess is present?
In over 90 percent of cases in which subperiosteal abscesses had not formed eradication of infection was achieved with antibiotics alone.

Why is decompression of the bone being advocated in the later stages of acute osteomyelitis?
Although the need to decompress the bone is controversial, it is being advocated in the hope that the extent of damage to the endosteal blood supply can be minimized and, consequently, the extent of sequestration of the cortex would hopefully be reduced.

References

1. Gillespie WJ. The epidemiology of acute haematogenous osteomyelitis of childhood. *Int J Epidemiol* 1985; **14**: 600–6.
2. Gillespie WJ. Hematogenous osteomyelitis. In: Bulstrode C, Buckwalter J, Carr A *et al.* (eds). *Oxford Textbook of Orthopedics and Trauma*, vol. 2. Oxford: Oxford University Press, 2002: 1421–30.
3. Bergdahl S, Ekengran K, Eriksson M. Neonatal hematogenous osteomyelitis: risk factors for long-term sequelae. *J Pediatr Orthop* 1985; **5**: 564–8.
4. Gillespie WJ, Mayo KM. The management of acute haematogenous osteomyelitis in the antibiotic era. A study of the outcome. *J Bone Joint Surg Br* 1981; **63**: 126–31.

5. Trueta J. The three types of acute haematogenous osteomyelitis: a clinical and vascular study. *J Bone Joint Surg Br* 1959; **41**: 671–80.

6. Howard CB, Einhorn M, Dagan R, Nyska M. Ultrasound in the diagnosis and management of acute haematogenous osteomyelitis in children. *J Bone Joint Surg Br* 1993; **75**: 79–82.

7. Jaramillo D, Treves ST, Kasser JR *et al.* Osteomyelits and septic arthritis in children. *AJR Am J Roentgenol* 1995; **165**: 399–403.

8. Dormans JP, Drummond DS. Pediatric hematogenous osteomyelitis: new trends in presentation, diagnosis and treatment. *J Am Acad Orthop Surg* 1994; **2**: 333–41.

9. Mollan RAB, Piggot J. Acute osteomyelitis in children. *J Bone Joint Surg Br* 1977; **59**: 2–7.

10. Blockey NJ, Watson JC. Acute osteomyelitis in children. *J Bone Joint Surg Br* 1970; **52**: 77–87.

11. Cole WG, Dalziel RE, Leitl S. Treatment of acute osteomyelitis in childhood. *J Bone Joint Surg Br* 1982; **64**: 218–23.

Index

OPERATIVE OBSTETRICS

SECOND EDITION

EDITED BY

John P. O'Grady, MD

Professor, Department of Obstetrics and Gynecology
Tufts University School of Medicine, Boston, Massachusetts
Medical Director, Family Life Center for Maternity
Director, Mercy Hospital Perinatal Service
Department of Obstetrics and Gynecology
Mercy Medical Center, Springfield, Massachusetts

Martin L. Gimovsky, MD

Professor, Department of Obstetrics, Gynecology and Reproductive Science
Mount Sinai School of Medicine, New York, New York
Vice Chair and Program Director, Department of Obstetrics and Gynecology
Newark Beth Israel Medical Center, Newark, New Jersey

ASSOCIATE EDITORS

Lucy A. Bayer-Zwirello, MD

Associate Professor, Department of Obstetrics and Gynecology
Tufts University School of Medicine, Boston, Massachusetts
Chief, Maternal-Fetal Medicine, Department of Obstetrics and Gynecology
Director, Labor and Delivery Services
St. Margaret's Center for Women and Infants
Caritas St. Elizabeth's Medical Center, Brighton, Massachusetts

Kevin Giordano, JD

Partner, Keyes and Donnellan, PC
Springfield, Massachusetts

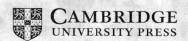

CAMBRIDGE
UNIVERSITY PRESS

WITHDRAWN

CAMBRIDGE UNIVERSITY PRESS
Cambridge, New York, Melbourne, Madrid, Cape Town, Singapore, São Paulo, Delhi

Cambridge University Press
32 Avenue of the Americas, New York, NY 10013-2473, USA

www.cambridge.org
Information on this title: www.cambridge.org/9780521862486

© John P. O'Grady 2008

This publication is in copyright. Subject to statutory exception
and to the provisions of relevant collective licensing agreements,
no reproduction of any part may take place without
the written permission of Cambridge University Press.

First published 2008

Printed in the United States of America

A catalog record for this publication is available from the British Library.

Library of Congress Cataloging in Publication Data

Operative obstetrics / edited by John P. O'Grady, Martin L. Gimovsky; associate editors,
Lucy Bayer-Zwirello, Kevin Giordano. – 2nd ed.
p. ; cm.
Includes bibliographical references and index.
ISBN 978-0-521-86248-6 (hardback)
1. Obstetrics–Surgery. I. O'Grady, John Patrick, 1945- II. Gimovsky, Martin L.
[DNLM: 1. Delivery, Obstetric. 2. Labor, Obstetric. 3. Pregnancy Complications–surgery. WQ 415 O61 2008]
RG725.O623 2008
618.8–dc22 2008002354

ISBN 978-0-521-86248-6 hardback

Every effort has been made in preparing this publication to provide accurate and up-to-date information that is in accord
with accepted standards and practice at the time of publication. Nevertheless, the authors, editors, and publisher can make
no warranties that the information contained herein is totally free from error, not least because clinical standards are
constantly changing through research and regulation. The authors, editors, and publisher therefore disclaim all liability for
direct or consequential damages resulting from the use of material contained in this publication. Readers are strongly
advised to pay careful attention to information provided by the manufacturer of any drugs or equipment that they
plan to use.

Cambridge University Press has no responsibility for the persistence or accuracy of URLs for external or third-party
Internet Web sites referred to in this publication, and does not guarantee that any content on such Web sites is, or will
remain, accurate or appropriate.

To JO: His son finally did become a surgeon. And to Molly for support and encouragement.

JPOG

For my family, Herakliusz, Stefania, Alexandria, and Madeline, for their patience and support during this endeavor.

LBZ

To Arlene, Alexis, and Matt. For your love and support.

MLG

To Marge and Bill, who sacrificed so much on my road to becoming an attorney.

KG

⎯⎯ ◦ ⎯⎯

ooking back over a long clinical lifetime, one tends to forget or take for granted one's successes; it is the failures which stand out like keloid scars, never to be forgotten and, hopefully, a warning to others. I have to recognise that if there is any classic mistake which I have not myself made it is simply because of the lack of time in which to commit it. It makes one wondrously sympathetic toward others in trouble. No apology is therefore made for the highly personal emphasis in this book.

Ian Donald (1910–1987)
Practical Obstetric Problems
London: Lloyd-Luke, 1979, p. viii.

Note to Readers

The advancement of medical science brings continuous changes in management, methods of diagnosis and evaluation, and drug therapy.

The editors of and contributors to *Operative Obstetrics* Second Edition, have closely reviewed the information included in this textbook, consulted appropriate literature, and conferred with experienced clinicians in the effort to provide accurate information and practice recommendations in accordance with the generally accepted standards of medical practice. The reader is cautioned, however, that owing to the rapid changes in the science of medicine and the possibility of human error, the authors of the various chapters, the editors, and the publisher cannot guarantee that all information included in this text is in every respect complete or accurate. We do not accept responsibility for errors, omissions, or results obtained from the use of these data. For these reasons, the reader is encouraged to confirm our practice suggestions with other standard sources. Relying on his or her experience, education, and unique knowledge of the individual patient, the attending physician or certified nurse midwife must determine the best treatment for a specific obstetric condition.

Recommended drugs and dosing schedules for various medical conditions do appear in this text. Before a drug is administered, however, clinicians should review standard compendia of drug information and package inserts for any changes in drug use or additional warnings of potential adverse reactions or other precautions. To ensure patient safety, caution is especially necessary when the drug in question is new to the practitioner, infrequently administered, or has the potential for serious side effects.

– The Editors

Contents

Part IV: SPECIAL ISSUES

APPENDIX

Foreword

THE PROCESS OF EVOLUTION affects not only the characteristics of a species but also the adaptive technology between a species and its environment. The practice of obstetrics is devoted to maximizing the ability of each human being to confront the environment and to be part of the creative, modulating path of evolution. It is almost, if not totally, impossible to discern evolutionary human changes within our own lifetimes; however, it is a different story with the technology of our interactions. Obstetrics has changed, and it has changed rapidly.

If the earth's lifetime were compressed into a single 24-hour day, humans would have appeared only 30 seconds ago. I cannot imagine what nanocalculation would be required to measure the history of operative obstetrics, yet that incredibly short measure of geologic time is packed with a geometrically increasing collection of events and stories. The interesting and comprehensive chapter on the history of operative delivery alone is worth the price of this book. Every contemporary obstetrician should know and learn from the history of obstetrics. Some might argue that this history is truly the past, and that operative obstetrics today is a matter of a few simple choices. Even that judgment, however, must be based on a critical analysis of the operative choices. Only then can the individual obstetrician understand the reasons behind modern decisions.

The modern focus on "evidence-based medicine" all too often fails to recognize the broad base of knowledge that is the foundation of clinical decision making. This book is an excellent example of the fact that medical knowledge is more than what we read in the literature. Although medicine tests the worth of specific procedures with appropriately designed clinical studies, physicians also learn from each and every clinical experience and modify their decisions according to an understanding of the individual patient's needs. Nowhere is this more important than in operative procedures. The authors of this book have solidified their recommendations with a comprehensive survey of the literature, but they have filtered this knowledge through the valuable experiences of multiple clinicians, finally offering clinical advice that is meaningful and useful.

Obstetric decisions today are not simpler. They are actually more complex, requiring an ever-expanding knowledge base. This book provides a knowledge base of operative obstetrics derived from the accomplishments of the past and the experiences of the present. In so doing, it serves an important purpose: to assist obstetricians in achieving the objective of a successful pregnancy and a healthy newborn.

Leon Speroff
Professor, Department of Obstetrics and Gynecology
Oregon Health and Science University
Portland, Oregon

Preface

*𝒪bstetrics is not one of the exact sciences, and, in our penury of truth
we ought to be accurate in our statements, generous in our doubts,
tolerant in our convictions.*

James Young Simpson (1811–1870)

MUCH TO OUR SURPRISE, more than ten years have passed since the publication of the first edition of *Operative Obstetrics*. Since the initial text appeared in 1995, new tests, surgical procedures, and novel methods of medical education have been introduced to the practice of obstetrics. In addition, there has been an expansion of roles for non-physician personnel in the provision of care to pregnant women. There remain important unresolved controversies in the specialty, including elective or patient-choice cesarean delivery, trials of vaginal birth after cesarean, patient safety during hospitalization, pregnancy termination, and the recruitment and training of new practitioners, to list only a few. The influx of new ideas and the development of new techniques over the last decade have accompanied increasing demands by institutions, third-party payers, and governmental agencies for evidence-based, cost-efficient, and safe practice. Clinicians are thus pressured from many directions to rapidly incorporate new scientific advances into their management, rethink traditional concepts of best practice, follow increasingly restrictive protocols and practice guidelines, and even revisit basic ethical concepts. Because of the unresolved issues concerning appropriate practice and the risks associated with adverse outcomes, it is inevitable that medicolegal risks in obstetrics remain high and that increasingly few clinicians, with a decade or more of active practice, now escape litigation.

The stated goal of all recent textbooks is to define best practice by employing the techniques of evidence-based medicine. In fact, there is now a growing body of evidence-based data concerning obstetric practice, much to the improvement of the specialty; however, many areas of management have never been subjected to such systemic study. Experienced practitioners rapidly discover that there are obstetric and surgical practices and clinical problems that have not proved amenable to the rigid demands of evidence-based analysis. These observations emphasize the limitations of current methodologies and serve as a constant reminder of the incompleteness of physicians' knowledge and the need for continuous improvement through appropriately designed prospective studies.

This new edition required the amalgamation of data derived from quite different sources. Working with the editors, our many collaborators have strived to reconcile current scientific knowledge and data from evidence-based clinical studies with the rich heritage available from the past. Philosophically, the editors remain unrepentant advocates of combining essential elements of the art of traditional obstetrics and the accumulated experience of our predecessors with new concepts and methods of management derived from meta-analysis and other prospective and randomized clinical investigations. Reflecting the realities of modern practice, this new edition includes legal commentaries on areas of special concerns, with recommendations for appropriate actions to help to avoid difficulty.

It is the editors' earnest anticipation that this new edition of *Operative Obstetrics* fulfills the demanding requirements of clinicians struggling with the many pressures of contemporary practice. Our aim is both to challenge and instruct our readers. The success of this endeavor will be measured by the extent to which we have constructively critiqued established ideas, fused the traditionally accepted with the scientifically proved aspects of practice, and sustained the reader's interest. Our measure of success is simple. If this textbook proves helpful in the management of a single case, our original expectations will be met, and we will consider our intense labors and those of our coworkers to have been amply rewarded.

John P. O'Grady
Martin L. Gimovsky
Lucy A. Bayer-Zwirello
Kevin Giordano

Acknowledgments

THE ASSISTANCE OF Zaya Duranian and Carolyn J. Taugher and the multiple and extensive labors of Shanna L. Burke, our research and editorial assistants, and the technical advice and help provided by Joanne Liebel in the preparation of this text are gratefully acknowledged.

Contributors

F. P. Bailey, MD
Assistant Professor
Department of Obstetrics and
   Gynecology
Tufts University School of Medicine
Boston, Massachusetts
Attending Physician
Pediatric and Adolescent
   Gynecology
Gynecology Division
Department of Obstetrics and
   Gynecology
Instructor
Department of Pediatrics
Baystate Medical Center
Springfield, Massachusetts

Lucy A. Bayer-Zwirello, MD
Associate Professor
Department of Obstetrics and
   Gynecology
Tufts University School of Medicine
Boston, Massachusetts
Chief
Maternal-Fetal Medicine
Director
Labor and Delivery Services
St. Margaret's Center for Women and Infants
Caritas St. Elizabeth's Medical Center
Brighton, Massachusetts

Shanna L. Burke
Social Worker
Florence, Massachusetts

Samantha F. Butts, MD, MSCE
Assistant Professor
Department of Obstetrics and Gynecology
Division of Infant and Reproductive Endocrinology
University of Pennsylvania Medical School
Philadelphia, Pennsylvania

Joanna M. Cain, MD
Professor and Chair
Department of Obstetrics and Gynecology
Director
Center for Women's Health
Oregon Health and Science University
Portland, Oregon

Wayne R. Cohen, MD
Professor
Department of Obstetrics and Gynecology
Weill Cornell Medical Center
New York, New York

Gabriel M. Cohn, MD
Assistant Professor
Department of Obstetrics and Gynecology
Tufts University School of Medicine
Boston, Massachusetts
Medical Director
Genetic Services

Chief
Clinical and Reproductive Genetics
Department of Obstetrics and Gynecology
Baystate Medical Center
Springfield, Massachusetts

Shad H. Deering, MD
Medical Director
Andersen Simulation Center
Staff Physician
Maternal-Fetal Medicine
Madigan Army Medical Center
Tacoma, Washington

Matthew A. Esposito, MD
Assistant Professor
Department of Obstetrics and Gynecology
University of Massachusetts Medical Center
Worcester, Massachusetts
Attending Physician
Division of Maternal-Fetal Medicine
Memorial Hospital
Worcester, Massachusetts

Reinaldo Figueroa, MD
Clinical Associate Professor
Department of Obstetrics, Gynecology and
 Reproductive Medicine
State University of New York at Stony Brook
Stony Brook University Medical Center
Stony Brook, New York

Timothy K. Fitzpatrick, MD
Fitzpatrick, Moran, Costa, and Haag-Rickert, PC
Obstetrics and Gynecology
Mercy Medical Center
Springfield, Massachusetts

Aileen M. Gariepy, MD
Clinical Instructor
Department of Obstetrics and Gynecology
Thomas Jefferson University
Philadelphia, Pennsylvania

Martin L. Gimovsky, MD
Professor
Department of Obstetrics and Gynecology
Mount Sinai School of Medicine
New York, New York
Vice Chair and Program Director

Residency Education Program
Department of Obstetrics and Gynecology
Newark Beth Israel Medical Center
Newark, New Jersey

Kevin Giordano, JD
Partner
Keyes and Donnellan, PC
Springfield, Massachusetts

Karen W. Green, MD
Associate Professor
Obstetrics and Gynecology
University of Massachusetts Medical Center
Worcester, Massachusetts
Chief
Maternal-Fetal Medicine
Division of Maternal-Fetal Medicine
Memorial Hospital
Worcester, Massachusetts

Daniel F. Grum, MD
Associate Professor
Department of Anesthesiology
The University of Tennessee School of Medicine
Chief
Department of Anesthesiology
Director
Resident Education
Department of Anesthesiology
The University of Tennessee Health Science Center
Memphis, Tennessee

Mat H. Ho, MD, PhD
Associate Professor
Department of Obstetrics and Gynecology
School of Medicine, Texas Tech University Health
 Sciences Center
Odessa, Texas
Associate Professor
Harbor-UCLA Medical Center
University of California at Los Angeles
Los Angeles, California
Associate Professor
Texas Tech University Health Sciences Center
Odessa, Texas

Russell W. Jennings, MD
Assistant Professor
Harvard Medical School
Boston, Massachusetts

Director
Advanced Fetal Care Center
Children's Hospital
Boston, Massachusetts
Attending Pediatric Surgeon
Children's Hospital
Boston, Massachusetts

Shaun M. Kunisaki, MD
Clinical Fellow
Department of Surgery
Harvard Medical School
Boston, Massachusetts
Resident Physician
Department of Surgery
Massachusetts General Hospital
Boston, Massachusetts

Alisa B. Modena, MD
Perinatologist
Division of Maternal-Fetal Medicine
Virtua Health
Voorhees, New Jersey

Munir A. Nazir, MD
Director
Maternal-Fetal Medicine Assessment
  Laboratory
Division of Maternal-Fetal Medicine
Department of Obstetrics and Gynecology
Newark Beth Israel Medical Center
Newark, New Jersey

James J. Nocon, MD, JD
Associate Professor
Department of Obstetrics and Gynecology
Indiana University School of Medicine
Indianapolis, Indiana

John P. O'Grady, MD
Professor
Department of Obstetrics and Gynecology
Tufts University School of Medicine
Boston, Massachusetts
Medical Director
Family Life Center for Maternity
Mercy Hospital Perinatal Service
Division of Obstetrics and Gynecology
Mercy Medical Center
Springfield, Massachusetts

J. Gerald Quirk, MD, PhD
Professor and Chair
Department of Obstetrics, Gynecology, and
  Reproductive Medicine
State University of New York at Stony Brook
Stony Brook University School of Medicine
Stony Brook, New York
Obstetrician/Gynecologist-in-Chief
Stony Brook University Medical Center
Stony Brook, New York

V. Ravishankar, MD
Clinical Assistant Professor
Department of Obstetrics, Gynecology, and
  Reproductive Sciences
State University of New York at Stony Brook
Stony Brook University School of Medicine
Stony Brook, New York

Heather Z. Sankey, MD
Assistant Professor
Department of Obstetrics and
  Gynecology
Tufts University School of Medicine
Boston, Massachusetts
Residency Program Director
Department of Obstetrics and Gynecology
Medical Director
Wesson Women's Clinic
Baystate Medical Center
Springfield, Massachusetts

Andrew J. Satin, MD
Chair
Department of Obstetrics and Gynecology
Johns Hopkins Bayview Medical Center
Vice Chair/Deputy Director
Department of Obstetrics and Gynecology
Johns Hopkins University School of Medicine
Baltimore, Maryland
Attending Physician
Walter Reed National Military Medical
  Center
Bethesda, Maryland

Barry S. Schifrin, MD
Director
Maternal-Fetal Medicine
Tarzana Regional Medical Center
Tarzana, California

Richard J. Scotti, MD
Clinical Professor
University of Southern California Keck School
 of Medicine
Los Angeles, California
President and CEO
Foundation for Medical Education, Research, and
 Care, Inc.
Long Beach, California

Margaret Sedensky, MD
Professor
Department of Anesthesiology and Department
 of Genetics
University Hospitals of Cleveland
Case Western Reserve University School
 of Medicine
Cleveland, Ohio

David B. Seifer, MD
Professor
Department of Obstetrics, Gynecology, and
 Reproductive Sciences
Mount Sinai School of Medicine
New York, New York
Co-Director
Genesis Fertility and Reproductive Medicine
Maimonides Medical Center
Brooklyn, New York

Leon Speroff, MD
Professor
Department of Obstetrics and Gynecology
Oregon Health and Science University
Portland, Oregon

Lisa Summers, CNM, PhD
Director
Professional Services
American College of Nurse Midwifery
Silver Spring, Maryland

Stuart Weiner, MD
Associate Professor
Department of Obstetrics and
 Gynecology
Thomas Jefferson University
Philadelphia, Pennsylvania
Director
Division of Reproductive Imaging and
 Genetics
Maternal-Fetal Medicine
Thomas Jefferson University/Jefferson
 Medical College
Philadelphia, Pennsylvania

Janice N. Young, MD
Medical Director
Woman to Woman Gynecology
 of Naples
Naples, Florida

Paul C. Youngstrom, MD
Staff Anesthesiologist
The Cleveland Clinic Foundation
Cleveland, Ohio
Affiliate Anesthesiologist
Wilford Hall Medical Center
Lackland Air Force Base, Texas

Part I

ANTEPARTUM

John P. O'Grady

Norwithstanding that I would use all my Endeavours to deter Men from the rash and imprudent Practice of instrumental Operations in Midwifery; yet it is not to be denied, but that such Operations are very useful and necessary, when undertaken with Caution, Skill and Prudence;...

Fielding Ould (1710–1789)
A Treatise of Midwifery in Three Parts
Dublin: O. Nelson & C. Connor,
1742: 111, pg 142.

Prolonged or obstructed labor, undeliverable fetal positions, maternal hemorrhage from retained products of conception, delivery of the second of twins, and the problematic extraction of large infants are among the recurring problems in human labor and delivery that do not resolve without intervention. Assistive techniques to manage these and other complications of human parturition are rooted deep in antiquity. Over many years, various manipulations and specialized instruments were developed to expedite delivery of viable infants or to remove the fetus and the other products of conception from the uterus in case of fetal demise or incomplete delivery. A brief historical review of the origins of operative delivery techniques increases the appreciation of modern practitioners for the complex roots of the science and art that have led to modern practice.

THE HISTORY OF CESAREAN DELIVERY

Myth and Legend

Reports of the surgical removal of the fetus from the mother are common in history and legend. Such tales figure in the origin myths for important personalities from many cultures. For example, Brahma is described as emerging from his mother's umbilicus, and in 5636 B.C.E., Buddha is reported to have been delivered from his mother Maya's right flank [1]. Tall tales of preternatural or miraculous births are also common in our western Greco-Roman cultural heritage. Classic Greek mythology includes several descriptions of what could be termed cesarean deliveries of various gods, demigods, and mortals [2]. A representative example is the case of the inconstant princess Coronis. Upon receiving proof of her infidelity with another male suitor, her enraged paramour Apollo (Phoebus Apollo), god of prophecy, music, and archery, dispatched her with an arrow. In some versions of

1

this tale it is Apollo's twin sister, Artemis (Diana), daughter of Zeus and Leto, who was responsible for this murderous archery. In any event, Apollo next placed the body of the newly dead Coronis on a funeral pyre. As the flames leaped up, Apollo's rage rapidly changed to consternation for the fate of his unborn child. At Apollo's urgent request, Hermes (Mercury), the messenger of the gods and the patron of heralds, thieves, travelers, and merchants, intervened, and the infant was delivered from his mother's body by means of an abdominal incision. This child, who was the product of this unique perimortem delivery, was subsequently tutored in the healing arts by Chiron the centaur, son of Coronos and the nymph Philyra, and eventually became the most famous physician of antiquity, Asclepius. This tale has an ending that should serve as a warning to overly ambitious physicians. In his later life, Asclepius developed his medical abilities to the point where he could resurrect the dead. For his presumption in using his medical talents to thwart the will of the gods, Zeus killed him with a thunderbolt!

In another setting, Zeus prematurely delivered Dionysus (Bacchus), god of wine and ecstasy, from the abdomen of the dying Semele, the daughter of Cadmus and Harmonia. Zeus had actually fathered this child. Unfortunately, complications with the pregnancy led to disaster. In the sixth month of the pregnancy, malevolent advice was given to the young woman by the jealous Hera, Zeus's wife, who was masquerading as Semele's elderly nurse, Beroe. Under this influence, Semele refused Zeus her bed unless he would come to her in his true form. Zeus, trapped by her request, resumed his accustomed form as a thunderbolt, a dramatic process that proved fatal to the hapless Semele. Through the intervention of the ever-present Hermes, however, the unborn and premature Dionysis was removed from Semele's womb, sewn into the thigh of Zeus, and, through this unusual mechanism, carried to maturity as a bizarre type of ectopic pregnancy [3].

There are other unusual tales of obstetric interventions in Greek and Roman mythology. Adonis, famous for his great beauty, was born of his mother, Myrrha of Smyrna, after her transformation into a tree. Myrrha had conceived following an incestuous relationship with her father, Cinyras. Cinyras was a Cypriot king and originally one of the lesser suitors to Helen before her abduction and the beginning of the Trojan War. This unusual relationship between father and daughter developed because of the enmity of Aphrodite, the goddess of love, who punished the unfortunate Myrrha because of her lack of devotion [2]. Aphrodite's intervention caused the poor Myrrha to fall in love with her own father. Under what proved to be a maleficient influence, Myrrha developed a subterfuge whereby she shared Cinyras' bed without his recognizing her. The god's punishment for Adonis's mother was her transformation into a myrrh tree, thus arresting her father's unacceptable advances. Her father's eventual fate was also severe. When he discovered that he had been tricked into impregnating his own daughter, Cinyras committed suicide.

In terms of drama, myth, and legend, classic theater also contains many stories of unusual births. Perhaps the most famous occurs in the denouement of the play *Macbeth*. Shakespeare's protagonist Macduff is free from mortal risk from Macbeth, because Macduff was "from his mother's womb untimely ripp'd...." [4] As he was not of woman born, Macduff fulfilled the prophecy of the witches and thus successfully defeated the regicidal Macbeth. This tale of ambition, greed, murder, and operative delivery has a long pedigree, with its origin well before the sixteenth century. Shakespeare had obtained the material for his tragedy from an earlier text, the *Chronicles of Holinshead*. From this reference, further sources for this Scottish tale can be traced to another text, *Scotorum, Historiae of Boece* (Paris, 1526); it can further be followed to a manuscript originally published in 1385! Doubtless, its roots are even earlier than the fourteenth century, in now lost sources.

History also includes many reports of unusual cesarean deliveries involving actural individuals. There are several well-documented cases in which women delivered themselves by conducting their own surgeries. Many if not most of these abdominal surgical deliveries would in current terminology be described as cesareans. Authentic reports from rural settings also describe traumatic deliveries when milkmaids were gored by cattle, the earliest dating back to 1647. In some of these latter cases, the mother, the infant, or both apparently survived [1].

Derivation of Terms *Cesarean* and *Section*

In common parlance transabdominal surgical deliveries are termed *cesareans*. How this nomenclature came to be employed for abdominal surgical delivery is a long and complex tale. The derivation of the term *cesarean* has been ascribed to several sources. Ancient historians, including Pliny the Elder are largely responsible for the widely believed myth that a Roman emperor or Caesar – either Scipio Africanus (237–183 B.C.E.) or more commonly, the most famous emperor, Gaius Julius Caesar (102?–44 B.C.E.) – was delivered from his mother via an abdominal incision. Unfortunately, it is unlikely that these historical figures or many of the other famous persons reputed to have been delivered by a surgical procedure were actually born in that manner. In reference to the historical Roman Emperor Gaius Julius Caesar, it is virtually certain he was *not* delivered surgically from his mother, since the term *cesarean* predates him by centuries. Furthermore, published letters of Julius Caesar indicate that he corresponded with his mother, Aurelia, while he was in Gaul. Finally, Aurelia is known to have lived until 54 B.C.E., when Caesar, who was then more than 40 years old, attended her funeral [5]. Her long-term survival after an unsterile abdominal surgery in the first century is distinctly improbable. The reports by Pliny and other classical writers of successful abdominal delivery of culturally important people such as the historical Emperor Julius Caesar lack historical support and are best viewed as political fables.

There are various interpretations but no clear evidence to explain how the family of Gaius Julius Caesar received the cognomen *caesar* and how this family name at some point became associated with a surgical procedure. The name of Caesar might derive from several literary sources, such as from the Latin *caedere/caedo*, meaning "to cut, fall, or kill; to cut down or to strike mortally as in conflict," [6] possibly reflecting a traumatic or surgical delivery sometime in the family's past [7]. It is also possible that a legend of an abdominal delivery became associated with the family name simply as an honor. Preternatural births were thought to confer on the child certain special virtues, powers, or abilities – exactly what might be expected of a world leader such as an emperor. After all, the Julian family was noble and from a patrician clan. Caesar's father, once the governor of Asia, had served as praetor, the second most important post after counsul [8].

Another possible origin of the term *cesarean* derives from legal responses to the problem of peri- or postmortem delivery. The first law relating to postmortem delivery is reputed to have been promulgated by the quasi-legendary king of Rome, Numa Pompilius (715–673 B.C.E.), and termed the *lex regia* (and subsequently *lex caesarea*) [1]. This edict concerned the abdominal delivery of a child during an acute life-saving effort in the unusual circumstance of a dying or recently dead mother. The statute was a type of Good Samaritan law, requiring delivery of the unborn child from its mother and forbidding the burial of the dead woman until this was accomplished. The law also protected the person who performed such a perimortem procedure from an accusation of murder or manslaughter, assuming that the amateur surgeon acted in good faith.

Some English words with specialized meaning have their origin in the Latin roots that originally gave us the term *cesarean*. In musical notation, a *caesura* is a set of closely approximated parallel lines in the score that mark a sudden stop, or cut, in the course of the program. This term is also used to indicate an interruption, break, or pause between words within a metrical foot in poetry, or in the middle of a line of text. In a social/political context, both the titles of *Kaiser* and *Tsar* (*Czar*) have their origin in the original Latin *Caesar*. In English, both Kaiser and Tsar either describe an authority figure, usually a tyrannical one, or are used in their historical sense as the traditional titles for a Holy Roman, Austrian-German, or Russian Emperor, respectively.

Whatever the origin of the term, by the mid-sixteenth century, the term *cesarean* was used to describe abdominal surgical deliveries in medical literature. One of the earliest commentators or medical editors to refer to the abdominal delivery of an infant as a cesarean was Richard Jonas, who translated, edited, and expanded one of the many editions of the obstetric textbook usually termed the *Roszgarten*, which was originally authored by Eucharius Rösslin of Frankfurt-am-Main (discussed later in this chapter). First published in 1540 in its English editions as *The Byrth of Mankynde*, this text was thereafter frequently reprinted. In one of these reprintings, Jonas commented in reference to abdominal delivery "...that are borne after this fashion be called cesares, for because they be cut of theyr mothers belly, whervpon also the noble Romane cesar...of that name in Rome toke his name..." [9].

The second part of the usual term for obstetric abdominal surgery, *section*, probably has its origin in the Latin verb *secare/seco*, meaning "to light, strike, or reach," or "to cut into, separate, divide, or part" [10]. Another possibility is *incidere/incido*, meaning "to fall or on, happen, or occur" [6,10].

At some indeterminate time in the past, the terms used to describe the surgical operation for abdominal delivery, *cesarean* and *section*, became inextricably linked. Over time, however, the terms used to describe the surgery for abdominal deliveries have changed. In modern times, such surgical delivery of the fetus was referred to as a *cesarean operation* until the early twentieth century, when the term *cesarean section* became popular [1]. Currently, the term *cesarean birth* is frequently used in both lay and professional literature. Because of the redundancy inherent in the term *cesarean section*, we prefer to describe the surgical operation for the abdomen delivery of a child as a *cesarean delivery*, a *cesearean operation*, or simply as a *cesarean*. These conventions are used in the current text.

Cesarean Delivery in the Historical Record

Beyond the mythology of the origins of the cesarean-related terms is also a long historical record of successful and not-so-successful abdominal deliveries. The oldest reliably recorded operations date back to the Sumerians in the second millennium B.C.E. More than 1,000 years later, Gorgias (483–375 B.C.E.), a famous orator from Sicily, is reputed to have been delivered by a cesarean Records from as early as the second century C.E. report the operation several times, and in early Jewish literature Maimonides (1135–1204) mentioned cesarean surgery and commented on technique. It was not until the seventeenth century, however, that thoroughly documented cesarean deliveries are known to have been performed on living women with occasional maternal or fetal survivals. Many of the earlier reports are incomplete, wildly improbable, or so warped and embellished by multiple retellings that they remain suspect.

Commentary concerning cesarean delivery appears early in obstetric literature; however, many of the classic medical authors fail entirely to mention the procedure, attesting to its rarity. As an example, Soranus of Ephesus (98–138 C.E.) does not include cesarean operations in his review of surgical procedures. Sonanus did describe the management of obstetric malpresentation by version and extraction but did not mention the use of instruments or abnormal surgery for delivery. Aurelius Cornelius Celsus (27 B.C.E.–50 C.E.) in his book *De Re Medica* (c. 30 C.E.) is also silent on abdominal delivery yet provided instructions for the extraction of dead infants by the use of a hook or crochet. Cesareans are also not a part of the corpus of Hippocratic writings. Eucharius Rösslin the Elder's (also Roeslin, Roesslyn, or Rhodion) important, early obstetric textbook *Der Swangern Frawen und Hebammen Rosegarten*, published in Strassburg in 1513 and widely known as *The Roszgarten* (also *Roszgarten* or *Rosengarten*) does not mention the cesarean operation. As earlier noted, however, one of the many later editors or revisers of this book, Richard Jonas, did make such a reference in a commentary included in one of the many subsequent English language reprintings of this remarkably long-lived textbook.

There are various reports of cesarean deliveries from numerous sources before the seventeenth century. Unfortunately, most simply document the danger of the procedure and the extreme risk to the mother's life. In Sweden, a postmortem cesarean operation was first recorded in 1360. Scipio Mercurio (1550–1616?), a surgeon of Padua, claimed several successful cesarean operations in his textbook *La Commare o Riccoglitrice*, published in 1596. In 1578, Giulio Cesari Aranzio (1530–1589) reported a successful postmortem cesarean delivery on a mother who had died late in the third trimester. Jacques Guillemeau (1544–1612) was surgeon to Henry and a student of the noted barber-surgeon Ambroise Paré (1510–1590). Guillemeau included a chapter on cesarean delivery in an obstetric text that was later translated into English by Thomas Hatfield in 1612 and entitled *Childbirth or, The Happie Deliverie of Women* [11]. Guillemeau stated that he had seen the operation carried out by various surgeons on a total of five women, all of whom had died. In his discussion of the procedure in this book, Guillemeau was among the first to introduce the word *section* into the medical literature.

The most controversial of the early reports of successful operative deliveries is that involving Jacob Nufer, a sow-gelder who is reputed to have performed a successful cesarean on his own wife circa 1500. The Jacob Nufer story was first related by Caspar Bauhin (1550–1624), more than 80 years after the supposed event, in the appendix and commentary to Bauhin's Latin translation of a text entitled *Traité Nouveau de l'hysterotomokie ou l'enfantement Caesarienne* printed in Paris in 1581 and originally authored by François Rousset (1535–1590?), physician to the Duke of Savoy [12]. Rousset, although not himself a surgeon, recounted cases of cesarean deliveries performed by others and claimed to have been an observer in still more, including several with maternal and fetal survivals. He argued that a cesarean was not only "a feasible operation" but also could preserve the lives of both mother and infant. As the title of his text reflects, Rousset termed the procedure a *cesarean delivery* or "enfantement Caesarienne" presumably in homage to the legend involving the birth of Julius Caesar [13]. The Nufer story was retold as late as the mid-eighteenth century by the reviewer and critic John Burton (1710–1771) in his textbook of obstetrics, *An Essay towards a Compleate New System of Midwifry*, published in 1751 [14].

As the Nufer tale is usually related, both lithotomists and midwives were called in consultation when the labor of Nufer's wife was obstructed. None of these attendants was able to bring the child forth, however. In desperation, Nufer himself performed a surgical delivery. His wife is supposed to have not only survived the operation but also later to have delivered other children vaginally. Although this entire story is suspect, it might contain a kernel of hidden truth. Because of the nature of his work in animal husbandry, Nufer would have had rough surgical and birthing experience. Such people with a functional knowledge of delivery mechanics were occasionally called on in the sixteenth century to help manage obstructed human labors. This might explain his active involvement in his wife's confinement. But, can the rest of this remarkable story be believed? Perhaps what Nufer's wife had was an advanced abdominal pregnancy. This could explain both her survival following an unsterile laparatomy and her subsequent unimpaired fertility. What actually happened in that Swiss hamlet in 1500, and the degree to which the Nufer story has been embellished and distorted over time, cannot now be determined as no new information is likely to be forthcoming.

In 1610, a physician in Wittenberg, Jeremias Trautmann, conducted the earliest well-documented cesarean delivery [15]. Although a surgery is known to have been performed and a child delivered, the clinical details remain confusing. It is possible that what Trautmann actually found was an anterior uterine sacculation or an abdominal pregnancy. In other accounts the pregnancy was normal and the reason for surgery was a large ventral hernia that precluded normal labor. In fact, whether a pregnancy was even diagnosed before the operation is uncertain, and the infant might have been an unexpected discovery during a surgical exploration to relieve acute abdominal symptoms. In any event, an abdominal procedure was conducted, a child was delivered and is presumed to have survived although the extant records are at best incomplete. Unfortunately, the mother died some 25 days after the original operation, presumably from infection.

From the inception of the operation, controversy concerning the propriety of cesarean delivery has characterized the medical literature. It was recognized very early that postmortem operations on mothers dying in labor or late in pregnancy would rarely result in a normal and surviving child. Owing to the state of development of surgical technique, a cesarean was a virtual death sentence for both mother and infant until the early nineteenth century. To operate on a living woman was thus shunned, owing to the profound maternal risk from surgery and the uncertainty of success in salvaging a living infant. When labor was obstructed, version and extraction, fetal destructive procedures, and later symphysiotomy were the accepted methods for delivery. Whereas the mother often survived these obstetric manipulations and destructive procedures for vaginal delivery, in almost all cases the infant did not.

With this background, including horrific reports in the literature and their own experience with disastrous cesarean results, most of the influential obstetric educators of the sixteenth and seventeenth centuries, including Ambroise Paré (1510–1590), Jacques Guillemeau (1550–1630), Pierre Dionis (1643?–1718), and François Mauriceau (1637–1709), advised strongly against performing a cesarean operation on living women. Mauriceau, the most celebrated obstetrician of the late seventeenth century, discussed known obstetric procedures in his textbooks, *Traité Les Maladies des Femmes Grosses, et Accouchées* (Figure 1.1) [16] and *Observations Sur la Grossesse et l'Accouchement des Femmes, et sur Leurs Maladies, &; celles des Enfans Nouveau – Nez* [17].

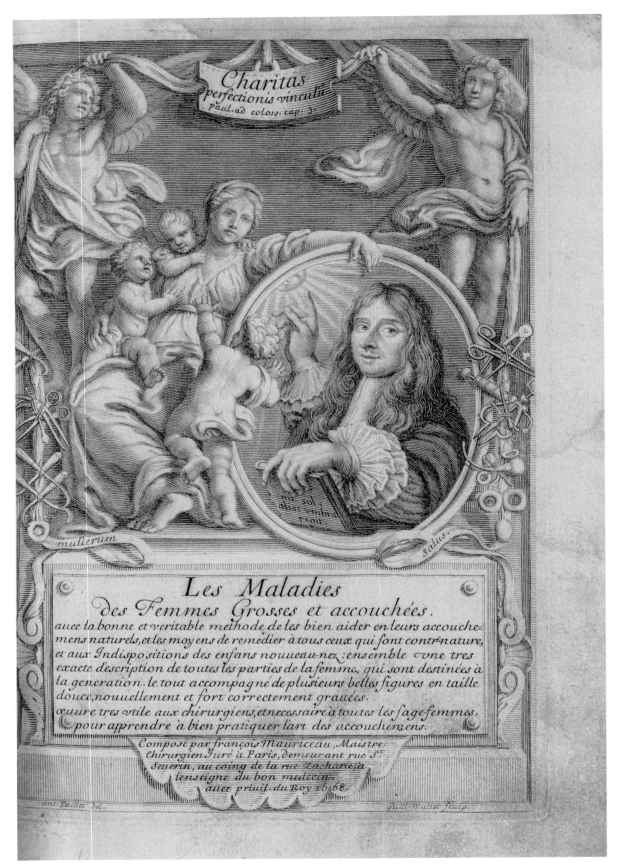

FIGURE 1.1.
Title page of the Traité *of François Mauriçeau (c. 1668).*

Mauriceau argued that only postmortem cesareans should be performed. He was well experienced in serious obstetric complications and knew firsthand of the limitations imposed by the inability of physicians to conduct abdominal deliveries. His own sister had experienced a serious antepartum hemorrhage from a placenta previa. When her attendants recoiled from intervention, Mauriceau had delivered her himself by version and extraction. Unfortunately, she did not survive this procedure [18].

In contrast, some early medical authors did support cesarean delivery. Jean-Louis Baudelocque (1746–1810) and André Levret (1703–1780) advocated cesareans for a contracted pelvis, in preference to the usual procedures of embryotomy, decapitation, or cranial decompression. The maternal and fetal results of most early cesarean operations were disastrous, however, reinforcing the argument for those who opposed such surgeries. According to Baskett [11], on one occasion, the noted French accoucheur Baudelocque was forced to defend himself in court when a contemporary called him an assassin because of Baudelocque's favorable opinions concerning cesarean delivery!

Cesarean deliveries were sporadically reported in the medical literature from the eighteenth through the mid-nineteenth century with generally poor results and often the loss of both mother and infant. In the early to mid-1700s cesarean deliveries were performed in Paris at a rate of approximately 1 per 4000 births. Unfortunately, the associated maternal mortality was 70% to 80%! A few successful abdominal deliveries did occur outside of the French capital between 1760 and 1814, however [19]. There were similarly grim statistics from the British Isles. There was not a cesarean delivery with documented maternal survival in Ireland until 1738, when a midwife, Mary Donally, operated on a 33-year-old multipara. In this case, Donally made a right paraumbilical incision with a razor; the incision subsequently closed with a tailor's needle and silk thread. The patient survived but later developed a ventral hernia. A cesarean delivery following a 6-day obstructed labor is also known to have occurred in England in 1737, but neither mother nor infant survived. In fact, a cesarean operation in England in which the mother is known to have survived did not occur until 1793 when the first case was reported. The mother in this instance had been in labor for three days when a surgeon, James Barlow delivered a dead child through a left paramedian incision [1]. From the same era there is an incompletely documented report of a successful cesarean delivery from America. Dr. Jesse Bennett (1769–1842) is supposed to have performed the procedure on his own wife in 1794 in Staunton, Virginia, following an unsuccessful effort at vaginal instrumental delivery. The details of this case are sketchy, and the documentation is poor. Thus, this claim is not generally considered credible. The first well-documented American report dates from 1827, when Dr. J. Cambert Richmond (1785–1855) performed an operation on a nulliparous eclamptic woman. Although the mother survived, the infant did not [20]. Another cesarean with maternal survival was performed before 1821 (exact date unknown) by the physician and surgeon James Miranda Barry in South Africa. Barry holds the unique distinction of being both an Edinburgh graduate and a woman who successfully masqueraded as a man from 1809 until her death in 1865 [18]. Africa is also the source for a report of another successful cesarean delivery performed by an unknown indigenous surgeon. In 1879, R. W. Felkin, a Scottish medical traveler in what later became Uganda in East Africa, witnessed and later published his observations concerning a cesarean delivery [21]. Preoperatively the surgeon cleansed his hands and the mother's abdomen with banana wine. The same fluid was administered orally to the mother before the surgery began, presumably to induce a degree of insensibility. After the delivery, which the surgeon performed through a midline incision, the uterus was not sutured. The abdominal incision was pinned together with iron needles and then secured by a bark-cloth string. Bleeding was controlled by cautery. Felkin claimed that the woman made a full recovery and noted the apparent expertise of the surgeon, concluding that the procedure was well established in that part of Africa.

In the late eighteenth century and into the early years of the nineteenth century, because of the serious risks of surgery, symphysiotomy vied with cesarean delivery as the best procedure for obstructed delivery. Intentional incision of the pubic symphysis was introduced to medical practice in 1768, when Jean René Sigault (1740–18??) described the technique in a single case [1,11,25]. Sigault successfully delivered a multiparous woman (a Madam Souchot), whose first child was lost owing to an obstructed labor and a fetal demise, eventually terminated by an embryotomy. Her other deliveries had been equally unfortunate, resulting in stillbirths. For his efforts, Sigault received both a medal from the Facility of Medicine in Paris, and a government pension. A medal was given to his assistant, Alphonse LeRoy (1742–1816), and to complete the awards, a pension was provided for the patient, who, despite a rocky postpartum course, including abscesses and a vesicovaginal fistula, survived! Despite such occasional successes, because of the manner in which symphysiotomy was performed, maternal morbidity and mortality were high. For these reasons, the procedure soon fell into disfavor and was not revived until the twentieth century. Symphysiotomy is still occasionally performed in parts of the nonindustrialized world as an alternative to a cesarean [23,24].

Prior to the late nineteenth century, several serious technical problems precluded safe cesarean deliveries. First, the operation was viewed as the last resort. It therefore usually was not performed until after prolonged labor, multiple examinations, manipulations, and various unsuccessful efforts at vaginal instrumental delivery. Inevitably, many of these women were exhausted and dehydrated, and most were infected. Surgical procedures at that time were also primitive. Before the invention of inhalation anesthesia in the late 1840s, surgery needed to be rapid. Only laudanum and alcohol were available as analgesic agents and the patient had to be actively restrained during the procedure. Furthermore, nothing was known concerning aseptic methods of surgery, ensuring a serious risk of infection. In the usual technique, the maternal abdomen was opened by a vertical incision, lateral to the rectus muscle. Attendants restrained the mother and, once the abdomen was entered, endeavored to hold back the intestines with their hands. The uterus was incised vertically and the child removed. Usually, the uterine wound was specifically not sutured because sutures were believed to predispose to complications, but the edges of the abdominal wound were usually reapproximated. Because of the timing of the operation, the absence of aseptic technique, and the failure to close the uterus, mothers usually rapidly died of hemorrhage or, if they lingered for several days, of peritonitis.

Progress was slow. The first reported instance of the successful use of uterine sutures at a cesarean was by the surgeon Jean LeBas (1717–1787). In a 1769 delivery, he applied silk thread sutures to a uterine incision to stop hemorrhage. The patient subsequently recovered. Inevitably, LeBas was heavily criticized by his contemporaries. After LeBas' report, several attempts at routine uterine suturing occurred in individual cases, usually with disastrous results [11].

From our vantage point, it is hard to understand why suturing of the uterine wound during a cesarean was considered inappropriate until almost the beginning of the twentieth century. This practice followed then-contemporary clinical experience and well-established surgical technique, however. A common reason given for not suturing the uterus routinely after a cesarean was the belief that rapid uterine involution would inevitably loosen any stitches, rendering them ineffective. Another problem was infection. In the eighteenth and well into the nineteenth century, sutures placed by a surgeon were routinely left long, protruding from the wound. This was believed necessary to facilitate drainage and to provide access for the eventual removal of the sutures, which usually were not absorbable and, of course, not sterile. Conventional wisdom and clinical observation held that deeply placed sutures invariably became infected, leading to abscess, cellulitis, or sepsis. A wound left open, with the suture ends exiting the skin, would eventually begin to develop what was termed laudable pus, however. With time, progressive tissue necrosis would eventually release the sutures. The usual practice was that several days after the surgery the surgeon would begin intermittently to pull gently on the suture ends. This process was subsequently repeated once or twice daily until local necrosis was sufficient to permit the extraction of the sutures without eliciting a hemorrhage. For patients who survived to the point of suture removal, eventual recovery was likely. After suture removal, the wound would slowly heal by secondary intention. Once the process of granulation was well advanced such wounds were quite resistant to infection and unlikely to lead to cellulitis or sepsis. Unfortunately, when such standard surgical techniques were used in cesarean deliveries, hemorrhage and infection were routine, with serious and usually fatal consequences for the mother.

When uterine reapproximation was finally introduced, silver wire became the initial suture material of choice, mirroring its use in nineteenth century gynecology. Frank E. Polin of Springfield, Kentucky, first reported the use of silver wire in the closure of a uterine wound in 1852. Other than silver wire, many other types of suture were in use, derived from a wide range of materials including silk, carbolized gut, horsehair, and even hemp. What would now be considered as appropriate uterine approximation with nonpermanent suture materials was not introduced until the early 1880s.

Many important surgical innovations begun in the mid-nineteenth century eventually made safe cesarean deliveries possible. Ether was first used during labor in Boston in 1847 and subsequently popularized by the socially prominent New England obstetrician Walter Channing (1786–1876). The anesthetic properties of chloroform were discovered by James Young Simpson (1811–1870) and first employed by him in deliveries in Edinburgh beginning in 1847 [11].

A major breakthrough in the technique of cesarean surgery occurred in the early 1880s. Max Sänger (1853–1903), then an assistant to Carl Siegmund Franz Credé (1819–1892) in Leipzig, introduced an operative procedure in 1882 that is now considered the classic cesarean operation. In doing so, Sänger revolutionized standard cesarean surgical technique [26]. In a general review for a monograph concerning the cesarean operation, Sänger had collected published case reports of prior deliveries that he carefully reviewed and critiqued. Based on these data from the literature and his own experience, Sänger argued that operative complications from cesareans would occur less frequently if the myometrium were closed and a concerted effort made to avoid the spillage of intrauterine secretions into the peritoneal cavity [26]. His procedure featured a meticulous, water-tight reapproximation of the uterine wound, employing buried sutures. Sänger also exteriorized the uterus before delivering the infant and attempted to improve postoperative drainage by passing a drain from the fundus out through the cervix.

Although maternal morbidity and mortality from cesarean deliveries remained high even with Sänger's improvements, statistics were substantially better with his technique than the levels previously experienced. It was only after Sänger's 1882 paper that closure of the uterus was finally recognized as both a feasible and necessary part of cesarean technique [1].

Horatio R. Storer, of Boston, Masschusetts, first performed a cesarean hysterectomy in 1868, on a woman with a large leiomyoma that obstructed the birth canal. He removed the uterine corpus and adnexa during this procedure. The child was stillborn and "in an advanced state of decomposition." The mother died three days later. The first maternal survivor following cesarean hysterectomy occurred in 1876, when a woman with rickets and pelvic contracture was delivered by Eduardo Porro (1842–1901) [1,27]. What later was termed the *Porro operation* was a unique surgical procedure originally suggested by the Florentine surgeon Joseph Cavallini in 1768. Cavallini and later Porro had experimented with pregnant hysterectomy in animal models. Cavallini had operated on dogs and sheep; Porro had used rabbits. Each had proved to his satisfaction that the uterus was not necessary for life and that its surgical removal was technically possible.

In early 1876, Porro encountered a 25-year-old nullipara with a rachitic pelvis and a true conjugate of 4 cm or less, precluding vaginal delivery. Following careful consideration and preparations, including preliminary handwashing with carbolic acid, Porro performed a classic cesarean delivery by means of a midline abdominal incision, with the patient under chloroform anesthesia. After delivery of the baby, an iron-wire snare was passed around the uterus, tubes, and ovaries. All these structures were then amputated and the remaining cervical stump was bought out of the abdomen through the lower end of the midline incision. Drainage tubes were inserted and the abdominal wall was then closed around the residual stump with silver-wire sutures. The snare was removed on the fourth day and the sutures on the seventh. The exterialized cervical stump and lower portion of the abdominal wound were then permitted to heal by secondary intention. Six weeks later, the woman left the hospital with her infant. Remarkably, she was the first to survive a cesarean delivery performed at that clinic!

The Porro operation rapidly gained acceptance in Europe because it radically solved the problems of both hemorrhage and infection. Maternal losses with the Porro operation remained high but were substantially below those experienced before the procedure was introduced. By 1884, approximately 140 of these operations had been reported in Europe, with a maternal mortality rate of 56%. After 1882, the classic cesarean operation without hysterectomy as popularized by Max Sänger began to replace Porro's operation as the surgical technique of choice because the rates of maternal morbidity and mortality were lower. By the onset of the twentieth century, the Porro operation had been entirely superseded.

Despite these and other innovations, cesarean delivery did not gain popularity with practitioners until well after the introduction of aseptic technique by Joseph Lister (1827–1912) and others in the latter decades of the nineteenth century. Drawing upon the new discoveries in bacteriology and the development of the germ theory of infection, the combination of improved anesthesia and new surgical methods finally blunted the horrific rates of maternal morbidity and mortality associated with cesarean operations [28]. The great safety of cesarean delivery still awaited changes introduced during the twentieth century.

The rapidly falling mortality rate of cesarean hysterectomy expanded the potential indications for the operation. Cesarean hysterectomy became progressively popular during the period from the late 1940s to the mid 1960s, and was often performed for sterilization. In recent decades, because of the substantial morbidity of the operation, cesarean hysterectomy has fallen from favor as an elective method of sterilization. At present, this procedure is generally restricted to management of uncontrolled hemorrhage, the rare case of nonreparable uterine injury, or for other reasons of severe uterine or cervical pathology. In recent years, the availability of potent uterotonics and broad-spectrum antibiotics, the development of embolization techniques, and new methods of vessel ligation have markedly reduced the need for emergency cesarean hysterectomy, although it still remains an important and potentially lifesaving procedure (See Chapter 18, Cesarean Delivery).

Other innovations in surgical technique lessened the risks of surgery. Maternal complications from cesarean deliveries were reduced by the development of the lower-segment cesarean operation, a procedure originally suggested by Johann F. Osiander of Goettingen (1759–1822). In 1805, Osiander opined that entry into the uterus through a vertical lower-segment incision could avoid the complications of the usual surgical technique, which then involved a vertical incision in the upper and thicker portion. More than a century later, Bernard Krönig (1912) revived this idea and proposed dissecting into the vesicouterine space and subsequently using the bladder serosa to cover the uterine incision, to protect the peritoneal cavity from exposure to the lochia. This combined technique of a lower-segment uterine entry and sequestration of the myometrial wound behind the peritoneum resulted in less immediate surgical morbidity and substantially reduced the risk of uterine rupture in subsequent pregnancies.

The extraperitoneal cesarean operation has an interesting history [20]. This procedure was first proposed by W. E. Horner in 1824. Such procedures were not performed until Alexander Johnston Chalmers Skene (1838–1900) successfully delivered a woman with a rachitic pelvis by this technique [7]. In 1909, the extraperitoneal operation gained support when Wilhelm Latzko of Vienna reported only two maternal deaths among thirty such procedures. Latzko's paravesical, extraperitoneal operation was later popularized in the years prior to World War by E. G. Waters [29] and J. F. Norton [30]. The theoretical advantage of this operation was to isolate the entire operative site retroperitoneally and thus potentially avoid the risk of peritoneal contamination. The progressively increasing safety of the transperitoneal approach, the rapidly decreasing incidence of protracted, dystocic labors, and the advent of antibiotics markedly reduced the importance and advantage of the extraperitoneal operation, however. It is now uncommonly attempted.

In recent decades, additional modifications in cesarean operative technique have been introduced. New and less tissue reactive suture materials are now available. In routine operations contemporary surgeons now frequently omit the serosal or vesicouterine flap closure and closure of the parietal peritoneum in an effort to reduce adhesion formation. The standard methods for both opening and closing both the fascia and uterus also have changed, at least for many surgeons, replacing the traditional sharp entry by techniques of blunt dissection and employing running as opposed to interrupted sutures for closure. Perhaps the most marked change in cesarean practice in the last 75 years has not been in surgical technique, however, but in the remarkable reduction in serious maternal morbidity and mortality associated with the operation by the administration of prophylactic antibiotics, the rapid development of medical therapies to treat complications, and general improvements in anesthesia. The overall mortality risk for unselected cesarean operations has fallen to 1 per 1,000 or less owing to these various advances and improvements.

INSTRUMENTAL DELIVERY

The development of atraumatic delivery instruments is a complex and fascinating part of the history of obstetrics [31–36]. Beginning 200 years ago, a remarkably small group of innovators developed and perfected new types of obstetric instruments. Their trials, false starts, occasional successes, and many failures make for a rousing tale that involves trade secrets, professional jealousy, true altruism, a touch of scandal, and inevitably, the search for profit and fame. Beyond technical considerations concerning instruments or technique, practitioners of the past were also well aware of the potential risks and benefits of the use of instruments in obstetric practice and of the classic alternatives, either a cesarean or a destructive operation. They sought to develop vaginal delivery devices that were safe, effective, and ultimately lifesaving. The different approaches that contemporary accoucheurs have toward instrument-assisted delivery mirrors a two-century-old tension between contending philosophies of obstetric practice. This persisting and irresolvable controversy is between those willing to intervene versus those whose preferences are to wait and observe. The balance in the relative ascendancy between these positions is influenced by various advances in the field of obstetric practice, including the periodic publication of critical reevaluations of traditional obstetric procedures, the introduction of new instruments, the popularity of novel techniques or procedures, the complex pressures of society, and medicolegal trends.

Prior to the introduction of safe delivery instruments, intravenous fluid therapy, blood transfusion, potent antibiotics, and potent uterotonics, the options available to birth attendants when labor was obstructed were starkly limited. The mother could be permitted to continue to labor at high risk for her own injury and for the loss of her child in the hope of an eventual vaginal delivery. Alternatively, version and extraction, symphysiotomy, or a procedure destructive to the fetus could be performed. Such procedures might save the mother but often did so

at the cost of severe or fatal fetal injuries. Furthermore, before the late nineteenth century, attempts at any intervention were often delayed until the situation was nearly hopeless, effectively determining the outcome. Abdominal operations such as cesareans were uncommon prior to the latter part of the nineteenth century. Surgery was brutal, far from safe, and performed without anesthesia. As discussed in the previous section, cesarean delivery did not become an acceptable option until after the mid 1880s owing to the horrific risks of hemorrhage and infection and the limitations of anesthesia. It was in this formidable setting that nondestructive delivery instruments were first invented.

Modern obstetric delivery forceps are the highly modified descendants of instruments destructive to the fetus that date from antiquity [31,32,34]. The term *forceps* most likely takes its origin from a contraction of a Latin root word, either *ferricepes* (*ferum*, meaning "iron," and *capio*, meaning "I take") or *formus* (meaning "hot") combined again with *capio*.

Although destructive instruments including hooks and other extraction devices are accepted as ancient, the date of invention for nontraumatic obstetric forceps is the subject of debate. Atraumatic instrumental delivery devices were unknown to the Greeks and probably to the Romans as well, although the latter is not completely certain. If the Romans ever had a nondestructive delivery forceps in their armamentarium, this device was lost over time and did not influence later developments. Destructive instruments, including cranial perforators, hooks and various cranial grasping devices, however, date to antiquity.

Various two-bladed, scissor-like metal instruments designed for obstetrical applications were in use by approximately 1000 C.E. and were known to Albucasis (1013–1106) and his contemporaries, Avicenna (c. 980–1037) and Maimonides (1135–1204). Jacob Rueff's (1500–1558) textbook *De Conceptu et Generatione Hominis* from 1544 illustrates such instruments (Figure 1.2). A surgeon and obstetrician in Zurich, Rueff drew his information largely from Soranus and from the previously mentioned text by Rösslin, usually entitled the *Rosengarten*, initially published in 1513. Unfortunately, devices depicted in this text were quite clearly designed for the destruction and removal of the fetus from the uterus and not to assist in the delivery of living infants. Atraumatic delivery required the

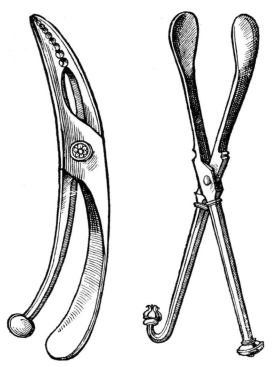

FIGURE 1.2.
Delivery instruments illustrated by Jacques Rueff in De Conceptu et Generatione Hominis *(1554). (Courtesy of the Historical Division/ Cleveland Health Sciences Library, Cleveland, OH.)*

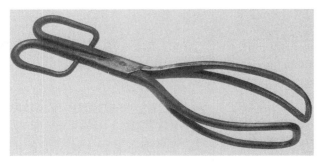

FIGURE 1.3.
Chamberlen delivery forceps c. 1610 (facsimile). (Courtesy of the Dittrick Museum of Medical History, Historical Division/Cleveland Health Sciences Library, Cleveland, OH.)

development of instruments capable of two different but related tasks: grasping the fetal head securely and permitting cranial rotation and traction. Both of the tasks also had to be accomplished without resulting in serious maternal injury. Neither technical limitations nor the lack of surgeons delayed the development of safe delivery instruments, however. Europe had many talented medical fabricators in the flourishing armament industry of the sixteenth and seventeenth centuries who could easily have produced metal scissor-like instruments like forceps on demand. The problem was twofold: first, the requirement to identify the need for such instruments, and second, the recruitment of sufficiently skilled practitioners to direct the transformation of initially destructive instruments into atraumatic delivery instruments. These changes awaited the Chamberlens.

During the reign of Charles , religious persecution drove many Protestants from France, including William Chamberlen (c. 1540–1596), a medical practitioner who subsequently established his

family in England [22,31,34,37]. By the late sixteenth century, the two sons of William Chamberlen were actively practicing medicine in London, working as barber surgeons and heavily involved in midwifery. Which of the brothers, Peter Chamberlen "the elder" (1560–1631) or Peter Chamberlen "the younger" (1572–1626) was the inventor of obstetric forceps is not clear, although Peter the Elder is usually give the credit. Although the process that led to the development of the Chamberlen instrument is unknown, it is believed that a practical forceps model was first developed after 1610 and then later modified several times based on clinical experience (Figure 1.3).

The Chamberlen delivery forceps were not released for general use after their invention, and for decades the instruments remained closely guarded as a family trade secret. The Chamberlen brothers and many of their descendants held themselves out as obstetric consultants. As such, they provided the public access to their secret method of delivery (the forceps) for a fee. Once they had been called in consultation, their "secret instrument" was delivered to the lying-in site in a large, gilded box [37]. All of the original birth attendants were then excluded from the room. The forceps were then removed from the box in such a fashion so as not to be seen by the parturient. As was usual continental practice, the delivery was conducted under the cover of a sheet that covered the parturient's bed and was tied behind the accoucheur's neck. His drape in place, the surgeon would sit at the end of the bed, grasp the forceps, and commence the procedure. Thus, both his manipulations and the delivery forceps were hidden under the sheet. After the delivery, the instrument was replaced in its box and the delivery fee claimed. Because of this process, neither the woman nor her family or friends could attest to what had actually occurred, and thus the secret remained secure.

A later and somewhat unsavory member of the Chamberlen family, Hugh the Elder (1630–17??) was a notable entrepreneur and self-styled deal-maker. In 1670, hoping to raise money he went to Paris and offered to sell the family secret to the noted French obstetrician François Mauriceau for what was then a large sum of money [3,33]. Mauriceau provided a test case, a woman with a markedly deformed pelvis in obstructed labor. Despite Chamberlen's prolonged and heroic efforts, both the women and infant died. At a later postmortem examination, the uterus was found to be ruptured. Not surprisingly, this sale fell through. Despite this debacle, Chamberlen managed to secure an agreement from his French colleague to translate Mauriceau's textbook, the *Traité*, into English. On his return to London, Chamberlen published a version of this book in English, initially entitled *The Accomplish't Midwife* (1672). The text proved highly successful and at least eight subsequent editions were printed. This literary and professional coup was a substantial contribution to midwifery practice in England and improved Chamberlen's prominence in his profession while also helping to attract a large clinical practice, thus improving both his social and financial position [22].

Forever embroiled in political affairs and financial schemes, Hugh the Elder subsequently encountered sufficient difficulty in England to induce him to flee to Holland. During his five years on the Continent, it is suspected that he sold obstetric instruments to either Hendrik van Roonhuysen [also Roon-Huyse, Roonhuyse] (1615–1672) or more likely his son and successor Rogier van Roonhuysen (c. 1650–1709), both surgeons in Amsterdam [33,36]. This sale probably occurred after 1693 or perhaps 1695. Although details of this transaction are extremely sketchy, this commercial deal could have first introduced an atraumatic delivery device to Europe. It is also possible that no sale of an instrument actually occurred. The Amsterdam forceps might have been an independent invention. It is also possible that what van Roonhuysen received from Chamberlen was only the *idea* for a delivery instrument that he later independently refined, rather than an actual working model. Paralleling the example set

by the Chamberlen family, the sale also permitted Roonhuysen and his successors to hold the use of this instrument (or perhaps instruments) as a local monopoly for more than 50 years. With the payment of a substantial fee, practitioners who passed the examination for the Amsterdam Surgeon's Guild were permitted introduction to this secret delivery instrument.

Various modifications to the original Chamberlen design or one or more vectus blades independently developed either by Roonhuysen or his close associates, Jean (or Joannes) de Bruin (1681–1753), Paulus deWind of Middleburg, and Regner Bloom of Amsterdam, eventually came to public notice in the Netherlands after 1747. This occurred partly because several practitioners, including a disgruntled applicant to the Amsterdam Surgeons Guild, John Peter (or Jan) Rathaw (also, Rathlaw, Rathlauw; 1720–1791), and Van der Suam (or Swam), a former pupil of Rogier van Roonhuysen, wished to finally break the Amsterdam monopoly [33,36]. As published by Rathaw and later independently by another surgeon in 1747, Daniel Schlichtingting (1703–1765), the revealed van Roonhuysen secret instrument consisted of a type of forceps, quite different from the known Chamberlen models, with thin, bandike parallel blades and no pelvic curve. This instrument was articulated only at the distal end of the handles.

On his deathbed in 1753, van Roonhuysen's closest pupil, Jean de Bruin, gave his original delivery instruments as a legacy to two friends, J. de Vischer and H. van de Poll. They subsequently published a description of one of these instruments in a text entitled *The Obstetric Secret of the Roonhuysens Discovered* (Leiden, 1753). What they revealed in this paper was a single-bladed device slightly curved at both ends and covered with dog leather. This instrument is best described as a modified lever or vectus blade.

The entire story of the van Roonhuysen's secret instrument(s), including what these instruments actually were, who was involved in the various transactions concerning these devices, and whether any of the "revealed" instruments were actually obtained from Hugh Chamberlen remains cloudy [36,38]. It is also uncertain if these forceps and vectus blades were actually invented independently by the van Roonhuysens or somehow inspired by their viewing an earlier model of the Chamberlen forceps.

Apparently, the Amsterdam group used two instruments, a vectus blade and a type of forceps. Part of the confusion lies in separating the "release," or publication of the description of these separate delivery instruments, from their actual invention (or modification?). Owing to the various claims and counterclaims by the people involved and our distance from the actual events, no resolution concerning what the Amsterdam cartel either purchased from Chamberlen or independently invented seems likely. Apart from the quibbles concerning its origin, the van Roonhuysen extractors proved to be poor competition for the Chamberlen forceps. Forceps based on the Amsterdam model never became popular and had little influence on future developments. While possibly representing a true independent invention, the van Roonhuysen forceps remain now as a historical curiosity only. Of interest, the use of levers or vectus blades remained common in the Netherlands well into the nineteenth century. These instruments might be the only lasting obstetric contribution that can be ascribed to the Amsterdam group (Figure 1.4).

Other delivery instruments also became available in the early to mid-eighteenth century. Independently of the Chamberlens, Johannes Palfyn of Ghent (1650–1730), a surgeon and anatomist with an uncertain interest in midwifery, developed a two-bladed delivery instrument, his *tire-tête* or *mains de fer* [11,22,36]. This device was demonstrated in Paris, probably in 1720, at a meeting of the Academie Royale de Sciences. This instrument was also presented to the Medical Faculty of Paris in

1723. Unfortunately, Palfyn never published anything on either the construction of this instrument or its clinical use. All information about his forceps comes from the comments of his contemporaries and his critics. Palfyn might have derived the inspiration for his invention from a vectus blade instrument originally developed by the noted French surgeon Ambroise Paré (1510–1590). Palfyn's innovation was to employ two blades, each with cephalic curve fitted to the sides of the fetal head. These blades were neither crossed nor otherwise articulated together, and they also lacked a pelvic curve. In its original description, the device was likened to a pair of "artificial hands" designed to assist the delivery of the fetal head. Thus their name, "iron hands" or *mains de fer*. Later, other practitioners including Guilles Le Doux of Ypres (c. 1710) and Grégoire the Elder (?–1730?) bound the two parallel blades together with a cloth tape or strap to try to increase their clinical utility. Parallel blades have a technical advantage over other forceps' designs since they avoid the cranial compression inherent in the scissor-like articulated blades of most instruments, including those of the Chamberlens. As a parallel-blade device, however, the Palfyn instrument had major technical problems. The lack of a pelvic curve restricted its potential use. Even with the wrapping of the shanks, the instrument proved unstable and was largely ineffective in clinical use.

Palfyn's device never achieved popularity owing to its technical limitations, marginal utility, and professional opposition from distinguished contemporaries. One of the most vocal critics, the noted accoucheur Guillaume-Manquest de la Motte (1665–1737), publicly denounced the *mains de fer* as both impractical and dangerous, which they most likely were. After this unfortunate trial presentation, nothing further was heard concerning Palfyn's instrument, and it disappeared from obstetric history.

Instability is a design problem for all parallel-blade instruments because traction immediately drives the blades laterally, predisposing them to slippage. In addition, if parallel blades are unsupported by a firm locking mechanism they can be easily twisted, risking lacerations of the birth canal. Following redesign and crossing of the blades and the fitting of a screw-based lock (Duseé modification) a later modification of the Palfyn instrument actually was made clinically usable. This instrument never

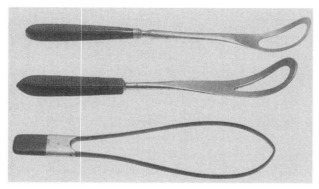

FIGURE 1.4.
Vectis blades and whale bone fillet c. 1850. (Courtesy of the Dittrick Museum of Medical History, Historical Division/Cleveland Health Sciences Library, Cleveland, OH.)

gained popularity and had little influence on subsequent forceps design, however [36]. Many years later, once the problems of blade articulation and stability had been solved, Laufe, Shute, and others successfully revived the parallel-blade design for obstetric forceps [39–41].

In the mid-1730s, following the publication of several case reports and informal exchanges between several practitioners, obstetric forceps of varying types rapidly came into general use in England. Thus in 1733, in his text *A Treatise on the Improvement of Midwifery*, Edmund Chapman (1680–1756) mentioned that forceps were instruments well known to his contemporaries [22]. Other practitioners, including William Giffard (?–1731) and Benjamin Pugh (c. 1710–1775) also reported using forceps before 1750 [33,36]. Exactly how the secret of the forceps was revealed to these accoucheurs remains unknown. It cannot be simply a coincidence that the several physicians most involved in popularizing these early, Chamberlen-like instruments all worked in Essex, England, in reasonable proximity to the Chamberlen estate. Unfortunately, the details of this potentially fascinating part of the forceps story are now irretrievably lost.

Modifications to these early delivery instruments were required before they achieved popularity and utility. Both the Chamberlen and Palfyn forceps were short and straight and lacked a pelvic curve. Owing to these design limitations, they would have been useful only as low or outlet instruments. To improve performance, André Levret (1703–1780), William Smellie (1697–1763), and Benjamin Pugh (c. 1710–1775) independently added a pelvic curve [11]. This helped to accommodate the forceps blades to the birth canal, and the new instruments that incorporated this modification were capable of more accurate and less traumatic applications. This improvement was introduced at the same time as the French obstetrician Jean Louis Baudelocque (1746–1810) developed a technique for estimating pelvic capacity by taking external measurements with a large caliper or pelvimeter. His studies of pelvimetry demonstrated the importance of pelvic shape and various pelvic dimensions in the mechanism of labor, thus improving the understanding of how instruments should be used [22].

The newly modified cross-bladed forceps that incorporated the pelvic curve provided an attractive alternative to the dreary triad of heroically prolonged labors, attempted version and extraction, and destructive operations that had characterized earlier practice. Unfortunately, the indiscriminate use of instruments, often by the inexperienced, led to abuse. Knowledge of techniques for safe application and training to disseminate improvements in technique lagged well behind the enthusiastic application of these new devices.

Overuse of instruments provoked the expected response. An era of lively debate concerning the appropriate use of instruments ensued, much of which was strikingly similar to modern discussions. The result was that several of the best eighteenth century English practitioners, including William Smellie (1697–1763) and his student William Hunter (1718–1783), taught the conservative use of instruments. Although Hunter clearly knew how to use forceps, he took pride in noting that his pair was so little used that they were covered in rust. Practitioners of an even more conservative school of obstetric management, including Thomas Denman (1733–1815), William Osborn (1736–1808), and Richard Croft (1762–1818), favored extreme prolongations of labor rather than any resort to instrumental assistance [11]. In their view, the risks attendant to instrumentation outweighed any potential. The general guidelines for appropriate forceps use as designated by the conservative school would be quite unacceptable by modern standards [36]. These included

- No intervention is to be performed if any progress is noted, no matter how slowly, unless fetal demise is diagnosed;

- No intervention may be considered until the head has been on the perineum for >6 hours;

- Forceps are to be used only for the most urgent occasions, and then sparingly.

A famous and poignant reminder of the potentially serious error of failing to intervene despite strong indication was the childbirth death of George IV's only heir, Princess Charlotte, in 1817 [42]. The royal obstetrician, Sir Richard Croft, was a socially prominent and fashionably conservative practitioner. The Princess' labor lasted 50 hours, and the child was stillborn. Six hours following the delivery, Princess Charlotte died from what is now presumed to have been exhaustion, dehydration, and hemorrhage. Forceps were available but never used. Later, in the face of intense public and professional criticism concerning his obstetric management, Croft committed suicide. Beyond the tragedy of these three related deaths, the event also presented a major political crisis. With the death of Charlotte, there was no legitimate heir for George. If no legitimate heir could be produced, the English crown would pass to a distant Hanoverian relative, the Duke of Brunswick, a young cousin of George. Eventually, after active intervention, a suitable bride of proven fertility for the king's brother was found. A successful pregnancy and delivery followed in 1819. Through this somewhat unusual mechanism, the English crown passed to the King's niece. In 1837, this woman assumed the English throne and was crowned as Queen Victoria, who proved to be the longest reigning of the English monarchs. The Princess Charlotte debacle and other similar events eventually discredited the ultraconservative school of obstetric management, and by the middle decades of the nineteenth century led to a more balanced view of the role of assisted delivery.

The extensive use of instrumental delivery was an event of the latter part of the nineteenth and the early twentieth century. Before the late 1840s, the incidence of forceps use both in England and the continent was 1% or less in large clinical services (Tables 1.1 and 1.2). Fleetwood Churchill was among the first practitioners to publish birth statistics. In his *Research on Operative Midwifery* (1841), he presented data summarizing experience in the late eighteenth and early nineteenth century (Table 1.1) [36]. These data indicate that both forceps and operations destructive to the fetus occurred in substantially fewer than 1% of all deliveries.

In 1875, T. More Madden of the Rotunda or Dublin Lying-in Hospital reported delivery data collected from 1787 to 1874 during the directorship of seven hospital masters (Table 1.2). As had been reported by Churchill, instrumental delivery was uncommon (0.5%) until midcentury. Thereafter, the rate rose from 1.6% for the interval 1847–1854 to 9.2% by 1868–1874.

During the interval from the eighteenth century until the latter decades of the nineteenth century, the percentage of procedures destructive to the fetus remained relatively stable, at approximately 0.4%. The increase in operative forceps deliveries probably reflects several factors:

TABLE 1.1 Frequency of Forceps Use and Craniotomy or Operations Destructive to the Fetus in the Late Eighteenth and Early Nineteenth Centuries*

Instrument Employed	Deliveries	Operations Performed (%)
Forceps		
British 1781–1840	42,196	120 (0.28)
French 1797–1831	44,736	277 (0.62)
German 1801–1837	261,224	1,702 (0.65)
Total	348,156	2,099 (0.60)
Perforator and Crotchet		
British 1781–1819	41,434	181 (0.45)
French 1797–1811	36,169	30 (0.08)
German 1801–1837	256,655	132 (0.05)
Total	334,258	343 (0.10)

*As reported by Churchill, 1841. *Modified from* Hibbard [36], reprinted with permission.

TABLE 1.2 Operative Deliveries at the Dublin Lying-in Hospital Under Various Masters: 1787–1874*†

Mastership	Deliveries	Forceps (%)	Perforator (%)
Joseph Clarke 1787–1794	10,387	14 (0.13)	49 (0.47)
Samuel Labatt 1815–1822	21,867	0	0
Robert Collins 1826–1833	16,654	24 (0.14)	118 (0.71)
Charles Johnson 1842–1833	6,702	18 (0.27)	54 (0.80)
Total	55,610	56 (0.10)	221 (0.40)
Robert Shekleton 1847–1854	13,748	220 (1.60)	54 (0.39)
A. H. McClintock 1854–1861	3,700	76 (2.05)‡	5 (0.14)
George T. Johnston 1868–1874	7,027	639 (9.1)	29 (0.41)
Total	24,475	935 (3.82)	88 (0.36)

*As reported by More Madden, 1875.
†From Hibbard [36], with permission.
‡Includes vectis blade operations.

the availability of anesthetic agents after 1849, the development of new delivery instruments, and changing concepts of obstetric management. The rate of destructive procedures remained unaltered because of technical problems in ascertaining fetal condition and the inability of clinicians to perform cesarean delivery without extreme maternal risk.

Of interest, and as a reflection of the difficult cases presented to these practitioners, Hibbard [36] reports that the maternal mortality from forceps procedures varied from 4.8% (14/294; England) to 7.3% (35/479; Germany and France). In comparison, maternal losses from destructive operations to the fetus (predominantly perforation) were an astounding 21% (52/251)!

In the middle and late nineteenth century, obstetrics underwent rapid changes. Advances in therapeutics accompanied the development of many new delivery instruments and techniques. The introduction of anesthesia in the late 1840s and the development of new instruments and aseptic practices in the 1880s profoundly changed obstetric practice, permitting both sufficient time and relative safety for various surgical procedures.

In the latter part of the nineteenth century, instrumental delivery by forceps became more common and the procedures more extensive. Both more difficult and ever-higher procedures were progressively attempted, including operations performed before full cervical dilation. Hibbard [36] suggests that this more aggressive use of forceps arose from a then general belief that once the membranes ruptured, uterine inertia was common. In this setting some type of intervention was therefore thought to be appropriate.

The English obstetrician James Young Simpson (1811–1870) and his American contemporary George T. Elliot (1827–1871) were among the most prominent practitioners of the mid-nineteenth century [11,43,44]. Simpson, a highly regarded and influential obstetrician working in Edinburgh, developed not only a type of forceps but also the first effective obstetric vacuum extractor. His specially designed forceps were introduced in 1848, rapidly became popular, and are still in use. A man of many interests, Simpson authored papers on hospital design, mesmerism, acupressure, and homeopathy, among other subjects. He also played a pivotal role in obstetric anesthesia, discovering the anesthetic properties of chloroform, which by 1848 he

had employed during deliveries and in the treatment of eclamptic seizures.

George T. Elliot (1827–1871) introduced his midwifery forceps in 1858. To limit compression of the fetal head, he included a setscrew in the instrument handle to control the degree to which the handles of the forceps could be approximated. Both his instrument and Simpson's remain among the most popular designs and are in common use today [32].

In the waning years of the nineteenth century, awakening interest in the mechanism of labor was reflected in the design of new instruments. Following earlier designs of Louis Joseph Hubert of Louvain (1810–1876) and his son E. Hubert and others, Etienne Stephene Tarnier (1828–1897) and Charles P. Pajot (1816–1896) introduced axis-traction forceps. These devices were developed to align the vector of traction with the pelvic curve, thus improving success and using force in a more judicious and less traumatic manner.

Friedrich Wilhelm Scanzoni (1821–1891) popularized rotational maneuvers, especially for management of occiput posterior positions [11]. Modifications of his grand rotation are still occasionally performed today (see Chapter 17, Instrumental Delivery).

Following an idea originally proposed in 1799, by Friedrich Osiander (1759–1822), solid-bladed forceps were popularized by James Woods McLane (1839–1912). To facilitate rotations, these forceps were modified with the addition of longer shanks by Ervin A. Tucker (1862–1902). Later, Ralph Herbert Luikart (1889–19??) modified these blades by selectively thinning the inner portion [45]. Such pseudo-fenestrated forceps blades retained the advantages of easy rotation inherent in the solid design yet maintained a firm grip on the fetal head. This modification remains popular and has been applied to several forceps types.

Rather than an inventor, the most important influence on American delivery practices in terms of instrumentation in the early part of the twentieth century was the medical educator, Joseph Bolivar DeLee (1869–1942). In the 1920s he described the prophylactic forceps operation [46]. Despite the lack of supporting data, DeLee championed the routine use of forceps combined with episiotomy for shortening the second stage once the fetal head had reached the pelvic floor, as a means of avoiding intracranial injury. This concept of routine operative delivery for both maternal and fetal reasons – even though unsupported by data and based on theoretic concerns – was widely followed and strongly influenced North American practice for more than four decades.

Many other clinicians practicing in the early twentieth century designed modified forceps for specific clinical indications. These included the instruments introduced by Lyman Guy Barton (1866–1944) for transverse arrest, Arthur Holbrook Bill (1877–1961) for axis traction, Edmund Brown Piper (1881–1935) for breech delivery, and Christian Casper Gabriel Kielland (1871–1941) for midpelvic rotations. Recent years have seen the development of various new forceps designs, such as those of Laufe, Hays, Nargolkar, and Salinas, among others. These new devices attempt to improve maternal and fetal safety through specific aspects of their design.

HISTORY OF THE VACUUM EXTRACTOR

Vacuum delivery instruments have their origin in the very old practice of cupping [38,47]. In cupping, a metal or glass cup or globe is heated over an open flame and then pressed against the skin. As the cup cools, suction develops, extracting blood or other fluids. A century of experimentation with modifications of the vacuum principle inherent in cupping, combined with various technical advances of the nineteenth and twentieth centuries led to the development of modern obstetric vacuum extractors. Applications of cupping for assistance at deliveries were first reported in the late seventeenth century, when James Younge (1646–1721) and other surgeons performed vacuum deliveries using glass or metal cups [48]. These practitioners failed to publicize their successes, however, and nothing is known about either the construction of these instruments or the techniques used for application or traction [32].

Cupping faced serious technical limitations when the technique began to be applied to vaginal delivery. As this procedure was commonly performed, the cups were initially heated over an open flame before their application. Obstetric use, however, required both a vaginal application of the vacuum cup and a method for traction. Thus, a different technology was needed. Several important features had to be incorporated: easy insertion into the birth canal, the ability to form a firm seal to the fetal head,

a means of continuous regeneration of the vacuum as a result of imperfections of the seal, and finally, a practical method for applying traction.

The vacuum principle was the subject of both experimentation and speculation in the early nineteenth century. It was recognized that evacuating either glass or metal globes could result in substantial pressure and that such devices could be used for traction in several important applications. It was not long before medical applications were suggested [49]. Based on contemporary experimentation and crude commercial vacuum-based devices, James Young Simpson, who developed a several obstetric devices, including the forceps that bear his name, invented the first practical obstetric vacuum extractor in 1849 [44,50,51]. His new device, which he termed an *air* or *suction tractor*, was proposed as an alternative to forceps for use in both cephalic and breech presentations when assisted delivery was required [44,50,51]. Simpson's device consisted of a piston syringe, probably derived from a breast pump, attached to a deep and flexible rubber cup (Figure 1.5). In use, the cup was placed firmly against the fetal head and the syringe was rapidly evacuated. Once suction was achieved, traction was applied by simply grasping the pump cylinder and pulling downward. The extractor was simple and, despite its limitations, successfully employed in several cases. Technical problems with traction, maintaining the vacuum, and the inability of the instrument to accommodate the pelvic curve as a result of its design eventually proved insurmountable, however. After a brief trial Simpson abandoned his vacuum device. Thereafter, despite the occasional introduction of various new designs, vacuum extraction essentially disappeared as an obstetric technique for nearly 100 years.

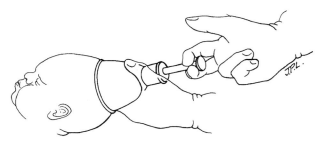

FIGURE 1.5.
Simpson's "air tractor" vacuum extractor (1849).
(Reprinted from O'Grady JP: Modern Vacuum Extraction. Parthenon, 1995; with permission.)

Several vacuum extractors were invented in the century following Simpson's original report, but none achieved either popularity or commercial success until the 1950s, when Malmström introduced his stainless steel cup [52]. The Malmström extractor rapidly became popular, especially in Europe. The device was rugged, successful, and could be used as an alternative to forceps [52–54]. Despite European success, metal cup extractors had a variable reception in the United States. After widespread interest in the early 1960s, vacuum extraction promptly fell into disfavor, largely because of reports of serious scalp injuries and other complications. The popularity of vacuum extraction resumed two decades later only when the soft-cup devices were introduced. At this time clinicians proved more receptive to an alternative for forceps, new instruments were available, and better techniques had been developed for vacuum-assisted delivery.

Malmström's device incorporated several important features now found on all vacuum devices. A protective disk was fitted into the interior of the cup to avoid injury to the fetal scalp. There was a separate vacuum source capable of continuous vacuum production, protected by a collecting bottle or trap. In addition, a pressure gauge was fitted to determine the degree of force generated. Finally, a metal chain firmly attached the cup to an easily grasped handle, permitting easy traction. In later years, other obstetricians including Bird, Lovset, Party, O'Neil, Halkin, and others invented, modified, and improved metal vacuum cups [55–57]. These modified instruments were intended to reduce the likelihood of detachment, facilitate application, or better protect the fetal scalp. Among the rigid metal cups, Bird's modification, in which the vacuum tube is attached to a lateral suction port independent of the traction chain, has proved to be the most popular and useful [55,57]. New models of rigid plastic extractors largely reprise the construction of the Malmström cup, extending the popularity of the original design.

An unknown number of Malmström-type metal cup extractors, predominantly of Bird's modified design, still remain in use. For several reasons, however, most American practitioners prefer to use the plastic cups that have been introduced in recent years [58]. These new designs are disposable single-use devices, constructed of polyethylene and/or

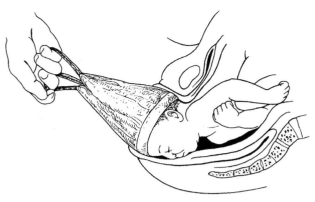

FIGURE 1.6.
Elliot's obstetric bonnet (1992). (From Elliott B, Ridgway LF, Berkus MD, Newton ER, Peairs W: The development and testing of new instruments for operative vaginal delivery. Am J Obstet Gynecol, 1992 Oct; 167(4 Pt 1): 1121–4; with permission.)

Silastic polymer plastic. They are easy to use and have proven effective in most cases. As is always true when new devices become a commercial success, currently too many vacuum cup designs are available, with little if any significant difference between them.

Experimentation with various types of vacuum traction devices has not ceased. Elliot recently described a vacuum-based instrument consisting of a rubber or plastic "bonnet" that lacks either a suction or vacuum port [59]. This unusual-appearing device is designed to be unrolled or fitted onto the fetal head like an inverted parachute. Tension on the handle flattens the membrane around the fetal cranium, providing the force necessary to assist parturition (Figure 1.6). The concept of inserting a net or bag to grasp the fetal head is certainly not new, as strikingly similar examples have appeared fleetingly in the obstetric literature for over two centuries, the earliest perhaps being the *tire-tête* of Pierre Amand from 1715 [36].

An important development in the use of vacuum extraction has been major improvements in practitioner education. These efforts reflect the increasing use of vacuum devices, an appreciation of their potential risks, and the need to better train practitioners in best techniques. Vacuum extraction has become increasingly popular in recent years, and instrumental delivery by vacuum extraction is now more common in the United States than forceps operations [60].

In recent years a greater appreciation of the risks and benefits of all types of assisted delivery has developed. This has prompted increased clinical study to define the best obstetric practices. The continued requirement for some means to accelerate or assist parturition in selected circumstances short of cesarean delivery ensures the continued use of vaginal delivery instruments for the foreseeable future (See Chapter 17, Instrumental Delivery).

REFERENCES

1. O'Dowd M, Phillip EE: The History of Obstetrics and Gynaecology. 1994, New York: The Parthenon Publishing Group.

2. Houtzager G: The Complete Encyclopedia of Greek Mythology. 2003, Edison, New Jersey: Chartwell Books, Inc.

3. Gottschalk W: Dystocia on Mount Olympus. Obstet Gynecol 1959 Mar; 13(3): 381–2.

4. Shakespeare W: *Macbeth*, 1606; V. vii. 44.

5. http://heraklia.fwsl.com.

6. http://www.perseus.Tufts.edu, 2006.

7. http://catholic.archives.nd.edu, 2006.

8. Grant M: Julius Caesar. 1992, New York: M. Evans and Company.

9. http://www.wordorigins.org/wordorc.htm, 2006.

10. http://catholic.archives.nd.edu, 2006.

11. Baskett TF: On the Shoulders of Giants: Eponyms and Names in Obstetrics and Gynecology. 1996, London: RCOG Press.

12. Rousset F: Traité Nouveau de l'Hystérotomokie ou l'Enfantement Caesarienne, qui Est Extraction de l'Enfant par Incision Laterale de Ventre et Matrice de la Femme Grosse. Pouvant Autrement Accoucher, et ce sans Préjudicer a la Vie de l'un de l'autre ni l'Empecher la Fécondité Maternelle par aprés. 1581, Paris: Demeys Duval.

13. Pottiee Sperry F: Biography: François Rousset. Hist Sci Med 1996; 30(2): 259–68.

14. Burton J: An Essay towards a Compleat New System of Midwifry. 1751, London: James Hodges.

15. Gordon BL: Medieval and Renaissance Medicine. 1959, New York: Philosophical Library.

16. Mauriceau F: Les Maladies des Femmes Grosses et Accouchées. 1668, Paris: Henavlt, D'Hovary, De Ninville and Coignard.

17. Mauriceau F: Observations sur La Grossesse et L'Accouchement des Femmes, et sur leurs Maladies, & celles des Enfants nouveau-nez. 1715, Paris: La Compagnie des Libraires Associez.

18. Drife J: The start of life: A history of obstetrics. Postgrad Med J 2002 May; 78(919): 311–15.

19. Huard P: sciences, Medicine, Pharmacie de la Revolution a l'Empire (1790–1815). 1970, Paris: Les Editions Roger Dacosta.

20. Speert H: Obstetrics and Gynecology in America. 1980, Washington, D.C.: American College of Obstetricians and Gynecologists.

21. Chipfakacha V: Abdominal deliveries in Africa: Food for thought to scholars of the history of medicine. Cent Afr J Med 1989 Feb; 35(2): 333–6.

22. Cutter IS, Viets HR: A Short History of Midwifery. 1964, Philadelphia: W.B. Saunders Company.

23. Mola G: Symphysiotomy or caesarean section after failed trial of assisted delivery. P N G Med J 1995 Sep; 38(3): 172–7.

24. Van Roosmalen J: Symphysiotomy – a reappraisal for the developing world. In Progress in Obstetrics and Gynaecology, J. Studd Editor. 1991, Edinburgh: Churchill-Livingstone. pp. 149–62.

25. Lauverjat T-E: Nouvelle Méthode de Practiquer L'Opération Césarienne, et Parallèlel de cette Opération & de la Section de la Symphyse des Os Pubis. Paris, 1788: pp. 150–1.

26. Sänger M: Der Kaiserschmitt. Arch Gynakol 1882; 19: 370.

27. Porro E: Della amputazione utero-ovarica come complemento di taglio Cesario. Ann Univ Med Chirurg 1876; 273: 289–350.

28. Lurie S, Glezerman M: The history of cesarean technique. Am J Obstet Gynecol 2003 Dec; 189(6): 1803–06.

29. Waters E: Retrovesical extraperitoneal cesarean section. Am J Obstet Gynecol 1940; 39: 423.

30. Norton J: Latzko extraperitoneal caesarean section. Am J Obstet Gynecol 1935; 30: 209.

31. Das K: Obstetric Forceps: Its History and Evolution. 1929, Calcutta: The Art Press.

32. O'Grady J: Modern Instrumental Delivery. 1988, Baltimore: Williams & Wilkins.

33. Radcliffe W: Milestones in Midwifery and the Secret Instrument. 1989, San Francisco: Norman Publishing.

34. Speert H: The obstetric forceps. Clin Obstet Gynecol 1960 Sep; 3: 761–6.

35. Drinkwater K: The midwifery forceps: Historical sketch. Med Chir J 1913; 64: 451–65.

36. Hibbard B: The Obstetrician's Armamentarium. 2000, San Anselmo, CA: Norman Publishing.

37. Speert H: Obstetrics and Gynecology: A History and Iconography. 1994, San Francisco: Norman Publishing.

38. Thiery M: Obstetric forceps and vectus: The roots. Acta Belg Hist Med 1992 Mar; 5(1): 4–20.

39. Shute W: Management of shoulder dystocia with the Shute parallel forceps. Am J Obstet Gynecol Oct 1; 84: 936–9.

40. Seidenschnur G, Koepcke E: Fetal risk in delivery with the Shute parallel forceps: Analysis of 1,503 forceps deliveries. Am J Obstet Gynecol 1979 Oct 1; 135(3): 312–7.

41. Shute W: An obstetrical forceps which uses new principle of parallelism. Am J Obstet Gynecol 1959 Feb; 72(2): 442–6.

42. Dewhurst J: Royal Confinements: A Gynaecological History of Britain's Royal Family. 1980, New York: St. Martin's Press.

43. Duns S: A Memoir of Sir James Y. Simpson. 1873, Edinburgh: Edmonston and Douglas. p. 288.

44. Chalmers J: James Young Simpson and the "suction tractor." J Obstet Gynaecol Br Commonw 1963; 70: 94–100.

45. Luikart R: A modification of the Kielland, Simpson and Tucker-McLane forceps to simplify their use and improve function and safety. Am J Obstet Gynecol 1937; 34: 686.

46. DeLee J: The prophylactic forceps operation. Am J Obstet Gynecol 1920; 1: 34–44.

47. O'Grady J, Gimovsky ML, McIlhargie CJ: Vacuum Extraction in Modern Obstetric Practice. 1995, New York: Parthenon Publishing Group Inc.

48. Younge J: An account of balls of hair taken from the uterus and ovaria of several women. Philos Trans R Soc (London) 1706–1707; 25: 2387.

49. Arnott N: Elements of Physics, or Natural Philosophy, General and Medical, Explained Independently of Technical Mathematics, and Containing New Disquisitions and Practical Suggestions, Vol 1. p. 543. 1831, Philadelphia: Carey and Lea.

50. Simpson J: On suction tractor or new mechanical power as a substitute for forceps in tedious labours. Edinburgh Monthly J Med Sci 1849; 32: 556–8.

51. Eustace D: James Young Simpson: The controversy surrounding the presentation of his Air Tractor (1848–849). J R Soc Med 1993 Nov; 86(11): 660–3.

52. Malmström T: The vacuum extractor: An obstetrical instrument. I. and the parturiometer, a tokographic device. . Acta Obstet Gynecol Scand 1957; 36(Suppl): 5–82.

53. Malmström T, Jansson I: Use of vacuum extractor. Clin Obstet Gynecol 1965; 8: 893–913.

54. Sjostedt J: The vacuum extractor and forceps in obstetrics: A clinical study. Acta Obstet Gynecol Scand 1967; 46(Suppl 10): 1–208.

55. Bird G: Modification of Malmström vacuum extractor. Br Med J: Online 1969; 3: 526–9.

56. Vacca A: Handbook of Vacuum Extraction in Obstetric Practice. 1992, London: Edward Arnold.

57. O'Neil A, Skull E, Michael C: A new method of traction for the vacuum cup. Aust N Z J Obstet Gynaecol 1981 Feb; 21(1): 24–5.

58. O'Grady J, Pope CS, Patel SS: Vacuum extraction in modern obstetric practice: A review and critique. Curr Opin Obstet Gynecol 2000 Dec; 12(6): 475–80.

59. Elliott B, Ridgway LF, Berkus MD, Newton ER, Peairs W: The development and testing of new instruments for operative vaginal delivery. Am J Obstet Gynecol 1992 Oct; 167(4 Pt 1): 1121–4.

60. Demissie K, Rhoads GG, Smulian JC, Balasubramanian BA, Gandhi K, Joseph KS, Kramer M: Operative vaginal delivery and neonatal and infant adverse outcomes: Population-based retrospective analysis. Br Med J 2004 Jul 3; 329(7456): 24–9.

Chapter 2 PRENATAL GENETIC TESTING

Gabriel M. Cohn

To some extent it may be said that the etiology of the transmitted foetal diseases is within our knowledge, and their diagnosis not altogether outside our grasp; with perseverence and skill their treatment will yet be hopefully undertaken by the well-informed physician.

John William Ballantyne (1861–1923)
Antenatal Pathology and Hygiene: The Embryo and the Foetus
Edinburgh: William Green and Sons, 1902.

The importance of genetics in clinical perinatal medicine has increased rapidly over the last three decades. Now, more than 6,000 genetic traits or disease entities have been identified (Figure 2.1) [1]. It is estimated that the incidence of genetic disease among newborns is 5%–6% [2]. Genetic disease has profound medical, financial, and societal consequences far greater than its actual numbers. With the progressive disappearance of many infectious and other diseases that in the past accounted for most hospital admissions, genetic disorders remain a serious contemporary social and medical problem. Studies examining inpatient pediatric admissions reveal that 33% to 52% of all pediatric hospitalizations result from complications of genetic disease [3]. If multifactorial disorders are eliminated, purely genetic diseases account for more than one in ten pediatric admissions [4]. Among adults, up to 11.5% of all inpatient admissions are due to genetically related abnormalities [5]. The contribution of genetic disorders to childhood mortality is edge with a substantial number of all pediatric deaths ascribed to genetic disease. Unfortunately, despite enhanced prenatal diagnostic capabilities and aggressive perinatal management, significant reductions in perinatal mortality associated with congenital malformations have not occurred [6].

In addition to its medical importance, genetic disease also has major financial and societal impact. Studies of patients with genetic diseases indicate that inpatient admissions for these patients are on average more common, more expensive, greater in duration, and, owing to geographic limitations of genetic services, require greater travel than similar treatment for persons with other types of illness. The loss of insurability following the diagnosis onset of genetic diseases doubles the likelihood that patients will pay out of pocket for medical services [3]. The societal cost is equally burdensome. Both years of work lost to impairment and years of life lost to disease span decades among persons afflicted with genetic disorders. In sum, the emotional, psychological, and financial impact of productivity lost

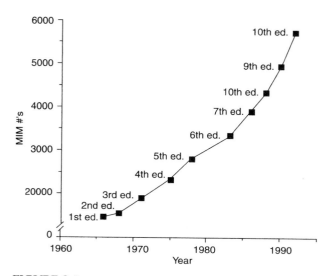

FIGURE 2.1.
Total number of entries in Mendelian Inheritance in Man.
Since 1966 there has been a 3.8-fold increase in
recognized human genetic traits and disorders.

to genetic disorders is extensive and often poorly appreciated.

With the improvement and automation of techniques in the fields of cyto- and molecular genetics and the identification of many genetic diseases, an understanding of the molecular pathophysiology of many disorders is now possible. Several molecular genetic assays have been developed in kit form to assist clinicians in the early diagnosis of genetic disease. It is believed that with this increased understanding of the mechanisms underlying many genetic entities and with the increasing accuracy of case identification, both pharmacogenetic and gene transfer interventions will progressively evolve. The introduction of such enhanced diagnostic and treatment capabilities will place increased reliance on prenatal diagnosis techniques as the basis for the *prevention* of genetic disease through termination of pregnancy or as the basis for the *treatment* of genetic disease through in-utero medical or surgical interventions. The questions of best practices in genetic screening as well as potential treatment for congenital disorders remain both complex and controversial. [7–10].

This chapter focuses on the procedures and techniques currently available to clinicians to evaluate genetic disorders. As our knowledge in molecular and clinical genetics progressively expands and as more potential therapies become available, the

obstetrician plays a greater role in the identification of at-risk cases and in the prenatal diagnosis of genetic disease. Several currently investigative procedures that could become available for clinical use in the near future are also reviewed and their importance is discussed. For those desiring more extensive information, several excellent genetics resources are available free of charge.[1]

HISTORY

The development of prenatal diagnostic techniques has closely paralleled the advances in clinical genetics. Amniocentesis was first introduced in the 1880s as a treatment for hydramnios [11–14]. It was not until 1960, however, that amniocentesis for X-chromatin evaluation was first described [15–17]. Amniotic fluid sampling subsequently proved useful for the diagnosis and management of Rh isoimmunization and more recently as a technique for direct evaluation of fetal pulmonary maturity [18]. With the advent of X-chromatin analysis, amniocentesis was demonstrated to identify fetal sex acccurately, providing a technique for identifying fetuses at risk for X-linked recessive disorders, such as Duchenne muscular dystrophy and hemophilia [19,20]. In 1966, Steel and Berg [21] were successful in culturing and karyotyping amniocytes, suggesting that prenatal diagnosis of chromosomal aneuploidies was feasible. Jacobsen and Barter [22] subsequently introduced the first report of a fetal chromosomal anomaly identified on amniocentesis, a D/D translocation. In 1968, Valenti and coworkers [23] and Nadler [24] described the prenatal diagnosis of Down syndrome identified on amniocytes obtained by amniocentesis. A biochemical disorder, galactosemia, was similarly identified prenatally by

---

[1]Two invaluable Web sites include Online Mendelian Inheritance in Man (OMIM) (http://www.ncbi.nlm.nih.gov/entrez/query. fcgi?db = OMIM) and the GeneTest Web site (http://www. genetests.org). OMIM is an extensive database searchable by disease, gene, or by clinical feature(s). This database can be particularly useful in generating a differential diagnosis based on ultrasound or other clinical findings, or alternatively in providing a synopsis of the key clinical features associated with a given genetic diagnosis. In addition, an extensive review of the literature is provided for approximately 6,000 known phenotypes, as well as several thousand genetic markers. The GeneTest Web site provides an up-to-date listing of genetic tests that are clinically available, labs and clinical centers that provide genetic services, as well as extensive reviews of several hundred common genetic disorders.

Nadler [24], indicating that prenatal diagnosis by amniocentesis was not strictly limited to chromosomal abnormalities. The first report of a clinical trial of genetic amniocentesis was published by Nadler and Gerbie [25] in 1970. This study demonstrated that prenatal diagnosis by amniotic fluid analysis was an accurate and a low-risk procedure when performed between 16 and 20 weeks.

Fetal visualization was another significant advance. In the 1930s, amniotic infusion of contrast media for amniography was introduced, a procedure used to visualize the fetus and the placenta. Further development of various radiographic and radioactive tracer techniques over the following decades assisted in utero diagnosis. These tests and procedures were promptly abandoned with the advent of high-resolution ultrasonography, however.

Despite its introduction into medicine soon after the Second World War, ultrasound scanning did not make a major impact on obstetric management until real-time machines of high resolution became widely available in the 1970s. Today, ultrasound scan is the primary screening method for many fetal abnormalities and is considered a necessity in many obstetric procedures (e.g., version, amniocentesis, and cordocentesis).

The initial experience with amniocentesis was performed without the benefit of ultrasonography. "Blind" procedures were performed by arbitrarily inserting a spinal needle 3 cm above the pubis symphysis, at no earlier than 15 weeks' gestation. Although considered a reliable technique, midtrimester amniocentesis had the disadvantage of relatively late timing and hence late diagnosis. Societal pressures limiting pregnancy termination for genetic indications and medical considerations of the enhanced complications associated with midtrimester abortions stimulated interest in methods of first-trimester prenatal diagnosis. Unfortunately, initial attempts at transvaginal amniocentesis at ≤10 weeks of gestation and first-trimester endoscopic chorion biopsy resulted in significant pregnancy loss as well as high failure rates [25, 26]. New methods were needed.

In 1968, the technique of chorionic tissue biopsy (i.e., chorionic villous biopsy [CVS]) for prenatal diagnosis was introduced by Mohr [27]. In this procedure, an endoscope of 6 mm in diameter was introduced by way of one of the vaginal fornices or transcervically. The endoscope was positioned against the chorion, the optical device removed, and suction applied. A tubular knife was next introduced and used to biopsy tissue captured by the endoscopic suction. Success proved elusive, as only one half of the samples obtained were chorionic tissue, and many samples were found to contain amniotic membrane. Modifications of this technique were introduced, and a series of studies were performed on pretermination patients with only modest success [27–29]. Clinicians at Teitung Hospital in China [30] subsequently demonstrated that simple first-trimester placental biopsy was indeed feasible. In their original procedure, a 3-mm diameter metal cannula was blindly introduced through the cervix and advanced until "soft resistance" was encountered. A smaller-diameter inner catheter was then introduced to approximately 1 cm beyond the cannula tip, and tissue was then aspirated by syringe suction. This procedure was attempted in 100 pregnancies to determine fetal sex. In ninety-three patients, the appropriate fetal sex was assigned based on X-chromatin analysis. Of seventy continuing pregnancies, 4% were subsequently lost. Unfortunately, attempts to repeat this technique by other groups proved unsuccessful [31,32]. Attempts at procedure modification (e.g., endocervical lavage) were similarly without great success [33–35]. CVS remained investigational until new biopsy techniques and modified equipment were combined with modern ultrasonic visualization to improve both safety and success.

Direct ultrasonic visualization proved important in the development and acceptance of both amniocentesis as well as CVS. Combined with high-resolution ultrasonography, amniocentesis was directed either at a site identified as most suitable by a sonogram performed prior to the procedure (*ultrasound guided*) or by a sonogram performed during the procedure (*ultrasound monitored*). These modifications permitted localization of the placenta and allowed prenatal diagnosis prior to 14 weeks of gestation – the limit previously established by blind amniocentesis. In the early 1980s, Kazy [36] used ultrasonography to direct thin biopsy forceps (1.7 mm in diameter) at the chorion frondosum and successfully sampled a series of pregnancies. Among the patients studied were women carrying fetuses at risk for genetic disease. Thirteen such women who elected to continue their pregnancies after sampling experienced a successful pregnancy outcome and the birth of a normal infant. Subsequently, Ward [37] and his London-based group introduced a method in which a blunt stainless steel malleable obturator served as a guide over which a 1.5-mm polyethylene catheter was threaded. Using continuous ultrasonographic guidance, this apparatus was introduced to abut the edge of the chorion frondosum. Once in position, the obturator was removed and a syringe applied. Chorionic villi were aspirated with negative pressure. Ward and coworkers [37] demonstrated that in pregnancies sampled between seven and 14 weeks, a 90% success in chorionic villus sampling was possible. Simoni and coworkers [38] subsequently compared four methods of villus biopsy, including blind insertion of the flexible catheter developed by Ward, blind insertion of an intravascular catheter, endoscopic sampling, and ultrasonographic introduction of the flexible Ward catheter. Using the first three approaches, maximal sampling success was limited to 76%, with bleeding occurring in 17% of attempts. With the Ward catheter used in conjunction with continuous ultrasonographic guidance, sampling success rates improved to 96%. In 1984, the technique of transabdominal CVS was introduced by Smidt-Jensen and coworkers (39) and proved to be a valuable alternative to transcervical sampling methods.

The role of CVS in early pregnancy diagnosis is developing. This issue is discussed in greater detail later, and the risk/benefit ratio is in the process of reconsideration. Recent evidence concerning possible fetal limb defects as a rare procedure-related complication continues to be closely analyzed.

Interest in transabdominal amniocentesis before 16 weeks was reawakened with the advent of improved ultrasound equipment. Subsequent evaluations have indicated, however, that early amniotic fluid sampling procedures (≤14 weeks) entail more complications and these have largely been abandoned. The technologic advances that have had the most important influence on prenatal diagnosis, however, include new molecular and cytogenetic testing such as the polymerase chain reaction (PCR) and fluorescent in situ hybridization (FISH) studies. These and similar study methods, as well as other noninvasive techniques for the detection of genetic disease, are in the process of development. Such innovations include detection of fetal cells in maternal circulation, preimplantation diagnosis, polar body biopsy, and oocyte typing.

AMNIOCENTESIS

Transabdominal Procedures

Genetic amniocentesis usually is performed after 15 completed weeks of gestation. After ultrasonic study to confirm dates, fetal viability, fetal number, fetal anatomic survey and placentation, the patient is requested to empty her bladder. The abdomen is aseptically cleansed with a povidone-iodine or another antiseptic solution, and sterile drapes are applied. Ultrasound gel is applied to a transducer, which is subsequently inserted into a sterile surgical glove or sleeve. The sterile cover is tightly wrapped around the transducer and sterile surgical lubricant is applied onto the exterior of the gloved transducer. This permits the transducer to be applied to the maternal abdomen with minimal risk of contamination. A pocket of fluid free of fetus and placenta is next identified. If an area free of placenta cannot be found, an area containing the thinnest section of the placenta away from the cord insertion is localized. Once an ideal target is noted, the skin can be infiltrated with a local anesthetic, although the author has generally found this to be unnecessary. Thereafter, under direct visualization, a 22-gauge disposable spinal needle with stylet is passed through the patient's skin and into the amniotic cavity (see Figure 2.2) [40]. The length of the standard needle is 9 cm. A needle insertion of approximately 3.5 to 4.5 cm will usually suffice to tap fluid. Thus the standard needle is appropriate for most patients. In selected obese patients, however, a longer needle might be required. In these special circumstances, evaluation by an initial scan serves as a guide to estimating the required needle length. Once the sac is entered, 20 milliliters of fluid are generally withdrawn, using at least two separate syringes. The first few milliliters are discarded to avoid maternal cell contamination [41]. This initial aliquot can be used for alpha-fetoprotein evaluation, however. Once the complete sample is obtained, the needle is promptly withdrawn. The puncture site is then observed under real-time ultrasound for fetal hemorrhage and normal fetal cardiac activity confirmed. If all is normal, this author subsequently discharges patients to home, requesting that they report any fluid loss, lower abdominal pain, cramping, contractions, or fever. Strenuous activity or coitus is discouraged for the following 24 hours, and thereafter routine activity

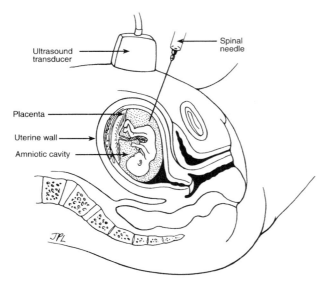

FIGURE 2.2.
Ultrasound-guided amniocenteses. Following aseptic preparations, a 5-gauge needle is guided into the amniotic cavity with the aid of real-time ultrasonography. (See text for details.)

may be resumed. Rh-negative patients subsequently receive Rh immunoglobulin (RhIG).

If, during the initial attempt, free-flowing amniotic fluid is not obtained, rotating the needle to reposition the bevel or minimal repositioning of the needle is often successful in achieving flow. Negative pressure should not be applied to the syringe during repositioning. If needle rotation or repositioning under ultrasonographic observation proves unsuccessful, a second tap attempt with a new needle is warranted. Whether repeat skin preparation is required for the second tap depends on the clinical circumstances. If a second attempt is unsuccessful, additional efforts are best postponed for 1 week [42,43]. Failure to obtain amniotic fluid is commonly due to needle misdirection, leiomyomas, uterine contractions, or membrane tenting [44,45]. The last problem problem occurs more frequently prior to 15 weeks of gestation.

Complications

The recent review by Alfirevic and Sundberg has examined the fetal loss rate associated with mid-trimester amniocentesis and CVS [46]. To evaluate the clinical relevance of such studies, the baseline loss rate for ultrasonographically diagnosed viable

pregnancies at that same gestation, for woman of the same age, must be known. Maternal age is a major factor in the incidence of spontaneous miscarriage. In established pregnancies, the overall spontaneous fetal loss rate is 13.6% among women 40 years of age and older, 4.5% in women in the 35- to 39-year-old group, and 1.5% among women younger than 35 years of age [47–50]. Further, *preamniocentesis maternal-serum alpha-fetoprotein* (MSAFP) elevations, if present, are associated with a significantly higher pregnancy loss rate. Read and coworkers [51] compared the outcome of 212 pregnant women undergoing amniocentesis for MSAFP elevation to the outcome of 219 pregnant women in whom a prior pregnancy had resulted in a fetus with an open neural tube defect (ONTD). The spontaneous loss rate following amniocentesis among patients with MSAFP elevation was 8% versus 2.8% among patients with prior ONTD fetus. These data suggest that many patients who undergo prenatal diagnosis (i.e., advanced maternal age and elevated MSAFP) are at increased risk for spontaneous pregnancy loss *independent* of the procedure-related risk.

Most spontaneous losses occur early in gestation. Evaluation of pregnancy loss rate by gestational age indicates that, of patients awaiting preamniocentesis counseling, 1.2% spontaneously aborted between 12 and 16 weeks. Sant-Cassia and coworkers [52] reported a 1% pregnancy loss rate between 16 and 28 weeks among controls for an amniocentesis study. These data should be included when counseling patients prior to any invasive prenatal testing.

Based on these data presented above, to evaluate studies examining procedure-related loss rates, study designs must incorporate appropriately matched control patients *not* undergoing amniocentesis. There are a number of studies addressing amniocentesis [46]. In 1976, the National Institute of Child Health and Human Development (NICHD) reported a prospective study of 1040 subjects undergoing amniocentesis compared with 992 controls matched for race, socioeconomic conditions, parity, and age [53]. The results suggested no significant differences in the fetal loss rate (3.2% in the control group versus 3.5% in the amniocentesis group), elective second-trimester termination (2.1% in the control group versus 2.3% in subjects), birthweight, 5-minute Apgar Scores, congenital anomalies, neonatal complications, or developmental problems. Immediate maternal complications (e.g., vaginal bleeding, leakage of amniotic fluid) were reported in 2.4% of patients undergoing amniocentesis. In this series, the risk of vaginal bleeding was significantly related to the number of needle insertions. The authors concluded that mid-trimester amniocentesis was both accurate and "highly safe" and did not significantly increase the risk of pregnancy loss. Interestingly, the loss rate observed in the control group was higher than that observed in other large series, suggesting the recruitment of a high-risk control population or perhaps imperfect matching of the control group.

Simpson and coworkers [54] reported the results of the Canadian Collaborative Group Study. A pregnancy loss rate of 3.2% was observed among 1,020 pregnancies in 900 women who underwent 1,223 amniocenteses. The immediate amniocentesis complication rate was 3.6%. A significantly higher fetal loss rate was observed in pregnancies sampled with needles of 19 gauge or larger, or when more than two needle insertions were undertaken in a single day. The authors concluded that amniocentesis was "... safe, accurate and reliable..." at about 16 weeks of gestation when carried out by an experienced clinician and monitored by ultrasound scan. This study lacked a control group, however.

The Working Party on Amniocentesis (U.K. Collaborative Study Group) [55] demonstrated a 2.4% spontaneous abortion rate among patients undergoing amniocentesis versus a 1.2% loss rate among matched controls. Furthermore, an increased risk of infantile respiratory difficulties and orthopedic abnormalities were seen among test subjects. There were, however, problems with study design; specifically, patient matching was imperfect. A significant fraction of patients in the amniocentesis group were selected on the basis of MSAFP elevation and were significantly older than the controls. In addition, in the data analysis, matched controls who spontaneously aborted were replaced with controls who had not aborted. Some controls also entered the study at older gestational ages than their matched subjects. These selection biases alone probably account for the observed differences between this study and the others previously described, and these data are to be interpreted with care.

Tabor and coworkers [56] performed a randomized, controlled study of amniocentesis on over 4,500 women aged between 24 and 34 years. Subjects and controls were matched for gestational age at entry, maternal age, prior induced and spontaneous abortions, stillbirths, low-birthweight infants, live births, smoking history and socioeconomic status. The loss rate was 0.7% in the control group and 1.7% in the subject group ($p \leq 0.01$). The study suggested an increased pregnancy loss rate in patients estimated at approximately 1% undergoing amniocentesis.

Many smaller studies of the risk of amniocentesis also have been conducted, with findings suggestive of no minimal differences between patients undergoing amniocentesis and controls. Unfortunately, not all subjects were appropriately matched with controls, rendering these results difficult to interpret. The recent comprehensive review and meta-analysis of Mujezinovic and Alfirevic [57], which appeared in September of 2007, summarized MEDLINE data published after January 1, 1995, concerning both amniocentesis and CVS. These authors noted a wide range in reported risk for pregnancy complications from these diagnostic procedures. The pooled estimate for a pregnancy loss within 14 days of an amniocentesis was 0.6% (95% CI 0.5–0.7). This provides a reasonable benchmark for clinicians to use in counseling [58].

Blood-tinged amniotic fluid is detected in 2% of amniocentesis. This event is associated with an increased fetal loss rate and can be due to either maternal or fetal bleeding. Documentation of maternal blood in the sample is associated with an increased pregnancy loss rate from 1.7% (control population) to 6.6% (hemorrhage population) [59]. Fetal blood in amniotic fluid is associated with a loss rate of up to 14.3% [60]. Perhaps not surprisingly, transplacental amniocentesis has a significantly higher loss rate than non-transplacental amniocentesis (2.9% vs. 1.2% respectively, with the control group significantly lower than both at 0.4%) [56]. MSAFP elevation following amniocentesis is more common in sampled pregnancies with anterior placentas. Such elevations are believed to result from subclinical maternal-fetal hemorrhage and, if present, are associated with an increased fetal loss rate (14% vs. 1%) [59, 60].

Following second-trimester amniocentesis, Rh sensitization is a potential complication [61]. Both

Khalil and coworkers [62] and Golbus and coworkers [63] reported a decreased risk of sensitization in Rh-negative women who routinely received RhIG following amniocentesis. Tabor and coworkers [64] could not demonstrate a significant increase to Rh sensitization following amniocentesis in Rh-negative patients who had not received RhIG. Although there is no uniformity of opinion concerning RhIG administration following midtrimester amniocentesis, the consensus is that RhIG administration is indicated in at-risk pregnancies to prevent Rh sensitization. The American College of Obstetricians and Gynecologists recommends the administration of 300 μg of RhIG following the procedure [65]. It has been this author's practice in the past to treat at-risk pregnancies (i.e., Rh negative and a negative maternal indirect Coomb's test), and such treatment remains the current recommendation of this author.

Up to 6% of the specimens resulting from mid-trimester amniocentesis have green or brown discoloration of the fluid (53,67–69). Biochemical analysis of the pigment found in the discolored fluid reveals it to be breakdown products of hemoglobin [70]. It is highly unlikely that this fluid discoloration is from meconium passage, an event virtually restricted to late gestation. A more plausible explanation is that the staining results from occult intrauterine hemorrhage, with subsequent transmembranous passage of heme pigments.

Several studies have investigated the association between amniotic fluid discoloration and pregnancy loss. In a case-controlled study, Hankins and coworkers [68] could demonstrate no increased risks among patients found to have discolored amniotic fluid at the time of genetic amniocentesis. Nevertheless, several other studies have demonstrated a significant increase in risk of pregnancy loss in instances in which amniotic fluid discoloration is noted during mid-trimester amniocentesis [64,67,65–70]. In these studies, the spontaneous abortion rates in the control groups ranged from 1.5% to 1.6%, whereas pregnancy loss rates in the stained-fluid group ranged from 9% to 100%. Thus, amniocentesis specimens complicated by fluid discoloration (i.e., fresh blood or green/brown discoloration presumably from chronic or occult bleeding) identifies a group at increased risk for pregnancy loss. Patients with this finding should be so counseled.

Although amniocentesis is frequently performed in conjunction with real-time ultrasonography, no adequately designed prospective study has been performed to assess the value of ultrasound use in this procedure. Nonetheless, there are substantial amounts of data reflecting clinical experience. Several studies have demonstrated a reduction in the number of dry taps, needle insertions, bloody taps, failed cultures, and pregnancy losses when ultrasonography is used routinely [40,67,69–77]. Other studies have demonstrated no benefit to amniocentesis [55,78,79]. Unfortunately, most of these studies are flawed in their design, with inadequate controls, improper randomization, inappropriate crossing over, or different operators performing amniocentesis with or without ultrasound scan. Although the benefits of ultrasonographically monitored amniocentesis have not been scientifically demonstrated, in this setting the rule of reason must apply. No reports of an *increased* incidence of adverse outcomes of ultrasonically directed procedures have been published. The important assistance of direct ultrasonic guidance for intrauterine procedure is clearly recognized by clinicians. The ability of scanning to localize the pocket to be entered by the sampling needle makes the procedure easier and the operator more confident. It is this author's firm opinion that amniocentesis should *always* be ultrasound monitored.

Maternal infection following amniocentesis is rare. The risk of amnionitis has been estimated to range between 1 in 1,000–8,000 procedures. One maternal death following amniocentesis has been reported [80]. Given the extreme low risk, the use of prophylactic antibiotics for this procedure is not warranted [81].

Vaginal leakage or spotting is reported in approximately 3% of patients who undergo mid-trimester amniocentesis. Although fluid leakage can result in either oligohydramnios or pregnancy loss, successful pregnancy outcome following conservative measures and monitoring of such pregnancies is also possible. Patients must be made aware of the potential risks of such management [82].

Accidental needling of the fetus potentially resulting in skin dimpling and minor scars is believed to occur in up to 2% to 9% of procedures [83]. The magnitude of the risk for resulting skin lesions is unknown, but it is believed to be very low. Rarely, more significant anomalies have been reported